Soft Tissue and Bone Tumours

WHO Classification of Tumours Editorial Board

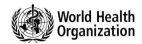

World Health Organization

Suggested citation

WHO Classification of Tumours Editorial Board. Soft tissue and bone tumours.
Lyon (France): International Agency for Research on Cancer; 2020.
(WHO classification of tumours series, 5th ed.; vol. 3).
https://publications.iarc.fr/588.

Sales, rights, and permissions

Print copies are distributed by WHO Press, World Health Organization, 20 Avenue Appia, 1211 Geneva 27, Switzerland
Tel.: +41 22 791 3264; Fax: +41 22 791 4857; email: bookorders@who.int; website: https://whobluebooks.iarc.fr

To purchase IARC publications in electronic format, see the IARC Publications website (https://publications.iarc.fr).

Requests for permission to reproduce or translate IARC publications – whether for sale or for non-commercial distribution – should be submitted
through the IARC Publications website (https://publications.iarc.fr/Rights-And-Permissions).

Third-party materials

If you wish to reuse material from this work that is attributed to a third party, such as figures, tables, or boxes, it is your responsibility to determine
whether permission is needed for that reuse and to obtain permission from the copyright holder. See *Sources*, pages 537–543. The risk of claims
resulting from infringement of any third-party-owned component in the work rests solely with the user.

General disclaimers

The designations employed and the presentation of the material in this publication do not imply the expression of any opinion whatsoever on the
part of WHO or contributing agencies concerning the legal status of any country, territory, city, or area, or of its authorities, or concerning the
delimitation of its frontiers or boundaries. Dotted and dashed lines on maps represent approximate border lines for which there may not yet be full
agreement.

The mention of specific companies or of certain manufacturers' products does not imply that they are endorsed or recommended by WHO or
contributing agencies in preference to others of a similar nature that are not mentioned. Errors and omissions excepted, the names of proprietary
products are distinguished by initial capital letters.

All reasonable precautions have been taken by WHO to verify the information contained in this publication. However, the published material is
being distributed without warranty of any kind, either expressed or implied. The responsibility for the interpretation and use of the material lies with
the reader. In no event shall WHO or contributing agencies be liable for damages arising from its use.

First print run (10 000 copies)

Updated corrigenda can be found at https://publications.iarc.fr

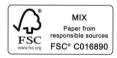

IARC Library Cataloguing-in-Publication Data

Names: WHO Classification of Tumours Editorial Board.
Title: Soft tissue and bone tumours / edited by WHO Classification of Tumours Editorial Board.
Description: Fifth edition. | Lyon: International Agency for Research on Cancer, 2020. | Series: World Health Organization classification of tumours.
    | Includes bibliographical references and index.
Identifiers: ISBN 9789283245025 (pbk.) | ISBN 9789283245032 (ebook)
Subjects: MESH: Bone neoplasms. | Neoplasms, connective and soft tissue.
Classification: NLM QZ 340

The WHO classification of soft tissue and bone tumours presented in this book reflects the views of the WHO Classification of Tumours Editorial Board that convened at the International Agency for Research on Cancer, Lyon, France, 6–8 May 2019.

The WHO Classification of Tumours Editorial Board

For the complete list of all contributors and their affiliations, see pages 528–534.

The WHO Classification of Tumours
Editorial Board (continued)

For the complete list of all contributors and their affiliations, see pages 528–534.

WHO Classification of Tumours
Soft Tissue and Bone Tumours

Edited by	The WHO Classification of Tumours Editorial Board
IARC Editors	Dilani Lokuhetty
	Valerie A. White
	Ian A. Cree
Epidemiology	Ariana Znaor
Project Assistant	Asiedua Asante
Assistants	Anne-Sophie Hameau
	Laura Brispot
Technical Editor	Jessica Cox
Database	Alberto Machado
Layout	Meaghan Fortune
Printed by	Naturaprint
	74370 Argonay, France
Publisher	International Agency for Research on Cancer (IARC)
	150 Cours Albert Thomas
	69372 Lyon Cedex 08, France

Contents

List of abbreviations

aCGH	array comparative genomic hybridization
AIDS	acquired immunodeficiency syndrome
AJCC	American Joint Committee on Cancer
ATP	adenosine triphosphate
bp	base pair
cAMP	cyclic adenosine monophosphate
cDNA	complementary DNA
CI	confidence interval
CNS	central nervous system
CT	computed tomography
DNA	deoxyribonucleic acid
EBV	Epstein–Barr virus
ER	estrogen receptor
ESR	erythrocyte sedimentation rate
EUS	endoscopic ultrasonography
FDG	18F-fluorodeoxyglucose
FDG PET	18F-fluorodeoxyglucose positron emission tomography
FISH	fluorescence in situ hybridization
FNA	fine-needle aspiration
FNCLCC	French Fédération Nationale des Centres de Lutte Contre le Cancer
GCB	germinal-centre B cell
H&E	haematoxylin and eosin
HAART	highly active antiretroviral therapy
HIV	human immunodeficiency virus
HPV	human papillomavirus
IARC	International Agency for Research on Cancer
ICD-11	International Classification of Diseases, 11th Revision
ICD-O	International Classification of Diseases for Oncology
Ig	immunoglobulin
IRSG	Intergroup Rhabdomyosarcoma Study Group
ITD	internal tandem duplication
kb	kilobase
kDa	kilodalton
LC	Langerhans cell
lincRNA	long intervening/intergenic non-coding RNA
M:F ratio	male-to-female ratio
MRI	magnetic resonance imaging
mRNA	messenger ribonucleic acid
N:C ratio	nuclear-to-cytoplasmic ratio
NCI	United States National Cancer Institute
NSAID	non-steroidal anti-inflammatory drug
NSE	neuron-specific enolase
PAS	periodic acid–Schiff
PASD	periodic acid–Schiff with diastase
PCR	polymerase chain reaction
PET	positron emission tomography
PET-CT	positron emission tomography–computed tomography
PET-MRI	positron emission tomography–magnetic resonance imaging
PR	progesterone receptor
RNA	ribonucleic acid
RT-PCR	reverse transcriptase polymerase chain reaction
SEER Program	Surveillance, Epidemiology, and End Results Program
SNP	single-nucleotide polymorphism
TNM	tumour, node, metastasis
UV	ultraviolet

Foreword

The WHO Classification of Tumours, published as a series of books (also known as the WHO Blue Books) and now as a website (https://tumourclassification.iarc.who.int), is an essential tool for standardizing diagnostic practice worldwide. The WHO classification also serves as a vehicle for the translation of cancer research into practice. The diagnostic criteria and standards that make up the classification are underpinned by evidence evaluated and debated by experts in the field. About 200 authors and editors participate in the production of each book, and they give their time freely to this task. I am very grateful for their help; it is a remarkable team effort.

This third volume of the fifth edition of the WHO Blue Books has, like the preceding two volumes, been led by the WHO Classification of Tumours Editorial Board, which is composed of standing members nominated by pathology organizations and expert members selected on the basis of informed bibliometric analysis. The diagnostic process is increasingly multidisciplinary, and we are delighted that several radiology and clinical experts have joined us to address specific needs.

The most conspicuous change to the format of the books in the fifth edition is that tumour types common to multiple systems are dealt with together. Because soft tissue tumours occur in all regions of the body, the current volume will serve as the basis for the information on soft tissue tumours in all upcoming volumes of the fifth edition. The other volumes will include site-specific features of soft tissue tumours. Similarly, this volume contains the main discussion and classification of bone tumours for the entire fifth edition. There is also a chapter on genetic tumour syndromes; genetic disorders are of increasing importance to diagnosis in individual patients, and the study of these disorders has undoubtedly informed our understanding of tumour biology and behaviour over the past decade.

We have attempted to take a more systematic approach to the multifaceted nature of tumour classification; each tumour type is described on the basis of its localization, clinical features, epidemiology, etiology, pathogenesis, histopathology, diagnostic molecular pathology, staging, and prognosis and prediction. We have also included information on macroscopic appearance and cytology, as well as essential and desirable diagnostic criteria. This standardized, modular approach makes it easier for the books to be accessible online, but it also enables us to call attention to areas in which there is little information, and where serious gaps in our knowledge remain to be addressed.

The organization of the WHO Blue Books content now follows the normal progression from benign to malignant – a break with the fourth edition, but one we hope will be welcome.

The volumes are still organized by anatomical site (digestive system, breast, soft tissue and bone, etc.), and each tumour type is listed within a taxonomic classification that follows the format below, which helps to structure the books in a systematic manner:

- Site; e.g. soft tissue and bone
- Category; e.g. soft tissue tumours
- Family (class); e.g. adipocytic tumours
- Type; e.g. pleomorphic liposarcoma
- Subtype; e.g. epithelioid pleomorphic liposarcoma

The issue of whether a given tumour type represents a distinct entity rather than a subtype continues to exercise pathologists, and it is the topic of many publications in the scientific literature. We continue to deal with this issue on a case-by-case basis, but we believe there are inherent rules that can be applied. For example, tumours in which multiple histological patterns contain shared truncal mutations are clearly of the same type, despite the differences in their appearance. Equally, genetic heterogeneity within the same tumour type may have implications for treatment. A small shift in terminology in the fifth edition is that the term "variant" in reference to a specific kind of tumour has been wholly superseded by "subtype", in an effort to more clearly differentiate this meaning from that of "variant" in reference to a genetic alteration.

The WHO Blue Books are much appreciated by pathologists and of increasing importance to practitioners of other clinical disciplines involved in cancer management, as well as to researchers. The new editorial board and I certainly hope that the series will continue to meet the need for standards in diagnosis and to facilitate the translation of diagnostic research into practice worldwide. It is particularly important that cancers continue to be classified and diagnosed according to the same standards internationally so that patients can benefit from multicentre clinical trials, as well as from the results of local trials conducted on different continents.

Dr Ian A. Cree

Head, WHO Classification of Tumours Group
International Agency for Research on Cancer
December 2019

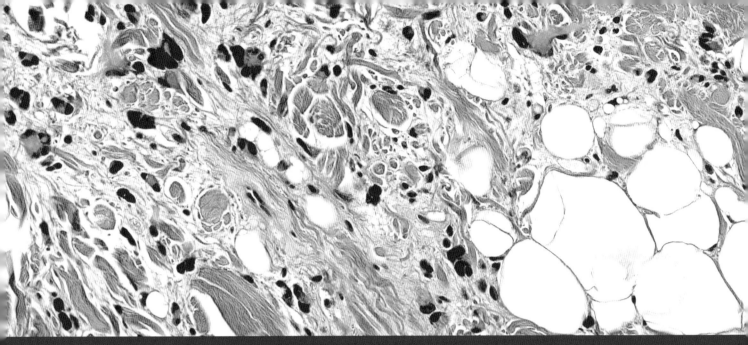

1

Soft tissue tumours

Edited by: Antonescu CR, Bridge JA, Cunha IW, Dei Tos AP, Fletcher CDM,
Folpe AL, Goldblum JR, Hornick JL, Miettinen M, Oda Y

Adipocytic tumours
Fibroblastic and myofibroblastic tumours
So-called fibrohistiocytic tumours
Vascular tumours
Pericytic (perivascular) tumours
Smooth muscle tumours
Skeletal muscle tumours
Gastrointestinal stromal tumour
Chondro-osseous tumours
Peripheral nerve sheath tumours
Tumours of uncertain differentiation

WHO classification of soft tissue tumours

Adipocytic tumours

Benign
8850/0 Lipoma NOS
8856/0   Intramuscular lipoma
            Chondrolipoma
            Lipomatosis
                Diffuse lipomatosis
                Multiple symmetrical lipomatosis
                Pelvic lipomatosis
                Steroid lipomatosis
                HIV lipodystrophy
            Lipomatosis of nerve
8881/0 Lipoblastomatosis
            Localized (lipoblastoma)
            Diffuse (lipoblastomatosis)
8861/0 Angiolipoma NOS
            Cellular angiolipoma
8890/0 Myolipoma
8862/0 Chondroid lipoma
8857/0 Spindle cell lipoma
8857/0 Atypical spindle cell / pleomorphic lipomatous tumour
8880/0 Hibernoma

Intermediate (locally aggressive)
8850/1 Atypical lipomatous tumour

Malignant
8851/3 Liposarcoma, well-differentiated, NOS
8851/3   Lipoma-like liposarcoma
8851/3   Inflammatory liposarcoma
8851/3   Sclerosing liposarcoma
8858/3 Dedifferentiated liposarcoma
8852/3 Myxoid liposarcoma
8854/3 Pleomorphic liposarcoma
            Epithelioid liposarcoma
8859/3* Myxoid pleomorphic liposarcoma

Fibroblastic and myofibroblastic tumours

Benign
8828/0 Nodular fasciitis
            Intravascular fasciitis
            Cranial fasciitis
8828/0 Proliferative fasciitis
8828/0 Proliferative myositis
            Myositis ossificans and fibro-osseous pseudotumour of
                digits
            Ischaemic fasciitis
8820/0 Elastofibroma
8992/0 Fibrous hamartoma of infancy
            Fibromatosis colli
            Juvenile hyaline fibromatosis
            Inclusion body fibromatosis
8813/0 Fibroma of tendon sheath
8810/0 Desmoplastic fibroblastoma
8825/0 Myofibroblastoma
8816/0 Calcifying aponeurotic fibroma
            EWSR1-SMAD3–positive fibroblastic tumour (emerging)
8826/0 Angiomyofibroblastoma
9160/0 Cellular angiofibroma
9160/0 Angiofibroma NOS
8810/0 Nuchal fibroma
8811/0 Acral fibromyxoma
8810/0 Gardner fibroma

Intermediate (locally aggressive)
8815/0 Solitary fibrous tumour, benign
8813/1 Palmar/plantar-type fibromatosis
8821/1 Desmoid-type fibromatosis
8821/1   Extra-abdominal desmoid
8822/1   Abdominal fibromatosis

8851/1 Lipofibromatosis
8834/1 Giant cell fibroblastoma

Intermediate (rarely metastasizing)
8832/1 Dermatofibrosarcoma protuberans NOS
8833/1   Pigmented dermatofibrosarcoma protuberans
8832/3   Dermatofibrosarcoma protuberans,
                fibrosarcomatous
            Myxoid dermatofibrosarcoma protuberans
                Dermatofibrosarcoma protuberans with myoid
                    differentiation
            Plaque-like dermatofibrosarcoma protuberans
8815/1 Solitary fibrous tumour NOS
            Fat-forming (lipomatous) solitary fibrous tumour
            Giant cell–rich solitary fibrous tumour
8825/1 Inflammatory myofibroblastic tumour
            Epithelioid inflammatory myofibroblastic sarcoma
8825/3 Myofibroblastic sarcoma
8810/1 Superficial CD34-positive fibroblastic tumour
8811/1 Myxoinflammatory fibroblastic sarcoma
8814/3 Infantile fibrosarcoma

Malignant
8815/3 Solitary fibrous tumour, malignant
8810/3 Fibrosarcoma NOS
8811/3 Myxofibrosarcoma
            Epithelioid myxofibrosarcoma
8840/3 Low-grade fibromyxoid sarcoma
8840/3 Sclerosing epithelioid fibrosarcoma

So-called fibrohistiocytic tumours

Benign
9252/0 Tenosynovial giant cell tumour NOS
9252/1   Tenosynovial giant cell tumour, diffuse
8831/0 Deep benign fibrous histiocytoma

Intermediate (rarely metastasizing)
8835/1 Plexiform fibrohistiocytic tumour
9251/1 Giant cell tumour of soft parts NOS

Malignant
9252/3 Malignant tenosynovial giant cell tumour

Vascular tumours

Benign
9120/0 Haemangioma NOS
9132/0 Intramuscular haemangioma
9123/0 Arteriovenous haemangioma
9122/0 Venous haemangioma
9125/0 Epithelioid haemangioma
            Cellular epithelioid haemangioma
            Atypical epithelioid haemangioma
9170/0 Lymphangioma NOS
            Lymphangiomatosis
9173/0 Cystic lymphangioma
9161/0 Acquired tufted haemangioma

Intermediate (locally aggressive)
9130/1 Kaposiform haemangioendothelioma

Intermediate (rarely metastasizing)
9136/1 Retiform haemangioendothelioma
9135/1 Papillary intralymphatic angioendothelioma
9136/1 Composite haemangioendothelioma
            Neuroendocrine composite haemangioendothelioma
9140/3 Kaposi sarcoma
            Classic indolent Kaposi sarcoma
            Endemic African Kaposi sarcoma
            AIDS-associated Kaposi sarcoma
            Iatrogenic Kaposi sarcoma
9138/1 Pseudomyogenic (epithelioid sarcoma–like)
            haemangioendothelioma

Malignant
9133/3 Epithelioid haemangioendothelioma NOS
           Epithelioid haemangioendothelioma with
           WWTR1-CAMTA1 fusion
           Epithelioid haemangioendothelioma with
           YAP1-TFE3 fusion
9120/3 Angiosarcoma

Pericytic (perivascular) tumours
Benign and intermediate
8711/0 Glomus tumour NOS
8712/0   Glomangioma
8713/0   Glomangiomyoma
8711/1   Glomangiomatosis
8711/1   Glomus tumour of uncertain malignant potential
8824/0 Myopericytoma
8824/1   Myofibromatosis
8824/0   Myofibroma
8824/1   Infantile myofibromatosis
8894/0 Angioleiomyoma

Malignant
8711/3 Glomus tumour, malignant

Smooth muscle tumours
Benign and intermediate
8890/0 Leiomyoma NOS
8897/1 Smooth muscle tumour of uncertain malignant potential
Malignant
8890/3 Leiomyosarcoma NOS

Skeletal muscle tumours
Benign
8900/0 Rhabdomyoma NOS
8903/0   Fetal rhabdomyoma
8904/0   Adult rhabdomyoma
8905/0   Genital rhabdomyoma

Malignant
8910/3 Embryonal rhabdomyosarcoma NOS
8910/3   Embryonal rhabdomyosarcoma, pleomorphic
8920/3 Alveolar rhabdomyosarcoma
8901/3 Pleomorphic rhabdomyosarcoma NOS
8912/3 Spindle cell rhabdomyosarcoma
           Congenital spindle cell rhabdomyosarcoma with
           VGLL2/NCOA2/CITED2 rearrangements
           MYOD1-mutant spindle cell / sclerosing
           rhabdomyosarcoma
           Intraosseous spindle cell rhabdomyosarcoma (with
           TFCP2/NCOA2 rearrangements)
8921/3 Ectomesenchymoma

Gastrointestinal stromal tumours
8936/3 Gastrointestinal stromal tumour

Chondro-osseous tumours
Benign
9220/0 Chondroma NOS
           Chondroblastoma-like soft tissue chondroma
Malignant
9180/3 Osteosarcoma, extraskeletal

Peripheral nerve sheath tumours
Benign
9560/0 Schwannoma NOS
9560/0   Ancient schwannoma
9560/0   Cellular schwannoma
9560/0   Plexiform schwannoma
           Epithelioid schwannoma
           Microcystic/reticular schwannoma

9540/0 Neurofibroma NOS
           Ancient neurofibroma
           Cellular neurofibroma
           Atypical neurofibroma
9550/0   Plexiform neurofibroma
9571/0 Perineurioma NOS
           Reticular perineurioma
           Sclerosing perineurioma
9580/0 Granular cell tumour NOS
9562/0 Nerve sheath myxoma
9570/0 Solitary circumscribed neuroma
           Plexiform solitary circumscribed neuroma
9530/0 Meningioma NOS
           Benign triton tumour / neuromuscular choristoma
9563/0 Hybrid nerve sheath tumour
           Perineurioma/schwannoma
           Schwannoma/neurofibroma
           Perineurioma/neurofibroma

Malignant
9540/3 Malignant peripheral nerve sheath tumour NOS
9542/3   Malignant peripheral nerve sheath tumour, epithelioid
9540/3 Melanotic malignant peripheral nerve sheath tumour
9580/3 Granular cell tumour, malignant
9571/3 Perineurioma, malignant

Tumours of uncertain differentiation
Benign
8840/0 Myxoma NOS
           Cellular myxoma
8841/0 Aggressive angiomyxoma
8802/1 Pleomorphic hyalinizing angiectatic tumour
8990/0 Phosphaturic mesenchymal tumour NOS
8714/0 Perivascular epithelioid tumour, benign
8860/0 Angiomyolipoma

Intermediate (locally aggressive)
8811/1 Haemosiderotic fibrolipomatous tumour
8860/1 Angiomyolipoma, epithelioid

Intermediate (rarely metastasizing)
8830/1 Atypical fibroxanthoma
8836/1 Angiomatoid fibrous histiocytoma
8842/0 Ossifying fibromyxoid tumour NOS
8940/0 Mixed tumour NOS
8940/3 Mixed tumour, malignant, NOS
8982/0 Myoepithelioma NOS

Malignant
8990/3 Phosphaturic mesenchymal tumour, malignant
           NTRK-rearranged spindle cell neoplasm (emerging)
9040/3 Synovial sarcoma NOS
9041/3   Synovial sarcoma, spindle cell
9043/3   Synovial sarcoma, biphasic
           Synovial sarcoma, poorly differentiated
8804/3 Epithelioid sarcoma
           Proximal or large cell epithelioid sarcoma
           Classic epithelioid sarcoma
9581/3 Alveolar soft part sarcoma
9044/3 Clear cell sarcoma NOS
9231/3 Extraskeletal myxoid chondrosarcoma
8806/3 Desmoplastic small round cell tumour
8963/3 Rhabdoid tumour NOS
8714/3 Perivascular epithelioid tumour, malignant
9137/3 Intimal sarcoma
8842/3 Ossifying fibromyxoid tumour, malignant
8982/3 Myoepithelial carcinoma
8805/3 Undifferentiated sarcoma
8801/3   Spindle cell sarcoma, undifferentiated
8802/3   Pleomorphic sarcoma, undifferentiated
8803/3   Round cell sarcoma, undifferentiated

These morphology codes are from the International Classification of Diseases for Oncology, third edition, second revision (ICD-O-3.2) {1471}. Behaviour is coded /0 for benign tumours; /1 for unspecified, borderline, or uncertain behaviour; /2 for carcinoma in situ and grade III intraepithelial neoplasia; /3 for malignant tumours, primary site; and /6 for malignant tumours, metastatic site. Behaviour code /6 is not generally used by cancer registries.
This classification is modified from the previous WHO classification, taking into account changes in our understanding of these lesions.
* Codes marked with an asterisk were approved by the IARC/WHO Committee for ICD-O at its meeting in January 2020.

TNM staging of tumours of soft tissues

Soft Tissues

(ICD-O-3 C38.1, 2, 3, C47-49)

Rules for Classification

There should be histological confirmation of the disease and division of cases by histological type and grade.

The following are the procedures for assessing T, N, and M categories:

T categories	Physical examination and imaging
N categories	Physical examination and imaging
M categories	Physical examination and imaging

Anatomical Sites
1. Connective, subcutaneous, and other soft tissues (C49), peripheral nerves (C47)
2. Retroperitoneum (C48.0)
3. Mediastinum: anterior (C38.1); posterior (C38.2); mediastinum, NOS (C38.3)

Histological Types of Tumour
The following histological types are not included:
- Kaposi sarcoma
- Dermatofibrosarcoma (protuberans)
- Fibromatosis (desmoid tumour)
- Sarcoma arising from the dura mater or brain
- Angiosarcoma, an aggressive sarcoma, is excluded because its natural history is not consistent with the classification.

Note
Cystosarcoma phyllodes is staged as a soft tissue sarcoma of the superficial trunk.

Regional Lymph Nodes
The regional lymph nodes are those appropriate to the site of the primary tumour. Regional node involvement is rare and cases in which nodal status is not assessed either clinically or pathologically could be considered N0 instead of NX or pNX.

TNM Clinical Classification
T – Primary Tumour
TX   Primary tumour cannot be assessed
T0   No evidence of primary tumour

Extremity and Superficial Trunk
T1   Tumour 5 cm or less in greatest dimension
T2   Tumour more than 5 cm but no more than 10 cm in greatest dimension
T3   Tumour more than 10 cm but no more than 15 cm in greatest dimension
T4   Tumour more than 15 cm in greatest dimension

Retroperitoneum
T1   Tumour 5 cm or less in greatest dimension
T2   Tumour more than 5 cm but no more than 10 cm in greatest dimension
T3   Tumour more than 10 cm but no more than 15 cm in greatest dimension
T4   Tumour more than 15 cm in greatest dimension

Head and Neck
T1   Tumour 2 cm or less in greatest dimension
T2   Tumour more than 2 cm but no more than 4 cm in greatest dimension
T3   Tumour more than 4 cm in greatest dimension
T4a   Tumour invades the orbit, skull base or dura, central compartment viscera, facial skeleton, and/or pterygoid muscles
T4b   Tumour invades the brain parenchyma, encases the carotid artery, invades prevertebral muscle or involves the central nervous system by perineural spread

Thoracic and Abdominal Viscera
T1   Tumour confined to a single organ
T2a   Tumour invades serosa or visceral peritoneum
T2b   Tumour with microscopic extension beyond the serosa
T3   Tumour invades another organ or macroscopic extension beyond the serosa
T4a   Multifocal tumour involving no more than two sites in one organ
T4b   Multifocal tumour involving more than two sites but not more than 5 sites
T4c   Multifocal tumour involving more than five sites

N – Regional Lymph Nodes
NX   Regional lymph nodes cannot be assessed
N0   No regional lymph node metastasis
N1   Regional lymph node metastasis

M – Distant Metastasis
M0   No distant metastasis
M1   Distant metastasis

pTNM Pathological Classification
The pT and pN categories correspond to the T and N categories.

pM – Distant Metastasis*
pM1   Distant metastasis microscopically confirmed

Note
* pM0 and pMX are not valid categories

Stage – Extremity and Superficial Trunk and Retroperitoneum

Stage IA	T1	N0	M0	G1,GX Low Grade
Stage IB	T2,T3,T4	N0	M0	G1,GX Low Grade
Stage II	T1	N0	M0	G2,G3 High Grade
Stage IIIA	T2	N0	M0	G2,G3 High Grade
Stage IIIB	T3,T4	N0	M0	G2,G3 High Grade
	Any T	N1*	M0	Any G
Stage IV	Any T	Any N	M1	Any G

Note
* AJCC classifies N1 as stage IV for extremity and superficial trunk.

Stage – Head and Neck and Thoracic and Abdominal Viscera
There is no stage for soft tissue sarcoma of the head and neck and thoracic and abdominal viscera.

The information presented here has been excerpted from the 2017 *TNM classification of malignant tumours*, eighth edition {423,3126}. © 2017 UICC. A help desk for specific questions about the TNM classification is available at https://www.uicc.org/tnm-help-desk.

TNM staging of gastrointestinal stromal tumours

Gastrointestinal Stromal Tumour (GIST)

Rules for Classification
The classification applies only to gastrointestinal stromal tumours. There should be histological confirmation of the disease.

The following are the procedures for assessing the T, N, and M categories.

T categories	Physical examination, imaging, endoscopy, and/or surgical exploration
N categories	Physical examination, imaging, and/or surgical exploration
M categories	Physical examination, imaging, and/or surgical exploration

Anatomical Sites and Subsites
- Oesophagus (C15)
- Stomach (C16)
- Small intestine (C17)
  1. Duodenum (C17.0)
  2. Jejunum (C17.1)
  3. Ileum (C17.2)
- Colon (C18)
- Rectosigmoid junction (C19)
- Rectum (C20)
- Omentum (C48.1)
- Mesentery (C48.1)

Regional Lymph Nodes
The regional lymph nodes are those appropriate to the site of the primary tumour; see gastrointestinal sites {423} for details.

TNM Clinical Classification
T – Primary Tumour
TX	Primary tumour cannot be assessed
T0	No evidence for primary tumour
T1	Tumour 2 cm or less
T2	Tumour more than 2 cm but not more than 5 cm
T3	Tumour more than 5 cm but not more than 10 cm
T4	Tumour more than 10 cm in greatest dimension

N – Regional Lymph Nodes
NX	Regional lymph nodes cannot be assessed*
N0	No regional lymph node metastasis
N1	Regional lymph node metastasis

Note
* NX: Regional lymph node involvement is rare for GISTs, so that cases in which the nodal status is not assessed clinically or pathologically could be considered N0 instead of NX or pNX.

M – Distant Metastasis
M0	No distant metastasis
M1	Distant metastasis

pTNM Pathological Classification
The pT and pN categories correspond to the T and N categories.

pM – Distant Metastasis*
pM1   Distant metastasis microscopically confirmed

Note
* pM0 and pMX are not valid categories

G Histopathological Grading
Grading for GIST is dependent on mitotic rate.*
Low mitotic rate:	5 or fewer per 50 hpf
High mitotic rate:	over 5 per 50 hpf

Note
* The mitotic rate of GIST is best expressed as the number of mitoses per 50 high power fields (hpf) using the 40× objective (total area 5 mm^2 in 50 fields).

Stage
Staging criteria for gastric tumours can be applied in primary, solitary omental GISTs. Staging criteria for intestinal tumours can be applied to GISTs in less common sites such as oesophagus, colon, rectum, and mesentery.

Gastric GIST

				Mitotic rate
Stage IA	T1,T2	N0	M0	Low
Stage IB	T3	N0	M0	Low
Stage II	T1,T2	N0	M0	High
	T4	N0	M0	Low
Stage IIIA	T3	N0	M0	High
Stage IIIB	T4	N0	M0	High
Stage IV	Any T	N1	M0	Any rate
	Any T	Any N	M1	Any rate

Small Intestinal GIST

				Mitotic rate
Stage I	T1,T2	N0	M0	Low
Stage II	T3	N0	M0	Low
Stage IIIA	T1	N0	M0	High
	T4	N0	M0	Low
Stage IIIB	T2,T3,T4	N0	M0	High
Stage IV	Any T	N1	M0	Any rate
	Any T	Any N	M1	Any rate

Note: The mitotic rates (counts) listed under the "G Histopathological Grading" heading above are based on a field area of 0.1 mm^2 as used in the original paper; modern microscopes are likely to have a field area of 0.2 mm^2, but measurement of field area is advisable, because instruments vary.

The information presented here has been excerpted from the 2017 *TNM classification of malignant tumours*, eighth edition {423,3126}. © 2017 UICC.
A help desk for specific questions about the TNM classification is available at https://www.uicc.org/tnm-help-desk.

Soft tissue tumours: Introduction

Fletcher CDM   Lazar AJ
Baldini EH   Messiou C
Blay JY   Pollock RE
Gronchi A   Singer S

Epidemiology

Incidence

Benign mesenchymal tumours outnumber sarcomas by a factor of at least 100. The annual clinical incidence (number of new patients consulting a doctor) of benign tumours of soft tissue has been estimated to be as high as 3000 cases per 1 million population {2232}, whereas the annual incidence of soft tissue sarcoma is about 50 cases per 1 million population {1123,1262, 1122}, i.e. < 1% of all malignant tumours (but more frequent in children). There are no data to indicate a change in the incidence of sarcoma, nor are there significant geographical differences.

Age and anatomical site distribution

At least 30% of the benign tumours of soft tissue are lipomas, 30% are fibrohistiocytic and fibrous tumours, 10% are vascular tumours, and 5% are nerve sheath tumours. There is a relationship between the tumour type, symptoms, and location and the patient age and sex. Lipomas are painless; rare in the hand, lower leg, and foot; and very uncommon in children {2232}. Angiolipomas are often painful and most common in young men. Angioleiomyomas are often painful and common in the lower leg of middle-aged women. Half of the vascular tumours occur in patients aged < 20 years {1794,2697}. Of the benign tumours, 99% are superficial and 95% are < 5 cm in diameter {2697}. Soft tissue sarcomas may occur anywhere, but 75% are located in the extremities (most commonly in thigh) and 10% each in the trunk wall and retroperitoneum. There is a slight male predominance. Of the extremity and trunk wall tumours, 30% are superficial with a median diameter of 5 cm, and 60% are deep-seated with a median diameter of 9 cm {1262}. Retroperitoneal tumours are often much larger before they become symptomatic. The ICD-O topographical coding for the main anatomical sites covered in this chapter is presented in Box 1.01.

About 10% of patients with sarcoma have detectable metastases (most commonly in the lungs) at diagnosis of the primary tumour. Overall, at least one third of patients with soft tissue sarcoma die from tumour-related disease, most of them from lung metastases. About 65% of soft tissue sarcomas are histologically classified as undifferentiated pleomorphic sarcoma (UPS; previously known as malignant fibrous histiocytoma [MFH]), liposarcoma, leiomyosarcoma, myxofibrosarcoma, synovial sarcoma, or malignant peripheral nerve sheath tumour (MPNST), and three quarters are highly malignant (see *Grading and staging of sarcomas*, p. 10) {2484}. The distribution of histotypes varies over time and between researchers, probably because of changing definitions of histotypes (as, for example, malignant fibrous histiocytoma in the 1990s).

Age-related incidences vary: embryonal rhabdomyosarcoma occurs almost exclusively in children, and synovial sarcoma mostly in young adults, whereas UPS, liposarcoma,

Box 1.01 ICD-O topographical coding for the main anatomical sites covered in this chapter (sarcomas arising in parenchymatous organs should be coded to those organs) {1077}

C47 Peripheral nerves and autonomic nervous system
C47.0 Peripheral nerves and autonomic nervous system of head, face, and neck
C47.1 Peripheral nerves and autonomic nervous system of upper limb and shoulder
C47.2 Peripheral nerves and autonomic nervous system of lower limb and hip
C47.3 Peripheral nerves and autonomic nervous system of thorax
C47.4 Peripheral nerves and autonomic nervous system of abdomen
C47.5 Peripheral nerves and autonomic nervous system of pelvis
C47.6 Peripheral nerves and autonomic nervous system of trunk NOS
C47.8 Overlapping lesion of peripheral nerves and autonomic nervous system
C47.9 Autonomic nervous system NOS

C48 Retroperitoneum and peritoneum
C48.0 Retroperitoneum

C49 Connective, subcutaneous, and other soft tissues
C49.0 Connective, subcutaneous, and other soft tissues of head, face, and neck
C49.1 Connective, subcutaneous, and other soft tissues of upper limb and shoulder
C49.2 Connective, subcutaneous, and other soft tissues of lower limb and hip
C49.3 Connective, subcutaneous, and other soft tissues of thorax
C49.4 Connective, subcutaneous, and other soft tissues of abdomen
C49.5 Connective, subcutaneous, and other soft tissues of pelvis
C49.6 Connective, subcutaneous, and other soft tissues of trunk NOS
C49.8 Overlapping lesion of connective, subcutaneous, and other soft tissues
C49.9 Connective, subcutaneous, and other soft tissues NOS

leiomyosarcoma, and myxofibrosarcoma dominate in the elderly. Like almost all other malignancies, soft tissue sarcomas become more common with increasing age; the median age at diagnosis is 65 years.

Etiology

The etiology of most benign and malignant tumours of soft tissue is unknown. In rare cases (< 10%), genetic and environmental factors, irradiation, viral infections, and immunodeficiency have been found to be associated with the development of usually malignant soft tissue tumours. There are also isolated reports of sarcomas arising in scar tissue, at fracture sites, and close to surgical implants {1642}. Some angiosarcomas arise in chronic lymphoedema. However, the large majority of soft tissue sarcomas seem to arise de novo, without an apparent causative factor. Some malignant mesenchymal neoplasms occur in the setting of familial cancer syndromes (see below and Chapter 4: *Genetic tumour syndromes of soft tissue and bone*, p. 501). Multistage tumorigenesis sequences with gradual accumulation of genetic alterations and an increasing histological degree of malignancy have not yet been clearly identified in most tumours of soft tissue. Four main types of etiological agents have been implicated in the literature: chemical carcinogens, radiation, viral infection and immunodeficiency, and genetic susceptibility.

Chemical carcinogens

Several studies, many of them from Sweden, have reported an increased incidence of soft tissue sarcoma after exposure to phenoxy herbicides, chlorophenols, and their contaminants (dioxins) in agricultural or forestry work {926,1301}. Other studies have not found this association. One explanation for the different findings may be the use of herbicides that are contaminated with dioxins at different levels {2036,3383}.

Radiation

About 5% of soft tissue sarcomas are radiation-associated {2161}. The reported incidence of radiation-associated osteosarcoma ranges from a few cases per 1000 person-years to nearly 1 case per 100 person-years. Most incidence estimates are based on patients with breast cancer treated with radiation as adjuvant therapy {1587}. The risk increases with dose; most patients have received ≥ 50 Gy, and the median time between exposure and tumour diagnosis is about 10 years, although there is some evidence that this latency interval is decreasing. More than half of these tumours have been classified as UPS, most often being highly malignant. In skin, angiosarcoma is by far most common. Patients with a germline mutation in the retinoblastoma gene (*RB1*) have a significantly elevated risk of developing radiation-associated osteosarcoma {1653}, usually osteosarcoma. Similarly, patients with a germline mutation in *TP53* (Li–Fraumeni syndrome) have a significantly higher risk of developing radiation-associated osteosarcoma {1359}, as do patients with neurofibromatosis type 1 (NF1) {2827}.

Viral infection and immunodeficiency

HHV8 infection plays a key role in the development of Kaposi sarcoma {338}, and the clinical course of the disease is dependent on the immune status of the patient {824}. EBV infection is associated with smooth muscle tumours in patients with immunodeficiency {811}.

Genetic susceptibility

Several types of benign soft tissue tumours have been reported to occur on a familial or inherited basis. However, these reports are rare and comprise an insignificant number of tumours. The most common example is probably hereditary multiple lipoma (or angiolipoma) {1,1182}. Desmoid tumours occur in patients with the Gardner syndrome subtype of familial adenomatous polyposis {1259}. NF1 and neurofibromatosis type 2 (NF2) are associated with multiple benign nerve sheath tumours (and sometimes also non-neural tumours). In as many as 5–10% of patients with NF1, MPNSTs develop, usually in a benign nerve sheath tumour {3286}. Moreover, 5–7% of these patients may develop one or more gastrointestinal stromal tumours. Li–Fraumeni syndrome {1375} is a rare autosomal dominant disease caused by germline mutations in the *TP53* tumour suppressor gene, which predispose individuals to the development of sarcoma {1187}. By the age of 30 years, half of all patients with Li–Fraumeni syndrome have already developed malignant tumours, of which > 30% are sarcomas of soft tissue or bone. The inherited (or bilateral) form of retinoblastoma, with a germline mutation of the *RB1* gene, may also be associated with development of sarcoma. One large study suggested that as many as 50% of sarcoma patients may have potentially pathogenic germline variants

{216}, but this remains to be validated, and the clinical significance of this finding remains uncertain.

Clinical features

Clinical features are only occasionally sufficient to distinguish benign from malignant tumours of soft tissue. Most soft tissue sarcomas of the extremities and trunk wall present as a large, painless, incidentally noted mass that patients sometimes associate with an episode of injury. Conversely, some patients present with rapidly growing tumours that are occasionally painful, leading to a rapid medical opinion. Most patients with intra-abdominal or retroperitoneal sarcomas present with an asymptomatic abdominal mass that is confirmed on abdominal imaging. On occasion, nonspecific abdominal pain is present. Less common symptoms include gastrointestinal bleeding, incomplete obstruction, neurological or systemic symptoms (e.g. fever, fatigue, and anaemia), and occasionally also alterations of liver function tests. The seemingly innocent presentation and the rarity of sarcomas often lead to their initial misinterpretation as benign conditions. All superficial soft tissue lesions measuring > 5 cm, and all deep-seated lesions, are statistically likely to be sarcoma. Patients with such lesions should therefore be referred to specialized centres for a diagnostic biopsy and expert pathology review followed by treatment {505,3206}.

Biopsy

A biopsy is mandatory to establish malignancy and assess histological type, subtype, and grade, and is recommended in clinical practice guidelines for all deep-seated tumours > 5 cm. Possible exceptions, most often in expert centres, are what appear radiologically to be pure well-differentiated fatty tumours in the limbs or trunk. Most limb and superficial trunk masses are best sampled through multiple Trucut core biopsies obtained through a single tract, which should be placed so that it can be completely excised during definitive resection with minimal sacrifice of overlying skin. If biopsy is performed with at least 2 or 3 adequate cores, the accuracy of histological classification, grading, and prognostication is very high {1355,2964}. Additional sampling may be required for specific research protocols. When the Trucut core approach fails, an alternative for most extremity masses is an incisional biopsy with minimal extension into adjacent tissue planes. Excisional biopsy should be avoided, particularly for lesions > 2 cm, because the contamination of surrounding tissue planes renders definitive re-excision more extensive. Frozen section diagnosis and FNA are not generally recommended. FNA is proposed by some expert centres with specific cytological expertise and the capability for careful clinicoradiological correlation.

Biopsy is important for decisions regarding neoadjuvant therapy because sensitivity to chemotherapy and radiation therapy varies among histological types and grades of sarcoma. Histological type may also inform the surgical approach and selection of chemotherapy agents. However, although the histological type is concordant with final pathology in 80% of cases, given the heterogeneity and large size of these tumours at presentation, grade can be underestimated in 40% of retroperitoneal tumours {82}. In experienced centres, pretreatment core biopsy is not required if the diagnosis is clear on imaging (liposarcoma and leiomyosarcoma of the inferior vena cava), no neoadjuvant therapy is planned, and complete resection of the tumour is likely with minimal morbidity.

Management

Once the histological diagnosis, size, and grade have been established and the work-up for distant metastasis performed, a multidisciplinary team of surgeons, radiation oncologists, and medical oncologists can design the most effective treatment plan for the patient. The plan must balance the goal of minimizing recurrence with preservation of function and quality of life. Surgery remains the principal therapeutic modality in soft tissue sarcoma, while the optimal combination of chemotherapy and radiotherapy must be tailored to the individual patient and the risk of local and distant recurrence.

Surgery

In principle, appropriate surgery for extremity and truncal sarcomas should consist of wide en bloc removal of the tumour with a cuff of healthy tissue all around. Every attempt should be made to avoid microscopically positive surgical margins, which are associated with higher risk of local recurrence, distant metastasis, and death {1225,1229,2954,3382}. However, in certain situations a microscopically positive margin may be unavoidable because of the need to preserve critical neurovascular structures; such cases should always be assessed by reference centres. When focal microscopically positive margins are planned in advance, the use of preoperative radiotherapy or chemotherapy plus radiotherapy may offset their negative prognostic impact on local recurrence and outcome {1252,1234}. The scope of the excision is generally dictated by the tumour size, histological subtype, anatomical relation to normal structures (e.g. major vessels and neurovascular bundles), and degree of morbidity and functional loss expected. Amputation is only indicated for soft tissue sarcoma on rare occasions and should be reserved for tumours that cannot be resected by any other means in patients without evidence of metastatic disease and with potential for good long-term functional rehabilitation.

Low-grade sarcomas of the extremities and trunk wall may be treated by surgery alone if negative margins are achieved. High-grade, large (> 5 cm) sarcomas most often receive preoperative or postoperative radiotherapy according to clinical practice guidelines, because randomized clinical trials have demonstrated reductions in the risk of local recurrence with radiation {3349}. For subcutaneous or intramuscular high-grade soft tissue sarcomas < 5 cm, or for low-grade sarcomas of any size, surgery alone should be considered if the tumour can be excised with a 1–2 cm cuff of surrounding fat and muscle. If the excision margin is close or there is extramuscular involvement, adjuvant radiotherapy should be added. However, preoperative or postoperative radiotherapy is probably used more often than strictly necessary, irrespective of grade. In fact, a substantial subset of subcutaneous and intramuscular sarcomas can be treated by wide-margin excision alone, with a local recurrence rate of only 5–10% {2519,211,1007}.

Retroperitoneal sarcomas tend to present at a later stage, often as very large tumours. As such, they have a tendency to invade adjacent organs, making the achievement of clean margins at the time of resection uncommon. Accordingly, the survival rate for retroperitoneal sarcomas is much lower than that for extremity soft tissue sarcomas. The most important prognostic factors for survival in retroperitoneal sarcoma are completeness of surgical resection, histological grade, and histological type/subtype {1233,3037,723,2867}. The utility of preoperative radiotherapy for these tumours remains controversial, but the soon-to-be-published results of the European Organisation for Research and Treatment of Cancer (EORTC) Soft Tissue and Bone Sarcoma Group (STBSG) 62092-22092 prospective randomized trial should help to address this question. Well-differentiated and dedifferentiated liposarcomas, which account for the majority of retroperitoneal sarcomas, frequently recur locally and multifocally {2867,894,1349}. Even with an aggressive surgical approach, locoregional recurrence is a substantial problem that leads to unresectable local disease and death in about 60% of patients {3037,2443}. However, dedifferentiated liposarcoma classified as grade 3 according to the French Fédération Nationale des Centres de Lutte Contre le Cancer (FNCLCC) Sarcoma Group system has a 30–50% risk of distant metastasis {1233,1231,1226}. In contrast, high-grade leiomyosarcoma has a lower 10-year cumulative incidence of local recurrence (25%), but it often gives rise to liver or lung metastases, with a 60% 10-year cumulative incidence of distant recurrence {3037}.

Complete gross resection is the cornerstone of management of retroperitoneal sarcomas, most achievable at the time of primary presentation. The extent of resection is affected by the tumour's proximity to important structures. Resection of the primary tumour should aim to achieve a macroscopically complete resection as a single specimen with contiguous organs when they are directly invaded or encased by the sarcoma. For well-differentiated and dedifferentiated liposarcomas, all of the retroperitoneal fat on the side of the sarcoma should be removed, because it is often difficult to distinguish normal retroperitoneal fat from well-differentiated liposarcoma. Preservation of specific organs (e.g. kidney, pancreas, duodenum, and bladder) should be considered on an individualized basis and mandates specific expertise in the disease to appropriately judge the overall tumour extent and expected biology, as well as the individual patient's characteristics. Decisions regarding which neurovascular structures to sacrifice, as well as the appropriateness of en bloc resection of liver and pancreas, must weigh the potential for local control against the potential surgical morbidity and potential for long-term dysfunction.

The management of desmoid-type fibromatosis has recently undergone a paradigm shift. Desmoids are now most often treated conservatively by initial observation, avoiding ablative surgery because of the substantial rate of spontaneous growth arrest and regression {1009,2719}. Prognostic factors predictive of indolent behaviour or spontaneous regression are lacking. However, a recent study found that the percentage of tumour volume characterized by hyperintense T2 signal on MRI is associated with desmoid progression during observation and may help distinguish patients who would benefit from early intervention from those who may simply be observed {509}. For patients who become increasingly symptomatic or exhibit progressive disease at multiple assessments, consideration should be given to systemic therapy such as sorafenib {1197,1198}, surgical resection, or local ablative treatment (e.g. cryotherapy).

Radiotherapy

The benefit of radiotherapy for extremity sarcoma was first established by a US National Cancer Institute (NCI)-sponsored randomized trial comparing amputation and conservative surgery with radiation {2661}. Two subsequent landmark randomized trials confirmed that adding radiation to conservative surgery improves local control, and this remains the standard approach for most intermediate- and high-grade soft tissue sarcomas of the extremities and trunk {3349,2517}. Adjuvant radiation is not routinely recommended after surgery for low-grade soft tissue sarcoma unless there are special circumstances such as large tumour size, positive resection margins, or local recurrence after initial surgery alone.

Radiation may be delivered preoperatively or postoperatively. The relative efficacy of preoperative versus postoperative radiation has been extensively studied, and a Canadian randomized trial demonstrated similar rates of local control, regional control, and distant metastases for both approaches {2395}, although postoperative radiation was associated with more-frequent fibrosis {740}. The advantages of preoperative radiation include delivery of a lower radiation dose (50 Gy compared with 60–66 Gy for postoperative treatment) and treatment to a smaller volume of tissue. Preoperatively, the radiation volume includes gross tumour plus margins, whereas postoperatively the radiation field must include not only the tumour bed with margins, but also all tissues handled at surgery, including the incision and drain sites. For these reasons, preoperative radiation is associated with less late radiation morbidity {740}. The main disadvantage of preoperative radiation is a higher rate of acute wound complications: 35% versus 17% with postoperative radiation according to the Canadian trial {2395,212}. The advent of intensity-modulated radiation therapy has enabled delivery of more-conformal dose distributions with maximal sparing of adjacent uninvolved normal tissues, shown in one study to improve local control compared with conventional 3D techniques {1043}. Careful implementation of intensity-modulated radiation therapy will also hopefully further reduce wound complication rates.

Finally, in some patients with high-grade sarcoma, radiation may be omitted without increasing risk of recurrence. One prospective and several retrospective studies of resection without radiation have shown excellent local control rates of > 85% {2519,211,2699}. However, it is not always clear which patient subsets can be safely treated with this approach. Those most likely to benefit include patients with unequivocally wide negative margins ≥ 1 cm or with an intact fascia. In our opinion, this approach should rarely be considered for initial unplanned excisions, in patients in whom salvage treatment of a local recurrence would be associated with substantial morbidity, or in patients who would not be compliant for close follow-up.

For retroperitoneal sarcoma, the role of preoperative radiation is less clear. Further study is warranted to optimally define the potential role of preoperative radiation therapy for the treatment of primary or locally recurrent retroperitoneal sarcoma.

Adjuvant and neoadjuvant chemotherapy

The value of chemotherapy for sarcoma depends on the tumour's specific histological type and location. Because of their very high risk of metastasis and sensitivity to chemotherapy, Ewing sarcoma and alveolar/embryonal rhabdomyosarcoma should always be treated with neoadjuvant chemotherapy. For other histological types of high-grade sarcoma, the choice to use chemotherapy depends on the risk of metastasis (governed by size, grade, and histology and computable by personalized nomograms, also available as a free app) {459}, the sensitivity of the histological type/subtype to neoadjuvant chemotherapy, and the patient's age and comorbidities.

Many randomized trials (and one meta-analysis of these trials' data) of soft tissue sarcoma have shown that chemotherapy improves disease-free survival, with improved local and locoregional control {88,398,2741,122}. An improvement in overall survival has been demonstrated in a single randomized trial, which involved an anthracycline (epirubicin) plus ifosfamide, although the trial had relatively short follow-up {1080}. This overall survival benefit was confirmed in a second meta-analysis, with a hazard ratio of 0.77 ($P = 0.01$) {2497}, and in another recent reanalysis of the largest randomized trial {2457}. However, other randomized trials have failed to demonstrate a benefit for chemotherapy, and thus its role remains controversial. Given the relatively small benefit, preoperative chemotherapy with an anthracycline and ifosfamide can be justified for large, high-grade tumours in carefully selected patients and for the histological types most likely to respond (synovial sarcoma, myxoid / round cell liposarcoma, pleomorphic liposarcoma, and UPS). A recent trial has shown that 3 cycles of full-dose anthracycline and ifosfamide have an equivalent outcome to 5 cycles {1228}; the more prolonged treatment may merely increase toxicity. Agents with activity against particular histological subtypes include gemcitabine and docetaxel for UPS and leiomyosarcoma {1950}, trabectedin for myxoid / round cell liposarcoma and leiomyosarcoma {1236}, gemcitabine and taxanes for angiosarcoma {2483,2932}, and ifosfamide for myxoid / round cell and pleomorphic liposarcoma {888} and synovial sarcoma {473,886}. However, none of these regimens was found to be superior to 3 cycles of full-dose anthracycline and ifosfamide for the management of high-risk localized soft tissue sarcoma in another recent randomized study {1227}.

Multimodal treatment

Surgery preceded or followed by radiotherapy, without preoperative or postoperative chemotherapy, remains the treatment of choice for most soft tissue sarcomas. For patients at high risk of distant metastases and death, chemotherapy may be considered in addition to the standard treatment of surgery and radiation therapy. Chemotherapy is most likely to benefit fit patients with large, rapidly growing, grade 3 tumours when the likelihood of R0 or R1 resection is uncertain. Because the efficacy of chemotherapy has not been clearly established, and this treatment has substantial toxicities, it is best proposed by an experienced multidisciplinary team expert in sarcoma management. For the multimodal treatment of large, high-grade sarcomas at high risk of distant metastasis, several sequencing schedules have been developed, and their application should be selected on an individual case basis by an interdisciplinary team {2868}: (1) neoadjuvant chemotherapy, then surgery, then postoperative radiotherapy; (2) neoadjuvant concurrent or interdigitated chemotherapy and preoperative radiotherapy, then surgery, then optional adjuvant chemotherapy; and (3) neoadjuvant sequential chemotherapy, then preoperative radiotherapy, then surgery, possibly followed by adjuvant chemotherapy. An advantage to the first and third approaches for patients with measurable disease is the ability to determine at an early stage whether the sarcoma is progressing on chemotherapy and, if so, to avoid further treatment with an agent that appears ineffective.

Imaging of tumours of soft tissue

Accurate clinical history is crucial to guide the choice of imaging modality and differential diagnosis, although final diagnosis in most cases rests on biopsy {2197}. The sarcomas most commonly recognizable on imaging include UPS, liposarcoma, leiomyosarcoma, gastrointestinal stromal tumour, synovial sarcoma, and MPNST.

For masses that are clinically fixed to bone or extremely firm, plain film may be helpful to distinguish between a primary bone and soft tissue mass and to identify calcifications. Ultrasound is cost-effective and readily available, and therefore often the first-line imaging investigation for an extremity soft tissue lump. Although diagnostic accuracy is limited, ultrasound serves as a triage tool for further investigations {1737,2256}.

MRI offers soft tissue contrast superior to that of other imaging modalities and is thus the imaging method of choice, particularly when tumours arise in the limbs or superficial tissue of the trunk. This is helpful not only for diagnosis but also surgical and radiotherapy planning and assessing response after radiotherapy. For patients in whom radiotherapy is considered, MRI can be useful for assessing local tumour extent as well as surrounding oedema, which is optimally included in the treatment volume. For limb sarcomas, a combination of axial T2-weighted, T1-weighted, T1-weighted with fat saturation, T1-weighted fat-saturated contrast-enhanced, and coronal short-tau inversion recovery (STIR) and coronal T1-weighted sequences should be used. These sequences can be supplemented by diffusion-weighted MRI sequences depending on local expertise {2104}. This complement of sequences allows for accurate staging of tumour margins; relationship to neurovascular structures; presence of macroscopic fat, myxoid elements, haemorrhage, and necrosis; and bone invasion and oedema. The apparent diffusion coefficient map from diffusion-weighted MRI may help assess the tumour's response to systemic or local treatments. For patients with absolute contraindications to MRI, contrast-enhanced CT can be used.

Contrast-enhanced CT is the most useful and widely available primary imaging method for possible soft tissue sarcoma of the thorax, abdomen, or pelvis, and it also allows staging of distant sites of disease. Relationships of the tumour with viscera, bowel, and vascular structures are usually well demonstrated. MRI is reserved for patients with allergy to iodinated contrast agents or for problem-solving when, for example, muscle, bone, or neural foraminal involvement is equivocal on CT. MRI may also be useful for delineating disease in the pelvis.

Although FDG PET has shown some ability to differentiate low-grade from high-grade sarcomas, the technique is not helpful for diagnosis, because it cannot reliably distinguish low-grade from benign lesions {826}. However, for extremely heterogeneous tumours, FDG PET-CT may be used to target biopsy to the most FDG-avid component, because GLUT1 expression and glucose metabolism have been shown to correlate with tumour grade in sarcoma {3054}. FDG PET-CT may also be able to detect malignant transformation in NF1, where increased glucose metabolism may indicate sarcomatous change of a neurofibroma to an MPNST {653}. FDG PET-CT or whole-body MRI is useful for problem-solving or staging before radical surgery and can also be helpful for sarcoma subtypes such as angiosarcomas and myxoid liposarcomas where metastatic disease may be occult on standard CT.

Terminology used to reflect biological potential

Soft tissue tumours are divided into four categories: benign, intermediate (locally aggressive), intermediate (rarely metastasizing), and malignant, which were defined in the third edition of the WHO Classification of Tumours series in 2002 as follows.

Benign: Most benign soft tissue tumours do not recur locally. Those that do recur do so in a non-destructive fashion and are almost always readily cured by complete local excision. Exceedingly rarely (almost certainly in < 1 in 50 000 cases and probably much less than that), a morphologically benign lesion may give rise to distant metastases. This is entirely unpredictable on the basis of conventional histological examination and to date has been best documented in cutaneous benign fibrous histiocytoma.

Intermediate (locally aggressive): Soft tissue tumours in this category often recur locally and may be associated with an infiltrative and locally destructive growth pattern. Lesions in this category very rarely if ever metastasize but typically require wide excision with a margin of normal tissue in order to ensure local control. The prototypical lesion in this category is desmoid fibromatosis.

Intermediate (rarely metastasizing): Soft tissue tumours in this category are often locally aggressive (see above) but, in addition, show the well-documented ability to give rise to distant metastases in occasional cases. The risk of such metastases appears to be < 2% and is not reliably predictable on the basis of histomorphology. Metastasis in such lesions is usually to lymph node or lung. Prototypical examples in this category include plexiform fibrohistiocytic tumour and angiomatoid fibrous histiocytoma.

Malignant: In addition to the potential for locally destructive growth and recurrence, malignant soft tissue tumours (known as soft tissue sarcomas) have a substantial risk of distant metastasis, ranging in most instances from 20% to almost 100%, depending on histological type and grade. Some (but not all) histologically low-grade sarcomas have a metastatic risk of only 2–10%, but such lesions may advance in grade in a local recurrence and thereby acquire a higher risk of distant spread (e.g. myxofibrosarcoma and leiomyosarcoma).

It is important to note that in this classification scheme, the intermediate categories do not correspond to histologically determined intermediate grade in a soft tissue sarcoma (see below), nor do they correspond to the ICD-O /1 behaviour category described as uncertain whether benign or malignant. The locally aggressive subset of entities with no metastatic potential, as defined above, are generally given ICD-O /1 codes, and the rarely metastasizing lesions are given ICD-O /3 codes.

Grading and staging of sarcomas

Grading

Except in a subset of sarcomas, histological typing alone does not provide sufficient information for predicting the clinical course of disease; thus, this must be achieved by grading and/or staging. Grading is based only on intrinsic qualities of the untreated primary tumour, whereas staging also takes into account tumour extent {1328,101}. Nomograms can assess multiple clinical and histological parameters to calculate the probability of recurrence for a given patient {887}.

Grading of sarcomas of soft tissue was first proposed in 1939 by Broders et al., but the first large-scale effort to use grade and stage in sarcomas was published in 1977 by Russell et al. {2692}. This study showed the prominent role of grade in predicting outcome for patients with sarcomas, although the grade used was determined subjectively. In the early 1980s, several grading systems based on various histological parameters were reported and demonstrated to correlate with prognosis {664, 2233,3104,3169}.

Most grading systems rely on mitotic activity and necrosis. An important change in this edition of the WHO Classification of Tumours series is the conversion of mitotic count from the traditional denominator of 10 high-power fields to a defined area expressed in mm². This serves to standardize the true area over which mitoses are enumerated, because different microscopes have high-power fields of different sizes. This change will also be helpful for anyone reporting using digital systems. The approximate number of fields per 1 mm² based on the field diameter and its corresponding area is presented in Table 1.01.

The two most widely used grading systems are those proposed by NCI {664} and the FNCLCC {3104}. The FNCLCC system appears to be more precisely defined and potentially more reproducible, and it is therefore the most widely used {814}. In accordance with College of American Pathologists (CAP) and American Joint Committee on Cancer (AJCC) recommendations, the FNCLCC system is preferred over the NCI system, at least in adults {2681,101}. Moreover, a comparison of the two systems showed greater efficiency of the FNCLCC system in terms of prognostic prediction and minimization of cases assigned to the intermediate category {1246}. Three independent prognostic factors are used for defining the grade: necrosis, mitotic activity, and degree of differentiation. A score is attributed independently to each parameter and the grade is obtained by summing the three attributed scores {3104}. The most challenging component of the system lies in the definition of differentiation score, which depends on histological type and subtype.

The main value of grading is its ability to indicate the probability of distant metastasis and overall survival in the whole group of sarcomas considered as a single entity, but also in individual types such as UPSs and synovial sarcomas {642}. On the other hand, grading is of little value for predicting local recurrence, which is strongly influenced by the quality of surgical margins.

Because of the pitfalls and limitations of grading, some rules must be respected: grading is not a substitute for an accurate histological diagnosis; it requires representative and well-processed material that must be obtained before administration of neoadjuvant therapy. Grading is less informative than histological type in some tumours (e.g. dedifferentiated and round cell liposarcomas, rhabdomyosarcoma, Ewing sarcoma, alveolar soft part sarcoma, epithelioid sarcoma, and clear cell sarcoma), and it should not be used in tumours that rarely metastasize {637,814}. The merits of grading in some tumours (e.g. MPNST and parenchymal breast angiosarcoma) continue to be debated {2265,2254}.

Table 1.01 Approximate number of fields per 1 mm² based on the field diameter and its corresponding area

Field diameter (mm)	Field area (mm²)	Approximate number of fields per 1 mm²
0.40	0.126	8
0.41	0.132	8
0.42	0.138	7
0.43	0.145	7
0.44	0.152	7
0.45	0.159	6
0.46	0.166	6
0.47	0.173	6
0.48	0.181	6
0.49	0.188	5
0.50	0.196	5
0.51	0.204	5
0.52	0.212	5
0.53	0.221	5
0.54	0.229	4
0.55	0.237	4
0.56	0.246	4
0.57	0.255	4
0.58	0.264	4
0.59	0.273	4
0.60	0.283	4
0.61	0.292	3
0.62	0.302	3
0.63	0.312	3
0.64	0.322	3
0.65	0.332	3
0.66	0.342	3
0.67	0.352	3
0.68	0.363	3
0.69	0.374	3

Several criticisms have been made of histological grading. A universal grading system is not possible for all sarcomas given their diversity, but it is unrealistic to develop a grading system for every specific histological type of sarcoma. However, the systems currently in use perform correctly for the most frequent sarcoma types and represent an acceptable alternative. The reproducibility of the same grading system among pathologists and of different grading systems for the same tumours is not ideal. Most grading systems are three-grade systems with an intermediate grade that in practice corresponds to undetermined prognosis (cannot be definitively classified as either high or low grade), and this category can subsume up to half of cases. The almost universal use of core needle biopsies is another important limitation for grading. Although grading on core needle biopsies has been reported to show an acceptable degree of accuracy {1385}, grade can be determined with certainty for high-grade sarcomas only, because low and intermediate grades must be applied as provisional "at least" designations, due to the possibility of sampling error. Histological grading can be aided by imaging procedures for evaluating necrosis and by MIB1 or PHH3 scores instead of mitotic count {1315}. Despite these clear limitations, grade remains the most important prognostic factor in most sarcomas, and it is evident that clinicians will continue to expect pathologists to provide a grade for most sarcomas to guide treatment selection.

Grading can be thought of as a morphological translation of molecular events that determine tumour aggressiveness; therefore, molecular parameters could eventually complement or even replace histological parameters. A molecular grading system based on the expression profile of 67 genes related to chromosome complexity and mitosis management, called CINSARC (Complexity Index in Sarcomas), has been described on a large series of sarcomas and other non-mesenchymal cancers with complex genomic profiles {1828}. This molecular grading system outperformed histological grading in this category of sarcomas, as well as in gastrointestinal stromal tumours {575, 1734,1784}, but independent validation is still lacking.

Staging

Staging of soft tissue sarcomas is based on histological and clinical information. The major staging systems used were developed by the Union for International Cancer Control (UICC) and AJCC and are clinically useful and of prognostic value. The TNM system incorporates histological grade as well as tumour size and depth, regional lymph node involvement, and distant metastasis {882}. Important prognostic factors for relapse and death include patient characteristics (e.g. sex and age), tumour characteristics (histology, grade, size, site, depth, and presence of metastasis at diagnosis), and management by the medical team (biopsy and review, unplanned surgery, and quality of resection). Nomograms incorporating non-anatomical and sometimes continuous rather than discrete variables, including those based on tumour type, site of involvement, and/or treatment regimen, have been proposed to guide patient management {3037,456,1175,459,1232}.

Lipoma

Fritchie KJ
Goldblum JR
Mertens F

Definition
Lipoma is a benign tumour composed of mature adipocytes.

ICD-O coding
8850/0 Lipoma NOS

ICD-11 coding
2E80.0Y Lipoma

Related terminology
None

Subtype(s)
Intramuscular lipoma; chondrolipoma

Localization
Lipomas are most common in the upper back, proximal extremity, and abdominal region, and the majority present as a superficial (subcutaneous) soft tissue mass. A smaller subset are deep-seated, arising within skeletal muscle (intramuscular lipoma), on the surface of bone (parosteal lipoma), or within the tendon sheath, or they may involve the gastrointestinal tract, oral cavity, or bronchial tree {1024,1635,2049,1599,2646,355,529,3056, 898,2955,440}. Intramuscular lipomas most frequently involve the thigh (40–50%), followed by the shoulder, chest wall, and upper limb {1635,2301}. Rare examples of retroperitoneal lipomas with cytogenetic and molecular confirmation have also been reported {1459,1924}. Synovial lipomatosis (lipoma arborescens) is a lipomatous proliferation of subsynovial connective tissue often associated with chronic joint disease, and recent work has shown that this adipocytic proliferation lacks HMGA2 overexpression, supporting a non-neoplastic reactive process {2381,2581}.

Clinical features
Lipomas typically present as a painless mass; however, larger tumours may compress peripheral nerves and result in pain or tenderness. Gastrointestinal lipomas may cause abdominal discomfort, melaena, or obstruction {529}. Approximately 5% of patients have multiple tumours, most often males in the back / posterior shoulder region {2698}. Individuals with *PTEN* hamartoma tumour syndrome, an autosomal dominant syndrome that includes Cowden syndrome and Bannayan–Riley–Ruvalcaba syndrome, may also have multiple lipomas {520,906}.

Imaging
Lipomas have characteristic features on both CT and MRI, presenting as discrete encapsulated masses with imaging features similar to those of the subcutaneous fat on both modalities. On CT, lipomas demonstrate homogeneous low attenuation (–120 to –65 Hounsfield units). On MRI, lipomas are homogeneous and isointense with subcutaneous fat on all pulse sequences. Lipomas may contain a few subtle thin internal striations that

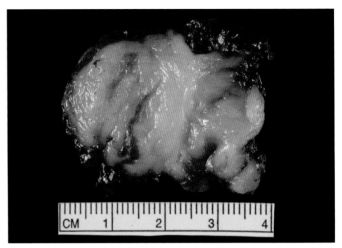

Fig.1.01 Lipoma. Gross examination shows a glistening yellowish-tan cut surface.

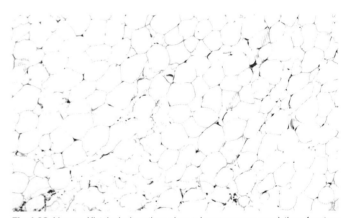

Fig.1.02 Lipoma. Histological sections show a homogeneous population of mature adipocytes.

measure < 2 mm due to muscle fibres, blood vessels, or fibrous septa, but they typically show no substantial internal enhancement on CT or MRI.

Epidemiology
Lipoma is the most common mesenchymal neoplasm in adults, is slightly more common in males, and tends to be associated with obesity {2698}. These tumours usually present in the fifth to seventh decades of life and are rare in the paediatric population.

Etiology
Unknown

Pathogenesis
The pathogenesis of lipomas is related to reactivated expression of the HMGA2 protein, which plays a role in the development of the mesodermal lineage during embryogenesis {169,1858,1388}.

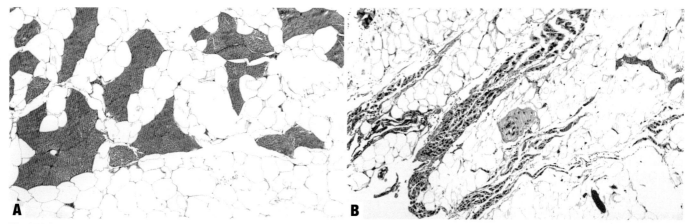

Fig. 1.03 Intramuscular lipoma. **A** These often show skeletal muscle fibres surrounded by mature adipocytes. **B** Atrophic skeletal muscle in intramuscular lipoma can mimic the atypical hyperchromatic stromal cells of atypical lipomatous tumour / well-differentiated liposarcoma.

Cytogenetics

Aberrant karyotypes, the vast majority of which are pseudodiploid or near-diploid, have been reported for close to 500 lipomas, most of which were deep-seated. Four major cytogenetic subgroups have emerged: (1) structural rearrangements of chromosome bands 12q13-q15 (two thirds of abnormal cases), (2) loss of material from chromosome arm 13q (15%), (3) structural rearrangements of band 6p21 (5%), and (4) supernumerary ring chromosomes (5%); about 5% of the cases display various combinations of these aberrations {2926,230}. Structural rearrangements involving 12q13-q15 are usually translocations, the most common of which is t(3;12)(q27-q28;q13-q15). Lipomas with ring chromosomes and amplified sequences from 12q most likely represent well-differentiated subtypes of atypical lipomatous tumour; lipomas with ring chromosomes are more often deep-seated, are larger, occur in older patients, and relapse more often than lipomas with other aberrations {230, 319}.

Molecular genetics

Chromosomal rearrangements of 12q target the *HMGA2* gene, encoding an architectural transcription factor. Typically, the break in *HMGA2* occurs in the large intron 3, either fusing the

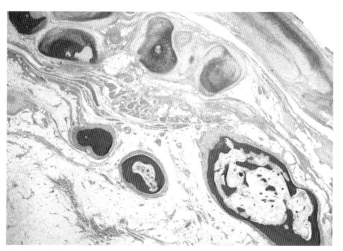

Fig. 1.04 Osteolipoma. These tumours contain nodules of metaplastic bone and cartilage.

first three AT-hook–encoding exons in-frame or out-of-frame with ectopic sequences or simply removing regulatory sequences from the 3′ untranslated region {177,2776,2503,1819}. The most common chimeric transcript is *HMGA2-LPP*, resulting from a t(3;12), but seven other fusion partners to *HMGA2* have been reported {309,2418}. The HMGA2 protein is important during embryogenesis, particularly in the development of the mesodermal lineage, but it is usually not expressed in differentiated adult tissues. The finding that reactivated expression of full-length, truncated, or fused HMGA2 is essential for lipoma development has been demonstrated not only through studies of lipomas, showing near-universal upregulation, but also by studies on mice and men with constitutional *HMGA2* rearrangements, as well as by the lack of other somatic mutations in lipomas {169,1858,1388}. The deletions affecting chromosome 13, with a minimal deleted region in 13q14, overlap with those in spindle cell lipoma, but the molecular outcome remains unclear {231}. Rearrangements of 6p21 affect *HMGA1*, a gene closely related to *HMGA2* {230,309}.

Macroscopic appearance

Lipomas, including intramuscular lipomas, are well-circumscribed tumours with a uniform glistening yellow to pale-tan cut surface. Superficial lipomas are typically < 5 cm, whereas those that are deep-seated may reach sizes > 20 cm. Osteolipomas and chondrolipomas harbour areas of grossly identifiable bone and cartilage, respectively. Chalky white foci of fat necrosis and dystrophic calcification, especially in large deep-seated tumours, may be present.

Histopathology

Histological examination reveals a well-differentiated lipomatous proliferation composed of mature adipocytes. Variably sized paucicellular fibrous septa may be present, but cytological atypia (atypical hyperchromatic stromal cells) is absent. Areas of fat necrosis are not uncommon, especially in larger or deep-seated lipomas. Intramuscular lipomas may show infiltration into surrounding skeletal muscle, and this finding has no clinical significance. However, atrophic skeletal muscle cells, a potential mimic of the atypical hyperchromatic stromal cells characteristic of atypical lipomatous tumour / well-differentiated liposarcoma, are often seen in these areas. Lipomas containing nodules of metaplastic bone or cartilage are termed osteoli-poma or chondrolipoma {1076}.

Cytology
Aspiration specimens show adipocytes containing a single large lipid droplet with a compressed rim of cytoplasm and a flattened inconspicuous nucleus.

Diagnostic molecular pathology
Diagnostic molecular pathology is not usually required, with the exception of retroperitoneal tumours and deep-seated fatty tumours > 10 cm, in which the exclusion of *MDM2* amplification is required.

Essential and desirable diagnostic criteria
Essential: circumscribed yellowish-tan mass; uniform prolifera-tion of mature adipose tissue without atypical hyperchromatic stromal cells.
Desirable (in selected cases): absence of giant marker/ring chromosomes / *MDM2* amplification.

Staging
Not clinically relevant

Prognosis and prediction
The recurrence rate of lipomas is < 5%. Deep-seated lipomas are more difficult to completely excise, leading to a higher rate of local recurrence.

Lipomatosis

Rosenberg AE
Nielsen GP

Definition
Lipomatosis is diffuse overgrowth of adipose tissue. Subclassification is based on clinical findings and anatomical distribution.

ICD-O coding
None

ICD-11 coding
EF02.1 Subcutaneous lipomatosis

Related terminology
Not recommended: Madelung disease; Launois–Bensaude syndrome.

Subtype(s)
Diffuse lipomatosis; multiple symmetrical lipomatosis; pelvic lipomatosis; steroid lipomatosis; HIV lipodystrophy

Localization
Diffuse lipomatosis involves the trunk, a large portion of an extremity, head and neck, abdomen, pelvis, or intestines. Macrodactyly or gigantism of a digit may be present {1217,2026}. Symmetrical lipomatosis manifests as symmetrical deposition of fat in the upper body, particularly the neck. In pelvic lipomatosis there is diffuse overgrowth of fat in the perivesical and perirectal areas. Steroid lipomatosis is characterized by accumulation of fat in the face, sternal region, or upper-middle back (buffalo hump). HIV lipodystrophy shows accumulation of visceral fat, breast adiposity, and cervical fat pads {2147,661}.

Clinical features
Patients present with massive accumulation of fat in affected areas that may mimic a neoplasm. Patients with symmetrical lipomatosis can have neuropathy and involvement of the CNS {2259,2524}. Accumulation of fat in the lower neck can cause laryngeal obstruction and compression of the vena cava. Pelvic lipomatosis causes urinary frequency, perineal pain, constipation, and abdominal and back pain. Bowel obstruction and hydronephrosis can develop. Imaging in lipomatosis shows the extent of fat accumulation and excludes other processes. Patients with HIV treated with antiretroviral medications may develop hyperlipidaemia, insulin resistance, and fat wasting in the face and limbs {1005}.

Epidemiology
Lipomatosis is rare. Diffuse lipomatosis usually occurs in children aged < 2 years, but it may affect adults. Pelvic lipomatosis often affects black males aged 9–80 years; the incidence

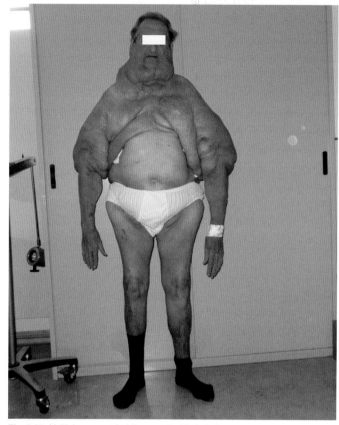

Fig. 1.05 Multiple symmetrical lipomatosis. Clinical photograph of an adult male patient with multiple symmetrical lipomatosis.

is 0.6–1.7 cases per 100 000 hospital admissions in the USA {3351}. Multiple symmetrical lipomatosis develops in middle-aged men (M:F ratio: 15:1) of Mediterranean descent, and the incidence is 1 case per 25 000 person-years {1350}. Patients have a history of liver disease or excessive alcohol consumption. Steroid lipomatosis manifests in patients on hormone therapy or who have increased endogenous production of adrenocortical steroids. Lipodystrophy is seen in HIV-positive patients treated with antiretroviral therapy.

Etiology
Multiple symmetrical lipomatosis is associated with liver disease or excessive alcohol consumption. Steroid lipomatosis manifests in patients on hormone therapy or who have increased endogenous production of adrenocortical steroids. HIV-infected patients treated with nucleoside reverse transcriptase inhibitors and protease inhibitors often develop lipodystrophy {1005}.

Pathogenesis
Patients with multiple symmetrical lipomatosis have mutations in mitochondrial DNA genes; familial subtypes are recognized {2230,2489}.

Macroscopic appearance
Grossly, lipomatosis appears as poorly circumscribed, soft, yellow fat identical to normal fat. The differences are the site and distribution of the fat.

Histopathology
All of the different types of lipomatosis have identical morphological features, consisting of lobules and sheets of mature adipocytes that may infiltrate other structures such as skeletal muscle.

Cytology
Not clinically relevant

Diagnostic molecular pathology
Not clinically relevant

Essential and desirable diagnostic criteria
Essential: diffuse overgrowth of mature adipose tissue.

Staging
Not clinically relevant

Prognosis and prediction
Idiopathic forms of lipomatosis tend to recur after surgery. Treatment is palliative surgical removal of excess fat. Massive accumulation of fat in the neck region may cause death due to laryngeal obstruction. Fat in steroid lipomatosis regresses after steroid levels are lowered. Patients with HIV treated with antiretroviral medications may experience metabolic disturbances.

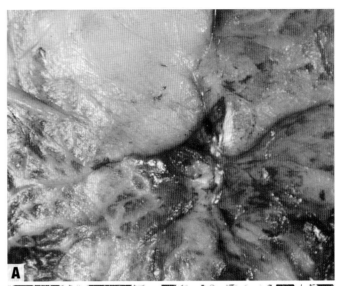
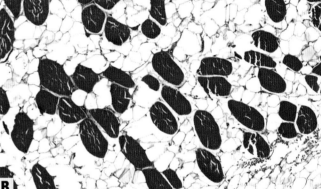

Fig. 1.06 Lipomatosis. **A** Adipose tissue infiltrating and replacing much of the involved skeletal muscle. **B** Mature white fat infiltrating skeletal muscle in diffuse lipomatosis.

Lipomatosis of nerve

Giannini C

Definition
Lipomatosis of nerve is a tumour characterized by overgrowth of mature fibroadipose tissue within the epineurium, surrounding and separating nerve fascicles.

ICD-O coding
None

ICD-11 coding
2E80.0Y Lipoma, other specified site

Related terminology
Acceptable: fibrolipomatous hamartoma; lipofibromatous hamartoma; macrodystrophia lipomatosa.

Subtype(s)
None

Localization
Lipomatosis of nerve occurs more frequently in the upper extremities (74%) than in the lower extremities (17%). The peripheral nerves most frequently affected include the median nerve (> 60%), ulnar nerve (7%), and plantar nerve (11%) {3022, 1977,1976}. Occasionally lipomatosis of nerve can be bilateral, affect multiple terminal nerves, or be restricted to the plexuses.

Clinical features
Sensory loss and paraesthesias are the most common symptoms (accounting for nearly half of patients' reported symptoms),

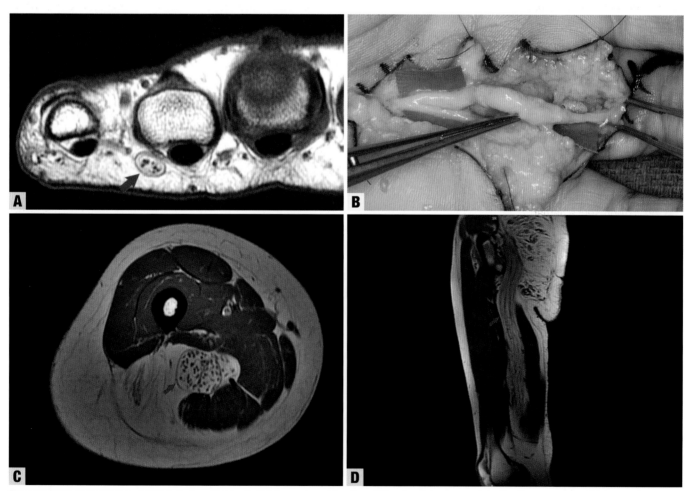

Fig. 1.07 Lipomatosis of nerve. **A** MRI. Left ulnar-sided fourth digital nerve (arrow) is enlarged (6 mm) and shows a coaxial cable–like appearance. **B** Intraoperative appearance. The fourth digital nerve is enlarged (6 mm) and shows a yellow lobulated appearance over a 2 cm length, typical of lipomatosis of nerve. **C** MRI. The sciatic nerve (arrow) is markedly enlarged (4 cm) and shows a typical coaxial cable–like appearance in this cross-section at the level of the thigh. **D** Longitudinal MRI. The sciatic nerve (arrow) is markedly enlarged (4 cm) and shows a typical spaghetti-like appearance in this longitudinal section at the level of the thigh.

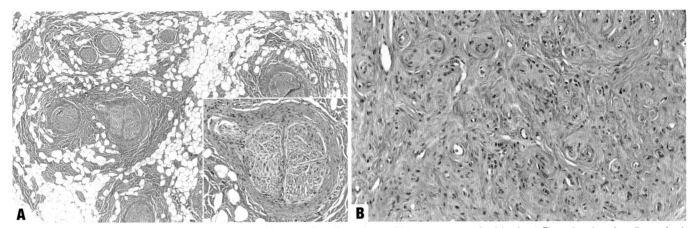

Fig. 1.08 Lipomatosis of nerve. **A** The endoneurium is expanded by mature fibroadipose tissue, which separates nerve fascicles. **Inset:** The perineurium of small nerve fascicles is markedly thickened. **B** Endoneurial pseudo–onion bulb–like hypertrophic change.

followed by pain and muscle weakness {1977}. Median nerve entrapment at the carpal tunnel most commonly accounts for neurological symptoms in median nerve lipomatosis of nerve. Overgrowth in the nerve distribution territory has been reported in > 60% of cases, especially in the upper extremities, with digital enlargement due to increase of soft tissue and skin and frequently true macrodactyly with enlargement of bone {1977}. On MRI, characteristic imaging features include a so-called coaxial cable–like appearance on the cross-sectional and spaghetti-like appearance on the longitudinal plane.

Epidemiology
A recent literature review identified 618 definite cases of lipomatosis of nerve {1977}. Patients typically present in the first decade of life (> 60%), with only 10% of cases coming to clinical attention after the fourth decade. Sex distribution was balanced between male (49%) and female (51%).

Etiology
Thought to represent a hamartomatous fibroadipose tissue overgrowth, lipomatosis of nerve is often progressive and behaves in a benign tumour–like fashion. It is sporadic. There are no syndromic associations except rare cases reported in association with Klippel–Trénaunay syndrome {89,2011} and Proteus syndrome {584}. Associated nerve-territory overgrowth seems to occur most frequently when lipomatosis of nerve occurs in motor and sensory nerve territory, suggesting that distal overgrowth may be influenced by the type of axons carried by the nerve {1976}.

Pathogenesis
PIK3CA mutations have been reported in patients with lipomatosis of nerve–associated macrodactyly {2637,3316}.

Macroscopic appearance
Lipomatosis of nerve causes a yellow lobulated fusiform enlargement of a peripheral nerve and at times its branches.

Histopathology
On transverse section, the epineurium is markedly expanded by mature adipose tissue and to a lesser extent by fibrous tissue; the nerve fascicles are widely spaced. Fascicles show frequently perineurial thickening and at times endoneurial septation with pseudo–onion bulb–like hypertrophic change mimicking intraneural perineurioma and probably representing reactive changes to nerve compression. Moderate to severe nerve fibre loss may be present. Immunohistochemical studies for EMA, S100, and NFP may help in characterizing nerve fibre pathology.

Cytology
Not clinically relevant

Diagnostic molecular pathology
Not clinically relevant

Essential and desirable diagnostic criteria
Essential: coaxial cable–like appearance on cross-sectional imaging; epineurial expansion by mature adipose tissue with widely spaced nerve fascicles; perineurial thickening and pseudo–onion bulb–like hypertrophic change.

Staging
Not clinically relevant

Prognosis and prediction
A benign condition, lipomatosis of nerve may require symptomatic treatment, including nerve decompression (e.g. carpal tunnel release for distal median nerve lipomatosis of nerve) or variable degrees of excision, balancing preservation of nerve function and soft tissue debulking and/or bony procedures to address functional and cosmetic issues.

Lipoblastoma and lipoblastomatosis

Black JO
Bridge JA
Pedeutour F

Definition
Lipoblastoma is a benign neoplasm of embryonal white fat, which may be a localized or diffuse tumour with a tendency for local recurrence if incompletely excised.

ICD-O coding
8881/0 Lipoblastomatosis

ICD-11 coding
2E80.1 & XH8L55 Lipoblastoma & Lipoblastomatosis

Related terminology
Not recommended: fetal lipoma; fetal fat tumour; fetocellular lipoma; embryonal lipoma; congenital lipomatoid tumour; lipoblastic tumour of childhood.

Subtype(s)
Localized (lipoblastoma); diffuse (lipoblastomatosis)

Localization
The trunk and extremities are the most common sites {629,3000, 1288}. Lipoblastoma may arise in the abdomen, mesentery, retroperitoneum, pelvis, inguinoscrotal or labial region, perineum, mediastinum, and head/neck (including the retropharynx and oral submucosa) {953,1288}. Lung, heart, colon, and parotid gland lipoblastoma have also been described {828,1556,1572, 2010,2828,1288}.

Clinical features
Superficial circumscribed lipoblastoma simulates lipoma or occasionally a vascular malformation. Lipoblastomatosis originates in deep soft tissue and is more infiltrative. Truncal tumours may infiltrate through the chest wall into the thoracic cavity from extrathoracic locations, or into the spine, with reports of neuroforaminal or intraspinal invasion requiring laminectomy for complete excision {2471,2439,2498,1258,1288}. Since both types recur, the distinction between circumscribed and infiltrative

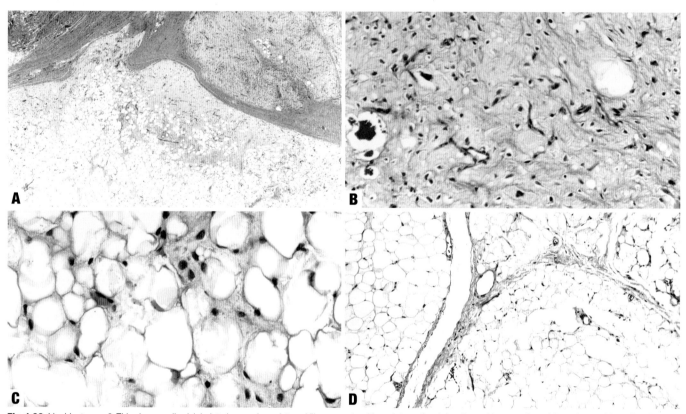

Fig. 1.09 Lipoblastoma. **A** This circumscribed, lobulated mass shows internal fibrous septa with a mixture of peripheral myxoid mesenchymal tissue in transition with adipocytic tissue, containing lipoblasts in various stages of maturation. **B** A myxoid area of lipoblastoma highlighting the delicate vasculature, myxoid matrix, and mesenchymal spindle cell component, which may occasionally include mild to moderate nuclear atypia. **C** Lipoblasts display a range of maturation, from multivacuolated lipoblasts to small signet-ring lipoblasts to mature adipocytes. **D** Mature lipoblastoma resembles fibrolipoma, with delicate internal fibrous septa, mostly mature adipocytes, and rare lipoblasts, most readily identified at the edges of the lobules, adjacent to foci of myxoid stroma.

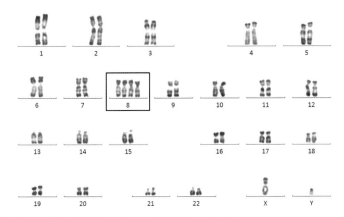

Fig. 1.10 Lipoblastoma. R-banded karyotype of a lipoblastoma showing polysomy of chromosome 8.

forms is not clinically relevant. Lipoblastoma can compress adjacent structures and interfere with function, particularly in large abdominal tumours, mediastinal tumours, or cervical tumours with stridor as a presenting symptom {629,2507,1501, 1923}. Colonic and mesenteric occurrences have been associated with intussusception and volvulus {439,2237}. Ultrasonography can detect tumours with high fluid content and vascularity in superficial tissues {1288}. MRI reveals a nodular mass with intensity similar to (or lower than) that of lipoma or subcutaneous fat on T1-weighted images {552,2440,2597,1288}. A subset of patients with lipoblastoma have developmental delays or abnormalities, seizures, congenital malformations, or familial lipomas, potentially related to larger chromosome 8q alterations that include the *PLAG1* gene {629,646,1368}.

Epidemiology
Lipoblastoma occurs predominantly in infancy and early childhood, with 75–90% of cases occurring before the age of 3 years {600,629,763,2919,1288}. Lipoblastoma is seen less frequently in older children and adolescents and rarely in adults. There is a slightly higher incidence in males {629,646,2078,3185,1288}.

Etiology
Unknown

Pathogenesis
Lipoblastomas typically exhibit simple, pseudodiploid, or hyperdiploid karyotypes that feature a structural alteration (translocation, inversion, insertion, or ring chromosome) of 8q11-q13 leading to rearrangement of *PLAG1*, a developmentally regulated zinc finger transcription factor gene, as characteristic {229,629,1158,958,704,2690}. The most common numerical change is one or more extra copies of chromosome 8, with or without concurrent rearrangement of 8q11-q13 {763,2070}. Reported *PLAG1* fusion gene partners in lipoblastoma include *HAS2* (8q24.13), *COL1A2* (7q21.3), *RAD51B* (14q24.1), *COL3A1* (2q32.2), *RAB2A* (8q12.1-q12.2), and *BOC* (3q13.2) {1362,2192, 428,771,3375,3248,2311}. *PLAG1* transcriptional upregulation leading to ectopic PLAG1 expression is the result of replacement of the *PLAG1* promoter element by constitutively active promoter regions from one of the partner genes. *PLAG1* rearrangements may be cytogenetically cryptic {2192}. Due to the close proximity of *RAB2A* and *PLAG1*, rearrangement of *PLAG1* may

be difficult to detect by FISH with this fusion event {3375}. It is unknown whether the excess copies of chromosome 8 that represent a potential alternative mechanism of tumorigenesis are wildtype or not {763,1158}. Lipoblastoma *PLAG1* fusion partners are distinct from those reported in pleomorphic adenoma; however, *RAD51B-PLAG1* has been identified in a subset of uterine myxoid leiomyosarcomas {166}.

Macroscopic appearance
Lipoblastomas are typically 2–5 cm in diameter, although they can exceed 10 cm {600,629,646,1288}. The soft; lobulated; yellow, white, or tan mass may display myxoid nodules, cystic spaces, or fat nodules separated by fine white fibrous trabeculae on the cut surface.

Histopathology
Lipoblastoma characteristically demonstrates lobular architecture with sheets of adipocytes separated by fibrovascular septa {357,600,629,646}. Myxoid areas display a plexiform vascular pattern with primitive mesenchymal cells. The fat cells show a spectrum of maturation, ranging from primitive stellate or spindled mesenchymal cells, to multivacuolated or small signet-ring lipoblasts, to mature adipocytes. The proportion of these cell types varies from case to case and from lobule to lobule. The fat lobule itself can occasionally exhibit a zonal pattern of maturation, with more immature myxoid cells at the periphery and adjacent to fibrous septa, with mature adipocytes in the centre of the lobule. The myxoid regions can occasionally show pooling of matrix similar to myxoid liposarcoma. Mature areas resemble lipoma or fibrolipoma with sparse lipoblasts {629, 646,2191}. Tumour maturation is documented, supported by reports of cases diagnosed by biopsy as lipoblastoma with later resection showing a fibrolipomatous appearance without

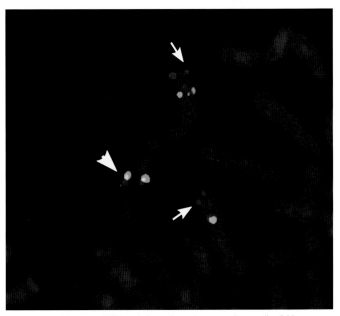

Fig. 1.11 Lipoblastoma. FISH analysis performed on metaphase cells of this case using a *PLAG1* break-apart probe set revealed the presence of two abnormal chromosome 8 homologues with a cytogenetically cryptic paracentric inversion resulting in *PLAG1* rearrangement (arrows). Normal chromosome 8 with juxtaposed orange/green signals (arrowhead).

lipoblasts {2831}. Mast cells are common. Other histological findings include fibroblastic proliferation with collagen deposition, chondroid metaplasia, extramedullary haematopoiesis, chronic inflammation, and sparse multinucleated or floret cells {629,646,675}. Hyperchromasia and mild nuclear atypia may be observed {2848}. Mitoses are very rare, and abnormal mitoses are absent.

The adipocytes of lipoblastoma demonstrate reactivity for S100, CD56, and CD34 {2164}. Nuclear p16 expression, which is frequently seen in liposarcoma, is observed in only a small subset of lipoblastomas, without correlation to macroscopic appearance or clinical behaviour {478}. The primitive mesenchymal cells are often reactive for desmin {629}.

Cytology

Cytological material from lipoblastoma varies according to the cellularity and the extent of the immature adipocyte, mature adipocyte, and myxoid matrix components {990,43,178}. Variation in adipocyte size is usually observed. Lipoblasts, fibrovascular network, and primitive spindled mesenchymal cells are also seen.

Diagnostic molecular pathology

In selected cases, the finding of *PLAG1* rearrangements / copy-number gain can support the diagnosis {704}.

Essential and desirable diagnostic criteria

Essential: lobulated mass formed of sheets of adipocytes with variable maturation separated by fibrovascular septa.

Staging

Not clinically relevant

Prognosis and prediction

Lipoblastoma is benign, with an excellent prognosis after excision {600,3185,629,2919,1288,3000}. The recurrence rate of 13–46% is usually due to incomplete excision, and recurrence can occur as late as 6 years after primary resection, supporting the practice of long-term follow-up, best evaluated with MRI or ultrasound for superficial tumours {2805}. Locally aggressive behaviour with multiple recurrences has been described, but re-excision is effective {1288}. There is no risk of metastasis.

Angiolipoma

Sciot R
Nielsen GP

Definition
Angiolipoma is a subcutaneous tumour consisting of mature fat cells intermingled with small and thin-walled vessels, a number of which contain fibrin thrombi.

ICD-O coding
8861/0 Angiolipoma NOS

ICD-11 coding
2E80.0Y & XH3C77 Other specified lipoma & Angiolipoma NOS

Related terminology
None

Subtype(s)
Cellular angiolipoma

Localization
The extremities (usually the forearm) are the most common site, followed by the trunk. Intramuscular haemangiomas and the so-called angiolipomas of parenchymal organs or of the CNS are different lesions, in that they contain larger vessels {2829,185}.

Clinical features
Angiolipomas most frequently present as multiple subcutaneous small nodules, usually tender to painful. There is no correlation between the intensity/occurrence of pain and the degree of vascularity {831}.

Epidemiology
Angiolipomas are relatively common and usually appear in the late second decade or early third decade of life. There is a male predominance, and an increased familial incidence has been described (5% of all cases) {1,831}. The mode of inheritance is autosomal dominant.

Etiology
Unknown

Pathogenesis
The vast majority of angiolipomas show a normal karyotype {2796,1965}, but rare cases have been reported to show rearrangements of chromosome 13 {2414}. The majority (80%) have been reported to have low-frequency *PRKD2* mutations {1388}.

Macroscopic appearance
Angiolipomas appear as encapsulated yellowish to reddish nodules.

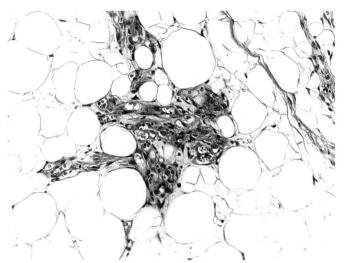

Fig. 1.12 Angiolipoma. The lesion consists of mature adipocytes and capillaries, some of which contain microthrombi.

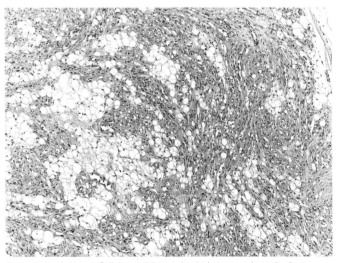

Fig. 1.13 Angiolipoma. Cellular angiolipoma, in which the vessels predominate.

Histopathology
Angiolipomas typically consist of two elements: mature adipocytes and branching capillary-sized vessels, which often contain fibrin thrombi. The vascularity is more prominent in the periphery {831}. The relative proportion of adipocytes and vessels varies, and some lesions are almost completely composed of vascular channels. These cellular angiolipomas should be distinguished from angiosarcoma and Kaposi sarcoma {1443}.

Cytology
Not clinically relevant

Diagnostic molecular pathology
Not clinically relevant

Essential and desirable diagnostic criteria
Essential: tender, often multiple subcutaneous nodules; mature fat with a variable amount of capillary vessels; fibrin micro-thrombi.

Staging
Not clinically relevant

Prognosis and prediction
Angiolipomas are always benign and show no tendency to recur.

Myolipoma of soft tissue

Fukushima M

Definition
Myolipoma of soft tissue is a benign extrauterine tumour composed of mature adipose tissue and well-differentiated smooth muscle cells.

ICD-O coding
8890/0 Myolipoma

ICD-11 coding
2E80.01 & XH4VB4 Deep subfascial lipoma & Angiomyolipoma

Related terminology
Acceptable: extrauterine lipoleiomyoma.

Subtype(s)
None

Localization
Myolipoma usually presents as a deeply situated mass within the retroperitoneum, abdominal cavity, pelvic cavity, or inguinal region. Less commonly it occurs in the trunk wall or extremities {1093,2059,2108}.

Clinical features
Lesions within the abdominal cavity are often found incidentally, whereas those involving the trunk or extremities are palpable {1093,2059}. MRI shows a fatty mass with associated signal-rich areas (corresponding to the smooth muscle component) that are heterogeneous on T1 postcontrast fat-suppressed images {3183}.

Epidemiology
Myolipoma is a rare tumour occurring chiefly in adult women. It is not associated with tuberous sclerosis {1093,2059,2108}.

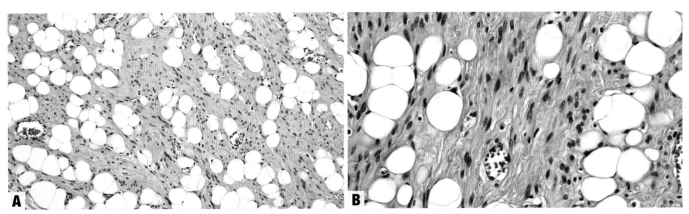

Fig. 1.14 Myolipoma. **A** The tumour is composed of an intimate admixture of adipocytes and smooth muscle cells. **B** No atypia or mitotic activity is observed in either adipocytes or smooth muscle cells.

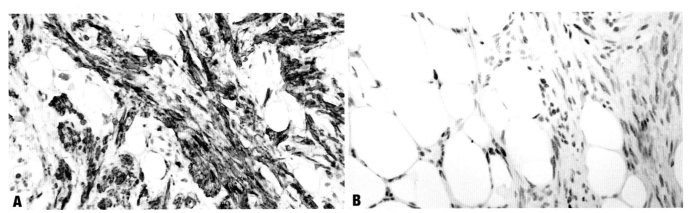

Fig. 1.15 Myolipoma. **A** Smooth muscle cells within the tumour show diffuse positivity for desmin. **B** Both smooth muscle cells and adipocytes often show nuclear positivity for HMGA2.

Etiology
Unknown

Pathogenesis
Cytogenetic alterations of the *HMGA2* gene have been reported in two cases {2413,1380}. Fusion of the *HMGA2* and *C9orf92* genes resulting from a t(9;12)(p22;q14) has been reported in one case of myolipoma {2413}.

Macroscopic appearance
Deep myolipomas are frequently large, often reaching 10–25 cm in size. Superficial lesions are smaller. The tumour is well circumscribed and usually surrounded by a thin capsule. The cut surface shows an admixture of yellowish adipose tissue and tan-whitish whorled nodules, depending on the amount and distribution of the smooth muscle component {1093,2059,2108}.

Histopathology
The lesions are composed of an intimate admixture of mature fat cells and spindled cells, in variable proportions. The spindled areas consist of well-differentiated smooth muscle, with intersecting fascicles of amitotic, cytologically bland cells having eosinophilic cytoplasm, cigar-shaped nuclei, and perinuclear vacuoles. The adipocytic component lacks any features to suggest atypical lipomatous tumour / well-differentiated liposarcoma (e.g. enlarged atypical nuclei, fibrous septation, lipoblasts) {1093,2059,2108}. The lesions usually contain variable numbers of small blood vessels and uterine thick-walled vessels {1093}. Immunohistochemically, desmin, caldesmon, and SMA positivity confirms smooth muscle differentiation. Nuclear positivity for HMGA2 is identified in 60% of cases. ER and PR are often positive. MDM2, CDK4, and HMB45 are negative {1093,2059,266,2464,3025}.

Cytology
Not clinically relevant

Diagnostic molecular pathology
Not clinically relevant

Essential and desirable diagnostic criteria
Essential: extrauterine location; admixture of well-differentiated, cytologically bland smooth muscle and mature fat.

Staging
Not clinically relevant

Prognosis and prediction
Complete resection is curative.

Chondroid lipoma

Bridge JA
Flucke U

Definition
Chondroid lipoma is a benign adipose tissue tumour composed of lipoblasts that intermingle with mature adipocytes in a myxo-hyaline chondroid matrix.

ICD-O coding
8862/0 Chondroid lipoma

ICD-11 coding
2E80.0Z & XH7WX8 Lipoma, unspecified & Chondroid lipoma

Related terminology
None

Subtype(s)
None

Localization
Tumours are typically deep-seated, involving skeletal muscle, deep fibrous connective tissue, or deep subcutaneous fat. Most

arise in the proximal extremities and limb girdles {2057}. Less common sites include distal extremities, trunk, and head and neck (including the oral cavity) {1095}.

Clinical features
Most patients present with a painless mass of variable duration, with some reporting a recent increase in size {2057}. Imaging studies typically show a well-defined, heterogeneous fatty and myxoid lesion, deviating from the appearance of lipoma but otherwise non-distinctive {1889}. Calcification is commonly present {2219}.

Epidemiology
Chondroid lipoma is a rare tumour that primarily affects adult women.

Etiology
Unknown

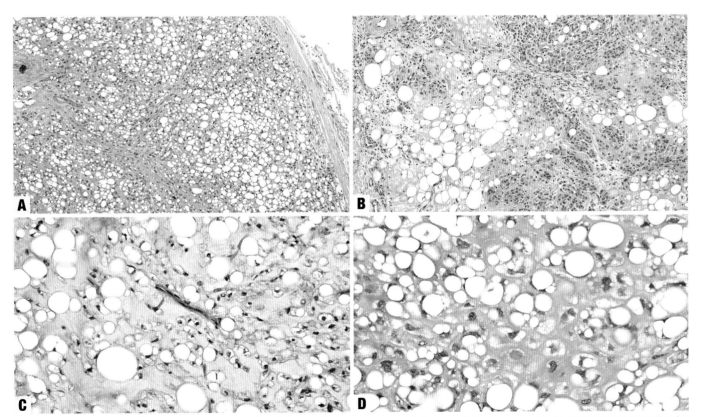

Fig. 1.16 Chondroid lipoma. **A** These tumours present as small, well-circumscribed or even encapsulated masses. **B** The tumour consists of a moderately cellular proliferation of epithelioid cells, lipoblasts, and mature fat, in a hyalinized, vaguely chondroid matrix. **C** Focally, chondroid lipomas can show arborizing capillaries, simulating myxoid liposarcoma. **D** High-power view of lipoblasts, mature fat, and hyalinized stroma in chondroid lipoma.

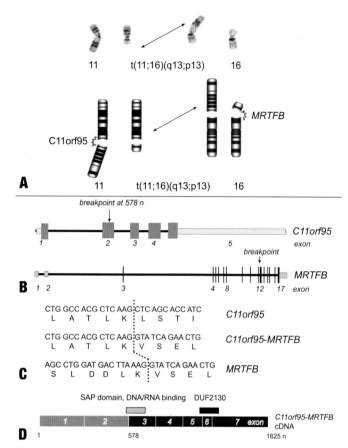

A

11   t(11;16)(q13;p13)   16

MRTFB

C11orf95

11   t(11;16)(q13;p13)   16

B

breakpoint at 578 n

C11orf95

1   2   3   4   5   exon

breakpoint

MRTFB

1 2   3   4 8   12 17   exon

C

CTG GCC ACG CTC AAG CTC AGC ACC ATC
 L   A   T   L   K   L   S   T   I   C11orf95

CTG GCC ACG CTC AAG GTA TCA GAA CTG
 L   A   T   L   K   V   S   E   L   C11orf95-MRTFB

AGC CTG GAT GAC TTA AAG GTA TCA GAA CTG
 S   L   D   D   L   K   V   S   E   L   MRTFB

D

SAP domain, DNA/RNA binding   DUF2130

1   2   3   4   5   6   7   exon   C11orf95-MRTFB cDNA

1   578   1625 n

Fig. 1.17 Genetics of chondroid lipoma. **A** Partial karyotype and schematic illustrating the characteristic 11;16 translocation. **B** Schematic of *C11orf95* and *MRTFB* showing corresponding breakpoints associated with the *C11orf95-MRTFB* fusion gene. **C** Nucleotide and amino acid sequences around the fusion point are presented. **D** The coding region of the fusion cDNA demonstrating the boundaries of exons and the position of conserved domains.

Pathogenesis

Chondroid lipoma is characterized by a recurrent t(11;16)(q13;p13) chromosomal translocation that results in fusion of the *C11orf95* (11q13.1) and *MRTFB* (previous alias *MKL2*; 16p13.12) genes {1425,1037}. MRTFB functions as a coactivator of the transcription factor SRF, which regulates a broad range of cellular processes such as organization of the cytoskeleton, cell migration, cell growth, and differentiation {2515}. *C11orf95* encodes for a hypothetical protein of unknown function.

Macroscopic appearance

Chondroid lipomas are well delineated, with yellowish-tan, gelatinous cut surfaces suggesting a mature fat component.

The tumour size ranges from 2 to 7 cm; those complicated by haemorrhage are usually larger {2057}.

Histopathology

Encapsulation and occasional lobulation may be seen. There are variable proportions of mature adipose tissue intermingled with nests and cords of small round vacuolated cells embedded in a myxoid-chondroid matrix. The small cells display a range of lipoblastic differentiation, consisting of undifferentiated bland cells with minimal cytoplasm to small univacuolated and multivacuolated lipoblasts with fat droplets scalloping bland nuclei. Cells with granular, eosinophilic cytoplasm may also be seen. PAS staining accentuates intracytoplasmic glycogen. Toluidine and Alcian blue staining at low pH indicates the presence of chondroitin sulfate. Owing to high vascularity, haemorrhage and fibrosis are common {1636,2057, 2284}; occasionally calcification or metaplastic bone formation is seen {1382}.

Immunohistochemistry for S100 is strongly positive in the mature fatty component, weaker in the lipoblastic elements, and usually negative in cells without apparent lipoblastic differentiation. Keratins may be detected rarely, and EMA is negative {1636}. Ultrastructural study confirms the presence of mature fat, as well as small embryonal cells with features of lipoblasts, chondroblasts, or both. The surrounding matrix consists of a network of thin filaments, thin collagen fibres, and abundant proteoglycan particles {1636,2284}.

Cytology

Cytologically, chondroid lipoma is composed of relatively cohesive clusters of mature adipocytes and variably sized lipoblasts in a chondromyxoid matrix {1157,3355}.

Diagnostic molecular pathology

Not clinically relevant

Essential and desirable diagnostic criteria

Essential: lobulated, circumscribed mass with variable admixture of mature adipocytes and lipoblasts embedded in a myxohyaline chondroid matrix.

Staging

Not clinically relevant

Prognosis and prediction

Surgical excision is usually curative and local recurrences are rare.

Spindle cell lipoma and pleomorphic lipoma

Billings SD
Ud Din N

Definition
Spindle cell lipomas and pleomorphic lipomas (SCL/PLs) represent the morphological spectrum of a single neoplasm. Spindle cell lipoma (SCL) is a benign adipocytic tumour composed of variable amounts of mature adipocytes, bland spindle cells, and ropy collagen {916}. Pleomorphic lipoma (PL) in addition contains pleomorphic and multinucleated floret-like giant cells.

ICD-O coding
8857/0 Spindle cell lipoma

ICD-11 coding
2E80.0Z & XH30M7 Lipoma, unspecified & Pleomorphic lipoma
2E80.0Z & XH4E98 Lipoma, unspecified & Spindle cell lipoma

Related terminology
Not recommended: dendritic fibromyxolipoma.

Subtype(s)
None

Localization
Approximately 80% of SCL/PLs arise within the subcutis of the posterior neck, back, and shoulders {916,2851}. The remaining 20% involve different sites, including the face, scalp, oral cavity, upper and lower limbs, and trunk {2851,117,1025,548,3122}. Cases in women are more likely to arise outside the typical locations {1659}. Rarely, intramuscular lesions and dermal-based lesions are seen {3122,1070}.

Clinical features
SCL/PLs typically present as a painless, slow-growing, solitary, mobile mass of the subcutis, often of several years' duration. Most tumours measure < 5 cm. Occasionally, multiple lesions are seen, and these cases may be familial {964,1309}.

Epidemiology
SCL/PLs most commonly affect men aged 45–60 years; < 10% of cases occur in females {916,2851,117,1025}. These tumours are relatively uncommon compared with conventional lipomas (ratio: 1:60) and account for approximately 1.5% of adipocytic neoplasms {1025}.

Etiology
Unknown

Pathogenesis
SCL/PL is characterized by partial or whole chromosome 13 and/or 16 deletions {722,709,1019}. Breakpoints in 13q deletions cluster around the region 13q14, where the *RB1* gene resides {709}. Loss of 13q14, including *RB1*, is characteristic of mammary and soft tissue myofibroblastomas, as well as of spindle cell / pleomorphic lipoma and cellular angiofibroma. In addition, the overlapping morphological and immunohistochemical features support the hypothesis that these tumours represent variations along a spectrum of genetically related lesions, the so-called 13q/*RB1* family of tumours {1941,1422,1040,26}.

Macroscopic appearance
Grossly, SCL appears as an oval or discoid mass. The cut surface is variably yellow, greyish-white, and myxoid, depending on the proportion of the constituent elements. The texture is often firmer than ordinary lipoma, but it can be gelatinous in extensively myxoid tumours.

Histopathology
SCL is usually well circumscribed and often encapsulated. Dermal and intramuscular tumours may have an infiltrative appearance. All are characterized by a triad of variable amounts of bland spindle cells, mature adipocytes, and ropy collagen (thick, refractile, eosinophilic) bundles. These components

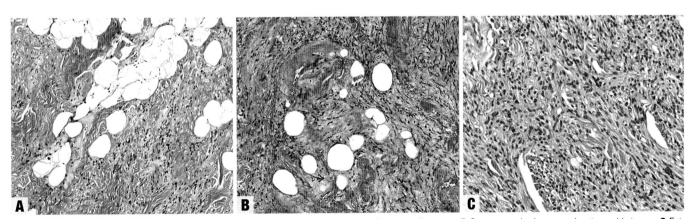

Fig. 1.18 Spindle cell lipoma. **A** This example contains bland spindle cells, ropy collagen, and mature adipocytes. **B** Some examples have prominent myxoid stroma. **C** Fat-free subtype of spindle cell lipoma with bland spindle cells and ropy collagen.

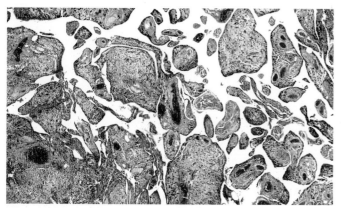

Fig. 1.19 Spindle cell lipoma. Pseudoangiomatous subtype of spindle cell lipoma.

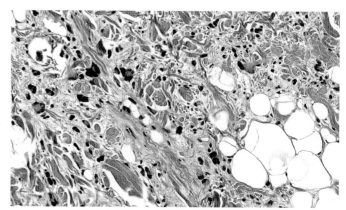

Fig. 1.20 Pleomorphic lipoma. Typical example with floret-like giant cells admixed with bland spindle cells, ropy collagen, and mature adipocytes.

are usually seen in a fibromyxoid stroma {916,117,1025}. Mast cells are a consistent finding. The adipocytes are variable in size, and occasional lipoblasts can be identified in as many as 50% of cases {2113}. The spindle cells are bland and randomly placed or arranged in short fascicles in a school-of-fish pattern, sometimes with nuclear palisading. Nuclei are uniform and elongated, with bipolar eosinophilic cytoplasmic processes. Some spindle cells may show small cytoplasmic vacuoles. Mitoses are rare and necrosis is absent. Some tumours may exhibit a vascular network composed of small to medium-sized thick-walled blood vessels, which may be hyalinized. PL in addition contains pleomorphic spindle cells and multinucleated floret-like giant cells. The latter cells have a ring of peripherally radially placed, hyperchromatic nuclei around central deeply eosinophilic cytoplasm (flower-petal arrangement) {2851,191}.

Morphological subtypes include fat-poor SCL, with little to no fat {320,2703}; the myxoid subtype, with abundant myxoid stroma {3306}; the (pseudo)angiomatous subtype, with branching and dilated vascular-like spaces that separate the spindle cells and stroma to form pseudopapillary projections {1326, 3385}; plexiform SCL {3391}; SCL with focal cartilaginous and osseous metaplasia {1025}; and SCL with extramedullary haematopoiesis {2797}. The spindle, pleomorphic, and floret-like giant cells characteristically stain for CD34 {3059,3001}, with loss of nuclear RB1 protein expression {550}.

Cytology

The smears show a mixture of adipocytes and clusters of or dispersed uniform spindle cells, often set in a myxoid stroma, which may contain mast cells. Fragments of brightly eosinophilic collagen fibres are also seen. PL, on the other hand, shows multinucleated giant cells with hyperchromatic nuclei and a moderate amount of cytoplasm {832}.

Diagnostic molecular pathology

Demonstration of loss of the *RB1* locus can be helpful in selected cases {709,231}.

Essential and desirable diagnostic criteria

Essential: bland spindle cells arranged in small, aligned groups; myxoid matrix; mature fat; ropy collagen; floret-like multinucleated giant cells in PL.

Staging

Not clinically relevant

Prognosis and prediction

SCL/PL is a benign tumour that is adequately treated with conservative excision. Local recurrence is rare, even with incomplete resection {916,2851,117}.

Hibernoma

Fanburg-Smith JC
Nord KH

Definition
Hibernoma is a rare, benign adipocytic tumour showing brown fat differentiation.

ICD-O coding
8880/0 Hibernoma

ICD-11 coding
2E80.0Z & XH1054 Lipoma, unspecified & Hibernoma

Related terminology
None

Subtype(s)
None

Localization
Hibernomas are most often located in the thigh, trunk, chest, upper extremity, and head and neck. Myxoid and spindle cell

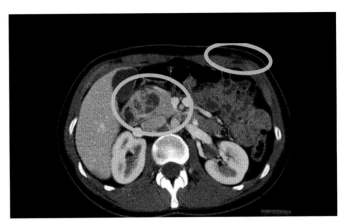

Fig. 1.22 Hibernoma. Multiple hibernomas (yellow ovals), in this instance arising in a patient with documented multiple endocrine neoplasia type 1.

subtypes often involve the posterior neck and shoulder {1096}. Fewer than 10% of cases occur in intra-abdominal, retroperitoneal, or thoracic locations. Very rare primary hibernomas of bone chiefly involve the axial skeleton {2906}.

Clinical features
Hibernomas typically present in young adults (mean age: 38 years; range: 2–75 years), as small, slow-growing, painless, mobile, subcutaneous masses {1096}. Fewer than 20% are intramuscular. They are slightly more common in males. On MRI, they are isointense or hypointense to fat on T1, isointense to hyperintense to fat on T2, and isointense to hyperintense to muscle on short-tau inversion recovery (STIR). They often contain low-signal internal strands and may be more heterogeneous, depending on their composition. Enhancement is common and more avid in lesions with a greater percentage of brown fat. Hibernomas are highly metabolically active and are frequently detected incidentally during FDG PET performed for the staging of various malignancies. There are two reports of hibernomas arising in patients with multiple endocrine neoplasia type 1 {1339,1974}.

Epidemiology
Hibernomas account for < 2% of benign and 1% of all adipocytic tumours.

Etiology
There is an association with multiple endocrine neoplasia type 1 {1339}.

Pathogenesis
Cytogenetically, almost all hibernomas have breakpoints in chromosome arm 11q, with a distinctive clustering to 11q13 {1159,1945,2098,2319}. FISH, SNP array, and multiplex ligation-dependent probe amplification analyses have revealed complex

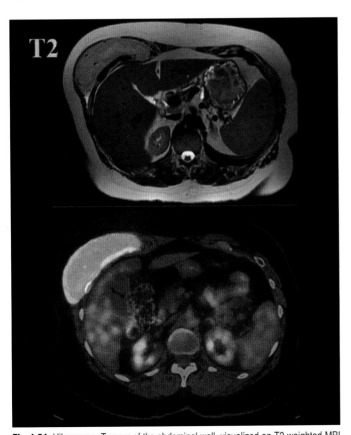

Fig. 1.21 Hibernoma. Tumour of the abdominal wall, visualized on T2-weighted MRI (top image) and FDG PET (bottom image). Hibernomas are very metabolically active and are often identified incidentally on FDG PET performed for the detection of metastatic disease in patients with known malignancies.

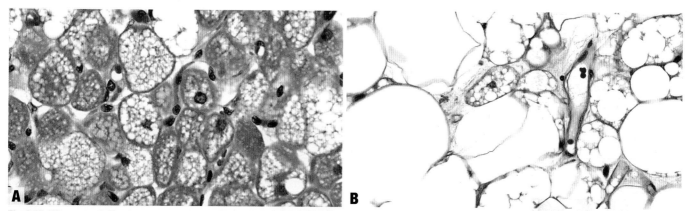

Fig. 1.23 Hibernoma. **A** Classic pattern, consisting of multivacuolated brown fat cells, with a centrally placed, normochromatic nucleus. **B** Lipoma-like subtype of hibernoma, consisting chiefly of white fat.

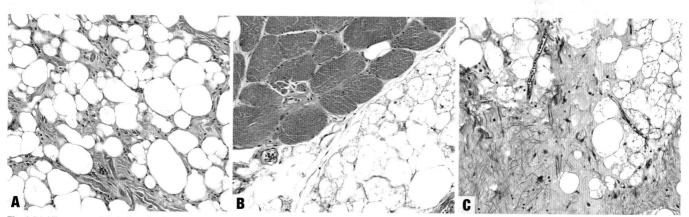

Fig. 1.24 Hibernoma. **A** Spindle cell subtype of hibernoma, with short spindled cells, wiry collagen, and scattered brown fat cells. **B** Rare hibernomas occur in an intramuscular location. **C** An example with stromal myxoid change and modestly atypical stromal cells. Such tumours are easily mistaken for atypical lipomatous tumour.

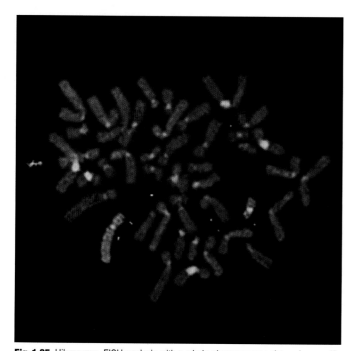

Fig. 1.25 Hibernoma. FISH analysis with a whole-chromosome paint probe specific for chromosome 11 reveals complex structural rearrangements involving this chromosome.

genomic rearrangements, with translocations and interstitial deletions that affect both homologues of chromosome 11 {1159, 1945,2319}. The ultimate consequence of these rearrangements is a set of deletions that cluster to a 3 Mb region in 11q13, with a preferential localization to regions covering the tumour suppressor genes *MEN1* and *AIP*. Somatic single-nucleotide variants in *MEN1* and *AIP* have not been detected in hibernoma {1938}. Hibernomas strongly express the brown fat marker gene *UCP1*; rearrangement, amplification, or increased expression of *HMGA2*, *CDK4*, or *MDM2* is not detected {232,67}.

Macroscopic appearance
Grossly, hibernomas are typically well circumscribed, vaguely lobular, and brown to yellow in appearance {1096}.

Histopathology
Hibernomas have a rich capillary network and are composed of eosinophilic and pale, polygonal, multivacuolated, granular, brown fat cells, with a variable component of univacuolated white fat. The nuclei of the brown fat cells are small, round, and centrally located, with small nucleoli. Classic hibernomas contain > 70% brown fat, with lipoma-like subtypes containing more white fat. Stromal myxoid change and an increased number of stromal spindled cells resembling those of spindle cell lipoma may be seen {1096}. Nuclear atypia and mitotic activity are absent {67}.

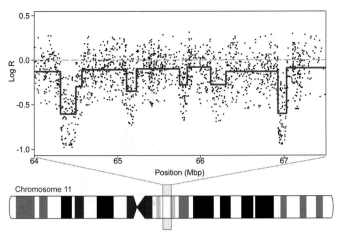

Fig. 1.26 Hibernoma. SNP array analysis shows hemizygous and homozygous deletions in chromosome band 11q13. The homozygous deletions contain the genes *MEN1* (64.3 Mb) and *AIP* (67.0 Mb).

Cytology
Cytology reveals uniform small multivacuolated brown fat cells with finely granular cytoplasm, bland round nuclei, and branching capillaries {1827}.

Diagnostic molecular pathology
Not clinically relevant

Essential and desirable diagnostic criteria
Essential: tumour composed of multivacuolated brown fat cells with small, normochromatic, centrally located nuclei.

Staging
Not clinically relevant

Prognosis and prediction
Hibernomas are entirely benign and typically do not recur after local excision {1096}.

Atypical spindle cell / pleomorphic lipomatous tumour

Creytens D
Marino-Enriquez A

Definition

Atypical spindle cell / pleomorphic lipomatous tumour is a benign adipocytic neoplasm, characterized by ill-defined tumour margins and the presence of variable proportions of mild to moderately atypical spindle cells, adipocytes, lipoblasts, pleomorphic cells, multinucleated giant cells, and a myxoid or collagenous extracellular matrix. It has a low tendency for local recurrence if incompletely excised. Unlike conventional atypical lipomatous tumours, there is no risk for dedifferentiation.

ICD-O coding

8857/0 Atypical spindle cell / pleomorphic lipomatous tumour

ICD-11 coding

2E80 & XH4E98 Benign lipomatous neoplasm & Spindle cell lipoma

Related terminology

Acceptable: atypical spindle cell lipoma.
Not recommended: spindle cell liposarcoma; fibrosarcoma-like lipomatous neoplasm.

Subtype(s)

None

Localization

Atypical spindle cell / pleomorphic lipomatous tumours arise in the subcutis slightly more frequently than in deep (subfascial) somatic soft tissues, and they only occasionally arise in intracavitary or visceral locations. The anatomical distribution is wide, predominating in the limbs and limb girdles {1983,678, 683}. The most common locations are the hand and foot and the thigh, followed by the shoulder and buttock, forearm, knee, lower leg, and upper arm. Less common locations are the head and neck, genital area, trunk, and back {1983,678,200}. Rare

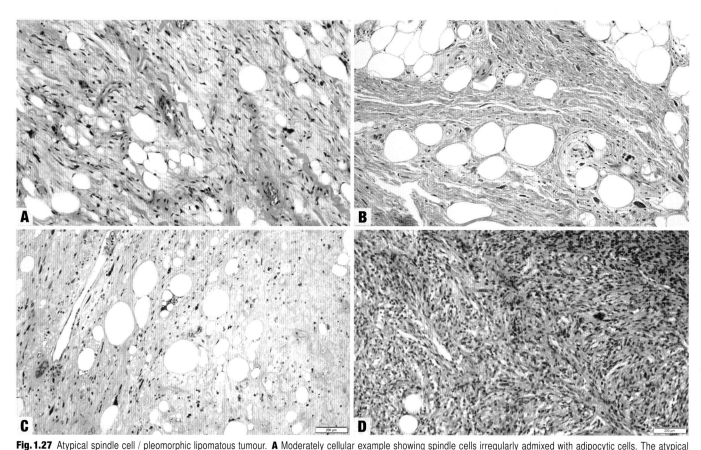

Fig. 1.27 Atypical spindle cell / pleomorphic lipomatous tumour. **A** Moderately cellular example showing spindle cells irregularly admixed with adipocytic cells. The atypical spindle tumour cells show an ill-defined, pale eosinophilic cytoplasm with hyperchromatic nuclei, set in a collagenous and myxoid stroma. **B** Area composed of atypical hyperchromatic spindle cells, adipocytes, multinucleated (floret-like) cells, and a collagenous extracellular matrix. **C** Bizarre pleomorphic cells and atypical spindle cells with enlarged, irregular, and hyperchromatic nuclei, irregularly admixed with lipoblasts. **D** Cellular example composed of moderately atypical hyperchromatic spindle cells.

sites of involvement include the larynx, mediastinum, retroperitoneum, trachea, and appendix {1983}.

Clinical features
The tumour manifests as a persistent or enlarging soft tissue mass, nodule, or swelling, sometimes with tenderness {1983}.

Epidemiology
Atypical spindle cell / pleomorphic lipomatous tumour occurs predominantly in middle-aged adults, with a peak incidence in the sixth decade of life, but it can affect patients of any age (cases have been described in patients aged 6–87 years {1983, 678,200}). The large majority of patients are > 30 years old. There is a slight male predominance.

Etiology
Unknown

Pathogenesis
Deletions or losses of 13q14, including *RB1* and its flanking genes *RCBTB2*, *DLEU1*, and *ITM2B*, have been identified in a substantial subset of cases {1983,678,683,200,677,2088}. In addition, monosomy 7 has been reported in some cases {1983,1487}.

Macroscopic appearance
Grossly, atypical spindle cell / pleomorphic lipomatous tumours are unencapsulated, show a nodular or multinodular growth pattern, and demonstrate ill-defined tumour margins. Tumour size is variable (range: 0.5–28 cm; median: 5–8.5 cm) {1983, 678}.

Histopathology
A wide range of microscopic appearances can be observed, even regionally within the same lesion, depending on the relative proportions of atypical spindle cells, adipocytes, lipoblasts, and pleomorphic (multinucleated) cells, as well as the variable amount of collagenous and/or myxoid extracellular matrix {1983,678}. The adipocytic component has a predominantly mature morphology, with variation in adipocytic size and shape. Patchy, often mild to moderate adipocytic atypia with chromatin coarsening, nuclear enlargement, and focal binucleation or multinucleation can be observed {21,679}. Morphologically, the lipoblasts can vary from small and univacuolated or bivacuolated to larger and multivacuolated (pleomorphic). Bizarre, hyperchromatic, and sometimes pleomorphic multinucleated cells are often scattered within the spindle cell or adipocytic components. Mitotic figures are often present but mostly scarce {678,680,681}. Tumour necrosis is absent. The morphology of these tumours can best be described as a broad spectrum defined by two morphological extremes {1983}. At one extreme, these tumours can be paucicellular, with few, cytologically bland spindle cells with minimal nuclear atypia set in a prominent extracellular matrix (the low-cellularity end of the spectrum, often described as atypical spindle cell lipoma morphology). These spindle cell–poor subtypes of atypical spindle cell / pleomorphic lipomatous tumour, which can have abundant myxoid matrix, tend to occur in the hands and feet and morphologically may resemble myxoid spindle cell lipoma, except for the presence of nuclear atypia / hyperchromasia and the anatomical location {1983,678,683,679,676}. At the other extreme, at the

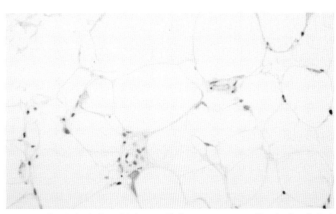

Fig. 1.28 Atypical spindle cell / pleomorphic lipomatous tumour. Neoplastic cells lack expression of RB1, while non-neoplastic endothelial cells and macrophages show intact nuclear RB1 expression.

high-cellularity end of the spectrum, atypical spindle cell / pleomorphic lipomatous tumours may be quite cellular, composed of numerous spindle cells showing diffuse, mild to moderate cytonuclear atypia, with easily identified lipoblasts and less extracellular matrix (spindle cell–rich subtypes, also described as fibrosarcoma-like lipomatous neoplasm morphology) {1983, 678,810,676}. A rare finding is heterologous (metaplastic) differentiation, including the presence of smooth muscle, cartilaginous, and/or osseous elements {1983,677}.

The tumour cells show variable expression of CD34, S100, and desmin {1983,678}. Weak and/or focal expression of MDM2 or CDK4 can be rarely seen {1983,683,2088}. The combination of MDM2 and CDK4 expression is not encountered {1983}. Loss of nuclear RB1 expression is observed in about 50–70% of cases {1983,678,200,683}.

Cytology
There are few reports, but FNA may show cells similar to those seen histologically {3366}.

Diagnostic molecular pathology
Molecular studies have shown a consistent absence of *MDM2* or *CDK4* amplification.

Essential and desirable diagnostic criteria
Essential: variable proportions of atypical spindle cells, adipocytes, univacuolated or bivacuolated to multivacuolated lipoblasts, pleomorphic (multinucleated) cells, and a myxoid to collagenous extracellular matrix.
Desirable (in selected cases): in a substantial subset of cases, RB1 expression is lost, correlating with *RB1* deletion; lack of *MDM2* or *CDK4* amplification.

Staging
Not clinically relevant

Prognosis and prediction
Atypical spindle cell / pleomorphic lipomatous tumour has a low rate of local recurrence (10–15%) for incompletely removed lesions. There is no documented risk for metastasis. Most patients will have an excellent prognosis if the lesion is completely excised {1983,678,200,2025,679}.

Atypical lipomatous tumour / well-differentiated liposarcoma

Sbaraglia M
Dei Tos AP
Pedeutour F

Definition

Atypical lipomatous tumour / well-differentiated liposarcoma (ALT/WDLPS) is a locally aggressive mesenchymal neoplasm composed either entirely or partly of an adipocytic proliferation showing at least focal nuclear atypia in both adipocytes and stromal cells. "Atypical lipomatous tumour" and "well-differentiated liposarcoma" are synonyms describing lesions that are morphologically and genetically identical. Amplification of *MDM2* and/or *CDK4* is almost always present.

ICD-O coding

8850/1 Atypical lipomatous tumour
8851/3 Liposarcoma, well-differentiated, NOS

ICD-11 coding

2F7C & XH0RW4 Neoplasms of uncertain behaviour of connective or other soft tissue & Atypical lipomatous tumour
2B5H & XH7Y61 Well-differentiated lipomatous tumour, primary site & Liposarcoma, well-differentiated

Related terminology

Not recommended: atypical lipoma.

Subtype(s)

Lipoma-like liposarcoma; inflammatory liposarcoma; sclerosing liposarcoma

Localization

ALT most frequently occurs in deep soft tissue of proximal extremities (thigh and buttock) and trunk (back and shoulder). The retroperitoneum and the paratesticular area are also commonly involved {919}. Rarer sites include the head and neck region, mediastinum, distal extremities, and skin {2253,1270,458,779}.

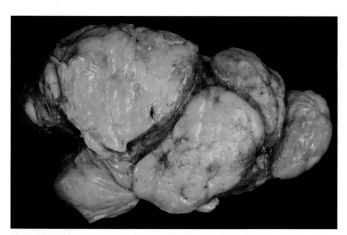

Fig. 1.29 Atypical lipomatous tumour / well-differentiated liposarcoma. Surgical specimen showing a well-circumscribed, lobulated, yellow mass.

Clinical features

ALT usually presents as a deep-seated, painless mass that can slowly attain a very large size, particularly in the retroperitoneum. Retroperitoneal lesions are often asymptomatic until the tumour has exceeded 20 cm in diameter.

Epidemiology

ALT/WDLPS represents the largest subgroup of adipocytic malignancies, accounting for approximately 40–45% of all liposarcomas. These lesions occur predominantly in middle-aged adults, with peak incidence between the fourth and fifth decades of life. Convincing examples in childhood are extremely rare but may be associated with Li–Fraumeni syndrome. Males and females are equally affected, with the obvious exception of those lesions affecting the spermatic cord {919,3312}.

Etiology

ALT/WDLPS may be associated with Li–Fraumeni syndrome, but nearly all cases are sporadic, and the etiology of these is unknown.

Pathogenesis

ALT is characterized by supernumerary ring and giant marker chromosomes, typically as the sole change or concomitant with a few other numerical or structural abnormalities {2728}. Telomeric associations are frequently observed and may give a false impression of complexity to ALT karyotypes {1966}. Both supernumerary rings and giant markers invariably contain amplified sequences originating from the 12q14-q15 region, *MDM2* (12q15) being the main driver gene. Several other genes located in the 12q14-q15 region, including *TSPAN31*, *CDK4* (12q14.1), *HMGA2* (12q14.3), *YEATS4* {224,1485,1486}, *CPM* {925}, and *FRS2* (12q15) {3245}, are frequently coamplified with *MDM2* {1530,1797,1570}. In addition to 12q14-q15–amplified sequences, they always contain coamplification of at least one other genomic segment {2472}. The chromosomal origin of these coamplified regions varies. The most frequent is 1q21-q25. Another striking feature of ALT supernumerary chromosomes is that they consistently contain a neocentromere {1491,1119}. Although generation of a neocentromere is a very rare event in tumour cells, it is a specific hallmark of ALT ring and marker chromosomes. The mechanism of formation of these peculiar chromosomes is not elucidated. They might be generated by chromothripsis {1119}. Overexpression of MDM2 protein resulting from genomic amplification inactivates p53; MDM2 targets p53 degradation towards the proteasome and inhibits p53-mediated transactivation.

Macroscopic appearance

ALT usually consists of a large, well-circumscribed, lobulated mass. Variable consistencies are present, from firm grey to gelatinous areas, depending on the proportion of fibrous and myxoid components. Larger retroperitoneal tumours appear

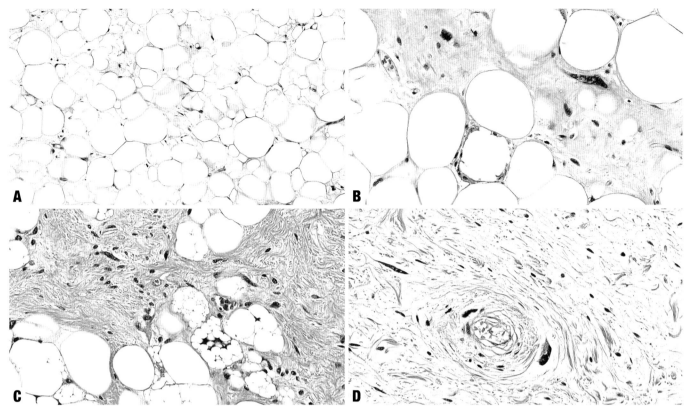

Fig. 1.30 Atypical lipomatous tumour / well-differentiated liposarcoma. **A** Striking variation in adipocytic size is a typical feature. **B** The presence of atypical, hyperchromatic stromal cells is an essential diagnostic feature. **C** A variable number of lipoblasts can be seen in atypical lipomatous tumour / well-differentiated liposarcoma; however, their presence neither makes nor is required for a diagnosis of liposarcoma. **D** The presence of scattered bizarre stromal cells exhibiting marked nuclear hyperchromasia set in a fibrillary collagenous background represents an important diagnostic feature of the sclerosing subtype.

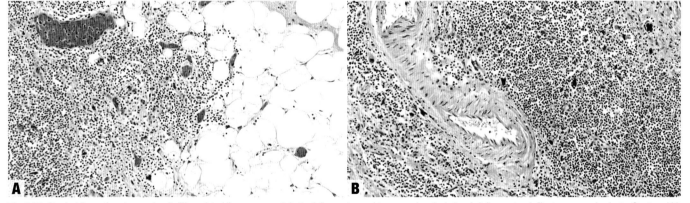

Fig. 1.31 Atypical lipomatous tumour / well-differentiated liposarcoma. **A** In the inflammatory subtype, an abundant chronic inflammatory infiltrate may predominate. Scattered bizarre stromal cells are present. **B** If the inflammatory component predominates, the identification of hyperchromatic, atypical stromal cells represents the most useful diagnostic clue.

more heterogeneous, often containing foci of fat necrosis and punctate haemorrhages.

Histopathology

ALT/WDLPS can be subdivided morphologically into three main subtypes: adipocytic (lipoma-like), sclerosing, and inflammatory {940}. The presence of more than one morphological pattern in the same lesion is common, particularly in retroperitoneal tumours. Lipoma-like ALT/WDLPS is composed of mature adipocytes in which, unlike in benign lipoma, substantial variation in cell size is appreciated alongside nuclear atypia in fat cells or stromal spindle cells. Scattered hyperchromatic stromal spindle cells

are easily identified within fibrous septa or blood vessel walls. Occasionally, fat cells assume hibernoma-like features {1276}. A varying number of lipoblasts (from many to none) may be found. Importantly, the mere presence of lipoblasts neither makes nor is required for a diagnosis of liposarcoma. Sclerosing ALT/WDLPS ranks second in frequency. This pattern is most often seen in retroperitoneum or spermatic cord. The main histological finding is the presence of scattered bizarre stromal cells, exhibiting marked nuclear hyperchromasia and set in an extensive fibrillary collagenous stroma. Multivacuolated lipoblasts can be observed. The fibrous component may overshadow lipogenic areas, which can therefore be easily missed in a small sample. Inflammatory

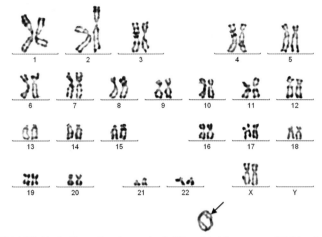

Fig. 1.32 Atypical lipomatous tumour / well-differentiated liposarcoma. RHG-banded near-diploid karyotype. The sole chromosomal anomaly is the presence of a supernumerary ring chromosome (arrow).

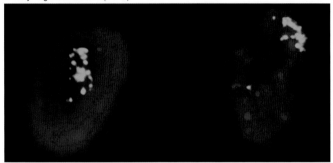

Fig. 1.33 Atypical lipomatous tumour / well-differentiated liposarcoma. Interphase FISH using probes for *MDM2* (green signal) and centromere of chromosome 12 (red signal) showing high-level amplification of *MDM2* grouped in clusters.

ALT/WDLPS represents the rarest subtype, occurring most often in retroperitoneum. A chronic inflammatory infiltrate predominates to the extent that the adipocytic nature of the neoplasm can be obscured {157,1697}. When dealing with cases in which the adipocytic component is scarce, the presence of bizarre multinucleated stromal cells represents a useful diagnostic clue. A rare finding in ALT/WDLPS is the presence of mature heterologous differentiation, which can be osseous or myogenic, but does not of itself imply dedifferentiation {3374,940,3003}. MDM2 and/or CDK4 nuclear immunopositivity is present in most cases {327,1485, 2875}. In lipoma-like ALT/WDLPS, MDM2 and CDK4 expression may prove difficult to evaluate, making FISH a valid alternative {611}. A major pitfall is represented by MDM2 nuclear positivity in histiocytes in fat necrosis. ALT/WDLPSs associated with Li–Fraumeni syndrome are MDM2-negative; however, they express p53.

Cytology
Cytology is not clinically relevant in most cases, with reported appearances in keeping with histology in 85% in one series {889}.

Diagnostic molecular pathology
Detection of *MDM2* (and/or *CDK4*) amplification {2875,684, 3047} serves to distinguish ALT from benign adipose tumours.

Essential and desirable diagnostic criteria
Essential: lipoma-like ALT/WDLPS: variation in adipocytic size associated with nuclear atypia in stromal and/or adipocytic cells; sclerosing ALT/WDLPS: hyperchromatic bizarre stromal cells set in a fibrillary sclerotic background; inflammatory ALT/WDLPS: scattered atypical stromal cells scattered in a chronic inflammatory background; lipoblasts are not required for diagnosis.
Desirable (in selected or challenging cases): MDM2 and/or CDK4 nuclear expression or evidence of *MDM2* and/or *CDK4* gene amplification.

Staging
Not clinically relevant

Prognosis and prediction
WDLPS shows no potential for metastasis unless it undergoes dedifferentiation, therefore justifying the introduction of the term "atypical lipomatous tumour" for lesions arising at anatomical sites for which complete surgical resection is curative. For lesions arising in anatomical sites such as retroperitoneum, spermatic cord, and mediastinum, which have shown greater potential for disease progression, retention of the term "well-differentiated liposarcoma" can be readily justified.

The most important prognostic factor is anatomical location. Lesions located in surgically amenable anatomical regions do not recur after complete excision. Tumours occurring in deep anatomical sites such as retroperitoneum, spermatic cord, or mediastinum tend to recur repeatedly and eventually cause death as a result of uncontrolled local effects or less often as a result of systemic spread subsequent to dedifferentiation. In retroperitoneum, multivisceral resections may increase relapse-free survival {366}. The ultimate risk of dedifferentiation varies according to site and lesional duration and is probably > 20% in the retroperitoneum but < 2% in the limbs. Overall, 10-year to 20-year mortality rates range from essentially 0% for ALT of the extremities to > 80% for WDLPS occurring in the retroperitoneum. The median time to death is 6–11 years {1904,3270}.

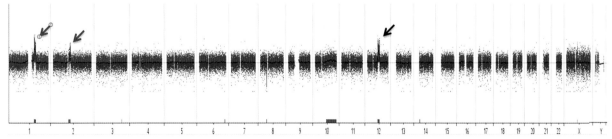

Fig. 1.34 Atypical lipomatous tumour / well-differentiated liposarcoma. Genomic quantitative profile obtained by array comparative genomic hybridization. The profile is simple, showing the characteristic 12q14-q15 amplification including *MDM2* (black arrow). Amplification of 1q23-q24 and 2q11-q13 is also observed in this case (blue arrows).

Dedifferentiated liposarcoma

Dei Tos AP
Marino-Enriquez A
Pedeutour F

Definition
Dedifferentiated liposarcoma (DDLPS) is an atypical lipomatous tumour / well-differentiated liposarcoma (ALT/WDLPS) showing progression, either in the primary or in a recurrence, to (usually non-lipogenic) sarcoma of variable histological grade. In most cases, there is amplification of *MDM2* and *CDK4*. A well-differentiated component may not be identifiable.

ICD-O coding
8858/3 Dedifferentiated liposarcoma

ICD-11 coding
2B59 & XH1C03 Liposarcoma, primary site & Dedifferentiated liposarcoma

Related terminology
None

Subtype(s)
None

Localization
Retroperitoneum is the most common location, outnumbering somatic soft tissue by at least 10:1. Other locations include the spermatic cord and (more rarely) mediastinum, head and neck, and trunk. Occurrence in subcutaneous tissue is extremely rare {778}. Recent molecular data suggest that the incidence of DDLPS at non-retroperitoneal sites may be underestimated {1782}.

Clinical features
DDLPS usually presents as a large painless mass, which may be found by chance (in particular in the retroperitoneum). In the limbs, a history of a longstanding mass exhibiting recent

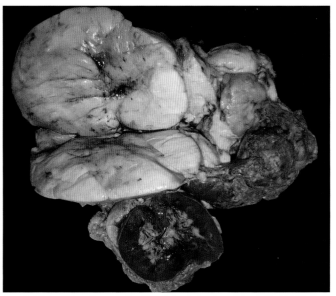

Fig. 1.35 Dedifferentiated liposarcoma. Multivisceral resection gross specimen featuring a large lipomatous mass associated with solid nodules representing the dedifferentiated component.

increase in size often indicates dedifferentiation. Radiological imaging often shows the coexistence of lipomatous and non-lipomatous solid components.

Epidemiology
DDLPS is a common form of liposarcoma, accounting for most pleomorphic sarcomas in the retroperitoneum. Dedifferentiation occurs in as many as 10% of WDLPSs, although the risk is higher for deep-seated (particularly retroperitoneal) lesions and significantly lower in the limbs. This is likely to represent a time-dependent more than a site-dependent phenomenon {3270}.

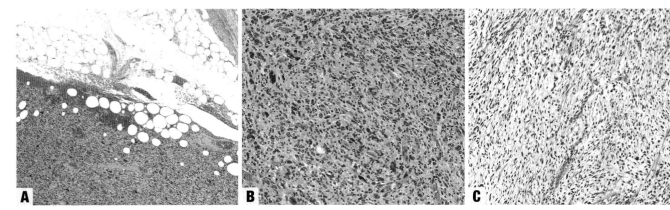

Fig. 1.36 Dedifferentiated liposarcoma. **A** Abrupt transition from well-differentiated liposarcoma to high-grade non-lipogenic pleomorphic sarcoma is seen. **B** The morphology of the dedifferentiated component most often overlaps with that of undifferentiated pleomorphic sarcoma. **C** The morphology of the dedifferentiated component may be identical to that of myxofibrosarcoma.

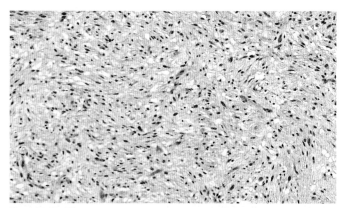

Fig. 1.37 Dedifferentiated liposarcoma. Low-grade dedifferentiation is characterized most often by the presence of uniform fibroblastic spindle cells with mild nuclear atypia.

DDLPS affects the same patient population as ALT/WDLPS and is equally frequent in males and females. About 90% of cases arise de novo, and 10% develop in recurrences {778}.

Etiology
Unknown

Pathogenesis
DDLPS genetically overlaps with ALT/WDLPS: both entities are characterized by consistent amplification of *MDM2* and *CDK4* (12q14-q15) {2702,1485}. As in ALT/WDLPS, many other genes from the 12q13-q21 region, as well as other chromosomal regions, are variably coamplified with *MDM2*. The amplicons are located in supernumerary ring or giant marker chromosomes with neocentromeres. Some genomic features appear to be more often related to DDLPS histology, although not restricted to DDLPS: amplification of *JUN* (1p32.1) {2899}, *TERT* (5p15.33), *CPM* {925}, *MAP3K5*, and other genes from the 6q21-q24 region {472,1978,1570}. Karyotypes and quantitative genomic profiles of DDLPS are often more complex than those of ALT/WDLPS. DDLPS shows *ATRX* deletion in 30% of cases {472}. In DDLPS, loss of 11q22-q24 (carrying several genes, e.g. *ATM*, *CHEK1*, *ZBTB16*, *PPP2R1B*, and *EI24*) is associated with genomic complexity {672}. In contrast to their high copy-number variations, DDLPSs present a low rate of mutations {1570,1391}.

Macroscopic appearance
DDLPS usually consists of large multinodular yellow masses containing discrete, solid, often tan-grey non-lipomatous (dedifferentiated) areas. Dedifferentiated areas may show necrosis. The transition between the lipomatous and the dedifferentiated areas may sometimes be gradual.

Histopathology
The histological hallmark of DDLPS is transition from ALT/WDLPS to non-lipogenic sarcoma, which in most cases is of high grade. The extent of dedifferentiation is variable. Transition is usually abrupt; however, in some cases it can be more gradual and, exceptionally, low- and high-grade areas appear to be intermingled. In some cases, a well-differentiated lipomatous component is hard to identify. Dedifferentiated areas exhibit a variable histological picture but most frequently resemble undifferentiated pleomorphic sarcoma or intermediate- to high-grade myxofibrosarcoma {2035,3270}. Although dedifferentiation was originally defined by high-grade morphology {942}, cases with low-grade dedifferentiation have increasingly been recognized {894,1349}. Low-grade dedifferentiation is characterized most often by the presence of uniform fibroblastic spindle cells with mild nuclear atypia, often organized in a fascicular pattern and exhibiting cellularity intermediate between well-differentiated sclerosing liposarcoma and usual high-grade areas. Low-grade DDLPS should not be confused with atypical spindle cell lipomatous tumours; the latter contain atypical adipocytes or lipoblasts, whereas dedifferentiated areas, both low- and high-grade, are generally non-lipogenic. Low-grade DDLPS is virtually indistinguishable from cellular WDLPS {940}. DDLPS may exhibit heterologous differentiation in about 5–10% of cases {948}. Most often the line of heterologous differentiation is myogenic or osteosarcomatous/chondrosarcomatous {3341}, but angiosarcomatous elements have also been reported. A peculiar neural-like or meningothelial-like whorling pattern of dedifferentiation has been described, which is often associated with ossification {969,2255}. Local recurrences of DDLPS may be entirely well differentiated {2035,3270}. Occasionally, the high-grade component may exhibit overt lipoblastic differentiation, either in the form of isolated lipoblasts scattered throughout the high-grade component or as sheets of atypical pleomorphic adipocytic cells resulting in areas morphologically

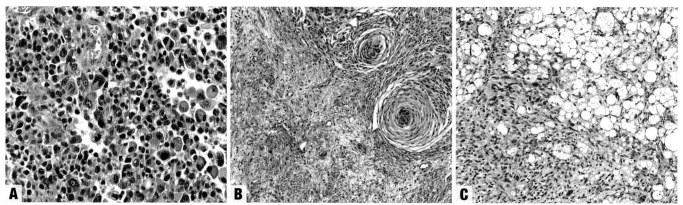

Fig. 1.38 Dedifferentiated liposarcoma. **A** Rhabdomyoblastic differentiation represents the most common type of heterologous differentiation in dedifferentiated liposarcoma. **B** Rarely, dedifferentiated liposarcoma may feature a distinctive whorled pattern reminiscent of neural or meningothelial structures. **C** Rarely, the dedifferentiated component exhibits striking lipogenic differentiation.

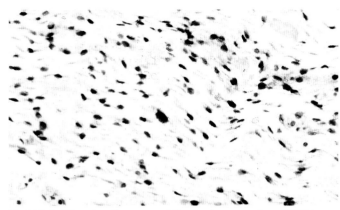

Fig. 1.39 Dedifferentiated liposarcoma. Diffuse nuclear expression of MDM2 is consistently observed in dedifferentiated liposarcoma.

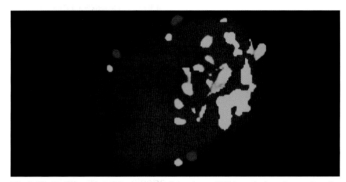

Fig. 1.40 Dedifferentiated liposarcoma. Interphase FISH analysis using probes for *MDM2* (green signals) and centromere 12 (red signals) showing high-level amplification of *MDM2*. The amplified signals are grouped in a large cluster, representative of the presence of a supernumerary ring or giant marker chromosome. The three coupled red-green signals indicate trisomy 12.

indistinguishable from pleomorphic liposarcoma. This phenomenon has been referred to as homologous lipoblastic differentiation or pleomorphic liposarcoma–like features {356,1349,1981}. Solitary fibrous tumour–like and inflammatory myofibroblastic tumour–like morphology can be rarely observed {1906}. The main role of immunohistochemistry is in the confirmation of divergent differentiation and exclusion of other tumour types. Diffuse nuclear expression of MDM2 and/or CDK4 is almost invariably observed {774} and also allows separation of homologous DDLPS from pleomorphic liposarcoma {2875,1981}.

Cytology
There are few reports, but cytology is likely to be challenging {889}.

Diagnostic molecular pathology
Detection of *MDM2* amplification by FISH {2875}, multiplex ligation-dependent probe amplification {684}, and array comparative genomic hybridization {3047} is helpful to distinguish DDLPS from other undifferentiated sarcomas in the appropriate clinical context.

Essential and desirable diagnostic criteria
Essential: transition (abrupt or gradual) from WDLPS (of any type) to spindle cell and pleomorphic non-lipogenic (rarely lipogenic) tumour (of low grade or high grade).
Desirable (in selected cases): expression of MDM2 or demonstration of *MDM2* gene amplification.

Staging
The American Joint Committee on Cancer (AJCC) and Union for International Cancer Control (UICC) TNM systems can be applied.

Prognosis and prediction
DDLPS is characterized by local recurrence in at least 40% of cases. However, almost all retroperitoneal examples seem to recur locally if patients are followed for 10–20 years. Distant metastases are observed in 15–20% of cases, with an overall mortality rate of 28–30% at 5-year follow-up, although this figure is undoubtedly much higher at 10–20 years {1349,2035,3270}. The most important prognostic factor is anatomical location, with retroperitoneal lesions exhibiting the worst clinical behaviour. The extent of dedifferentiated areas does not seem to predict outcome. DDLPS, despite its high-grade morphology, exhibits a less aggressive clinical course than other types of high-grade pleomorphic sarcoma, and an accelerated clinical course is observed in only a minority of patients. Recent data would indicate that a prognostic difference does exist based on grading when the French Fédération Nationale des Centres de Lutte Contre le Cancer (FNCLCC) grading system is used {1226}. Moreover, in contrast with previous observation {326}, myogenic (in particular rhabdomyoblastic) differentiation appears to be associated with worse outcome {1226}. Multivisceral resections appear to increase relapse-free survival {1230,366}.

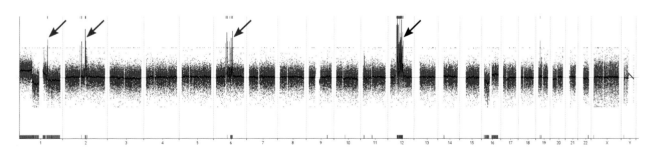

Fig. 1.41 Dedifferentiated liposarcoma. Array comparative genomic hybridization. Relatively simple quantitative genomic profile, showing characteristic high-level 12q amplification (black arrow) including *MDM2* (12q15). The 12q amplicon is large (from 12q12 up to q21) and discontinuous. It contains several genes frequently coamplified with *MDM2*, such as *CDK4*, *HMGA2*, and *FRS2*. A few other imbalanced alterations are also observed: amplification of 1q24, 2p11, 2q11, and 6p11-q16 regions (blue arrows), as well as gains and losses on chromosomes 1, 16, and 20.

Myxoid liposarcoma

Thway K
Nielsen TO

Definition
Myxoid liposarcoma (MLPS) is a malignant tumour composed of uniform, round to ovoid cells with variable numbers of small lipoblasts, set in a myxoid stroma with a branching capillary vasculature. Translocations producing *FUS-DDIT3* or rarely *EWSR1-DDIT3* fusion transcripts are pathognomonic. Included in this category are more-cellular, high-grade tumours formerly known as round cell liposarcoma.

ICD-O coding
8852/3 Myxoid liposarcoma

ICD-11 coding
2B59.Y & XH3EL0 Liposarcoma, other specified primary site & Myxoid liposarcoma

Related terminology
Not recommended: round cell liposarcoma.

Subtype(s)
None

Localization
MLPSs typically present within deep soft tissues of the extremities, most often the thigh {1624,1387}. Very rarely they arise as primary neoplasms of the subcutis or retroperitoneum {2816, 766}.

Clinical features
MLPSs typically present as large, painless masses. Retroperitoneal MLPS most often represents a metastasis {2816, 766}. Multifocal disease, either synchronous or metachronous, represents distant soft tissue metastases of monoclonal origin {130}. Surgical wide excision is the current treatment mainstay

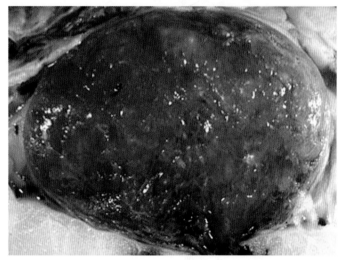

Fig. 1.42 Myxoid liposarcoma. Macroscopically, the tumour, present here within subcutaneous fat, has a soft, glistening reddish cut surface, due to old and recent haemorrhage.

{1008}. MLPS is extremely radiosensitive {241} and relatively sensitive to anthracyclines and trabectedin compared with other sarcomas {1546,1236}.

Epidemiology
MLPS accounts for approximately 20–30% of liposarcomas {2389} and 5% of adult soft tissue sarcomas, without significant sex predilection. Although peak incidence is in the fourth to fifth decades, MLPS is the most common liposarcoma subtype of children and adolescents {1438,58}.

Etiology
Unknown

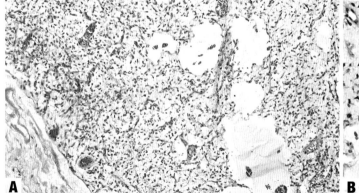 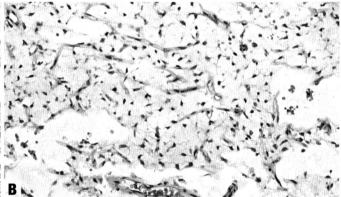

Fig. 1.43 Myxoid liposarcoma. **A** Low-grade myxoid liposarcoma, with abundant myxoid matrix, and lymphangioma-like cystic spaces. **B** Higher-power magnification of low-grade myxoid liposarcoma, illustrating the characteristic elaborate capillary vasculature of this tumour. The neoplastic cells are small, round to ovoid, and bland. Lipoblasts were very difficult to find in this particular tumour and are not required for diagnosis.

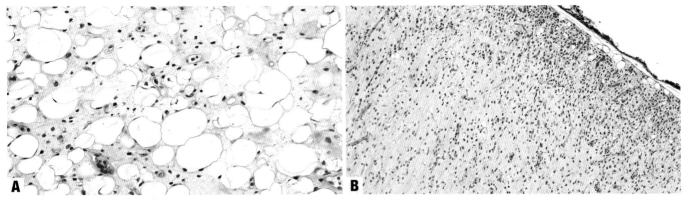

Fig. 1.44 Myxoid liposarcoma. **A** Differentiating myxoid liposarcoma, with a component of mature white fat. On occasion, myxoid liposarcomas may contain abundant mature fat, mimicking lipoma with myxoid change. **B** Myxoid liposarcomas typically show increased cellularity at the periphery of lobules. This should not be interpreted as round cell change, for purposes of grading.

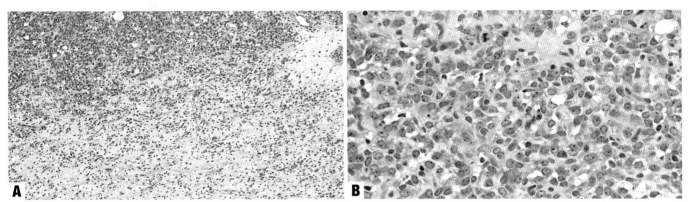

Fig. 1.45 High-grade myxoid liposarcoma. **A** This lesion shows an abrupt transition between typical low-grade histology (bottom) and high-grade, round cell morphology (top). **B** High-power view showing cellular overlap, elevated nuclear grade, mitotic activity, and obscuring of the underlying vascular pattern.

Pathogenesis

MLPS and its hypercellular subtype (formerly, round cell liposarcoma) harbour the same genetic abnormality. Most are characterized by the t(12;16)(q13;p11) translocation generating *FUS-DDIT3* fusion transcripts, translated into a chimeric oncoprotein that alters transcription and differentiation. DDIT3 (CHOP, GADD153) is a DNA-binding transcription factor normally induced under cell stress, which blocks adipocytic terminal differentiation {1287, 409}. Fusion transcripts always include the full coding sequence. In the fusion, *FUS*, a gene widely expressed in normal tissues, provides promoter sequences and its first 3–13 exons {2531}. Fusion protein variants consistently retain the FUS N-terminal transcriptional activation domain that is largely conserved across FET protein family members, including EWSR1 {2790}. *EWSR1* substitutes for *FUS* in about 3% of MLPSs, generating EWSR1-DDIT3 oncoproteins {2531}, without proven histological or prognostic differences. The net result is a block to terminal fatty differentiation {2490}. The genomic background shows a low mutation burden, with wildtype *TP53* {1550}. More than 50% of cases carry *TERT* promoter mutations {1667}, and about 25% have mutations activating PI3K/mTOR {3098}, but no other genetic events occur consistently at frequencies > 20%.

Macroscopic appearance

MLPSs are typically large (> 10 cm), circumscribed, multinodular intramuscular neoplasms {140}. The cut surface is smooth, gelatinous, and glistening. Higher-grade tumours show a firmer, fleshy tan surface. Macroscopic necrosis is uncommon. Adequate sampling to estimate the amount of hypercellularity is essential, because this is a major prognostic determinant {935,2922}.

Histopathology

At low magnification, MLPSs are moderately cellular, lobulated tumours with increased peripheral cellularity, comprising patternless arrays of uniform, small, ovoid cells without morphological adipocytic differentiation, with variable numbers of small lipoblasts. The tumours contain abundant, lightly basophilic, myxoid stroma with a striking plexiform, delicately arborizing, capillary network (chicken wire) {2389}, around which neoplastic cells often cluster. Paucicellular extracellular mucin pools may be present, imparting a microcystic / pulmonary oedema–like pattern. MLPS typically lacks atypia, substantial mitotic activity, or spindling. The lipoblasts are smaller than in other liposarcomas, and predominantly univacuolated/bivacuolated. Lipoblasts may be rare or even absent. A variable percentage of mature fat may be present. Chondroid and osseous elements are rare and are thought to be metaplastic in nature {3265}.

High-grade MLPSs show > 5% of the tumour to have cellular overlap, diminished myxoid matrix, less-apparent capillary vasculature, elevated nuclear grade, and increased mitotic activity. A corded or trabecular pattern is often present. Pure high-grade MLPS may be indistinguishable from other round cell sarcomas, requiring molecular genetic studies for diagnosis. The presence of > 5% hypercellularity is associated with significantly

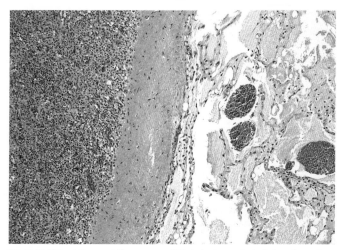

Fig. 1.46 Metastatic myxoid liposarcoma. This lesion is a metastasis from the surface of the spleen. Essentially all intra-abdominal and retroperitoneal myxoid liposarcomas represent metastases.

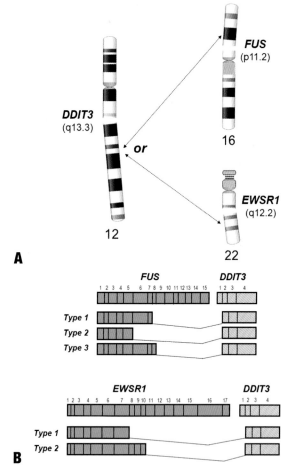

Fig. 1.47 Myxoid liposarcoma. **A** Schematic illustration of the breakpoints involved in the translocations t(12;16)(q13.3;p11.2) and t(12;22)(q13.3;q12.2) resulting in *FUS-DDIT3* and *EWSR1-DDIT3* fusions, respectively. **B** The N-terminal transcriptional activation domain of *FUS* or *EWSR1* is retained in the fusion to the entire coding region of *DDIT3*, which encodes an apparent DNA-binding and dimerization domain. There are at least 11 different isoforms of the *FUS-DDIT3* fusion transcript (with types 1–3 being most common) and 4 of *EWSR1-DDIT3* (with type 1 being most common in this rare molecular subtype).

poorer prognosis (French Fédération Nationale des Centres de Lutte Contre le Cancer [FNCLCC] grading system differentiation score of 3). The presence and percentage of hypercellular areas should be recorded. Some cases show so-called transitional areas with modestly increased cellularity without elevated nuclear grade and mitotic activity {2898}.

Immunohistochemistry plays little role in the diagnosis of MLPS, but it may be of some value in the distinction of high-grade tumours from other round cell sarcomas. MLPSs treated with either preoperative chemotherapy or radiotherapy often show a marked decrease in cellularity, with only scattered ovoid cells, extensive stromal hyalinization, and sometimes maturation into white adipose tissue.

Cytology

Cytological appearances consist of variable proportions of small round cells in myxoid matrix containing thin-walled branching vessels.

Diagnostic molecular pathology

Demonstration of the translocation/fusion transcript may be helpful in distinguishing MLPS from other myxoid sarcomas, and high-grade MLPS from various round cell sarcomas {1489}. *FUS* and *EWSR1* can substitute for each other and occur in other sarcomas, whereas *DDIT3* is unique to MLPS. Thus, FISH break-apart probes directed at *DDIT3* are a sensitive, specific strategy {2248}. Alternative diagnostic methods include RT-PCR with primers designed to cover all common fusion variants {2531}, massively parallel sequencing {3016}, and multiplexed colour-coded probe pair technologies {538}.

Essential and desirable diagnostic criteria

Essential: myxoid matrix containing delicately arborizing capillaries; bland round to ovoid cells; variable number of small non-pleomorphic lipoblasts, often adjacent to capillaries; hypercellularity, diminished myxoid matrix, obscured capillaries, and elevated nuclear grade and mitotic activity in high-grade MLPS.

Desirable: demonstration of *DDIT3* rearrangement (*FUS-DDIT3* or *EWSR1-DDIT3* fusion genes).

Staging

The American Joint Committee on Cancer (AJCC) and Union for International Cancer Control (UICC) TNM systems can be applied.

Prognosis and prediction

Local recurrence occurs in 12–25% of cases {1293,1008}. Distant metastases develop in approximately 30–60%, sometimes years after initial diagnosis, and may progress slowly {2922}. Unlike most sarcomas, MLPSs often metastasize to other soft tissue sites and can metastasize to bone (particularly spine) {2189}, in preference to lung {2922,935}. Histologically high-grade tumours (> 5% hypercellularity) have a statistically significant higher rate of metastasis or death from disease {2898,140, 1387,1008,2922,2189}. Necrosis and *TP53* and *CDKN2A* alterations have been associated with adverse prognosis {1008,140, 1293,2349}. The prognostic significance of transitional areas with more-limited hypercellularity is less certain. There is no association between different *FUS-DDIT3* transcript isoforms and grade or prognosis {140,347}.

Pleomorphic liposarcoma

Pedeutour F
Montgomery EA

Definition

Pleomorphic liposarcoma is a pleomorphic, high-grade sarcoma containing variable numbers of pleomorphic lipoblasts. No areas of atypical lipomatous tumour / well-differentiated liposarcoma or other lines of differentiation are present.

ICD-O coding

8854/3 Pleomorphic liposarcoma

ICD-11 coding

2B59.Y & XH25R1 Liposarcoma, other specified primary site & Pleomorphic liposarcoma

Related terminology

None

Subtype(s)

Epithelioid liposarcoma

Localization

Pleomorphic liposarcoma occurs on the extremities in two thirds of cases (more commonly in the lower than the upper limbs); the trunk wall, retroperitoneum, and spermatic cord are less frequently affected {848,1404,1126,2117}. Rare sites of involvement include the mediastinum, heart, pleura, breast, scalp, colon, and orbit {458,1126,1404}. Most cases arise in deep soft tissue, but about 25% develop in subcutaneous fat {1126,1404}; purely dermal cases are very rare {779, 848,1404,1126}.

Clinical features

Most patients report a rapidly growing painless mass, usually with a short preoperative duration (median: 3–6 months); a subset of patients report pain, and some patients have symptoms related to tumour location {1126,1404}.

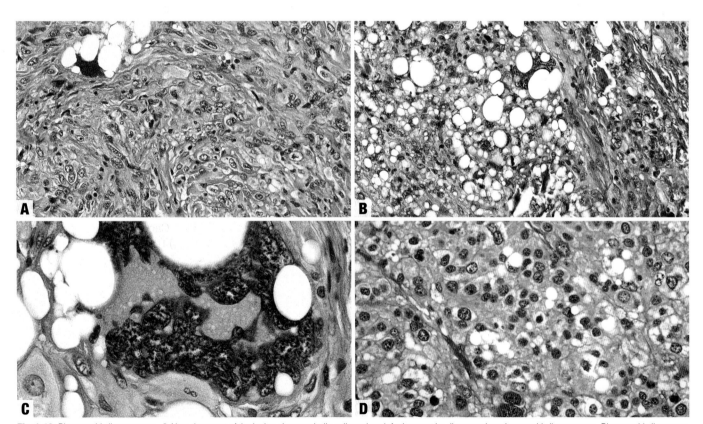

Fig. 1.48 Pleomorphic liposarcoma. **A** Note that most of the lesion shows spindle cells and such foci cannot be diagnosed as pleomorphic liposarcoma. Pleomorphic liposarcoma is diagnosed on H&E staining by identifying pleomorphic lipoblasts, as in the upper left of the image, in which lipid droplets crisply indent the pleomorphic nucleus. Sometimes examination of multiple tissue blocks is required to identify the diagnostic areas, which can be missed on needle biopsies. **B** This field shows numerous pleomorphic lipoblasts, each with nuclear indentations by cytoplasmic lipid droplets. **C** These neoplasms feature some of the most bizarre nuclei in human neoplasia and lack characteristic translocations and gene fusions. **D** This epithelioid pleomorphic liposarcoma shows lipid droplets but also shows many epithelioid cells with round nuclei and a rich vascular network.

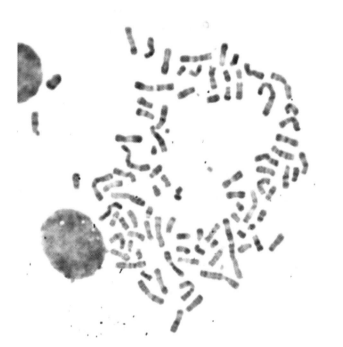

Fig. 1.49 Pleomorphic liposarcoma. Metaphase cell (RHG-banding) showing numerous quantitative and structural chromosomal alterations: near-tetraploidy and complex marker chromosomes.

Epidemiology

Pleomorphic liposarcoma is a rare subtype of liposarcoma, accounting for < 5% of all liposarcomas {1403,110}. Most cases occur in adults in later life, with peak incidence in the seventh decade of life and a slightly higher incidence in males than females. Paediatric cases are exceptional {58}.

Etiology

Unknown

Pathogenesis

The molecular profiles of pleomorphic liposarcomas more closely resemble those of other pleomorphic sarcomas than those of atypical lipomatous tumour / well-differentiated liposarcoma, dedifferentiated liposarcoma, or myxoid liposarcoma {472,1078}. Metaphase cells show high chromosomal counts and complex structural rearrangements. This complexity is represented by unidentifiable marker chromosomes, non-clonal aberrations, polyploidy, and intercellular heterogeneity. No pathognomonic structural rearrangement, such as recurrent translocation or consistent presence of supernumerary ring chromosomes, has been identified. Studies using array comparative genomic hybridization have shown complex profiles with numerous chromosomal imbalances {1078,1460,2623, 2768,3057}. The most frequent mutations involve *TP53* and *NF1* {224,2774,3057}. It has been noted that the genomic profiles of pleomorphic liposarcoma and myxofibrosarcoma are similar {224,1460}. Amplification of the 12q14-q15 region is absent in pleomorphic liposarcoma {1078,2869,3232}.

Macroscopic appearance

Most tumours are large, with a median size of 8–10 cm {1126, 1404}. They are well demarcated but non-encapsulated, or ill-defined and infiltrative and sometimes multinodular. On sectioning, most tumours are white to yellow. Myxoid changes and foci of necrosis are often observed.

Histopathology

Histologically, most cases have infiltrative margins, and all tumours contain a varying proportion of pleomorphic lipoblasts in a background of a high-grade, usually pleomorphic, undifferentiated sarcoma {501,778}. The presence of lipoblasts is necessary for the diagnosis, but their number varies considerably between cases and between areas within the same tumour, emphasizing the importance of adequate sampling. In most cases, the non-lipogenic component resembles undifferentiated pleomorphic sarcoma with spindle and multinucleated giant cells arranged in short fascicles, with some notable features: namely, the presence of extremely large tumour cells often showing clear or vacuolated cytoplasm, and the presence of extracellular and occasionally intracellular eosinophilic hyaline droplets. Almost half of cases contain at least focal areas similar to intermediate- to high-grade myxofibrosarcoma-like zones associated with pleomorphic lipoblasts. This myxofibrosarcoma-like component is predominant in some cases. Epithelioid morphology is seen in about one quarter of cases with areas resembling poorly differentiated carcinoma, renal clear cell carcinoma, adrenocortical carcinoma, or melanoma {1126, 1404,2117,455,1426}. Necrosis is present in more than half of cases.

Unlike in dedifferentiated liposarcoma with homologous differentiation, staining for MDM2 and CDK4 is typically negative in pleomorphic liposarcoma {858,1126,1404,1981}. The epithelioid subtype may be positive for keratins and melan-A {110}.

Cytology

There are few reports, but cytology is likely to be challenging {889}.

Diagnostic molecular pathology

Absence of amplification of *MDM2* can help distinguish pleomorphic liposarcoma from dedifferentiated liposarcoma.

Essential and desirable diagnostic criteria

Essential: pleomorphic spindle cell sarcoma containing a variable number of pleomorphic lipoblasts; myxofibrosarcoma-like morphology with pleomorphic lipoblasts; epithelioid subtype with sheets of carcinoma-like epithelioid cells with pleomorphic lipoblasts; tumours may consist only of pleomorphic lipoblasts.

Staging

The American Joint Committee on Cancer (AJCC) and Union for International Cancer Control (UICC) TNM systems can be applied.

Prognosis and prediction

Pleomorphic liposarcomas are aggressive sarcomas exhibiting local recurrence and metastatic rates of 30–50%, with an overall 5-year survival rate of about 60%. Metastases occur mostly in the lungs and pleura. Central location, increased tumour depth, greater size, and higher mitotic count have been associated with a worse prognosis {1126,1404}.

Myxoid pleomorphic liposarcoma

Alaggio R
Creytens D

Definition
Myxoid pleomorphic liposarcoma is an exceptionally rare, aggressive adipocytic neoplasm, typically occurring in children and adolescents. Myxoid pleomorphic liposarcoma shows mixed histological features of conventional myxoid liposarcoma and pleomorphic liposarcoma and lacks the gene fusions and amplifications of myxoid liposarcoma, atypical lipomatous tumour, and dedifferentiated liposarcoma.

ICD-O coding
8859/3 Myxoid pleomorphic liposarcoma

ICD-11 coding
2B59.Y & XH3EL0 & XH25R1 Liposarcoma, other specified primary site & Myxoid liposarcoma & Pleomorphic liposarcoma

Related terminology
Acceptable: pleomorphic myxoid liposarcoma.

Subtype(s)
None

Localization
Myxoid pleomorphic liposarcoma has a predilection for the mediastinum {58,623,352}. Other reported locations include the thigh, head and neck, perineum, abdomen, and back {58,682, 1389,2866}.

Clinical features
Myxoid pleomorphic liposarcoma generally manifests as a large, deep-seated soft tissue mass {682,1389}.

Epidemiology
Myxoid pleomorphic liposarcoma occurs predominantly in children and young adults. Patient age in the large majority of published cases is < 30 years {58,682,1389,2866}. There is a female predominance {58}.

Etiology
Unknown

Pathogenesis
Myxoid pleomorphic liposarcoma has been associated with Li–Fraumeni syndrome {2866}, numerical chromosomal aberrations, and inactivation of the *RB1* tumour suppressor gene {1389,676,110,2554,785}.

Macroscopic appearance
Grossly, myxoid pleomorphic liposarcomas are non-encapsulated tumours with ill-defined margins {682}.

Histopathology
Histologically, the tumours show variable proportions of myxoid liposarcoma–like areas, characterized by abundant myxoid matrix, scattered lipoblasts, relatively bland primitive round to oval cells, and a delicate curvilinear to plexiform capillary network {58,682}. Lymphangioma-like myxoid pools can be observed {682}. Pleomorphic spindle or ovoid cells with hyperchromatic nuclei may be scattered within the myxoid component, with a progressive transition into more-cellular, high-grade pleomorphic liposarcoma–like areas displaying severe cytological atypia, increased mitotic activity, atypical mitoses, pleomorphic lipoblasts, and occasional necrosis {58,682}. Myxoid pleomorphic liposarcomas have a nonspecific immunophenotype.

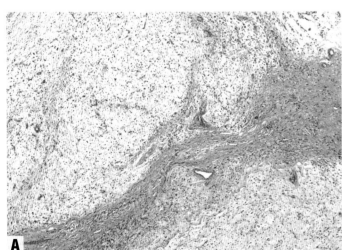
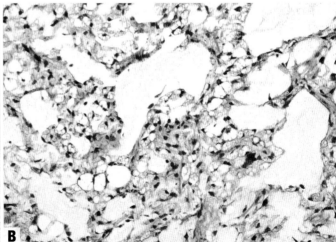

Fig. 1.50 Myxoid pleomorphic liposarcoma. **A** A fibrous, densely cellular area with pleomorphism is adjacent to a myxoid liposarcoma–like component. **B** Pseudocystic changes in myxoid areas with associated classic monovacuolated and multivacuolated lipoblasts. An isolated pleomorphic cell is seen.

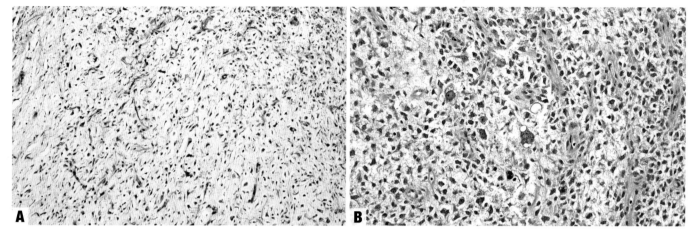

Fig. 1.51 Myxoid pleomorphic liposarcoma. **A** Delicate vaguely plexiform vascular pattern in the context of a myxoid background. Primitive cells and isolated cells with a hyperchromatic nucleus are seen. **B** Myxoid pleomorphic liposarcoma showing a myxoid liposarcoma–like arborizing capillary vasculature, marked nuclear atypia, and pleomorphic lipoblasts.

Cytology
Not clinically relevant

Diagnostic molecular pathology
FISH studies have shown that myxoid pleomorphic liposarcoma lacks the *FUS/EWSR1-DDIT3* gene fusions seen in conventional myxoid liposarcoma, as well as the *MDM2* amplification present in well-differentiated/dedifferentiated liposarcoma {58,682}.

Essential and desirable diagnostic criteria
Essential: distinctive admixture of relatively bland zones resembling conventional myxoid liposarcoma and much more cellular and atypical areas, resembling pleomorphic liposarcoma.
Desirable (in selected cases): absence of *FUS/EWSR1-DDIT3* gene fusions and *MDM2* amplifications.

Staging
The American Joint Committee on Cancer (AJCC) and Union for International Cancer Control (UICC) TNM systems can be applied.

Prognosis and prediction
Myxoid pleomorphic liposarcoma is an extremely aggressive tumour type with a high recurrence rate; metastasis to lung, bone, and soft tissue; and poor overall survival {58,623}.

Nodular fasciitis

Oliveira AM
Wang J
Wang WL

Definition
Nodular fasciitis is a self-limiting mesenchymal neoplasm that usually occurs in subcutaneous tissue. It is composed of plump, uniform fibroblastic/myofibroblastic cells displaying a tissue culture–like architectural pattern, and it usually harbours *USP6* rearrangement.

ICD-O coding
8828/0 Nodular fasciitis

ICD-11 coding
FB51.2 & XH5LM1 Pseudosarcomatous fibromatosis & Nodular fasciitis

Related terminology
Not recommended: pseudosarcomatous fasciitis.

Subtype(s)
Intravascular fasciitis; cranial fasciitis

Localization
Nodular fasciitis typically develops on the surface of fascia and extends into subcutis, although occasional cases are intramuscular {2066}. Dermal localization is rare {773,1707}. Any anatomical site can be involved, but the upper extremities, trunk, and head and neck are most frequently affected. Intra-articular involvement has been described {1410}. Intravascular fasciitis is usually subcutaneous. It occurs in small to medium-sized vessels, predominantly veins but occasionally arteries {2458}. Cranial fasciitis typically involves the outer table of the skull and contiguous soft tissue of the scalp and may extend downwards through the inner table into the meninges {1773}.

Clinical features
Nodular fasciitis typically grows rapidly and has a preoperative duration in most cases of not more than 2–3 months. Soreness or tenderness may be present. It usually measures ≤ 2 cm and almost always < 5 cm. Intravascular fasciitis may enlarge more slowly but is also normally not more than 2 cm. Cranial fasciitis expands quickly, like nodular fasciitis, and may become somewhat larger than the usual example of the latter. When the skull is involved, X-ray imaging shows a lytic defect, often with a sclerotic rim. In contrast, nodular fasciitis presents as a nondistinctive soft tissue mass on imaging studies.

Epidemiology
Nodular fasciitis is relatively common {76,280,1446,1683,2847, 2914,2543}. It occurs in all age groups but more often in young adults. Intravascular fasciitis {2458} and cranial fasciitis {1773} are rare. Intravascular fasciitis is found mostly in people aged < 30 years, whereas cranial fasciitis develops predominantly in infants aged < 2 years. Nodular fasciitis and intravascular fasciitis occur equally frequently in males and females, but cranial fasciitis is more common in boys.

Etiology
Unknown

Pathogenesis
The identification of recurrent *USP6* gene rearrangements in nodular fasciitis has firmly established its previously disputed clonal neoplastic nature {329,838,924,1679,2749,3184,3262, 2461}. *USP6* (17p13.2) is a deubiquitinating protease involved in cell trafficking, protein degradation, signalling, and inflammation. Multiple promoter partners have been described {924, 2461,1254}; the most frequent partner is *MYH9* (22q12.3), which encodes non-muscular myosin heavy chain 9 (MYH9), which is involved in cell-shape maintenance, cell motility, adhesion, differentiation, and development {2370,2461}. The *USP6* fusion causes transcriptional upregulation of the entire coding sequence of *USP6* driven by the active (usually *MYH9*) promoter in a classic promoter-swapping mechanism. As an example of

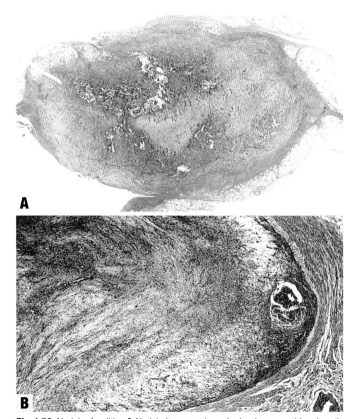

Fig. 1.52 Nodular fasciitis. **A** Nodularity, vague irregular borders, myxoid and cystic changes, and haemorrhagic areas are readily observed at low power in this typical example. **B** Occasional cases are intravascular.

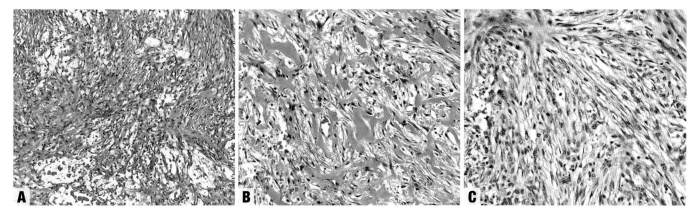

Fig. 1.53 Nodular fasciitis. **A** At medium power, the characteristic tissue culture–like appearance and cystic myxoid changes are virtually diagnostic. **B** Hyalinized areas are commonly encountered. **C** The tumour cells contain ovoid to tapering nuclei, fine chromatin, small nucleoli, and amphophilic cytoplasm. Note the loose fascicular architecture and prominent mitotic activity.

a consistently self-limited and regressing lesion with a recurrent fusion gene, the term "transient neoplasia" has been suggested {924}. *USP6* rearrangements are also found in aneurysmal bone cyst, myositis ossificans, cellular fibroma of tendon sheath, and fibro-osseous pseudotumour of digits, which share some histological features with nodular fasciitis, suggesting a possible biological relationship among these tumour types {2371,2375, 2373,1036,2980,496}. Recent mechanistic studies have identified the NF-κB and JAK-1/STAT3 pathways as critical mediators of tumorigenesis by USP6 {2560,2546}. Few cases of cranial fasciitis have been reported to have *USP6* rearrangement {2723}.

Macroscopic appearance
Macroscopically, nodular fasciitis may appear circumscribed or infiltrative, but it is not encapsulated. The cut surface varies from myxoid to fibrous, and occasionally there is central cystic change. Intravascular fasciitis ranges from nodular to plexiform, the latter contour resulting when there is extensive intravascular growth. Cranial fasciitis is typically circumscribed and rubbery to firm, and it may be focally myxoid or cystic in its centre.

Histopathology
Nodular fasciitis is composed of plump spindle-shaped cells lacking nuclear hyperchromasia or pleomorphism. Mitotic figures may be plentiful, but atypical forms are not observed. The lesion may be highly cellular, but typically it is partly discohesive and myxoid, with a torn, feathery, or tissue culture–like character. In more-cellular areas, there is often growth in S-shaped or C-shaped fascicles, or sometimes in a storiform pattern. There is normally little collagen, but collagen may be increased focally, and keloidal collagen bundles may be present and occasionally prominent. Microcystic stromal changes are also typical. Extravasated erythrocytes, lymphocytes, and osteoclast-like giant cells are frequently identified. The lesional border is typically infiltrative (at least focally), although it may be well delineated; peripheral extension is often seen between fat cells in the subcutis and between muscle cells in intramuscular locations. Small vessels are numerous, which may occasionally result in a resemblance to granulation tissue.

Intravascular fasciitis and cranial fasciitis are similar to nodular fasciitis histologically, although intravascular fasciitis often displays a greater number of osteoclast-like giant cells. Intravascular fasciitis ranges from predominantly extravascular, with only a minor intravascular component, to predominantly intravascular. Osseous metaplasia is occasionally seen in nodular fasciitis (fasciitis ossificans) and cranial fasciitis {734,1724}.

By immunohistochemistry, the neoplastic cells express SMA and MSA in a typical myofibroblastic (tram-track) pattern; desmin positivity is occasionally found, usually focally {2180}. Nuclear β-catenin may be seen in cranial fasciitis {2569}.

Cytology
Cytology preparations reveal bland spindle cells with unipolar curved to bipolar processes, round to oval elongated nuclei, and occasional small nucleoli. A tissue culture–like appearance and myxoid stroma can be appreciated {81,283}.

Diagnostic molecular pathology
Molecular testing is usually unnecessary in clinically and histologically typical cases. However, in challenging cases, breakapart *USP6* FISH or next-generation sequencing techniques may be used to confirm the diagnosis {2461,923,1739}.

Essential and desirable diagnostic criteria
Essential: bland, typically cellular myofibroblastic proliferation with a tissue culture–like growth pattern; variably myxoid stroma with microcystic changes; extravasated red blood cells.
Desirable: assessment of *USP6* rearrangement can be helpful in selected cases.

Staging
Not clinically relevant

Prognosis and prediction
Recurrence of nodular fasciitis after excision is rare, but occasional instances have been observed. An exceptional case of malignant nodular fasciitis harbouring the fusion transcript *PPP6R3-USP6* has been described in a patient with long-term recurrences and multiple metastases {1254,3061A}.

Proliferative fasciitis and proliferative myositis

Wang WL
Lazar AJ

Definition

Proliferative fasciitis is a mass-forming subcutaneous proliferation characterized by large ganglion-like cells and plump myofibroblastic/fibroblastic cells. Proliferative myositis has the same cellular composition but occurs within skeletal muscle.

ICD-O coding

8828/0 Proliferative fasciitis
8828/0 Proliferative myositis

ICD-11 coding

FB51.Y Other specified fibroblastic disorders (index term Fasciitis NOS)

Related terminology

None

Subtype(s)

None

Localization

Proliferative fasciitis develops most frequently in the upper extremities, particularly the forearms, followed by the lower extremities and trunk. Proliferative myositis arises predominantly in the trunk, shoulder girdles, and upper arms, and less often in the thighs. By definition, proliferative fasciitis is subcutaneous and proliferative myositis is intramuscular.

Clinical features

Both proliferative fasciitis and proliferative myositis characteristically grow rapidly and are usually excised within 2 months from the time they are first noted. Proliferative fasciitis almost always measures < 5 cm and is most often < 3 cm. Proliferative myositis may be slightly larger. Either lesion may be painful or tender; this is more common with proliferative fasciitis. The

imaging characteristics of proliferative myositis can be suggestive of the diagnosis; those of proliferative fasciitis are less well studied {2409}.

Epidemiology

Proliferative fasciitis and proliferative myositis are much less common than nodular fasciitis. Both occur predominantly in middle-aged or older adults, i.e. in an older age group than nodular fasciitis {606,915,1613}. A rare subtype of proliferative fasciitis is described in children {2060}.

Etiology

Unknown

Pathogenesis

Unlike in nodular fasciitis, a recurrent genomic abnormality or translocation has yet to be firmly established in proliferative fasciitis/myositis.

Macroscopic appearance

Proliferative fasciitis typically forms a poorly circumscribed mass in the subcutaneous tissue and may extend horizontally along fascia. The rare childhood subtype is often better circumscribed. Proliferative myositis is also poorly marginated and involves a variable proportion of the muscle.

Histopathology

Both proliferative fasciitis and myositis contain plump myofibroblastic/fibroblastic spindle cells similar to those seen in nodular fasciitis but also demonstrate large ganglion-like cells with rounded nuclei, prominent nucleoli, and abundant amphophilic to basophilic cytoplasm {606}. These cells usually have one nucleus but may have two or three. They may be evenly or irregularly distributed. Mitotic figures are found in both the spindle cells and the ganglion-like cells and may be relatively

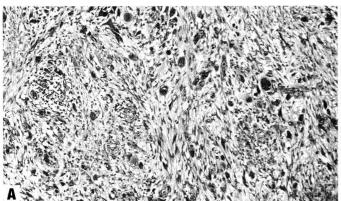 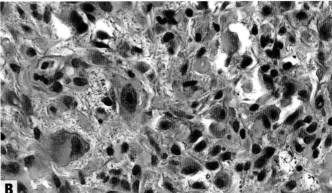

Fig. 1.54 Proliferative fasciitis. **A** Ganglion-like cells are admixed with spindle cells and lymphocytes in a loose myxoid matrix. **B** Ganglion-like cells at higher power.

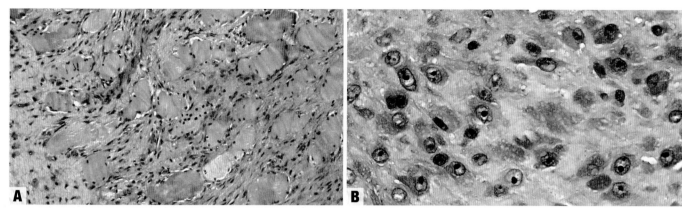

Fig. 1.55 Proliferative myositis. **A** Note the spindle cells. Ganglion-like cells sporting amphophilic cytoplasm are admixed. **B** Details of the cytological features of the ganglion-like cells with prominent nucleoli.

numerous but are not atypical. The stroma varies from myxoid to collagenous. The lesional borders are typically infiltrative or even ill defined. Proliferative fasciitis may grow laterally along fascial planes, whereas proliferative myositis extends between individual muscle fibres, creating the characteristic checkerboard pattern. The childhood subtype of proliferative fasciitis generally has better-delineated borders than the adult form, as well as greater cellularity, a predominance of ganglion-like cells, and more mitoses. Focal necrosis and acute inflammation may also be present. Proliferative myositis may contain metaplastic bone, demonstrating possible kinship to myositis ossificans. The immunohistochemical profile is similar to that of nodular fasciitis; the spindle cells usually express SMA and MSA and are negative for desmin {895,1914}. The ganglion-like cells are often negative for actins.

Cytology

On cytology, spindle cells with long cytoplasmic processes and round or oval nuclei can be appreciated in addition to variable numbers of large ganglion-like cells with prominent nucleoli, smooth nuclear membranes, and fine chromatin. Admixed skeletal muscle cells can be seen in proliferative myositis {3305}.

Diagnostic molecular pathology

Not clinically relevant

Essential and desirable diagnostic criteria

Essential: myofibroblastic/fibroblastic proliferation with ganglion-like cells; variable collagenous/myxoid stroma; subcutaneous/fascial involvement (proliferative fasciitis); intramuscular checkerboard growth pattern (proliferative myositis).

Staging

Not clinically relevant

Prognosis and prediction

Both proliferative fasciitis and proliferative myositis rarely recur after conservative local excision, but they do not metastasize.

Myositis ossificans and fibro-osseous pseudotumour of digits

Oliveira AM
Rosenberg AE

Definition
Myositis ossificans and fibro-osseous pseudotumour of digits (FP) are self-limited benign neoplasms composed of spindle cells and osteoblasts. Myositis ossificans, FP, and soft tissue aneurysmal bone cyst belong to the same neoplastic spectrum.

ICD-O coding
None

ICD-11 coding
FB31.Y Myositis ossificans
FB51.Y Fibro-osseous pseudotumour of digits

Related terminology
Not recommended: pseudomalignant osseous tumour of soft tissue; myositis ossificans circumscripta; myositis ossificans traumatica.

Subtype(s)
None

Localization
Myositis ossificans can develop anywhere in the body {12,802, 2116,2335,2658,2987}. Common locations are those susceptible to trauma, such as the elbow, thigh, buttock, and shoulder. Typically it develops within skeletal muscle, but similar lesions occur in the subcutis and in the tendons/fascia and are known as panniculitis ossificans and fasciitis ossificans, respectively. FP affects the subcutaneous tissues of the proximal phalanx of the fingers and less frequently the toes {545,2187}. Myositis ossificans–like lesions have also been reported in the mesentery {3388}.

Clinical features
The lesions grow rapidly and the clinical and radiological features evolve over time. In the early phase (1–2 weeks), there is swelling and pain. Soft tissue fullness and oedema are present on radiographs and CT; MRI reveals signal heterogeneity, with high signal intensity on T2-weighted images. Flocculent mineralization becomes evident at the periphery of the mass 2–6 weeks after onset of symptoms; it evolves into an eggshell-like layer of bone, and the centre is radiolucent. The mineralization is randomly distributed in FP. Over time, myositis ossificans and FP become hard and well demarcated and pain diminishes {12,802,2116,2335,2658,2987}.

Epidemiology
Myositis ossificans and FP develop from infancy to late adulthood; they usually occur in physically active young adults (mean age: 32 years) {12,802,2116,2335,2658,2987,2817,3218}. The M:F ratio is 1.5:1 for myositis ossificans; females are more commonly affected by FP.

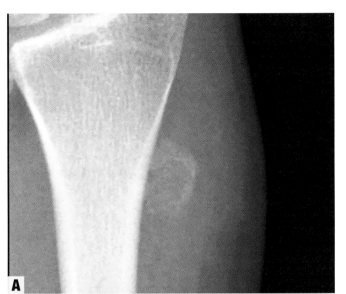

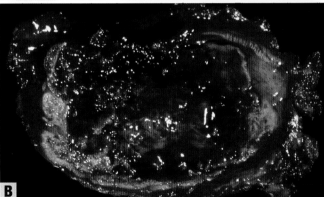

Fig. 1.56 Myositis ossificans. **A** Radiograph of a round mass in the soft tissues of the wrist showing a fine cloud-like pattern of mineralization, densest at the periphery. **B** Well-circumscribed tan haemorrhagic mass.

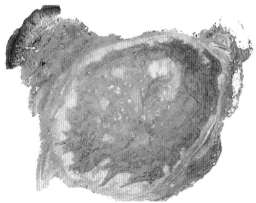

Fig. 1.57 Fibro-osseous pseudotumour of digits. The lesion presents as a well-circumscribed subcuticular mass.

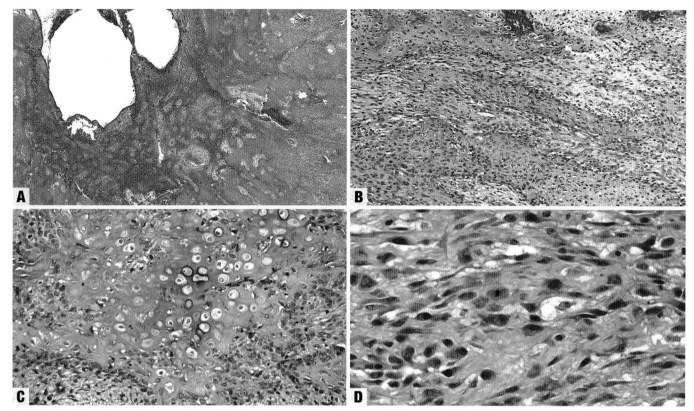

Fig. 1.58 Myositis ossificans. **A** Zonation pattern with focally cystic hypercellular centre surrounded by progressively maturing woven bone. **B** Poorly formed woven bone associated with osteoblasts merges with matrix that is well formed and trabecular in architecture. **C** Hypercellular hyaline cartilage undergoing enchondral ossification. **D** Fascicles of plump spindle cells with elongate nuclei that are mitotically active. The stroma is myxocollagenous with scattered extravasated red blood cells. Histological resemblance to nodular fasciitis is evident.

is extraskeletal osteosarcoma, which lacks zonation and shows malignant cytology.

Cytology
Cytology features a dual cell population of spindle cells and large ganglion-like cells set in a myxoid stroma {1649}.

Diagnostic molecular pathology
Molecular studies for *USP6* rearrangement may be useful in the appropriate clinicopathological context.

Essential and desirable diagnostic criteria
Essential: hypercellular fascicles of uniform spindle cells; admixed woven bone with zonation, being most mature at the periphery.

Staging
Not clinically relevant

Prognosis and prediction
Treatment of myositis ossificans and FP is usually simple excision. Prognosis is excellent; recurrence is uncommon.

Ischaemic fasciitis

Liegl-Atzwanger B

Definition
Ischaemic fasciitis is a reactive pseudosarcomatous fibroblastic/myofibroblastic proliferation, sometimes associated with physical immobility.

ICD-O coding
None

ICD-11 coding
FB51.2 Ischaemic fasciitis

Related terminology
Not recommended: atypical decubital fibroplasia; pseudosarcomatous fibromatosis.

Subtype(s)
None

Localization
Ischaemic fasciitis usually arises around the limb girdles, sacral region, and greater trochanter; the chest wall and back may also be affected. Ischaemic fasciitis usually develops in the deep subcutis, but involvement of the deep dermis, skeletal muscle, and tendinous tissue can also occur {1855}.

Clinical features
This lesion occurs as a painless mass with a median size of 4.7 cm. Ischaemic fasciitis may be associated with immobility or debilitation in some cases {1855}.

Epidemiology
Ischaemic fasciitis mainly affects elderly patients, with a peak incidence between the seventh and ninth decades of life, although the age range is wide. Males are affected slightly more often than females {2181,2491,1855}.

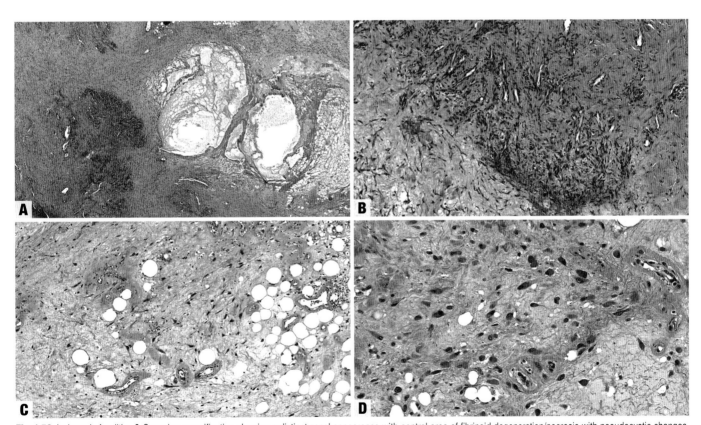

Fig. 1.59 Ischaemic fasciitis. **A** Scanning magnification showing a distinct zonal appearance with central area of fibrinoid degeneration/necrosis with pseudocystic changes, surrounded by granulation tissue–like vascular proliferation. **B** Ischaemic fasciitis with a vascular proliferation showing endothelial cells with reactive hyperchromatic nuclei (no endothelial multilayering), admixed with a reactive fibroblastic/myofibroblastic proliferation with extravasated erythrocytes. **C** Ischaemic fasciitis with focally myxoid stroma, infarcted fat, hyalinized vessel walls, and reactive fibroblasts/myofibroblasts with a ganglion cell–like appearance. **D** Ischaemic fasciitis with polygonal fibroblasts showing enlarged nuclei, prominent nucleoli, and amphophilic cytoplasm, similar to ganglion-like cells in proliferative fasciitis.

Etiology

Ischaemia caused by constant pressure or trauma to a predisposed region may contribute to the pathogenesis in some patients {2181,2491,3328}.

Pathogenesis

Unknown

Macroscopic appearance

Ischaemic fasciitis presents as a white fibrous to tan-yellow lesion with central necrosis or occasionally cystic change {1855}.

Histopathology

The histological hallmark of ischaemic fasciitis is a distinct zonal appearance. The central part of the lesion is characterized by a hypocellular area of fibrinoid degeneration/necrosis with or without pseudocystic degeneration or infarcted fat. The central area is surrounded by a granulation tissue–like vascular proliferation mixed with fibroblasts and myofibroblasts, some polygonal with amphophilic cytoplasm and a ganglion cell-like appearance, similar to proliferative fasciitis. The fibroblastic/myofibroblastic cells vary in size and shape. Fibrosis/fibrohyalinosis or myxoid stromal change, hyalinosis of vessel walls, vessels with fibrin thrombi, an inflammatory infiltrate, and extravasated erythrocytes may be observed. Mitotic activity can be seen, mainly in the granulation tissue–like areas, but is inconspicuous overall {2181,2491,1855}. By immunohistochemistry, variable expression of SMA, desmin, and CD34 may be observed {1855}.

Cytology

Not clinically relevant

Diagnostic molecular pathology

Not clinically relevant

Essential and desirable diagnostic criteria

Essential: mass-forming lesion mainly in the deep subcutis; zonal appearance with central fibrinoid degeneration/necrosis and cystic changes; periphery with granulation tissue–like vascular component; admixed plump activated fibroblasts/myofibroblasts (ganglion-like cells).

Staging

Not clinically relevant

Prognosis and prediction

Patients are usually cured by local excision even if incomplete. Recurrences may rarely develop in immobilized patients, due to persistence of the underlying cause.

Elastofibroma

Hisaoka M
Nishio J

Definition
Elastofibroma is a benign, ill-defined proliferation of fibroelastic tissue with excessive abnormal elastic fibres.

ICD-O coding
8820/0 Elastofibroma

ICD-11 coding
FB51.Y & XH3BQ8 Other specified fibroblastic disorders & Elastofibroma

Related terminology
Acceptable: elastofibroma dorsi.

Subtype(s)
None

Localization
Elastofibroma most often arises in the deep soft tissue between the lower scapula and the thoracic wall. It may rarely occur in extrascapular locations, including other parts of the thoracic wall, extremities, limb girdles, neck, eyes, and gastrointestinal tract or other viscera. Although elastofibroma is usually a unilateral and solitary mass, bilateral or multiple lesions have been reported.

Clinical features
Elastofibroma occurs almost exclusively in the elderly, with a peak incidence between the seventh and eighth decades of life. There is a striking female predominance (M:F ratio: ~0.08:1) {2236}. The lesion usually presents as a slow-growing asymptomatic mass or rarely causes pain, stiffness, scapular snapping, and impingement. CT and MRI show a poorly defined, heterogeneous soft tissue mass with tissue attenuation similar to that of skeletal muscle interlaced with fat strands {2261}. The lesion may be hypermetabolic on FDG PET-CT {2385}.

Epidemiology
Although elastofibroma was previously considered to be rare, its exact prevalence is unknown. The lesions are detectable in 2% of adults aged > 60 years by CT and in 16% of autopsy cases from adults aged > 55 years {400,1514}.

Etiology
Unknown

Pathogenesis
Elastotic degeneration of collagen or abnormal elastotic fibrogenesis may underlie the pathogenesis of elastofibroma {2942, 1713,1089}, and active neovascularization or endothelial–mesenchymal transition plays a potential pathogenetic role {1561, 816}. Elastofibroma often exhibits chromosomal instability

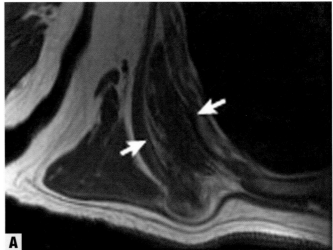

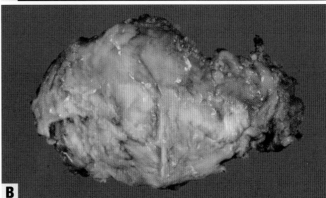

Fig. 1.60 Elastofibroma. **A** Axial T1-weighted MRI showing an inhomogeneous lesion with low and streaky high signal intensities (arrows) in the back. **B** An ill-defined mass comprising an admixture of greyish-white fibrous tissue and intervening yellow fat.

including gains of 6p25-q25 and Xq12-q22 and losses of 1p, 13q, 19p, and 22q {2310,1352}. Deletions of *CASR* (3q13.33-q21.1), *GSTP1* (11q13.2), and *BRCA2* (13q13.1), as well as gains of *APC* (5q22.2) and *PAH* (12q23.2), have also been described {1352}.

Macroscopic appearance
The lesion is poorly defined and rubbery, composed of grey or whitish fibrous tissue with variable intervening streaks of yellow fatty tissue. The diameter ranges from 2 to 15 cm.

Histopathology
Elastofibroma is composed predominantly of fibrocollagenous tissue containing a large number of abnormal elastic fibres and dispersed, bland-appearing spindle cells, admixed with a variable amount of adipose tissue and small blood vessels. A focally myxoid matrix is common. The elastic fibres are typically

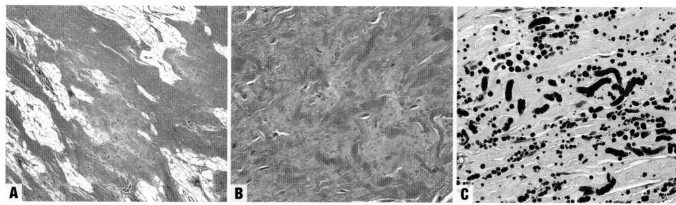

Fig. 1.61 Elastofibroma. **A** Hypocellular fibrocollagenous tissue with mature adipose tissue. **B** Thick or coarse, deeply eosinophilic elastic fibres arranged in beaded strings or globules. **C** Elastic-Masson staining highlights the abnormal elastic fibres.

thick or coarse, deeply eosinophilic, and fragmented into linearly arranged globular or serrated disc-like structures, simulating beads on a string, which are highlighted using elastic stains.

Cytology
Linear (braid-like), globular, or stellate structures of degenerated elastic fibres are cytological features in elastofibroma {833}.

Diagnostic molecular pathology
Not clinically relevant

Essential and desirable diagnostic criteria
Essential: a bland-appearing, hypocellular fibrofatty tumour with excessive abnormal elastic fibres.

Staging
Not clinically relevant

Prognosis and prediction
Elastofibroma is a benign lesion and is cured by simple excision. Local recurrence is exceptional.

Fibrous hamartoma of infancy

Al-Ibraheemi A
Folpe AL

Definition

Fibrous hamartoma of infancy is a benign soft tissue neoplasm of infants and young children, showing organoid, triphasic morphology with bundles of bland fibroblastic/myofibroblastic cells; nodules of primitive, rounded or stellate cells with myxoid stroma, and mature adipose tissue.

ICD-O coding

8992/0 Fibrous hamartoma of infancy

ICD-11 coding

LC2Y Other specified hamartomata derived from dermal connective tissue

Related terminology

Not recommended: subdermal fibromatous tumour of infancy.

Subtype(s)

None

Localization

Fibrous hamartoma of infancy commonly involves the axilla, trunk, upper extremities, and genital regions. This lesion has also been described in other locations, including scalp, foot, hand, orbit, and buttock {72,2701}.

Clinical features

Fibrous hamartoma of infancy typically presents as painless solitary subcutaneous masses, sometimes with overlying skin discolouration, oedema, hypertrichosis, and tethering {72}. There are rare reports of this tumour type presenting as multiple lesions in the same patient and in patients with tuberous sclerosis and Williams syndrome {72,1286,3080}.

Epidemiology

Fibrous hamartoma of infancy is rare and most often occurs in children aged < 2 years, with a male predominance. However, it can occur in older children {72}. About 15–25% of cases are congenital {2701}.

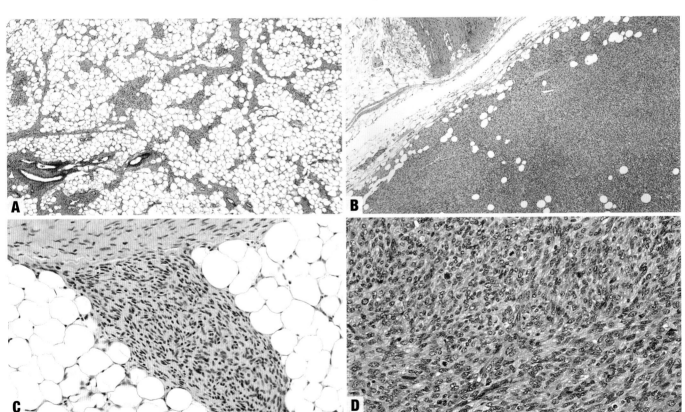

Fig. 1.62 Fibrous hamartoma of infancy. **A** Low-power view showing the triphasic organoid pattern with bundles of fibroblastic spindle cells, mature adipose tissue, and nodules of primitive mesenchyme. **B** Fibrous hamartoma of infancy with sarcomatous features. Typical triphasic fibrous hamartoma of infancy showing an abrupt transition to a highly cellular, sarcomatous spindle cell neoplasm. **C** Medium-power view showing the triphasic organoid pattern with bundles of fibroblastic spindle cells, mature adipose tissue, and nodules of primitive mesenchyme. **D** Fibrous hamartoma of infancy with sarcomatous features. High-power view of the sarcomatous area showing spindled to round cells with hyperchromatic nuclei and brisk mitotic activity.

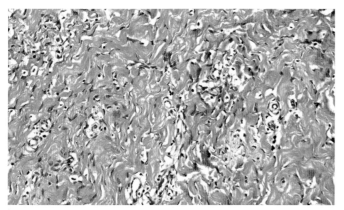

Fig. 1.63 Fibrous hamartoma of infancy. Giant cell fibroblastoma–like areas with abundant collagen with cracking artefact forming slit-like spaces lined by flattened tumour cells.

Etiology
Unknown

Pathogenesis
Although fibrous hamartoma of infancy was historically considered a hamartoma, the recent discovery of recurrent EGFR exon 20 insertion/duplication mutations in this lesion indicates a neoplastic process {2444}. Minimal to moderate EGFR (HER1) protein expression has been reported, mostly in the primitive mesenchyme {2444}.

Macroscopic appearance
The excised lesions are poorly circumscribed and of varying size (mean: 3 cm). The cut surfaces have a variable amount of adipose tissue and greyish-tan fibrous tissue.

Histopathology
Fibrous hamartoma of infancy has a triphasic organoid pattern with haphazardly arranged fascicles of cytologically bland fibroblastic/myofibroblastic cells, admixed with mature adipose tissue and myxoid nodules containing primitive mesenchymal cells with rounded to stellate nuclei. One quarter of cases show areas resembling giant cell fibroblastoma, composed of hyalinized zones containing collagen with cracking artefact forming slit-like spaces lined by flattened tumour cells. Mitotic figures are infrequent, and necrosis is typically absent. Interspersed inflammatory cells can be seen. Very recently, two tumours showing both typical and sarcomatous morphology were reported as part of a larger series {72}. By immunohistochemistry, fibrous hamartoma of infancy shows variable expression of SMA in the fibroblastic areas and occasionally in the primitive mesenchyme. CD34 is expressed within the primitive mesenchyme and in areas with giant cell fibroblastoma–like morphology.

Cytology
FNA shows bland-appearing fibroblasts in a collagenous matrix and mature fat without substantial nuclear atypia or mitoses {2818}.

Diagnostic molecular pathology
Not clinically relevant

Essential and desirable diagnostic criteria
Essential: organoid, triphasic morphology; variable prominence of bundles of bland fibroblastic/myofibroblastic cells, nodules of primitive mesenchyme, and mature adipose tissue.

Staging
Not clinically relevant

Prognosis and prediction
Most patients are cured with simple excision, although roughly 15% of cases have been reported to locally recur if incompletely excised. The clinical significance of sarcoma-like foci within fibrous hamartoma of infancy is unclear {72}.

Fibromatosis colli

Davis JL

Definition
Fibromatosis colli is a benign, self-limited fibrous proliferation occurring in the sternocleidomastoid muscle of infants. Some cases progress to shortening of the muscle, resulting in torticollis.

ICD-O coding
None

ICD-11 coding
FB51.Y Other specified fibroblastic disorders

Related terminology
Not recommended: sternocleidomastoid tumour of infancy; pseudotumour of infancy; congenital muscular torticollis.

Subtype(s)
None

Localization
Fibromatosis colli affects the sternocleidomastoid muscle, with a predilection for the right over the left. Most commonly the middle or distal third of the muscle body is involved; however, about 15% of cases involve the entire muscle {567,566}.

Clinical features
Fibromatosis colli presents as a mass within the sternocleidomastoid muscle, most often congenitally or within the first 2–4 weeks of life. Continued growth may occur over several weeks, followed by stabilization and then spontaneous resolution in the majority of cases {2528,566,567}. Approximately 10–20% of patients develop congenital muscular torticollis {2528,566}. These patients demonstrate head tilt towards the involved sternocleidomastoid muscle, with the chin directed towards the contralateral shoulder. Plagiocephaly may also occur. Fibromatosis colli is associated with other musculoskeletal congenital anomalies, including hip dysplasia, metatarsus adductus, talipes equinovarus, and prominent ears {2528,566, 567}. Ultrasound is the preferred imaging method, demonstrating an isoechoic to hypoechoic solid, well-defined ovoid mass in continuity with the sternocleidomastoid muscle {246,7}.

Epidemiology
Fibromatosis colli is uncommon; however, it is the most common cause of a neck mass in the perinatal period. The reported incidence is 0.3–2.0% of live births {568}. There is a slight male predominance (M:F ratio: 1.5:1) {566,1706}.

Etiology
Unknown

Pathogenesis
The pathogenesis is uncertain; however, a scar-like/reactive process due to injury of the sternocleidomastoid muscle is most likely, acquired either in utero or at the time of delivery {2298, 739,1706}. Possible mechanisms include fetal malposition/crowding, birth trauma, vascular compromise, and infection {1706,739,2528}.

Macroscopic appearance
If fibromatosis colli is excised, the gross appearance is that of a firm to hard, tan-white mass with associated skeletal muscle.

Histopathology
Surgical specimens are infrequent, obtained only in the minority of patients requiring tenotomy for persistent torticollis. When histology is obtained, sections demonstrate a paucicellular, scar-like fibroblastic proliferation entrapping skeletal muscle {1706}.

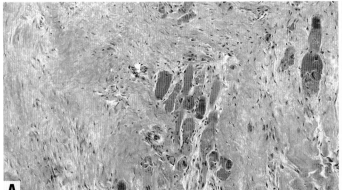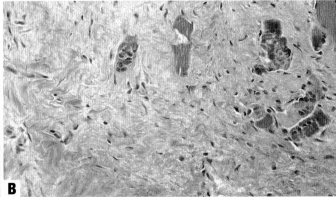

Fig. 1.64 Fibromatosis colli. **A,B** Paucicellular, scar-like fibroblastic proliferation entrapping atrophic skeletal muscle.

Soft tissue tumours   61

Cytology

FNA is a potential means of tissue diagnosis {3215,1706,1720, 1618}. Smears are typically scant to mildly cellular, composed of spindled to plump fibroblasts with associated collagen fibres and atrophic/degenerating skeletal muscle. The fibroblastic cells are singly or loosely cohesive, with bland oval to elongated nuclei and unipolar or bipolar tails of cytoplasm; bare nuclei may also be present. Atrophic, multinucleated myocytes are often admixed {3215,1706,1720,1618}.

Diagnostic molecular pathology

Not clinically relevant

Essential and desirable diagnostic criteria

Essential: infant with a fusiform mass associated with the sternocleidomastoid muscle; bland fibroblastic proliferation with associated atrophic skeletal muscle.
Desirable: clinical torticollis is variably present.

Staging

Not clinically relevant

Prognosis and prediction

The majority of fibromatosis colli lesions are self-limited, with resolution within the first 6 months of life; however, a subset of cases progress with continued tumour growth and/or the development of torticollis. If untreated, torticollis will worsen with patient growth and development {2528,568}. Within the first year of life, passive manual stretching/manipulations or physiotherapy is effective in about 95% of cases. However, in those cases that do not resolve by stretching/physiotherapy (< 10% of cases), operative management may be required {568,567, 1896}. Patients who present at an age > 1 year are more likely to require surgical intervention {566,1896,568}.

Juvenile hyaline fibromatosis

Davis JL

Definition
Juvenile hyaline fibromatosis / hyaline fibromatosis syndrome is an extremely rare autosomal recessive syndrome that typically presents in infancy. It is characterized by painful, disfiguring, abnormal deposits of hyalinized fibrous material (extracellular matrix) in the dermis, subcutaneous soft tissues, and gingiva.

ICD-O coding
None

ICD-11 coding
EE6Y Other specified fibromatous disorders of skin and soft tissue

Related terminology
Acceptable: hyaline fibromatosis syndrome; infantile systemic hyalinosis.

Subtype(s)
None

Localization
Hyaline fibromatosis syndrome is a multisystem disease (see below).

Clinical features
Hyaline fibromatosis syndrome typically presents in infancy but can occur later in childhood; more-severe cases present earlier {507,792}. The most common clinical manifestations are subcutaneous / soft tissue nodules and papules, gingival hypertrophy, and joint contractures (85–95% of cases), followed by other cutaneous and bone manifestations. Systemic/visceral involvement leading to failure to thrive, intractable diarrhoea (50% of cases), and recurrent infections (30% of cases) is defined as severe disease and is associated with early mortality {507,792,2313}.

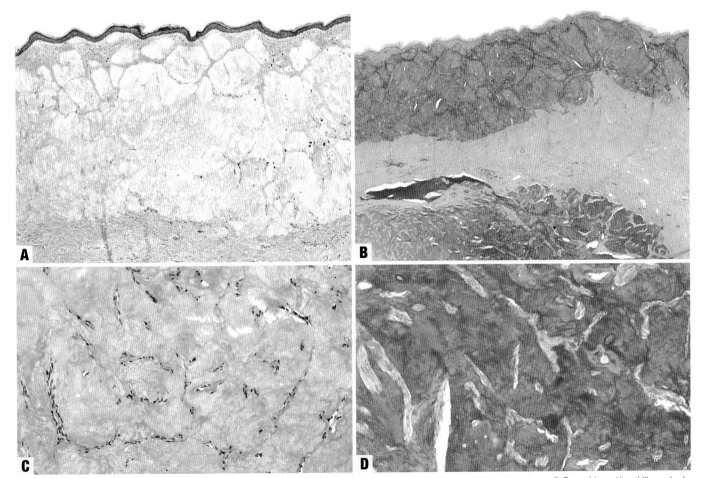

Fig. 1.65 Juvenile hyaline fibromatosis. **A** Dermal-based band-like deposits of hyaline matrix with obliteration of normal adnexal structures. **B** Dermal-based band-like and subcutaneous nodular deposits of avidly PAS-positive hyaline material (PASD staining). **C** Cords of fibroblasts in a background of abundant amorphous hyaline material. **D** Cords of fibroblasts in a background of abundant amorphous hyaline material (PASD staining).

Epidemiology

Hyaline fibromatosis syndrome demonstrates no sex predilection, following an autosomal recessive inheritance pattern.

Etiology

Juvenile hyaline fibromatosis is an autosomal recessive syndrome resulting from loss-of-function mutations, including inactivating homozygous or compound heterozygous mutations in the *ANTXR2* (*CMG2*) gene {3380,507}.

Pathogenesis

The *ANTXR2* gene encodes for a transmembrane protein that binds the extracellular proteins laminin and collagen VI; it also serves as a receptor for the anthrax toxin {806}. The nodules in hyaline fibromatosis syndrome patients are reported to contain collagen VI, suggesting that ANTXR2 may mediate its degradation. Therefore, in hyaline fibromatosis syndrome, given the loss of ANTXR2 function, collagen VI would accumulate in the extracellular matrix {447}.

Macroscopic appearance

The nodules are solid and homogeneous.

Histopathology

Hyaline fibromatosis syndrome is characterized by hyaline-like extracellular matrix deposits. The lesions show variable cellularity and are composed of plump to spindled uniform fibroblasts, often arranged in cords simulating vascular spaces, admixed with abundant extracellular eosinophilic non-fibrillar hyaline material, obliterating normal structures {792,3137}. The hyaline material stains strongly with PAS and is diastase-resistant {792,3137}.

Cytology

Not clinically relevant

Diagnostic molecular pathology

Germline sequencing of *ANTXR2* (4q21.21) can confirm the diagnosis.

Essential and desirable diagnostic criteria

Essential: subcutaneous nodules and gingival hypertrophy with abundant hyaline-like material.
Desirable: confirmation by germline sequencing of the *ANTXR2* gene.

Staging

Not clinically relevant

Prognosis and prediction

Age at presentation is a predictor of prognosis, with earlier presentation associated with more-severe disease. In systemic/severe disease, the median age at death is 15 months {507, 2313,792}. For patients with milder forms, wheelchair use may become necessary because of joint contractures. Phenotype–genotype correlations have demonstrated that *ANTXR2* missense mutations in exons 1–12 and mutations leading to a premature stop codon more commonly lead to severe disease, whereas missense mutations in exons 13–17 lead to a mild form of disease {507,3380,806,896}. Treatment is largely supportive. Surgical excision of subcutaneous nodules and/or gingivectomy for gingival hypertrophy is often performed; however, recurrences are common {507,792}.

Inclusion body fibromatosis

Laskin WB

Definition
Inclusion body fibromatosis is a benign, sometimes multicentric, myofibroblastic tumour with characteristic eosinophilic intracytoplasmic inclusions and potential for local recurrence.

ICD-O coding
None

ICD-11 coding
EE6Y Other specified fibromatous disorders of skin and soft tissue

Related terminology
Acceptable: infantile digital fibroma/fibromatosis; recurring digital fibrous tumour(s) of childhood; recurring digital fibroma(s) of childhood/infancy.

Subtype(s)
None

Localization
The classic subtype involves the dorsal or dorsolateral aspect of the distal or middle portion of the second, third, and fourth digits, followed by the fifth digit, while typically sparing the first digit, hand, and foot {245,599,1760}. Extradigital examples are reported on the extremities, tongue, and breast {1760}.

Clinical features
The classic subtype presents as an asymptomatic dome-shaped or polypoid cutaneous nodule, typically no larger than 2 cm {245,2700,1760}. Synchronous and/or metachronous lesions (sometimes affecting multiple digits) occur, but simultaneous involvement of both fingers and toes is rare {77, 245,2700}. Non-classic examples typically present as solitary masses or nodules {1760}.

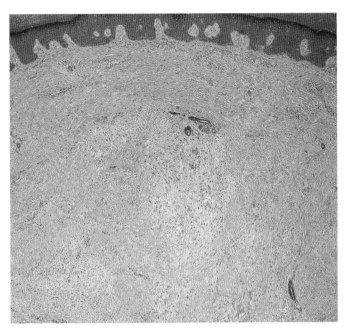

Fig. 1.67 Inclusion body fibromatosis. Spindled cells in short fascicles and whorls surrounding adnexa are a characteristic growth pattern.

Epidemiology
The classic subtype accounts for 0.1% of registered soft tissue tumours {77} and 2% of paediatric fibroblastic tumours {625}. Nearly all cases are reported before the age of 5 years {599}. Most tumours are documented during the first year of life, with about 30% present at birth {599,245,2700}. Rare cases occur in adults {3200,2743,2522}. No sex predilection exists.

Etiology
Unknown

Pathogenesis
Unknown

Macroscopic appearance
Tumours are firm or rubbery, ill-defined protuberant or polypoid dermal nodules. The cut surface is fibrous and off-white to grey in colour.

Histopathology
Spindle cells have lightly eosinophilic cytoplasm and an elongated, cytologically bland nucleus, and they exhibit low mitotic activity. Cells proliferate in whorls, interlacing short fascicles, or storiform arrays within a variably collagenous dermis, and they characteristically grow perpendicular to the epidermis, surround adnexa, and occasionally infiltrate deeper tissues {77,599}. Cells harbour a 1.5–24 μm, rounded, pale-pink to red

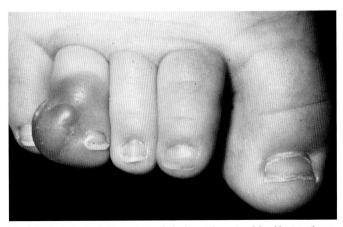

Fig. 1.66 Inclusion body fibromatosis. A single protuberant nodule with an erythematous surface on the lateral aspect of the distal toe.

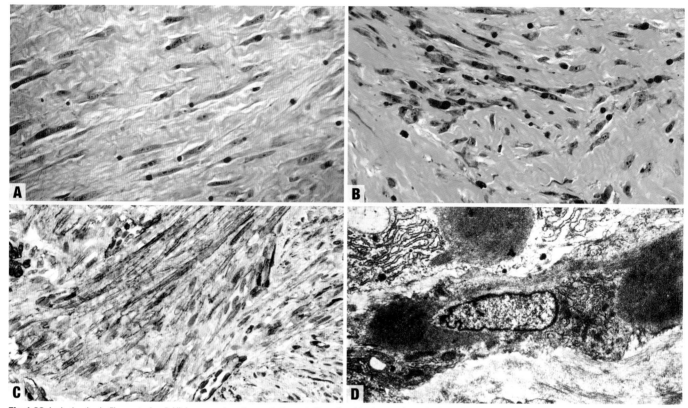

Fig. 1.68 Inclusion body fibromatosis. **A** High-power view demonstrates spindle cells with elongated, cytologically bland nuclei and rounded, eosinophilic, intracytoplasmic inclusions, some indenting the nucleus. **B** Gomori trichrome staining highlights intracytoplasmic inclusions (red). **C** Immunostaining for SMA demonstrates a peripheral (tram-track) pattern of expression. **D** Ultrastructurally, myofilamentous bundles at the periphery of a tumour cell merge with a dense intracytoplasmic inclusion.

intracytoplasmic inclusion, which is frequently paranuclear, indenting the nucleus {2618,599}, and is highlighted by trichrome (red), phosphotungstic acid–haematoxylin (dark purple), and Movat (pink) stains {1760}. Ultrastructurally, tumour cells contain intracytoplasmic bundles of actin-rich myofilaments with dense bodies, which are in continuity with a non–membrane-bound, rounded inclusion consisting of a dense core of tightly packed myofilaments {2211,306,1497}. The inclusions commonly mark with actin {2210} and calponin-1 {1348}, and occasionally with caldesmon {1760}.

Cytology
There are abundant plump spindle cells and few polygonal cells with a moderate cytoplasm set in a collagenous background. Scattered prominent intracytoplasmic inclusions are present {2362}.

Diagnostic molecular pathology
Not clinically relevant

Essential and desirable diagnostic criteria
Essential: dermal-based and cytologically bland myofibroblastic proliferation; eosinophilic intracytoplasmic and paranuclear inclusions.

Staging
Not clinically relevant

Prognosis and prediction
Recurrence rates between 61% and 75% are reported in large series and reviews for the classic subtype {2660,599,1760}. Lower recurrence rates are achievable with initial complete (preferably wide) excision {955,2633,3031}. Current treatment recommendations include function-preserving excision or intralesional steroid injection for symptomatic lesions and clinical observation after diagnosis for asymptomatic tumours {1985, 952}, because lesions may spontaneously regress {2274}. Approximately 25% of non-classic tumours recur {1760}.

Fibroma of tendon sheath

Sciot R
Cunha IW

Definition
Fibroma of tendon sheath is a benign fibroblastic/myofibroblastic nodular proliferation, usually attached to a tendon (sheath).

ICD-O coding
8813/0 Fibroma of tendon sheath

ICD-11 coding
EE6Y & XH0WB3 Other specified fibromatous disorders of skin and soft tissue & Fibroma of tendon sheath

Related terminology
Not recommended: tenosynovial fibroma.

Subtype(s)
None

Localization
The lesion typically occurs on the finger tendons. The thumb, index finger, and middle finger are the digits most frequently involved. Intra-articular locations (knee, elbow, wrist) have rarely been described {2446,1714,608}.

Clinical features
The tumour presents as a firm, small (≤ 3 cm), slow-growing nodule.

Epidemiology
Fibroma of tendon sheath is rare and typically occurs in patients aged 20–50 years {2549,84}.

Etiology
Unknown

Pathogenesis
A clonal chromosomal abnormality, t(2;11)(q31-q32;q12), has been described in two classic cases {720,2307}. Notably, an apparently identical translocation has also been observed in desmoplastic fibroblastoma, which can show morphological overlap with fibroma of tendon sheath {1926,277,2306}. Diffuse and strong nuclear FOSL1 expression seems to be characteristic of desmoplastic fibroblastoma and absent in fibroma of tendon sheath {1592,1926}. Some cellular subtypes of fibroma of tendon sheath are characterized by *USP6* rearrangement, as seen in nodular fasciitis {496}. In view of the similar morphological and molecular genetic features, some lesions diagnosed as cellular fibroma of tendon sheath are probably in fact tenosynovial nodular fasciitis {1410}.

Macroscopic appearance
Fibroma of tendon sheath has a lobular fibrous appearance, reminiscent of a localized tenosynovial giant cell tumour, except for the pigment, which is absent in fibroma of tendon sheath.

Histopathology
The lesion is well circumscribed and contains bland spindle cells in a collagenous background. The cellularity is usually low but can be variable and is often higher at the tumour edge. There are characteristic slit-like thin-walled vessels. Degenerative features such as myxoid/cystic changes, chondroid or osseous metaplasia, and bizarre pleomorphic cells can be seen. The morphological features of the cellular subtype are identical to those of nodular fasciitis.

Cytology
Not clinically relevant

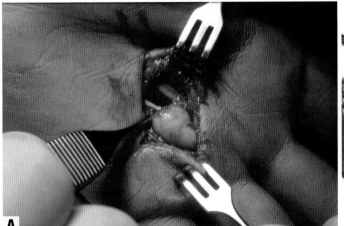
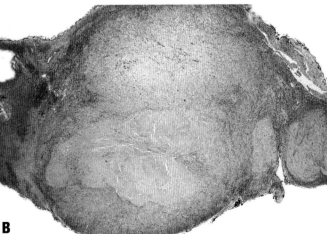

Fig. 1.69 Fibroma of tendon sheath. **A** Intraoperative photo showing the smooth nodular surface and attachment to a tendon. **B** This lower-power view shows characteristic variation in cellularity.

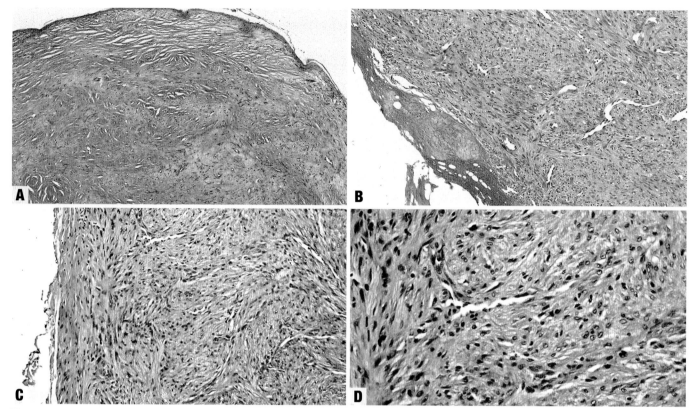

Fig. 1.70 Fibroma of tendon sheath. **A** Low-power view showing the highly sclerotic and hypocellular appearances. Note the small vessels and clefts. **B** Some cases can show increased cellularity, which is most obvious at the edge. **C** The tumour is well circumscribed and is composed of bland spindle cells with a prominent collagenous stroma and slit-like, thin-walled blood vessels. **D** The tumour cells contain fine chromatin and indistinct pale cytoplasm. Note the collagenous stroma and thin-walled blood vessel.

Diagnostic molecular pathology
Not clinically relevant

Essential and desirable diagnostic criteria
Essential: benign firm nodule most often on the finger tendons; usually a paucicellular collagen-rich lesion with slit-like vessels.

Staging
Not clinically relevant

Prognosis and prediction
Fibroma of tendon sheath is benign but can recur in 5–10% of cases.

Desmoplastic fibroblastoma

Miettinen M
Bridge JA

Definition
Desmoplastic fibroblastoma is a benign, paucicellular, soft tissue tumour with abundant collagenous or myxocollagenous matrix; low vascularity; and scattered, bland, stellate-shaped and spindled fibroblastic cells.

ICD-O coding
8810/0 Desmoplastic fibroblastoma

ICD-11 coding
EE6Y & XH2ZF3 Other specified fibromatous disorders of skin and soft tissue & Desmoplastic fibroblastoma

Related terminology
Acceptable: collagenous fibroma.

Subtype(s)
None

Localization
The most common sites are the upper arm, shoulder, lower limb, back, forearm, hand, and foot {941,2285,2120}.

Clinical features
The tumour typically presents as an asymptomatic, slow-growing subcutaneous mass, but fascial and skeletal muscle involvement is relatively common.

Epidemiology
Desmoplastic fibroblastoma is a rare tumour that predominantly affects adults, with a median age of 50–60 years.

Etiology
Unknown

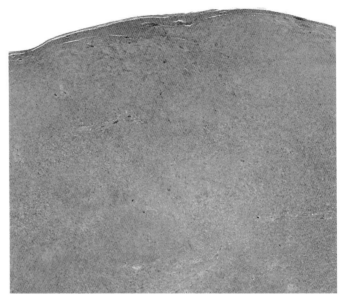

Fig. 1.72 Desmoplastic fibroblastoma. The lesion is well circumscribed with a smooth rounded border.

Pathogenesis
Most of the karyotypic studies of desmoplastic fibroblastoma have demonstrated a recurrent t(2;11)(q31;q12) {277,2306, 2715}. Deregulated expression of FOSL1 appears to be the functional outcome of 11q12 rearrangements in desmoplastic fibroblastoma, based on global gene expression profiling and quantitative real-time PCR {1926}. Notably, diffuse, strong FOSL1 nuclear immunoreactivity is seen in desmoplastic fibroblastomas with 11q12 rearrangement, in contrast to the absence of overexpression in 11q12-rearranged fibromas of tendon sheath {1592}.

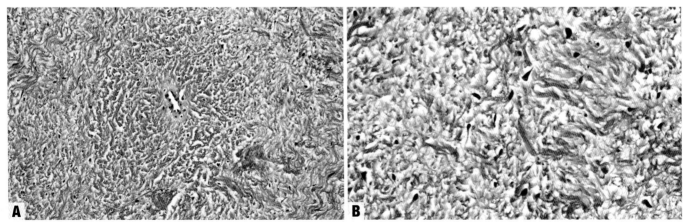

Fig. 1.71 Desmoplastic fibroblastoma. **A,B** The tumour is paucicellular and composed of uniform, often stellate-shaped, fibroblasts.

Macroscopic appearance

Desmoplastic fibroblastomas are usually relatively small, often measuring 1–4 cm in greatest dimension, but examples > 10 cm and as large as 20 cm have occurred. Grossly, the lesions appear well circumscribed and form oval, fusiform, or discoid masses. Some examples have an externally lobulated, cobblestone-like surface. The tumours have a firm, cartilage-like consistency, and on cut section they have a homogeneous pearl-grey colour.

Histopathology

Although often well demarcated grossly, most tumours microscopically infiltrate into subcutaneous fat, and approximately 25% extend into skeletal muscle {941,2285,2120}. Rare examples are purely intramuscular. The lesions have abundant collagenous or myxocollagenous matrix with low vascularity. Cellularity ranges from low to moderate, and the neoplastic cells tend to be uniformly distributed within the extracellular matrix. The lesional cells are stellate-shaped, bipolar, and spindled, and they have uniform, bland nuclei with distinct small nucleoli. Mitotic figures are uncommon. Rare examples have focal intravascular growth. The tumour cells may be focally positive for SMA.

Cytology

Not clinically relevant

Diagnostic molecular pathology

Not clinically relevant

Essential and desirable diagnostic criteria

Essential: hypocellular with abundant collagenous or myxocollagenous matrix; stellate, bipolar, and spindle cells with small nucleoli.

Staging

Not clinically relevant

Prognosis and prediction

The behaviour of this tumour is benign, and none of the published clinicopathological series have documented any recurrences.

Myofibroblastoma

Magro G
Howitt BE
Liegl-Atzwanger B
McMenamin ME

Definition

Myofibroblastoma of soft tissue is a benign neoplasm comparable to myofibroblastoma of breast, composed of myofibroblastic cells, bands of hyalinized collagen, and usually an adipocytic component.

ICD-O coding

8825/0 Myofibroblastoma

ICD-11 coding

EE6Y & XH3NQ0 Other specified fibromatous disorders of skin and soft tissue & Myofibroblastoma

Related terminology

Acceptable: mammary-type myofibroblastoma.

Subtype(s)

None

Localization

Approximately 50% of cases occur in the inguinal/groin area, including in the vulva/vagina, perineum, and scrotum; however, there is a wide anatomical distribution, including trunk/axilla, breast, extremities, abdominal cavity, retroperitoneum, and viscera {2047,1422}. The majority are superficial/subcutaneous. The remainder are deep-seated; intramuscular; or in the pelvis, abdomen, or retroperitoneum {1422}.

Clinical features

Tumours generally present as either painless masses or incidental lesions; occasional lesions are painful. Tumours may be present for > 20 years before clinical presentation {1422}.

Epidemiology

Lesions arise predominantly in adults in the fifth and sixth decades of life, but there is a wide age range (4–96 years; median age: 54 years) and a male predominance (M:F ratio: 2:1).

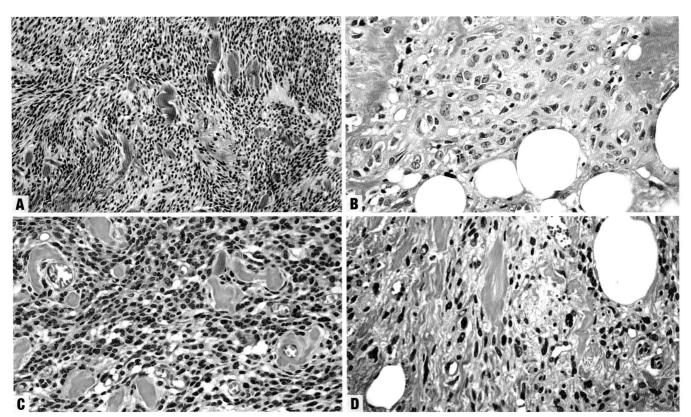

Fig. 1.73 Myofibroblastoma. **A** Proliferation of bland spindle cells with interspersed bands of hyalinized collagen. **B** Neoplastic cells may exhibit epithelioid cell morphology with a pseudoinfiltrative growth pattern. **C** Neoplastic cells showing round cell morphology: the presence of bands of hyalinized collagen and the absence of mitoses and nuclear atypia are helpful diagnostic features. **D** This tumour shows degenerative features, exhibiting cells with moderate nuclear atypia. Mitoses and necrosis are absent.

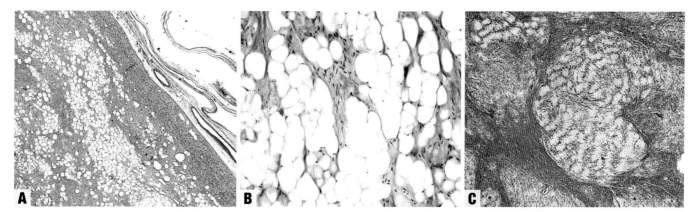

Fig. 1.74 Myofibroblastoma. **A** This tumour contains a lipomatous component. Low magnification showing well-circumscribed borders. **B** A fibrofatty tumour with spindle cell lipoma–like morphology: admixture of mature adipocytes with bland spindle cells set in a fibrous stroma. **C** Proliferation of spindle cells with formation of Verocay-like bodies, mimicking schwannoma.

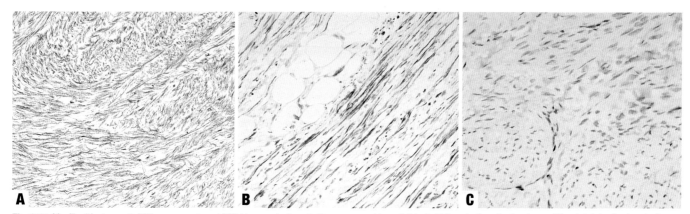

Fig. 1.75 Myofibroblastoma. **A** Diffuse expression of CD34 by neoplastic cells (immunoperoxidase staining). **B** Neoplastic cells showing multifocal staining for desmin (immunoperoxidase staining). **C** Loss of nuclear RB1, maintained in endothelial and inflammatory cells.

Etiology
Unknown

Pathogenesis
Loss of 13q14, including *RB1*, is characteristic of mammary and soft tissue myofibroblastomas, as well as of spindle cell / pleomorphic lipoma and cellular angiofibroma. In addition, the overlapping morphological and immunohistochemical features support the hypothesis that these tumours represent variations along a spectrum of genetically related lesions, the so-called 13q/*RB1* family of tumours {1941,1422,1040,26}.

Macroscopic appearance
Size ranges from < 1 cm to 22 cm (median: 6.6 cm). The tumours are generally well circumscribed, mobile, and rubbery to gelatinous. The colour can be variable (white/yellow/pink, grey, or tan). The cut surface may be whorled or nodular and variably fatty.

Histopathology
Tumours are unencapsulated and generally well circumscribed. They are usually composed of spindle cells with short stubby nuclei with finely dispersed chromatin, small or inconspicuous nucleoli, eosinophilic to amphophilic cytoplasm, indistinct cell borders, and sometimes elongated cytoplasmic processes. They are generally arranged in variably sized short fascicles, with interspersed broad bands of hyalinized collagen or (less commonly) ropy collagen. Scattered mast cells are generally present. Tumours may vary from markedly cellular to paucicellular and hyalinized. There is usually a variable admixture of mature adipocytes, which can range from rare to occasionally the dominant component. Schwannoma-like palisading, focal epithelioid or round cell morphology, or degenerative-type nuclear atypia (enlarged hyperchromatic nuclei and multinucleation) can occur {1422}. The blood vessels are generally inconspicuous, being small and often focally hyalinized and having a perivascular lymphocytic infiltrate.

By immunohistochemistry, myofibroblastoma typically shows diffuse coexpression of desmin and CD34 (each positive in 90% of cases). Rare cases are negative for both markers. Expression of SMA is present in one third of cases. About 90% of cases show loss of nuclear RB1 {550,1422}.

Cytology
Not clinically relevant

Diagnostic molecular pathology
Loss of *RB1* can be demonstrated by FISH, although this is usually not necessary to establish the diagnosis.

Essential and desirable diagnostic criteria

Essential: haphazardly intersecting short fascicles of bland, short or elongated spindle cells; bands of hyalinized collagen; variable adipocytic component; expression of CD34 and desmin.

Desirable: loss of *RB1* (demonstrated by immunohistochemistry or FISH).

Staging

Not clinically relevant

Prognosis and prediction

All tumours reported to date have followed a benign course after marginal local excision, with exceptional local recurrences.

Calcifying aponeurotic fibroma

Puls F
Kilpatrick SE

Definition
Calcifying aponeurotic fibroma is a rare benign tumour with potential for local recurrence that typically arises on the distal extremities of children and adolescents. It is characterized by bland spindle cells and less cellular zones of calcification with plump to epithelioid fibroblasts.

ICD-O coding
8816/0 Calcifying aponeurotic fibroma

ICD-11 coding
EE6Y & XH8ZE3 Other specified fibromatous disorders of skin and soft tissue & Calcifying aponeurotic fibroma

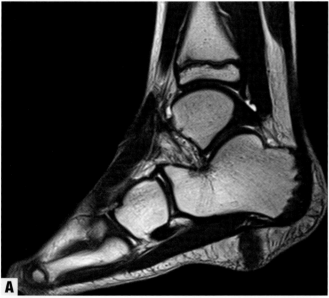

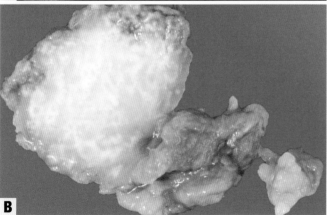

Fig. 1.76 Calcifying aponeurotic fibroma. **A** The MRI shows a 1.6 cm solid mass on the plantar aspect of the foot in an 8-year-old boy. **B** A resection specimen with an ill-defined greyish-white lesion with a gritty consistency.

Related terminology
Acceptable: juvenile aponeurotic fibroma; aponeurotic fibroma.

Subtype(s)
None

Localization
Calcifying aponeurotic fibroma arises most commonly on the palmar surfaces of the hands and fingers, followed by the plantar surfaces of the feet and toes {79}. Wrists and ankles are less commonly involved {998}. Unusual locations are proximal extremities and trunk {998}. Rare examples have been documented in the head and neck region {3063}. Most lesions arise in the subcutis, often connected to tendons and aponeuroses {79,998}.

Clinical features
Patients generally present with a painless, poorly circumscribed soft tissue mass or swelling, often of extended duration. Radiographic images often demonstrate calcifications.

Epidemiology
Calcifying aponeurotic fibroma is a rare neoplasm. Its peak incidence is between the ages of 5 and 15 years, although well-documented examples in adults have been reported {998}. Males are more often affected than females {998}.

Etiology
Unknown

Pathogenesis
A recurrent *FN1-EGF* gene fusion has been identified {2550}.

Macroscopic appearance
Resected specimens are usually 1–3 cm, appearing as ill-defined, greyish-white to gritty soft tissue masses.

Histopathology
Calcifying aponeurotic fibroma is characterized by a fibromatosis-like infiltrative component and a nodular calcified component {1603}. The former is moderately cellular, composed of uniform, plump spindle cells, without substantial nuclear atypia. The tumour often extends into adjacent soft tissues, where it may be attached to tendons or entrap peripheral nerves and blood vessels. Mitotic figures are rare. The nodular calcified areas are less cellular and appear hyalinized to chondroid, wherein cells often appear rounded and chondrocyte-like and may encircle or radiate from the calcium deposits. Osteoclast-type giant cells are usually present. Lesions typically contain both components to a varying degree, although non-calcified lesions showing only a fibromatosis-like pattern can be seen. There is evidence suggesting that lesions may evolve from a

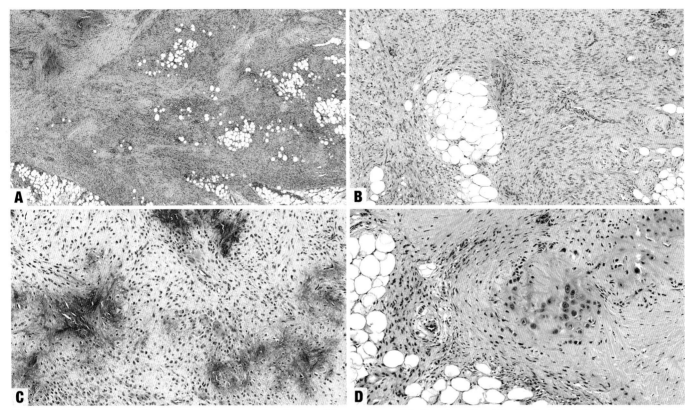

Fig. 1.77 Calcifying aponeurotic fibroma. **A** An infiltrative spindle cell lesion within subcutaneous fat with early matrix calcification (top left). **B** The infiltrative spindle cell component is reminiscent of fibromatosis. **C** Calcified areas contain epithelioid fibroblasts and scattered giant cells. **D** Chondroid areas may be present (decalcified specimen).

spindle cell–predominant morphology to a less cellular lesion with more-extensive calcifications {79,70}. By immunohisto-chemistry, lesional cells react with SMA, MSA, CD99, and (in the chondroid areas) S100. Nuclear staining for β-catenin is not seen {480}.

Cytology
Not clinically relevant

Diagnostic molecular pathology
Detection of the *FN1-EGF* gene fusion may be helpful in cases of calcifying aponeurotic fibroma lacking calcification {70}, although this is not required for routine diagnosis.

Essential and desirable diagnostic criteria
Essential: infiltrative lesion composed of bland, evenly spaced spindle cells lying in parallel within a collagenous matrix; islands or geographical areas of calcified matrix often surrounded by palisading epithelioid fibroblasts.
Desirable: FN1-EGF gene fusion (as needed in unusual cases).

Staging
Not clinically relevant

Prognosis and prediction
Largely due to the infiltrative features of calcifying aponeurotic fibroma, local recurrence, which may occur years after initial excision, is observed in as many as 50% of cases {79,998}. The risk of local recurrence seems to be higher in younger children (aged < 5 years). Calcifying aponeurotic fibroma typically has a limited growth potential, and multiple recurrences are rare {2228,998}. Conservative surgical management, with preservation of function, is typically recommended.

EWSR1-SMAD3–positive fibroblastic tumour (emerging)

Antonescu CR
Suurmeijer AJH

Definition
EWSR1-SMAD3–positive fibroblastic tumour is a benign neo-plasm with a strong predilection for the hands and feet. Tumour nomenclature is provisional.

ICD-O coding
None

ICD-11 coding
None

Related terminology
None

Subtype(s)
None

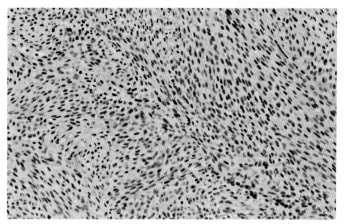

Fig. 1.79 *EWSR1-SMAD3* fibroblastic tumour. Diffuse nuclear staining for ERG by immunohistochemistry.

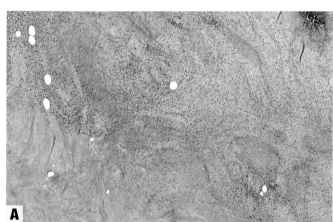

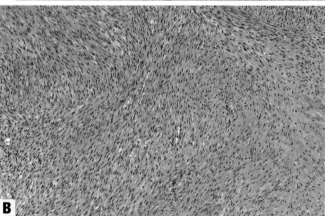

Fig. 1.78 *EWSR1-SMAD3* fibroblastic tumour. **A** Low-power view showing the char-acteristic zonation with an acellular hyalinized centre and peripheral areas composed of a cellular spindle cell component. Focal calcifications can also be noted. **B** Higher power of the peripheral area showing intersecting fascicles of monomorphic spindle cells with pale eosinophilic cytoplasm and uniform ovoid nuclei.

Localization
Tumours are superficially located within dermis and/or subcuta-neous fat. The large majority of these lesions occur in the hands and feet {2109,1574}.

Clinical features
Patients usually present with a small painless superficial tumour in acral sites.

Epidemiology
There is a wide age range (1–68 years), with female predilection {2109,1574}.

Etiology
Unknown

Pathogenesis
The tumour is defined by a fusion of exon 7 of *EWSR1* with exon 5 of *SMAD3* {2109,1574}. SMAD3 is an important signal transducer in the TGF-β/SMAD signalling pathway, which is involved in extracellular matrix synthesis by fibroblasts. By RNA sequencing, one case showed substantial upregulation of *FN1*, similar to other fibroblastic tumours, as well as ERG overexpres-sion {1574}.

Macroscopic appearance
The tumours are small, measuring 1–2 cm in greatest dimen-sion, and have a nodular appearance.

Histopathology
The tumours are typically well demarcated but show infiltration into subcutaneous fat. In particular in adult cases, the acellular centre of the tumour appears hyalinized, whereas the peripheral zones consist of intersecting cellular fascicles of fibroblastic spindle

cells lacking nuclear pleomorphism, hyperchromasia, prominent nucleoli, or mitotic activity. Focally stippled dystrophic calcification may be found. By immunohistochemistry, the fibroblastic tumour cells consistently show diffuse ERG nuclear expression, whereas staining for SMA and CD34 is negative.

Cytology
Not clinically relevant

Diagnostic molecular pathology
The *EWSR1-SMAD3* fusion may be confirmed by molecular methods.

Essential and desirable diagnostic criteria
Essential: small dermal and subcutaneous acral nodule; histological zonation with acellular hyalinized centre and peripheral fascicular spindle cell growth; immunoreactivity for ERG.
Desirable: EWSR1-SMAD3 fusion (if available).

Staging
Not clinically relevant

Prognosis and prediction
EWSR1-SMAD3–positive fibroblastic tumour is benign. Local recurrence may occur after incomplete excision.

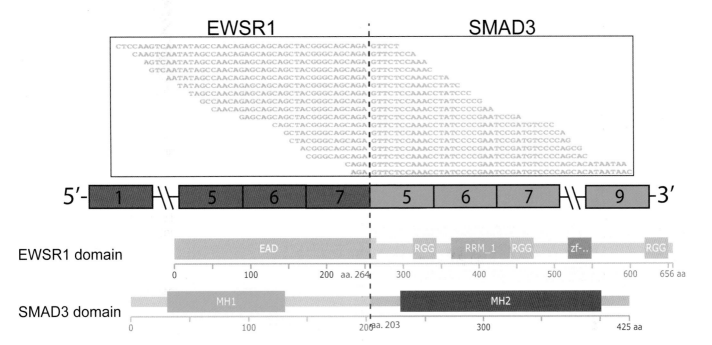

Fig. 1.80 *EWSR1-SMAD3* fibroblastic tumour. Diagrammatic representation of the *EWSR1-SMAD3* fusion and the predicted protein domains of the fusion oncoprotein.

Angiomyofibroblastoma

Fletcher CDM

Definition

Angiomyofibroblastoma is a benign, well-circumscribed myofibroblastic neoplasm, usually arising in the pelviperineal region, especially the vulva, and apparently composed of stromal cells distinctive of this anatomical region.

ICD-O coding

8826/0 Angiomyofibroblastoma

ICD-11 coding

EE6Y & XH8A47 Other specified fibromatous disorders of skin and soft tissue & Angiomyofibroblastoma

Related terminology

None

Subtype(s)

None

Localization

Virtually all cases arise in pelviperineal subcutaneous tissue, with the majority arising in the vulva. About 10–15% of cases are located in the vagina. Lesions in men occur in the scrotum or paratesticular soft tissue.

Clinical features

Most cases present as a slowly enlarging, painless, circumscribed mass. The most frequent preoperative diagnosis is Bartholin gland cyst.

Epidemiology

Angiomyofibroblastoma is uncommon, having an incidence comparable to that of deep (aggressive) angiomyxoma. These tumours arise predominantly in females, principally in adults between menarche and menopause {1026,1758,2288,1940}. About 10% of patients are postmenopausal. Convincing examples have not been described before puberty. Rare cases occur in males {1026,2341}.

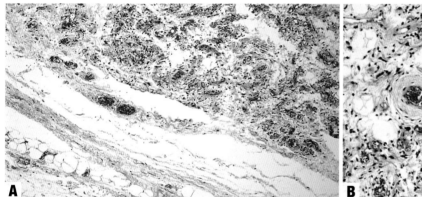

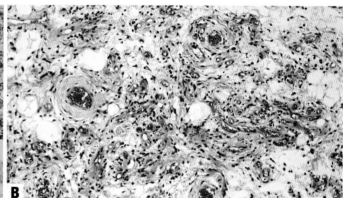

Fig. 1.81 Angiomyofibroblastoma. **A** Angiomyofibroblastoma is typically well circumscribed. **B** The tumour is more cellular and vascular than aggressive angiomyxoma. Note the adipocytic component.

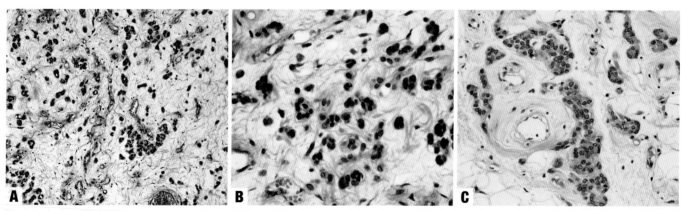

Fig. 1.82 Angiomyofibroblastoma. **A** Tumour cells and vessels are set in a loose oedematous stroma. **B** Binucleated and multinucleated cells are frequent and may have a plasmacytoid appearance. **C** In this example the tumour cells are focally clustered and have an epithelioid appearance.

Etiology
Unknown

Pathogenesis
Unknown

Macroscopic appearance
These lesions are well circumscribed but not encapsulated, with a tan/pink cut surface and a soft consistency. Necrosis is not seen. Most cases measure < 5 cm in maximum diameter, although rare examples as large as 10 cm have been recognized. Some cases may be pedunculated.

Histopathology
Tumours are generally well demarcated by a thin fibrous pseudocapsule and, at low power, show varying cellularity with prominent vessels throughout. Vessels are mostly small, thin-walled, and ectatic and are set in an abundant loose, oedematous stroma. The tumour cells are round to spindle-shaped, with eosinophilic cytoplasm, and they are typically concentrated around vessels. Mitoses are rare. Binucleated and multinucleated tumour cells are common. Some cases show plasmacytoid or epithelioid cytomorphology and rare examples show degenerative (ancient) nuclear hyperchromasia and atypia. About 10% of cases have a variably prominent well-differentiated adipocytic component, sometimes > 90% of the tumour {1911}. In postmenopausal patients, the stroma is often less oedematous and more fibrous, and there may be hyalinization of vessel walls. Rare cases show morphological overlap with aggressive angiomyxoma {1208}.

By immunohistochemistry, the majority of cases show strong and diffuse positive staining for desmin, whereas there is usually at most only focal positivity for SMA or pan-muscle actin {1026}. Desmin staining may be reduced or absent in postmenopausal cases. Tumour cells are consistently positive for ER and PR and occasionally positive for CD34.

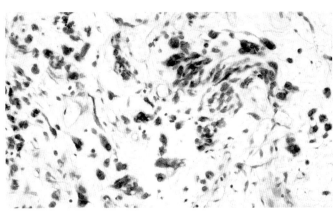

Fig. 1.83 Angiomyofibroblastoma. Immunopositivity for desmin is a typical feature in most cases.

Cytology
Not clinically relevant

Diagnostic molecular pathology
Not clinically relevant

Essential and desirable diagnostic criteria
Essential: well-circumscribed, prominent stromal vessels; round to spindle-shaped cells (often multinucleated) in a perivascular distribution.
Desirable: usually desmin-positive.

Staging
Not clinically relevant

Prognosis and prediction
Angiomyofibroblastoma is benign and recurrence appears to be rare, even after marginal local excision.

Cellular angiofibroma

Iwasa Y
Fletcher CDM
Flucke U

Definition
Cellular angiofibroma is a benign, cellular, and richly vascularized fibroblastic neoplasm that usually arises in the superficial soft tissues of the vulva or inguinoscrotal regions.

ICD-O coding
9160/0 Cellular angiofibroma

ICD-11 coding
EE6Y & XH4E06 Other specified fibromatous disorders of skin and soft tissue & Cellular angiofibroma

Related terminology
Not recommended: male angiomyofibroblastoma-like tumour.

Subtype(s)
None

Localization
Although these tumours typically arise in the superficial soft tissues of the vulvovaginal region and the inguinoscrotal or paratesticular region, rare examples have been described in other sites.

Clinical features
Patients usually present with a slow-growing painless mass. The most frequent preoperative diagnosis is (Bartholin) cyst {1040, 1496,2331}. In males, the mass may be associated with hernia or hydrocoele {1496,1757}.

Epidemiology
Cellular angiofibroma is a rare neoplasm arising in adults. Females and males are roughly equally affected, with a peak incidence in the fifth decade of life in women and the seventh decade in men {1040,1496,1757,2331}.

Etiology
Unknown

Pathogenesis
Partial or complete losses of chromosome 13 (including the *RB1* locus) and/or 16 are found in cellular angiofibroma {1937,1040, 550,2416}. Loss of 13q14, including *RB1*, is characteristic of mammary and soft tissue myofibroblastomas, as well as of spindle cell / pleomorphic lipoma and cellular angiofibroma. In addition, the overlapping morphological and immunohistochemical features support the hypothesis that these tumours represent variations along a spectrum of genetically related lesions, the so-called 13q/*RB1* family of tumours {1941,1422,1040,26}.

Macroscopic appearance
The tumours vary in size from 0.6 to 25 cm. Those in women are generally smaller (median: 2.8 cm) than those in men (median: 7.0 cm). The tumours appear as round, oval, or lobulated well-circumscribed nodules. The consistency of the lesion varies from soft to rubbery and the cut surface is solid with a greyish-pink to yellowish-brown colour {1496,1757}. Foci of haemorrhage or necrosis are exceptional {1496}.

Histopathology
The tumours are generally well circumscribed. Poorly marginated, more-infiltrative tumours occur rarely in men. Tumours are composed of uniform, short spindle-shaped cells in an oedematous to fibrous stroma containing short bundles of delicate collagen fibres and numerous small to medium-sized thick-walled blood vessels with rounded, irregularly ectatic or branching lumina.

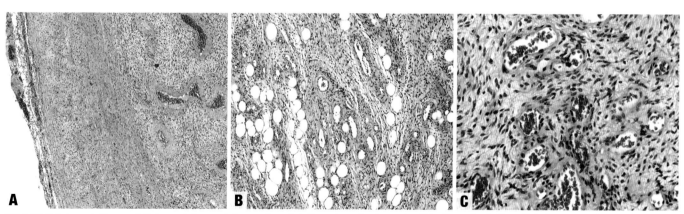

Fig. 1.84 Cellular angiofibroma. **A** Note usual circumscription, varying cellularity, and prominent vessels with hyaline walls. **B** About 50% of cases contain variably prominent mature adipocytes. **C** At high power, the spindle cells have short stubby nuclei and indistinct cytoplasm, resembling spindle cell lipoma. Note the admixed mast cells and rounded vessels.

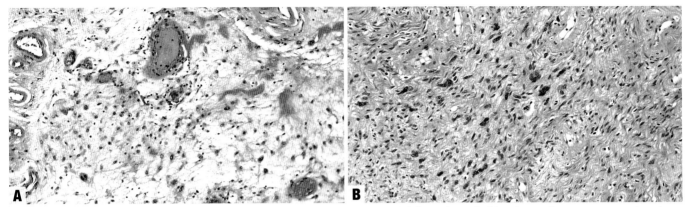

Fig. 1.85 Cellular angiofibroma. **A** Degenerative changes such as stromal oedema, patchy chronic inflammation, and mild nuclear atypia are more common in male patients. **B** Rare cases show small aggregates of highly atypical cells, as here, and occasional cases may show overtly sarcomatous morphology but appear to retain benign behaviour.

The spindle cell component is usually moderately to highly cellular and randomly distributed throughout the lesion, occasionally with a fascicular arrangement or nuclear palisading. Spindle cells have short, oval to fusiform nuclei with inconspicuous nucleoli and scant, palely eosinophilic cytoplasm with ill-defined borders. Mitoses are generally sparse, but they can be more frequent in some cases. The stroma consists primarily of wispy collagen, with occasional short bundles of densely eosinophilic collagen fibres. Variable stromal oedema, hyalinization, or myxoid change is often seen, especially in males. Perivascular lymphoid aggregates may be present. Mast cells are frequent. Small aggregates or individual adipocytes are observed in close to 50% of cases. Degenerative changes of slight nuclear enlargement and hyperchromasia, intravascular thrombi, and cystic change are seen in some cases {1496,1757,2031}.

Morphological sarcomatous transformation has been described rarely, mostly in the vulva {553,1040,1566}. Abrupt transition from cellular angiofibroma to a discrete sarcomatous nodule composed of multivacuolated lipoblasts, or pleomorphic and hyperchromatic spindle cells showing morphological features of pleomorphic liposarcoma, atypical lipomatous tumour, or pleomorphic spindle cell sarcoma, has been reported. Other rare cases show severely atypical cells scattered in conventional cellular angiofibroma. No necrosis or haemorrhage is observed. In sarcomatous areas there are few mitoses {553, 1040}. By immunohistochemistry, CD34 expression has been

documented in 30–60% of tumours. Variable expression of SMA and desmin is identified in a minority of cases. ER and PR are expressed in many cases {1496,1757,2031}. RB1 loss is frequently detected.

Cytology
Not clinically relevant

Diagnostic molecular pathology
Deletions of *RB1*, located in chromosome band 13q14, can be detected but are usually not required {1937,1040,2416}.

Essential and desirable diagnostic criteria
Essential: bland spindle cells, short bundles of delicate collagen fibres, and numerous small to medium-sized thick-walled vessels, with or without adipose tissue.
Desirable: usually in vulvovaginal or inguinoscrotal regions; loss of RB1 may be helpful.

Staging
Not clinically relevant

Prognosis and prediction
Local recurrence is very infrequent {1496,1757,2031}. The rare cases with atypia or sarcomatous transformation have not developed recurrence or metastasis so far {553,1040,1566}.

Angiofibroma of soft tissue

Marino-Enriquez A
Mertens F
Wang J
Yamada Y

Definition

Angiofibroma of soft tissue is a benign fibroblastic neoplasm composed of uniform spindle cells with abundant fibromyxoid stroma and a prominent network of innumerable branching, thin-walled blood vessels.

ICD-O coding

9160/0 Angiofibroma NOS

ICD-11 coding

EE6Y & XH1JJ2 Other specified fibromatous disorders of skin and soft tissue & Angiofibroma NOS

Related terminology

None

Subtype(s)

None

Localization

Angiofibroma of soft tissue typically arises in the extremities, mainly the legs, frequently involving or adjacent to large joints such as the knee. Unusual anatomical locations include the back, abdominal wall, pelvic cavity, and breast. The tumours are often subcutaneous but may be intramuscular and deep {1980,3330,261}.

Clinical features

The lesion presents most often as a slow-growing painless mass {1980,3330,261}. Preoperative duration may be long {1980}. Most lesions are sharply demarcated; however, infiltration into adjacent structures may be detected on imaging {1980,261}.

Epidemiology

Angiofibroma of soft tissue affects predominantly middle-aged adults, with a peak incidence in the sixth decade of life, but patients of any age may be affected {1980,3330,261}. There is a slight female predominance (M:F ratio: ~0.75:1) {1980,3330,261}.

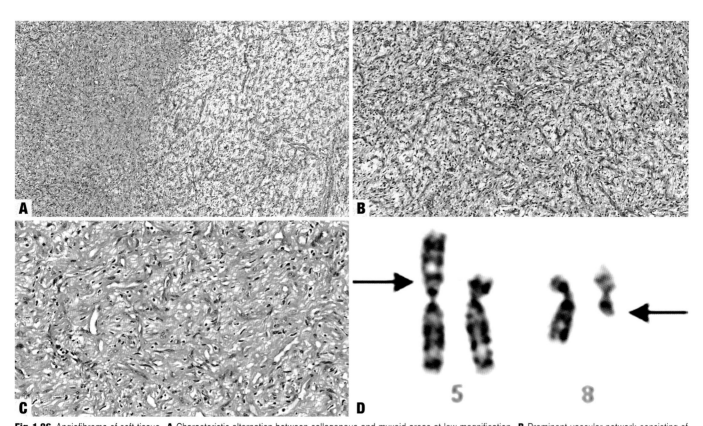

Fig. 1.86 Angiofibroma of soft tissue. **A** Characteristic alternation between collagenous and myxoid areas at low magnification. **B** Prominent vascular network consisting of innumerable thin-walled branching blood vessels. **C** Uniform proliferation of neoplastic spindle cells with inconspicuous palely eosinophilic cytoplasm and short ovoid or tapering nuclei. **D** Partial karyogram showing the characteristic t(5;8)(p15;q13) that results in the *AHRR-NCOA2* fusion. Arrows indicate breakpoints.

Etiology
Unknown

Pathogenesis
Soft tissue angiofibromas have near-diploid karyotypes with a recurrent t(5;8)(p15;q13), which results in fusion of *AHRR* in chromosome band 5p15 and *NCOA2* in 8q13 {1529}. The AHRR-NCOA2 chimera, including the basic helix-loop-helix and PAS domains of AHRR and the two transcriptional activation domains of NCOA2, is present in 60–80% of the tumours {1529,3330,261}; variant *GTF2I-NCOA2* or *GAB1-ABL1* fusions have been found in single cases {151,261}. The AHRR-NCOA2 chimera is expected to upregulate the AHRR/ARNT signalling pathway.

Macroscopic appearance
Most lesions are well-demarcated, nodular or multinodular solid tumours of variable size, with a white to yellow, often glistening, cut surface. Cystic or haemorrhagic areas may be present {1980,3330,261}.

Histopathology
Angiofibroma of soft tissue is composed of uniform bland spindle cells in a variably myxoid to collagenous stroma with a prominent vascular network. The lesions are well circumscribed. The architecture is vaguely lobulated, with alternating myxoid and collagenous areas and regional variation in cellularity. The neoplastic spindle cells have inconspicuous palely eosinophilic cytoplasm and short ovoid or tapering nuclei, with irregular nuclear contours, fine chromatin, and indistinct nucleoli. Cytological atypia and nuclear hyperchromasia are generally absent. Occasional cases show degenerative nuclear atypia. The prominent vascular network is composed of innumerable small thin-walled branching blood vessels evenly distributed throughout the lesion. Less prominent medium-sized or large blood vessels with variably thick walls are usually also present. Common additional features include perivascular collagen deposition and marked hyalinization or fibrinoid necrosis of medium-sized vessel walls. Degenerative changes may be focally present, including haemorrhage or aggregates of foamy histiocytes. A variably dense inflammatory infiltrate comprising mainly small lymphocytes is usually present, sometimes in a perivascular distribution. By immunohistochemistry, the neoplastic cells variably express EMA and CD34; sometimes desmin is seen in dendritic cells {1980,261}.

Cytology
Not clinically relevant

Diagnostic molecular pathology
Detection of *NCOA2* rearrangement or an *AHRR-NCOA2* fusion gene (or a variant fusion) supports the diagnosis of angiofibroma of soft tissue, but it is generally not required.

Essential and desirable diagnostic criteria
Essential: variably myxoid or collagenous stroma; bland and uniform short spindle cells; innumerable small thin-walled branching blood vessels.
Desirable: NCOA2 gene rearrangements (in selected cases).

Staging
Not clinically relevant

Prognosis and prediction
Angiofibroma of soft tissue pursues a benign clinical course, with rare local recurrences and no evident metastatic potential {1980,3330,261}.

Nuchal-type fibroma

Doyle LA

Definition
Nuchal-type fibroma is a rare benign collagenous lesion that usually arises in the neck.

ICD-O coding
8810/0 Nuchal fibroma

ICD-11 coding
EE6Y & XH0XH6 Other specified fibromatous disorders of skin and soft tissue & Nuchal fibroma

Related terminology
Acceptable: nuchal fibroma.
Not recommended: collagenosis nuchae.

Subtype(s)
None

Localization
Nuchal-type fibroma typically arises in the subcutaneous tissues of the posterior neck, but it can also occur at other sites {208,2111}. Most extranuchal tumours are located on the upper back, but tumours can also arise on the face and extremities.

Clinical features
As many as 50% of patients with nuchal-type fibroma have diabetes mellitus {2111}.

Epidemiology
Nuchal-type fibroma is significantly more common in men, with a peak incidence in the fourth and fifth decades of life.

Etiology
Unknown

Pathogenesis
Unknown

Macroscopic appearance
The mean tumour size is 3 cm. Nuchal-type fibroma is ill defined and has a firm consistency and a white cut surface.

Histopathology
Nuchal-type fibroma is a poorly circumscribed and paucicellular lesion composed of bland spindle cells, thick haphazardly arranged collagen fibres, and entrapped subcutaneous adipose tissue. Elastic fibres and small blood vessels are present between the collagen fibres. Many nuchal-type fibromas contain a localized proliferation of small nerves, in some cases similar to those seen in traumatic neuroma. This feature is usually absent from Gardner fibroma, which is often otherwise indistinguishable from nuchal-type fibroma. Compared with normal tissue from the nuchal area, nuchal-type fibroma shows similarly thick collagen fibres. However, in nuchal-type fibroma there is an expansion of collagenized dermis with encasement of adnexa, effacement of the subcutis with entrapment of adipocytes, and (in many cases) extension into underlying skeletal muscle. By immunohistochemistry, the spindled fibroblasts are CD34-positive and negative for β-catenin.

Cytology
Not clinically relevant

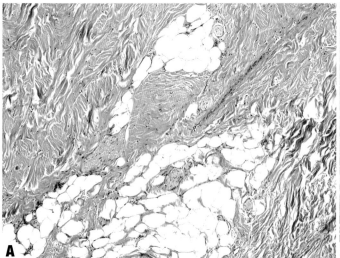 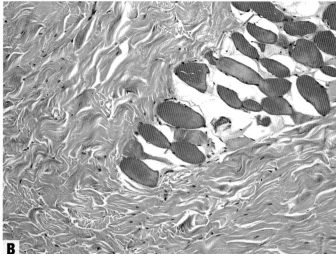

Fig. 1.87 Nuchal-type fibroma. **A** The tumour is paucicellular and contains thick haphazardly arranged collagen fibres entrapping adipose tissue and peripheral nerves. **B** The lesional cells are bland spindled fibroblasts. Extension into skeletal muscle is common.

Diagnostic molecular pathology
Not clinically relevant

Essential and desirable diagnostic criteria
Essential: paucicellular collagenous lesion usually with small nerve bundles; typically arising in the neck; bland CD34-positive spindle cells.

Staging
Not clinically relevant

Prognosis and prediction
Nuchal-type fibroma is benign. It often locally recurs but it does not metastasize.

Acral fibromyxoma

Brenn T
Agaimy A
Hollmann TJ

Definition

Acral fibromyxoma is a benign fibroblastic neoplasm with a marked predilection for the subungual and periungual aspects of the digits and potential for local recurrence.

ICD-O coding

8811/0 Acral fibromyxoma

ICD-11 coding

EE6Y & XH5XQ3 Other specified fibromatous disorders of skin and soft tissue & Fibromyxoma

Related terminology

Acceptable: superficial acral fibromyxoma; digital fibromyxoma.
Not recommended: cellular digital fibroma.

Subtype(s)

None

Localization

There is a strong predilection for the periungual and subungual aspects of the fingers and toes {691,1396,2536,66,997}. Other areas of the hands and feet, ankles, wrists, lower legs, and thighs may rarely be affected {1396,26}.

Clinical features

Acral fibromyxomas present as slowly enlarging and frequently painful solitary tumours, typically measuring 1–2 cm {691,1396, 2536,66}. The tumours may cause nail deformity, and erosive or lytic lesions of the underlying bone may be detected radiographically {1396}.

Epidemiology

A wide age range is affected, but most tumours present in middle-aged adults, with a median age of about 50 years. Males are more frequently affected than females {997,1396}.

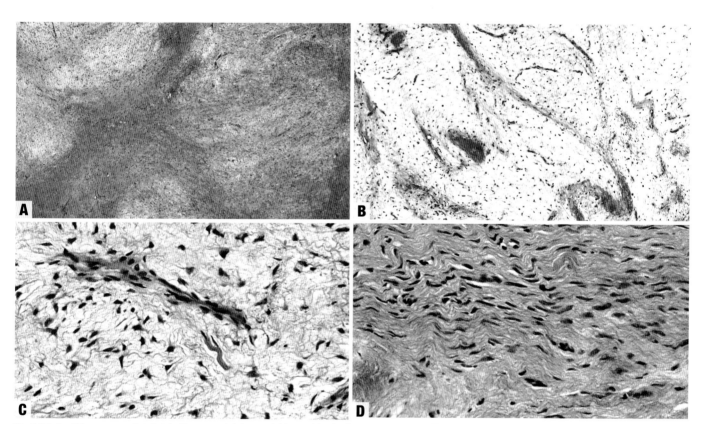

Fig. 1.88 Acral fibromyxoma. **A** Lobulated tumour containing a variably myxoid and collagenous stroma. **B** The tumours may be predominantly myxoid and show a proliferation of small delicate vascular channels. **C** The bland and uniform spindled and stellate tumour cells are loosely distributed in a fibromyxoid stroma. **D** This cellular area is characterized by a fascicular growth of uniform spindle cells in a collagenous matrix. Note the absence of cytological atypia.

Etiology
Unknown

Pathogenesis
RB1 deletions have been reported {26}.

Macroscopic appearance
On macroscopic examination, the tumours appear dome-shaped, polypoid, or verrucoid, with soft to firm consistency, an often lobulated aspect, and poorly defined borders.

Histopathology
Acral fibromyxomas present in dermis and subcutis as lobulated tumours, occasionally with a polypoid growth and surrounding epidermal collarette formation. The majority of tumours show an infiltrative growth pattern, with rare invasion of underlying bone. The tumours are composed of bland-appearing spindled or stellate cells arranged loosely in a variably myxoid or collagenous stroma. Scattered multinucleated cells may be admixed. A vaguely storiform or fascicular growth pattern may be seen, and a proliferation of small vascular channels is present in the myxoid areas. Cartilaginous or osseous metaplasia is rarely observed. Nuclear pleomorphism and tumour necrosis are absent, and mitoses are rare. By immunohistochemistry, the tumour cells express CD34 and occasionally EMA and SMA. There is loss of RB1 expression in the majority of tumours {26}.

Cytology
Not clinically relevant

Diagnostic molecular pathology
The tumours show deletion of the *RB1* gene {26}, but this is not required.

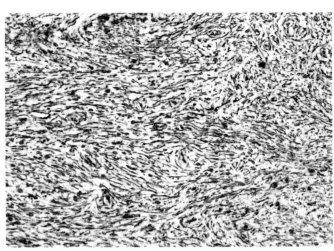

Fig. 1.89 Acral fibromyxoma. Strong and diffuse expression of CD34.

Essential and desirable diagnostic criteria
Essential: acral, usually periungual location; dermal-based tumour with infiltration of subcutis; lobulated architecture with vaguely storiform or fascicular growth; bland spindle cells in a variably myxoid or collagenous matrix.
Desirable: CD34 positivity and frequent loss of RB1 expression by immunohistochemistry.

Staging
Not clinically relevant

Prognosis and prediction
Acral fibromyxomas recur locally in as many as 22% of cases. Local recurrences are non-destructive and can be cured by re-excision. Metastases have not been reported {997,1396}.

Gardner fibroma

Cates JMM
Cunha IW

Definition
Gardner fibroma is a benign plaque-like mass composed of thick, haphazardly arranged collagen bundles with sparsely interspersed fibroblasts, and it is usually associated with familial adenomatous polyposis (FAP).

ICD-O coding
8810/0 Gardner fibroma

ICD-11 coding
EE6Y & XH7GT0 Other specified fibromatous disorders of skin and soft tissue & Gardner fibroma

Related terminology
Acceptable: Gardner-associated fibroma.
Not recommended: desmoid precursor lesion.

Subtype(s)
None

Localization
Gardner fibromas commonly arise in the superficial and deep soft tissues of the torso (usually the back or paraspinal region) or head/neck region, but almost any non-visceral anatomical site can be involved, including the mesentery {3259,627}.

Clinical features
These tumours typically present as painless masses {3259,627}.

Epidemiology
Gardner fibroma is diagnosed most often in children aged < 10 years but may present in young adults as well. There is no sex predilection {3259,627}.

Etiology
Approximately 80% of cases are associated with FAP, *APC* mutation, or familial desmoid fibromatosis {3259,627}.

Pathogenesis
Most cases arise in patients with germline *APC* mutations (see *Desmoid fibromatosis*, p. 93).

Macroscopic appearance
Gardner fibroma is a poorly circumscribed, rubbery, tan-white mass ranging in size from < 1 cm to > 10 cm {3259,627}.

Histopathology
The dominant histopathological feature is the haphazard arrangement of coarse collagen fibres with characteristic clefts or cracks and few inconspicuous spindle cells {3259,627}. A helpful diagnostic feature is entrapment of adjacent adipose tissue and neurovascular bundles at the edge of the lesion. By immunohistochemistry, CD34 is almost always positive, whereas SMA is negative {3259,627}. Nuclear accumulation of β-catenin is often observed, particularly in cases associated with FAP {627,708}.

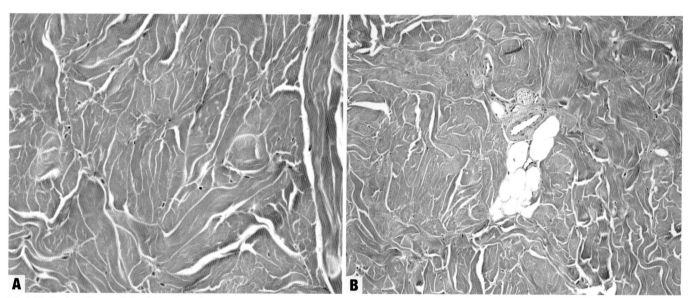

Fig. 1.90 Gardner fibroma. **A** Small bland spindle cells are dispersed in cracks between collagen fibres. **B** Entrapped mature adipose tissue and benign nerve fibres are frequently seen in Gardner fibroma.

Cytology
Not clinically relevant

Diagnostic molecular pathology
Not clinically relevant

Essential and desirable diagnostic criteria
Essential: plaque-like mass in the paraspinal region or trunk of young children; haphazard arrangement of coarse collagen fibres with clefts or cracks and few inconspicuous spindle cells; expression of CD34 and nuclear β-catenin.

Staging
Not clinically relevant

Prognosis and prediction
Gardner fibroma is benign but is associated with concurrent or subsequent development of desmoid fibromatosis in approximately 20% of cases {627,610}. Conversely, an associated Gardner fibroma or an area in the desmoid tumour resembling Gardner fibroma can be identified in as many as 37% of patients with desmoid fibromatosis {515,3408}. Given the close association between Gardner fibroma and FAP, a diagnosis of Gardner fibroma should prompt screening of the family for FAP.

Palmar fibromatosis and plantar fibromatosis

Thway K
Nascimento AF

Definition
Palmar and plantar fibromatoses are benign nodular fibroblastic/myofibroblastic proliferations typically arising in the volar aspect of the hands and fingers or involving plantar aponeuroses, respectively.

ICD-O coding
8813/1 Palmar/plantar-type fibromatosis

ICD-11 coding
FB51.Y & XH75J5 Other specified fibroblastic disorders & Palmar/plantar-type fibromatosis

Related terminology
Palmar fibromatosis
Acceptable: Dupuytren disease/contracture.

Plantar fibromatosis
Acceptable: Ledderhose disease.

Subtype(s)
None

Localization
Palmar fibromatosis preferentially involves the volar or flexor aspect of the hands and is bilateral in as many as 50% of cases. Plantar fibromatosis is typically located in non–weight-bearing areas, such as the aponeurosis of the medial plantar arch, from the region of the navicular bone to the base of the first metatarsal {3139}, and it is bilateral in as many as 35% of cases. Paediatric cases of plantar fibromatosis typically involve the anteromedial portion of the heel pad.

Clinical features
Palmar fibromatosis typically has an insidious onset, with development of small, painless nodules that slowly evolve to form cords or band-like indurations between nodules in the subcutis and underlying fascia, leading to digit contractures and puckering of overlying skin. In contrast, plantar fibromatosis does not typically cause contractures and is often asymptomatic, although mild pain may develop after prolonged standing or walking.

Epidemiology
Palmar fibromatosis predominantly affects adults, with a male predominance (M:F ratio: 3:1) and highest prevalence in white people {2664}. Its incidence increases with age, and it is rare among individuals aged < 30 years. Plantar fibromatosis is more common in younger patients (including those as young as 9 months), with almost half of all patients aged < 30 years {1170,996}. In paediatric cases, plantar fibromatosis shows a female predominance {996}. Palmar or plantar fibromatosis can be associated with synchronous or metachronous development of the other form (with 5–20% of patients developing both), but not desmoid fibromatosis {996,3139}. Associations with epilepsy and phenobarbital therapy, diabetes mellitus, cigarette smoking, and alcoholism with cirrhosis are reported but have not been widely validated {451}.

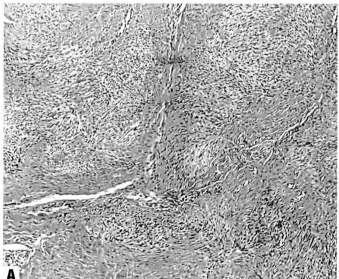
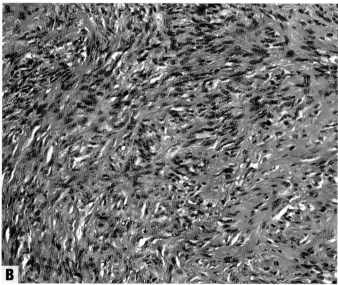

Fig. 1.91 Palmar fibromatosis. **A** In the early (proliferative) phase, palmar fascial or aponeurotic tissue is expanded by hypercellular spindle cell nodules. **B** This early-stage lesion is cellular and shows loose fascicles of uniform spindle cells within prominent collagenous stroma.

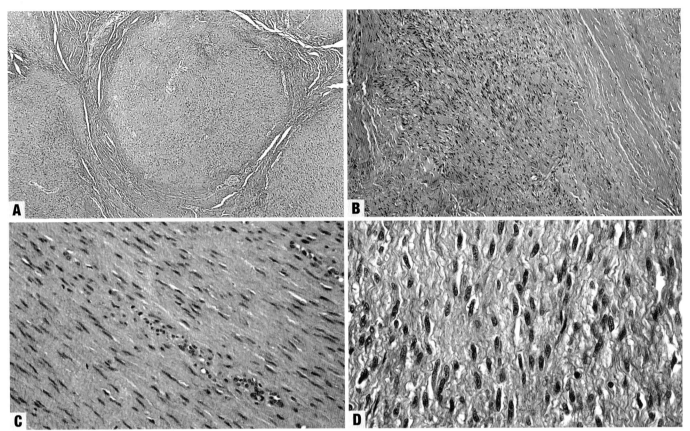

Fig. 1.92 Plantar fibromatosis. **A** Low-power view showing typically multinodular growth pattern (within tendoaponeurotic fibrous tissue), as is usually seen in plantar lesions. **B** Intimate association of the cellular, proliferative-phase lesional spindle cells with native fibrotendinous tissue is seen. **C** Spindle cells arranged in long, parallel fascicles in more-densely collagenous matrix. The cells are uniform and lack discernible atypia. There are associated mild chronic inflammation and rare mitotic figures. **D** In the proliferative phase, plump, bland-appearing spindle cells with elongated nuclei with vesicular chromatin and inconspicuous nucleoli are predominant.

Etiology

Unknown

Pathogenesis

Although still driven at least in part by the WNT/β-catenin signalling pathway, this tumour lacks the *CTNNB1* and *APC* mutations characteristic of desmoid fibromatosis {2178,3378,491}.

Macroscopic appearance

Tumours are small, poorly defined 0.5–3.0 cm nodules, intimately associated with a tendon or aponeurosis and extending into subcutaneous tissue. The cut surface is firm, greyish-yellow or white (depending on the collagen content), and slightly whorled.

Histopathology

Typically, tumours involve a thickened palmar/plantar aponeurosis and form single to multiple discontinuous, moderately cellular spindle cell nodules in collagenous stroma {996}. Morphologically, there are three phases of growth (proliferative, involutional, and late-stage). The proliferative phase comprises cellular, parallel fascicles of bland, plump, relatively uniform spindled fibroblasts with tapering nuclei, vesicular chromatin, and small or inconspicuous nucleoli, with minimal stromal collagen. Some plantar lesions are hypercellular and can mimic spindle cell sarcomas, but they lack atypia. There may be scattered,

often perivascular chronic inflammation and occasional typical mitotic figures, especially in early lesions. Mitotic activity may be particularly prominent in paediatric patients. Occasional, particularly plantar lesions show interspersed multinucleated cells. Late-stage histology is associated with increased

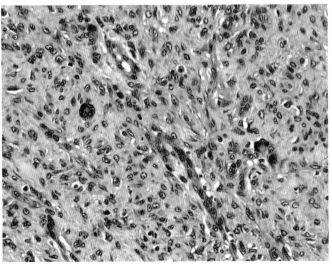

Fig. 1.93 Plantar fibromatosis. This lesion shows small numbers of osteoclast-type, multinucleated giant cells, interspersed among the plump, cellular fibroblastic cells.

collagenous matrix and decreased cellularity. Rarely, there is osseous or cartilaginous metaplasia. By immunohistochemistry, tumour cells are variably positive for SMA and occasionally for desmin. A subset show nuclear β-catenin expression, despite the absence of *CTNNB1* or *APC* gene mutations {2178,480}.

Cytology
Not clinically relevant

Diagnostic molecular pathology
Not clinically relevant

Essential and desirable diagnostic criteria
Essential: bland, variably cellular proliferation of spindled fibroblasts/myofibroblasts; collagenous stroma; involvement of aponeurosis and variably subcutis and dermis.

Staging
Not clinically relevant

Prognosis and prediction
The risk of local recurrence is mostly dependent on the extent of surgical resection, although this is reserved for patients who have failed conservative management {3378}.

Desmoid fibromatosis

Fritchie KJ
Crago AM
van de Rijn M

Definition
Desmoid fibromatosis is a locally aggressive but non-metastasizing deep-seated (myo)fibroblastic neoplasm with infiltrative growth and propensity for local recurrence.

ICD-O coding
8821/1 Desmoid-type fibromatosis

ICD-11 coding
2F7C & XH13Z3 Neoplasms of uncertain behaviour of connective or other soft tissue & Desmoid-type fibromatosis (aggressive fibromatosis)
2F7C & XH6116 Neoplasms of uncertain behaviour of connective or other soft tissue & Abdominal (mesenteric) fibromatosis

Related terminology
Acceptable: aggressive fibromatosis; desmoid tumour.
Not recommended: musculoaponeurotic fibromatosis.

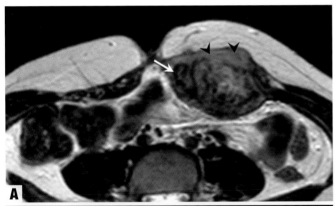

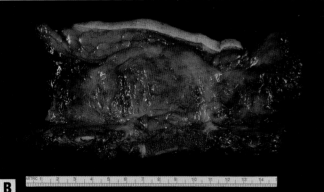

Fig. 1.94 Desmoid fibromatosis. **A** Axial T2-weighted MRI of the abdomen shows a mass within the rectus abdominis with mixed internal heterogeneity. Areas of low signal (arrow) correspond to fibrosis, whereas areas of high T2 signal (arrowheads) correspond to areas of increased cellularity. **B** Gross examination reveals a firm, tan surface with infiltration into surrounding fat and skeletal muscle.

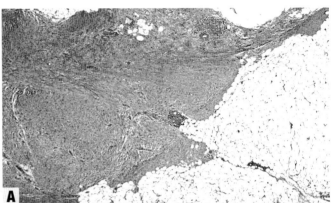

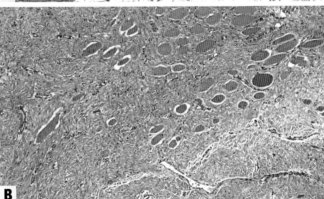

Fig. 1.95 Desmoid fibromatosis. **A** Low-power examination reveals an infiltrative lesion extending into surrounding adipose tissue with lymphoid aggregates at the advancing edge. **B** There is infiltration of adjacent skeletal muscle.

Subtype(s)
Extra-abdominal desmoid; abdominal fibromatosis

Localization
Desmoid fibromatosis is most commonly diagnosed in the extremities (30–40% of cases). Lesions also occur in the retroperitoneum or abdominal cavity (15%), abdominal wall (20%), and chest wall (10–15%). Less common sites include head and neck, paraspinal region, and flank {671,2719,1831}.

Clinical features
Desmoid fibromatosis generally presents as a painless mass localized to the deep compartments that is fixed on physical examination. Approximately 10% of patients report prior trauma or surgery in the region of the desmoid tumour, and 15% have a history of recent or current pregnancy (abdominal wall desmoids) within 5 years of diagnosis {3160}. Patients with familial adenomatous polyposis most often present with intra-abdominal tumours after abdominal surgery. MRI showing mixed hyperintense and isointense signals is suggestive of

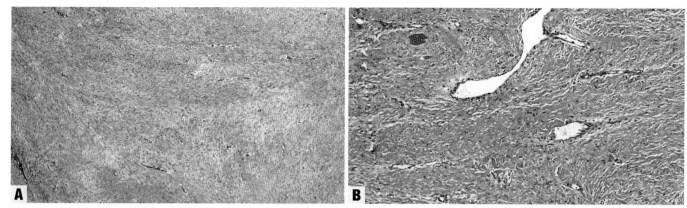

Fig. 1.96 Desmoid fibromatosis. **A** The fascicles of desmoid fibromatosis are long and sweeping. **B** Hyalinized area of a desmoid tumour showing gaping thin-walled blood vessels.

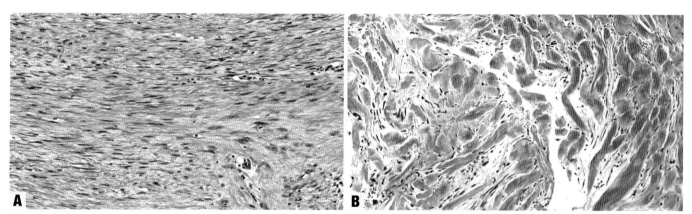

Fig. 1.97 Desmoid fibromatosis. **A** High-power examination reveals bland fibroblasts and myofibroblasts without cytological atypia or nuclear hyperchromasia. **B** Occasionally, desmoid tumours, especially those arising in the abdominal cavity, may show areas with keloid-type collagen deposition.

desmoid fibromatosis; this finding reflects variable content of tumour cellularity and fibrous stroma {3172,2992}.

Site-specific complications can occur due to local progression. Intra-abdominal lesions can cause intestinal obstruction or fistulization with infectious symptoms or gastrointestinal bleeding; in these cases, the tumour commonly involves the root of the mesentery. Extremity lesions can be multifocal (particularly in paediatric and young adult patients) and extensive, causing limb contracture and chronic pain. A small subset of desmoid tumours occur in the context of familial adenomatous polyposis (Gardner syndrome); in this setting, lesions are frequently intra-abdominal, multifocal, and diagnosed in children or young adults {2292}.

Epidemiology

Desmoid fibromatosis is estimated to affect < 4 patients per 1 million population per year {2598}. Patients tend to be young, with a median age of 37–39 years. The disease is more common in women than men (M:F ratio: 0.5:1), although in paediatric patients and patients past childbearing age, the disease shows an equal sex distribution {2598,671,2719}.

Etiology

The etiology of desmoid fibromatosis is multifactorial and includes genetic factors (most commonly sporadic somatic *CTNNB1* mutations and less frequently germline *APC* mutations

in Gardner syndrome) and physical factors (trauma, surgery, pregnancy) {1590}. Surgery increases the risk of tumour development {1200}.

Pathogenesis

The majority (90–95%) of sporadic desmoid tumours result from three different point mutations in two codons (41 and 45) of exon 3 of the gene that encodes β-catenin (*CTNNB1*): p.Thr41Ala, p.Ser45Pro, and p.Ser45Phe {98,1781,652,834,670}. p.Thr41Ala and p.Ser45Phe are the most common mutations {834,1781,98}. A smaller percentage of desmoid tumours arise in the setting of Gardner syndrome; affected patients harbour germline mutations in the *APC* tumour suppressor gene, specifically mutations at or beyond codon 1444, with subsequent loss of heterozygosity of the wildtype allele, and rare cases of desmoid tumours with sporadic *APC* mutations have also been described {1148,285,1259,1872,2293,1515,2969,2294, 508,3242}. The activating mutations in *CTNNB1* or inactivating mutations in *APC* interfere with β-catenin proteasomal degradation, leading to nuclear β-catenin accumulation {219}. Because β-catenin functions as part of the transcription apparatus in the nucleus, this increased activation of the WNT/β-catenin pathway is thought to ultimately promote cell proliferation and survival and appears to drive tumorigenesis {1780,2336,1687}. A subset of the neoplastic population of desmoid fibromatosis may harbour trisomies for chromosomes 8 and/or 20; however, these aberrations are unlikely to play a substantial role in pathogenesis or behaviour {419,767,1028,2100,2718}.

Macroscopic appearance

Gross examination reveals a solid mass with a wide size range and a whitish-tan, coarsely trabecular or whorled cut surface. Most lesions appear poorly circumscribed with ill-defined margins and infiltration into adjacent tissues. Intra-abdominal desmoid fibromatosis tends to present as a large mass, often as large as 10 cm in diameter, with a whorled cut surface.

Histopathology

Desmoid fibromatosis is characterized by long, sweeping fascicles of bland fibroblasts and myofibroblasts with infiltration into surrounding soft tissues. The fascicles often span an entire 10× objective field, and lymphoid aggregates are often appreciated at the advancing edge of the lesion. The tumour cells demonstrate pale eosinophilic cytoplasm and lack nuclear hyperchromasia or cytological atypia. Thin-walled blood vessels, occasionally with a gaping or staghorn appearance, are often prominent with variable perivascular oedema. Mitotic figures are typically absent or rare, and atypical mitoses are lacking. A subset of tumours harbour densely eosinophilic stromal keloidal-type collagen, a finding most common in intra-abdominal tumours. Other morphological patterns include myxoid change, paucicellular hyalinized areas, and zones resembling nodular fasciitis {3408,449}. By immunohistochemistry, the lesional cells are positive for SMA and MSA. The majority of tumours (~80%) show nuclear β-catenin expression, although definite nuclear reactivity can be difficult to appreciate {305, 480,2271}.

Cytology

FNA specimens are variably cellular and typically show loose clusters of bland or reactive-appearing fibroblasts and myofibroblasts without substantial cytological atypia or nuclear hyperchromasia {2564}. The relatively nonspecific findings make desmoid tumours difficult to diagnose by FNA.

Diagnostic molecular pathology

CTNNB1 mutation analysis may be helpful in small biopsy specimens, when diagnostic morphological features are not readily apparent, and/or when β-catenin immunostaining is equivocal or challenging to interpret {650,1785}.

Essential and desirable diagnostic criteria

Essential: long, sweeping fascicles of bland fibroblasts and myofibroblasts without substantial cytological atypia; infiltrative growth.
Desirable: nuclear β-catenin expression; characteristic *CTNNB1* mutation (in challenging cases or small biopsies).

Staging

Not clinically relevant

Prognosis and prediction

The natural course of desmoid fibromatosis in individual patients is variable, with unpredictable growth, stabilization, and regression. Tumour-related deaths are rare but seem to be more common in patients with familial adenomatous polyposis {804}. Although primary surgery with negative surgical margins was classically considered to be the standard of care, local recurrence does not consistently correlate with margin status {2719,651}. Approximately one third of patients experience recurrence after resection; extensive surgery can be morbid; and spontaneous regression has been observed in a subset of advanced, unresectable tumours. For these reasons, a watchful waiting approach with a period of initial observation has been advocated for asymptomatic patients {1590}. When surgery is considered for patients with desmoid tumours, higher rates of local recurrence are associated with extra-abdominal location, younger age, larger tumour size, and mutation status {2719, 671,1831}. Studies have suggested that tumours harbouring *CTNNB1* p.Ser45Phe mutations have a greater risk for local recurrence {346,652,834,1781}. It is unclear whether similar molecular or clinicopathological factors predict progression during active observation.

Lipofibromatosis

Miettinen M
Al-Ibraheemi A
Zambrano E

Definition

Lipofibromatosis is a rare, frequently recurring paediatric soft tissue tumour with a predilection for the hands and feet. It is composed of a distinctive admixture of mature fat, short fascicles of bland spindle cells, and lipoblast-like cells in the interface between the spindle cell and lipomatous components.

ICD-O coding

8851/1 Lipofibromatosis

ICD-11 coding

FB51.Y & XH4QB6 Other specified fibroblastic disorders & Lipofibromatosis

Related terminology

Not recommended: infantile/juvenile fibromatosis variant (non-desmoid type).

Subtype(s)

None

Localization

Lipofibromatosis preferentially involves the hands and feet, although it can also occur at other locations such as the trunk and the head and neck {1000}.

Clinical features

Lipofibromatosis typically presents as a slow-growing, poorly demarcated subcutaneous mass, which can also involve skeletal muscle {1000}.

Epidemiology

Lipofibromatosis occurs in children from birth to early in the second decade of life, with an M:F ratio of 2:1. Half of the cases are diagnosed by the age of 1 year, and 20% are congenital {1000, 70}.

Etiology

Unknown

Pathogenesis

Identification of fusions involving ligands (EGF, HBEGF, TGF-α) to EGFR (HER1) or EGFR itself, or other receptor tyrosine kinases (ROS1, RET, PDGFRB), suggests that activation of the PI3K/AKT/mTOR pathway might be implicated in the pathogenesis of lipofibromatosis {70}.

Macroscopic appearance

The firm, rubbery, poorly demarcated mass has a white or yellow cut surface; margins are difficult to discern. Most lesions are 1–7 cm in diameter, although larger tumours have been reported, with some involving the entire extremity {1000,70, 1215}.

Histopathology

Lipofibromatosis is composed of mature adipose tissue traversed by cellular fascicles of spindle cells with bland, uniform, elongated nuclei. Fat usually forms a major proportion of the lesion. In newborn patients, the fat lobules may have an immature appearance with myxoid matrix. Small collections of univacuolated cells may be present in the fibroblastic component,

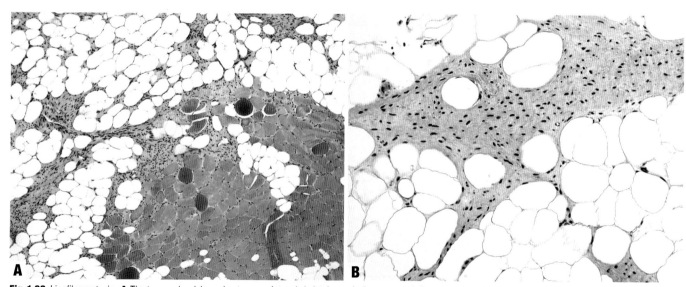

Fig. 1.98 Lipofibromatosis. **A** The tumour, involving subcutaneous fat and skeletal muscle, is composed of mature-appearing adipose tissue and cellular fibrous septa without atypia or mitotic activity, imparting a fibromatosis-like appearance. **B** The fibroblasts show a uniform appearance and are embedded in an abundant collagenous matrix.

where melanin-laden cells have occasionally been documented. Lipofibromatosis entraps subcutaneous tissue and sometimes skeletal muscle. Mitotic activity is rare and necrosis absent. Occasional recurrent lesions are indistinguishable from calcifying aponeurotic fibroma {70}. By immunohistochemistry, the fibroblasts show variable expression of CD34 and SMA. The spindle cells are negative for desmin, in contrast to the spindle cells in lipoblastoma.

Cytology
FNA smears show bland-appearing fibroblasts and mature fat.

Diagnostic molecular pathology
Not clinically relevant

Essential and desirable diagnostic criteria
Essential: painless subcutaneous mass; most often in the hands and feet of young children; admixture of mature fat, short fascicles of bland spindle cells, and lipoblast-like cells; infiltrative margins.

Staging
Not clinically relevant

Prognosis and prediction
Lipofibromatosis has a 70% local recurrence rate but no metastatic potential. Congenital onset, male sex, acral location, mitotic activity in the fibroblastic component, and incomplete excision may be risk factors for recurrence {1000}.

Giant cell fibroblastoma

Mentzel TDW
Pedeutour F

Definition

Giant cell fibroblastoma is a locally aggressive fibroblastic neoplasm, closely related to dermatofibrosarcoma protuberans (DFSP), arising primarily in children and characterized by the presence of multinucleated giant cells, pseudovascular spaces, and a *COL1A1-PDGFB* fusion.

ICD-O coding

8834/1 Giant cell fibroblastoma

ICD-11 coding

FB51.Y & XH9AV8 Other specified fibroblastic disorders & Giant cell fibroblastoma

Related terminology

None

Subtype(s)

None

Localization

The majority of cases of giant cell fibroblastoma arise in superficial soft tissues of the trunk, the groin and axillary region, and (more rarely) the extremities and the head and neck region {876, 1526,2852,3062}.

Clinical features

The affected patients usually report a slow-growing, painless cutaneous lesion that is most often plaque-like {1526,2852}.

Epidemiology

Giant cell fibroblastoma is a rare neoplasm arising predominantly but not exclusively in children, with a mean age of 6 years and a male predominance {1526,2852}.

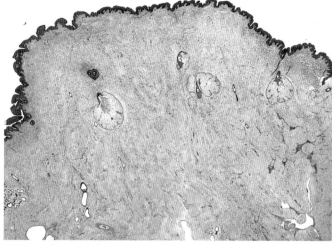

Fig. 1.100 Giant cell fibroblastoma. Low-power view shows a hypocellular dermal neoplasm with irregularly branching pseudovascular spaces.

Etiology

Unknown

Pathogenesis

Giant cell fibroblastoma and DFSP share chromosomal and molecular features, consisting of rearrangements of chromosomes 17 and 22 and formation of a chimeric gene that fuses *COL1A1* at 17q21.33 with *PDGFB* at 22q13.1 {2864}. The breakpoint in *COL1A1* is variable between patients (from exon 6 up to exon 49), whereas the breakpoint in *PDGFB* is consistently located in intron 1 {2876}. There is no evidence of a correlation between a specific breakpoint within *COL1A1* and either giant cell fibroblastoma or classic DFSP (or other DFSP-related tumours) {1143}. Giant cell fibroblastoma more frequently shows

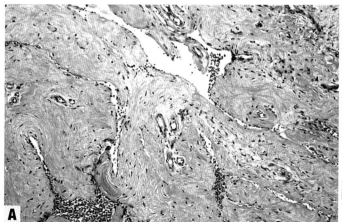

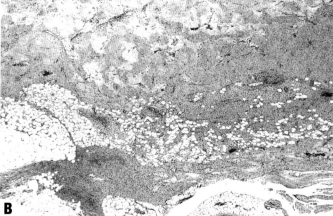

Fig. 1.99 Giant cell fibroblastoma. **A** The neoplasms are composed of spindle cells and scattered multinucleated giant cells that also line pseudovascular spaces. **B** Hybrid tumour with features of giant cell fibroblastoma (top) and dermatofibrosarcoma protuberans (bottom).

a balanced translocation without amplification than does DFSP (see *Dermatofibrosarcoma protuberans*, p. 100).

Macroscopic appearance
Grossly, giant cell fibroblastoma is an ill-defined, infiltrative lesion with greyish-yellow and mucoid cut surfaces. The size of the lesions ranges from 0.6 to 8 cm, with a mean of 3–4 cm {1526,2852,3062}.

Histopathology
Giant cell fibroblastoma is a mainly subcutaneous neoplasm with infiltration of the dermis and (more rarely) superficial skeletal muscle. Typical cases of giant cell fibroblastoma infiltrate the subcutis in honeycomb or parallel growth patterns, spare cutaneous adnexal structures, and show variable cellularity; however, hypocellular areas with myxoid or collagenous stroma often predominate. The neoplasms are composed of bland spindled and stellate tumour cells and scattered multinucleated giant cells with a wreath-like arrangement of nuclei, which also line irregularly branching pseudovascular spaces. Mitoses are rare, and areas of tumour necrosis are usually absent. In about 15% of cases, areas of conventional DFSP are present (hybrid cases) {1526,2852,3062}. Rarely, cases contain pigmented tumour cells, show prominent myxoid change, or contain fibrosarcomatous areas (representing tumour progression) {1526}. By immunohistochemistry, spindle-shaped cells and multinucleated tumour giant cells are positive for CD34 {1526,3062}.

Cytology
Not clinically relevant

Diagnostic molecular pathology
COL1A1-PDGFB fusion may be detected by various molecular approaches but is not generally required.

Essential and desirable diagnostic criteria
Essential: infiltrative margins within dermis and subcutis; hypocellular lesion with myxoid or collagenous stroma; bland spindled and stellate cells and scattered multinucleated giant cells, often lining pseudovascular spaces.
Desirable: *COL1A1-PDGFB* fusion (in selected cases).

Staging
Not clinically relevant

Prognosis and prediction
A local recurrence rate of about 50% has been reported {2852}; however, if widely excised, giant cell fibroblastoma locally recurs only rarely {3062}.

Dermatofibrosarcoma protuberans

Mentzel TDW
Pedeutour F

Definition
Dermatofibrosarcoma protuberans (DFSP) is a superficial, locally aggressive fibroblastic neoplasm, having a cellular storiform appearance and carrying a *COL1A1-PDGFB* or related fusion.

ICD-O coding
8832/1 Dermatofibrosarcoma protuberans NOS

ICD-11 coding
2B53.Y & XH4QZ8 Other specified fibroblastic or myofibroblastic tumour, primary site & Dermatofibrosarcoma NOS

2B53.Y & XH5CT4 Other specified fibroblastic or myofibroblastic tumour, primary site & Pigmented dermatofibrosarcoma protuberans

Related terminology
Not recommended: Bednar tumour.

Subtype(s)
Pigmented dermatofibrosarcoma protuberans; dermatofibrosarcoma protuberans, fibrosarcomatous; myxoid dermatofibrosarcoma protuberans; dermatofibrosarcoma protuberans with myoid differentiation; plaque-like dermatofibrosarcoma protuberans

Localization
These neoplasms occur most commonly on the trunk and the proximal extremities, followed by the head and neck region. A subset of cases are seen in the genital area, the breast, and at acral sites {1792,823,2821}.

Clinical features
DFSP typically presents as a nodular or multinodular cutaneous mass, often with a history of slow but persistent growth. Early lesions may show a plaque-like growth with peripheral red discolouration. These neoplasms may show rapid enlargement during pregnancy or due to tumour progression to fibrosarcomatous DFSP.

Epidemiology
DFSP usually presents in young to middle-aged adults, with a slight male predominance. However, a substantial number of cases are seen in children (including congenital presentations) {1478,3062} and in the elderly. Although it represents a rare neoplasm (< 1 case per 100 000 person-years), DFSP is one of the most common dermal sarcomas.

Etiology
Most of these tumours occur sporadically. DFSP with unique features, such as multicentricity, small size, and occurrence at early age, has been shown in children affected with adenosine

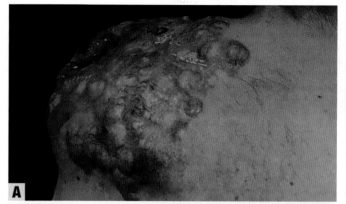
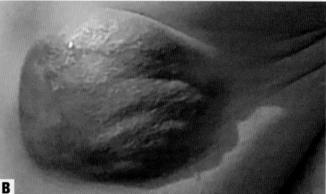

Fig. 1.101 Dermatofibrosarcoma protuberans. **A** Giant dermatofibrosarcoma protuberans presenting clinically as a huge exophytic, multinodular mass with focal ulceration. **B** A case containing numerous blood vessels mimicking a vascular lesion.

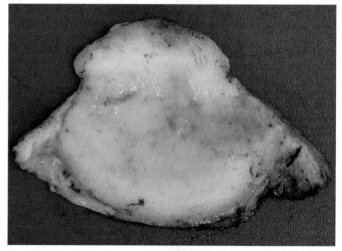

Fig. 1.102 Dermatofibrosarcoma protuberans. Cross-sectioning reveals a firm fibrous tumour.

deaminase–deficient severe combined immunodeficiency {1616}.

Pathogenesis

DFSP is characterized by the presence of supernumerary ring chromosomes {2876,2729} that contain the centromere of chromosome 22 and comprise interspersed sequences from chromosomes 17 and 22 {2473}. Additional aberrations, such as trisomy 5 and trisomy 8, are also observed {2876,2729}. Unbalanced t(17;22)(q21.3;q13.1) translocations are present in most children and rarely in adults {2876,2729}. Most DFSP cells harbour not only a structural rearrangement but also a gain of 17q21.3-17qter and 22q10-q31 sequences {1870,1593}. Both ring and der(22)t(17;22) chromosomes contain a chimeric gene fusing *COL1A1* at 17q21.33 with *PDGFB* at 22q13.1 {2864}. The breakpoint in *COL1A1* is variable: the chimeric gene is composed of at least the first 6 exons up to exon 49 of *COL1A1* and a consistent fragment retaining all but exon 1 of the *PDGFB* gene. Fewer than 5% of typical DFSP cases are negative for the *COL1A1-PDGFB* fusion gene by routine molecular testing; alternative *COL6A3-PDGFD* and *EMILIN2-PDGFD* fusion genes have been identified {705,823}, and in some cases, *COL1A1-PDGFB* rearrangement is cryptic {705}. The *COL1A1-PDGFB* fusion gene encodes a fusion protein that is proteolytically processed to normal *PDGFB* ligand. Because tumour cells express the PDGFRB receptor on their cell surfaces, autocrine stimulation of neoplastic cells drives tumorigenesis. This molecular pathway provides a rationale for targeted therapy with tyrosine kinase inhibitors for unresectable DFSP or metastatic fibrosarcomatous DFSP {2340,1885,2460,2694,3125,1082,2706}. Alteration of the PDGFRB/AKT/mTOR pathway is seen in fibrosarcomatous DFSP {1370}.

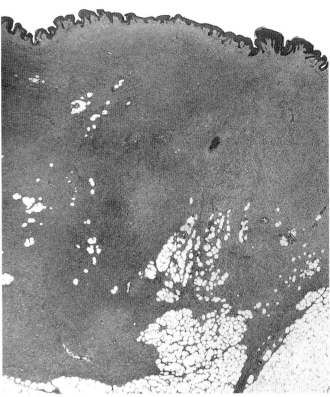

Fig. 1.104 Dermatofibrosarcoma protuberans. Tumour fills the dermis and expands into the subcutis, often along fibrous septa.

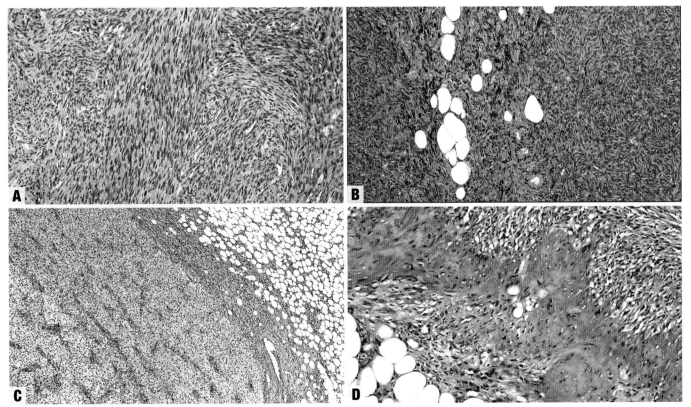

Fig. 1.103 Dermatofibrosarcoma protuberans. **A** Increased cytological atypia and increased proliferative activity are seen in fibrosarcomatous areas. **B** Pigmented cells are seen in addition to fibroblastic tumour cells. **C** A diffusely infiltrating myxoid neoplasm with numerous vessels with slightly fibrosed vessel walls is seen. **D** An example with focal myoid differentiation, showing a proliferation of eosinophilic spindled tumour cells set in a hyalinized stroma.

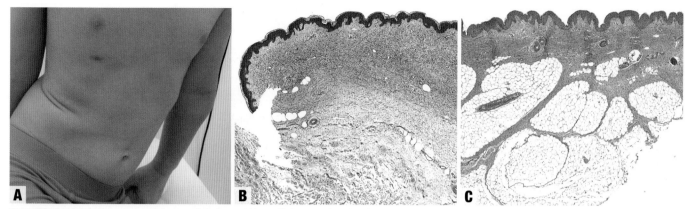

Fig. 1.105 Dermatofibrosarcoma protuberans. **A** A 4-year-old boy with known adenosine deaminase–deficient severe combined immunodeficiency developed multiple flat dermatofibrosarcoma protuberans. **B** Flat, plaque-like dermatofibrosarcoma protuberans mimicking a benign dermal neoplasm. **C** A hypocellular example of flat dermatofibrosarcoma protuberans is seen in this young patient with known adenosine deaminase–deficient severe combined immunodeficiency.

Macroscopic appearance

DFSP lesions are indurated plaques with one or multiple nodules. Multiple protuberant tumours are often seen in recurrent lesions. These ill-defined and infiltrative neoplasms have firm, greyish-white cut surfaces with occasional gelatinous areas, whereas areas of tumour necrosis are only rarely observed.

Histopathology

Classic DFSP

DFSP is characterized by a diffuse infiltration of dermis and subcutis. The neoplastic cells infiltrate the subcutaneous fat, resulting in a typical honeycomb appearance. The epidermis is usually uninvolved and tumour cells encase skin appendages without destroying them. DFSP is composed of cytologically uniform spindled tumour cells containing plump or elongated wavy nuclei arranged in storiform, whorled, or cartwheel growth patterns. Cytological atypia is minimal and mitotic activity is low. The collagenous stroma contains small blood vessels. The superficial portion of the neoplasm may be less cellular, causing considerable challenges in the differential diagnosis on small biopsies. Rarely, cases of DFSP present as a subcutaneous mass with infiltration of deep soft tissues {1886,199}. Rare cases

may show prominent vessels, granular cell change, prominent nuclear palisading, and Verocay body formation {3046,3260}.

Pigmented DFSP (also known as Bednar tumour)

Some cases of DFSP contain a variable number of pigmented, dendritic melanocytic cells {874}.

Myxoid DFSP

Rarely, DFSP may show prominent myxoid stroma with a more nodular growth and numerous vessels with slightly fibrotic vessel walls, often producing a more variable architecture, which may mimic other myxoid mesenchymal neoplasms {1072,2595}.

DFSP with myoid differentiation

In addition to a myointimal, non-neoplastic proliferation in entrapped vessels, bundles and nests of spindled myofibroblastic tumour cells are rarely observed {461}, more often in the fibrosarcomatous subtype {2077}.

Plaque-like DFSP

In rare cases, DFSP may show a flat, plaque-like growth resembling benign plaque-like CD34-positive dermal fibroma {1723}.

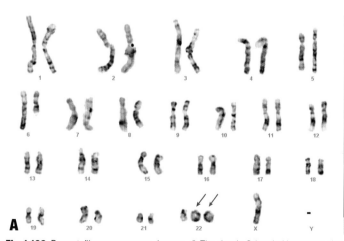
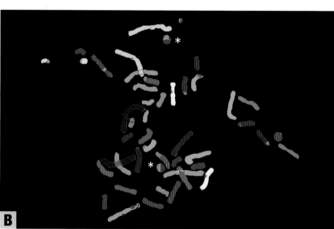

Fig. 1.106 Dermatofibrosarcoma protuberans. **A** The classic G-banded karyotype shows two supernumerary chromosomes (arrows). **B** Multiplexed spectral in situ hybridization of a chromosomal spread shows supernumerary chromosomes pseudocoloured to demonstrate material from both 22 and 17, in pink and blue, respectively (asterisks).

Fibrosarcomatous DFSP

Fibrosarcomatous DFSP
Fibrosarcomatous DFSP represents morphological progression to a usually fascicular pattern, with acquisition of metastatic potential. Fibrosarcomatous changes occur de novo or less commonly in local recurrences and either abrupt or more-gradual transformation can be encountered. The fibrosarcomatous component often shows a nodular, rather well-circumscribed growth and is composed of cellular spindle cell fascicles with a herringbone appearance. The neoplastic cells in fibrosarcomatous areas are characterized by increased atypia and proliferative activity {2077,1178,2}. Very rarely, transformation to pleomorphic sarcomatous areas has been reported {2077,3009}.

Immunohistochemistry
By immunohistochemistry, tumour cells stain positively for CD34 and may show expression of EMA {3386,3276}. Importantly, fibrosarcomatous DFSP can show loss of CD34 expression in about half of the cases {2077}. Tumour cells in myoid nodules and bundles stain strongly for SMA.

Cytology
Not clinically relevant

Diagnostic molecular pathology
For histologically challenging cases and for tumours composed entirely of fibrosarcomatous DFSP without a conventional component, detection of *COL1A1-PDGFB* can be used to confirm the diagnosis {1586,1489}. However, the *COL1A1-PDGFB* fusion may be cryptic in about 2% of cases, and another 2% of cases harbour alternative fusions involving *PDGFD* {705,823}.

Essential and desirable diagnostic criteria
Essential: a storiform architecture and uniform spindle cell morphology; diffusely infiltrative growth with a honeycomb pattern in the subcutis; expression of CD34; fibrosarcomatous DFSP: fascicular architecture with increased mitotic activity.
Desirable: COL1A1-PDGFB gene fusion or rarely alternative PDGFD rearrangements (in selected cases).

Staging
The American Joint Committee on Cancer (AJCC) or Union for International Cancer Control (UICC) TNM system can be applied for fibrosarcomatous DFSP.

Prognosis and prediction
DFSP is characterized by locally aggressive growth and frequent, often repeated local recurrences unless widely excised. The rate of local recurrences varies from 20% to 50% in the setting of inadequate margins {1178,2072,1299}. In contrast, ordinary DFSP almost never metastasizes. Higher-grade fibrosarcomatous progression is seen in 5% of cases. Fibrosarcomatous DFSP exhibits more-aggressive behaviour than ordinary DFSP, and 10–15% of patients develop distant metastases, most often to the lungs {390,1884,3208,1386,1848}. Histological grading has not been shown to be prognostic in fibrosarcomatous DFSP.

Solitary fibrous tumour

Demicco EG
Fritchie KJ
Han A

Definition
Solitary fibrous tumour (SFT) is a fibroblastic tumour characterized by a prominent, branching, thin-walled, dilated (staghorn) vasculature and *NAB2-STAT6* gene rearrangement.

ICD-O coding
8815/0 Solitary fibrous tumour, benign
8815/1 Solitary fibrous tumour NOS
8815/3 Solitary fibrous tumour, malignant

ICD-11 coding
2F7C & XH7E62 Neoplasms of uncertain behaviour of connective or other soft tissue & Solitary fibrous tumour NOS
2B5Y & XH1HP3 Other specified malignant mesenchymal neoplasms & Solitary fibrous tumour, malignant

Related terminology
Not recommended: haemangiopericytoma; giant cell angiofibroma; benign solitary fibrous tumour.

Subtype(s)
Fat-forming (lipomatous) solitary fibrous tumour; giant cell–rich solitary fibrous tumour

Localization
SFTs may occur at any anatomical site, including superficial and deep soft tissues and within visceral organs and bone, and they are more common at extrapleural locations. About 30–40% of extrapleural SFTs arise in the extremities; 30–40% arise in deep soft tissues, the abdominal cavity, the pelvis, or the retroperitoneum; 10–15% arise in the head and neck; and 10–15% arise in the trunk {1140,2456,2720,788,790, 1074,2784}. Deep tumours are more common than superficial tumours, accounting for 70–90% of cases {1140,2456}. In the head and neck, the sinonasal tract and orbit are the most common sites, followed by the oral cavity and salivary glands {2897}.

Clinical features
Most tumours present as slow-growing, painless masses. Abdominopelvic tumours may present with distention, constipation, urinary retention, or early satiety, whereas head and neck SFTs may present with nasal obstruction, voice changes, or bleeding {2270,1600}. Large SFTs may cause paraneoplastic syndromes such as Doege–Potter syndrome, with the induction of severe hypoglycaemia or (more rarely) acromegaloid changes due to tumour production of IGF2 {760,559}. The radiographic features of SFT are largely nonspecific. CT demonstrates a well-defined, occasionally lobulated mass that is isodense to skeletal muscle, with heterogeneous contrast enhancement due to the extensive tumour vasculature {3363,1611}. MRI shows intermediate

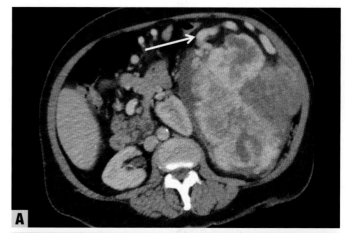

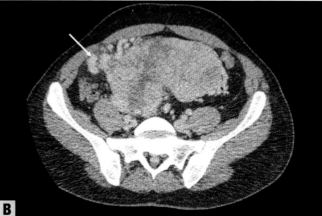

Fig. 1.107 Solitary fibrous tumour. **A** Axial contrast-enhanced CT shows a large, left-sided, peripherally enhancing retroperitoneal mass. Large feeding vessels (arrow) are seen anteriorly. **B** Axial contrast-enhanced CT shows a large central abdominal mass. Large feeding vessels (arrow) are seen anteriorly.

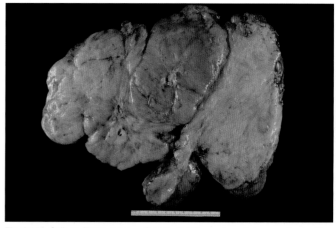

Fig. 1.108 Solitary fibrous tumour. Grossly, the tumour is well circumscribed, with a tan, fleshy, multilobular cut surface.

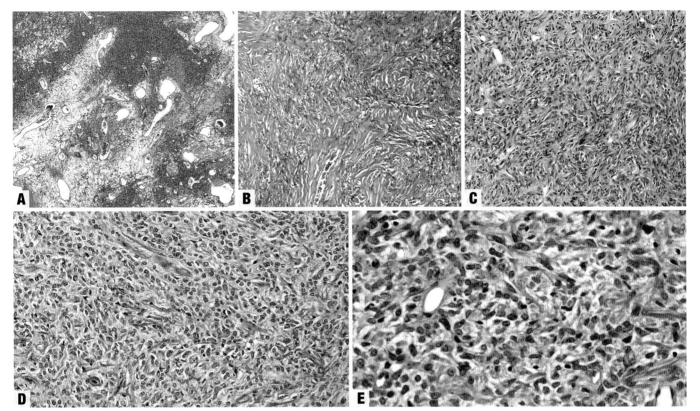

Fig. 1.109 Solitary fibrous tumour. **A** Tumours often have variable cellularity and a prominent ectatic, branching vasculature. **B** Hypocellular tumours often have a dense hyalinized collagenous stroma. Note the patternless architecture. **C** Cellular tumours may have little intervening stromal collagen, and the vascular network may be obscured by tumour cells. **D** Tumour cells may be spindled or ovoid, as in this example. **E** Tumour cells typically display scant to moderate amounts of indistinct, palely eosinophilic cytoplasm and bland nuclei with fine pale chromatin and inconspicuous nucleoli.

intensity on T1-weighted images and variable hypointensity to hyperintensity on T2-weighted images, corresponding to fibrous and cellular or myxoid areas, respectively {304,1611, 986}. Larger or aggressive cases may display increased heterogeneity due to fibrosis, haemorrhage, necrosis, myxoid and cystic degeneration, or calcifications {1611}.

Epidemiology
SFTs affect men and women equally and are most common in adults, with a peak incidence between 40 and 70 years {2720, 1140,788,790,1074,2784}.

Etiology
Unknown

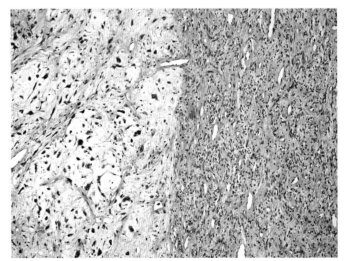

Fig. 1.110 Giant cell–rich solitary fibrous tumour. This lesion shows scattered multinucleated giant cells lining cystic spaces.

Fig. 1.111 Dedifferentiated solitary fibrous tumour. This field shows an abrupt transition from typical solitary fibrous tumour (right) to an undifferentiated sarcoma (left; this example shows a pleomorphic myxoid sarcoma).

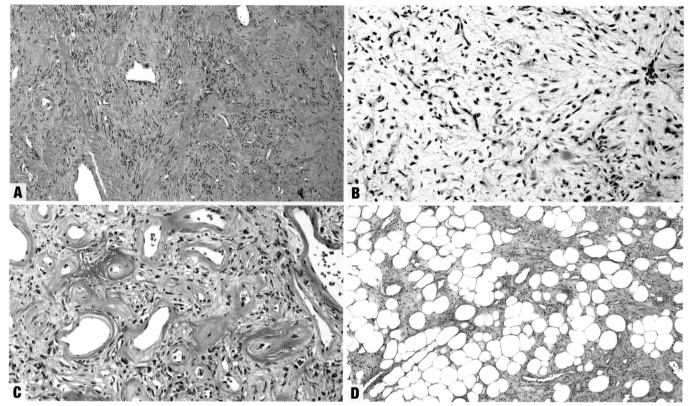

Fig. 1.112 Solitary fibrous tumour. **A** Some tumours may have a predominantly collagenous appearance with few cellular areas. **B** Myxoid change is common and may predominate in tumours that have received neoadjuvant radiation. **C** Stromal and perivascular hyalinization is common. **D** Fat-forming (lipomatous) solitary fibrous tumour shows typical features of solitary fibrous tumour with areas of mature adipose tissue or scattered adipocytes.

Pathogenesis

The genetic hallmark of SFT is a paracentric inversion involving chromosome 12q, resulting in the fusion of the *NAB2* and *STAT6* genes {577,2167,2640}. Some studies have shown a correlation between fusion types and histological features {52,227,1075}. The *NAB2-STAT6* fusion is thought to convert wildtype NAB2 from a transcriptional repressor of EGR1-mediated signalling into a transcriptional activator via replacement of the C-terminal repression domain by the transcriptional activation domain of STAT6, thereby resulting in a feedforward loop of constitutive EGR1-mediated transactivation of proliferation and survival-associated growth factors, including *IGF2* and *FGFR1* {2640}. Overexpression of *ALDH1A1* (*ALDH1*), *EGFR*, *JAK2*, histone deacetylases, and retinoic acid receptor may also contribute to tumorigenesis {1274,299}. Other alterations associated with aggressive behaviour and dedifferentiation include *TERT* promoter mutations {791,205,1868,52} and deletions or mutations of *TP53* {1716,707,52,2972}.

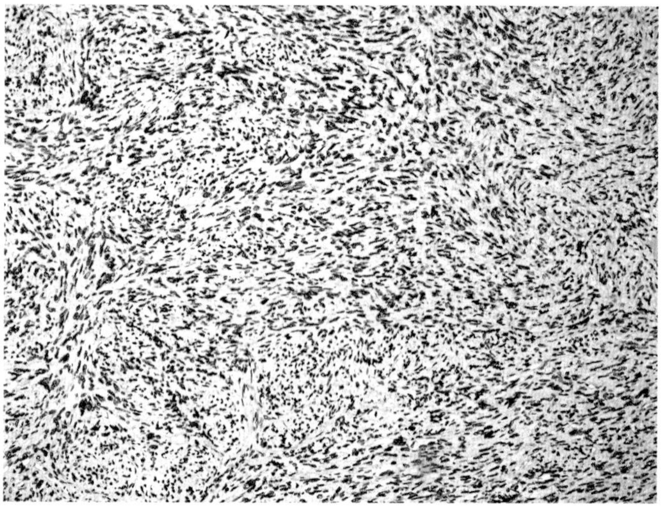

Macroscopic appearance

SFTs are well-circumscribed masses that typically measure 5–10 cm, although some lesions may exceed 25 cm in greatest dimension. The cut surface is nodular and tan to reddish-brown, and it occasionally shows haemorrhage, myxoid change, or cystic degeneration {1091,1312}.

Histopathology

SFTs are composed of haphazardly arranged spindled to ovoid cells with indistinct, pale eosinophilic cytoplasm within a variably collagenous stroma, admixed with branching and hyalinized staghorn-shaped (haemangiopericytomatous) blood vessels. There is a wide histological spectrum, ranging from paucicellular lesions with abundant stromal keloidal-type collagen to highly cellular tumours consisting of closely spaced cells with little or no intervening stroma. Myxoid change may be present {796}. SFTs most often have low mitotic counts, without substantial nuclear pleomorphism or necrosis. Tumours demonstrating a high mitotic

Fig. 1.113 Solitary fibrous tumour. Immunohistochemical expression of STAT6 is characteristic of the neoplastic cells of solitary fibrous tumour. Only strong and diffuse nuclear staining should be considered positive.

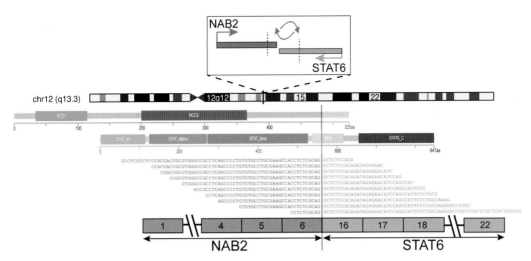

Fig. 1.114 Schematic *NAB2-STAT6* gene fusion in solitary fibrous tumour. The *NAB2* and *STAT6* genes are adjacent genes on chromosome 12q13 that are transcribed in opposite directions. This intrachromosomal fusion results from a genomic inversion at the 12q13 locus, fusing *NAB2* and *STAT6* in a common direction of transcription. The fusion transcript illustrated includes *NAB2* exon 6 fused to *STAT6* exon 16.

count with or without increased cellularity, atypia, necrosis, and infiltrative growth have traditionally been termed malignant, but new risk stratification models more accurately predict prognosis.

Fat-forming (lipomatous) SFT harbours a component of mature adipose tissue {1047,1247,2281,563}. Giant cell–rich SFT, formerly known as giant cell angiofibroma, shows features of conventional SFT with an admixed population of multinucleated giant cells within the stroma and lining pseudovascular spaces {777,1248}. Dedifferentiated (anaplastic) SFTs show transition to high-grade sarcoma with or without heterologous elements such as rhabdomyosarcoma or osteosarcoma {1939, 2008,2972,52,3071,2205,644,3048}. By immunohistochemistry, SFT typically shows strong and diffuse expression of CD34 and nuclear STAT6 {2793,854,787}, but expression may be lost in dedifferentiated SFT {644,2205,707,2771}.

Cytology

Cytological examination reveals oval, elongated, or rounded cells with wispy cytoplasm and eosinophilic collagenous stroma {3044}.

Diagnostic molecular pathology

NAB2-STAT6 gene fusions are pathognomonic for SFT. However, because *NAB2* and *STAT6* are in close proximity on chromosome 12q, detection of their fusion is difficult by conventional cytogenetic methods, and the diversity of breakpoints occurring in both exons and introns makes PCR-based detection of fusion variants difficult without multiplexed sequencing assays. STAT6 immunohistochemistry is a sensitive and specific surrogate for all fusions {854,1668,2793}.

Table 1.02 Three-variable and modified four-variable risk models for the prediction of metastatic risk in solitary fibrous tumours {788,790}

Risk factor	Cut-off	Points assigned	
		3-variable model	4-variable model
Patient age in years	< 55	0	0
	≥ 55	1	1
Mitoses/mm² (mitoses per 10 HPFs)	0 (0)	0	0
	0.5–1.5 (1–3)	1	1
	≥ 2 (≥ 4)	2	2
Tumour size in cm	0–4.9	0	0
	5–9.9	1	1
	10–14.9	2	2
	≥ 15	3	3
Tumour necrosis	< 10%	n/a	0
	≥ 10%	n/a	1
Risk	Low	0–2 points	0–3 points
	Intermediate	3–4 points	4–5 points
	High	5–6 points	6–7 points

HPF, high-power field; n/a, not applicable.

Essential and desirable diagnostic criteria

Essential: spindled to ovoid cells arranged around a branching and hyalinized vasculature; variable stromal collagen deposition; CD34 and/or STAT6 expression by immunohistochemistry.

Desirable (in selected cases): demonstration of *NAB2-STAT6* gene fusion.

Staging

Risk stratification models are preferred over anatomical staging.

Prognosis and prediction

Recurrence (distant or local) occurs in 10–30% of SFTs {788, 1140,2720,2456,1074}, with 10–40% of recurrences reported after 5 years {2041,3144} and rare recurrences seen after 15 years {1140}. *TERT* promoter mutations are more common in tumours with aggressive features, but they may also be seen in low-risk SFT {791,205,52}. Various single clinical or histological features have been reported to correlate with metastatic or local recurrence potential in large series, including high mitotic count (> 2 mitoses/mm^2, equating to > 4 mitoses per 10 high-power fields of 0.5 mm in diameter and 0.2 mm^2 in area) {788, 3161,2456,2720}, tumour size {3161,788,1140}, necrosis {788, 2456}, patient age {788,2720}, tumour cellularity and nuclear pleomorphism {2456}, and tumour site {1140,2720}. However, individual studies contradict one another regarding which specific features are important.

The development of multivariate risk models has resulted in improved prognostication over the traditional benign/malignant distinction. Of these models, the one most similar to the traditional definition of malignant SFT stratifies tumours into four risk tiers based on mitotic count, pleomorphism, and tumour cellularity {2456}. A set of risk calculators proposed by the French Sarcoma Group (FSG) incorporates clinical data (patient age, tumour site), pathological features (mitotic count), and history of radiotherapy to variously predict overall survival, local recurrence, and distant metastatic risk {2720}. The most widely used model for metastatic risk (see Table 1.02, p. 107) incorporates mitotic count (≥ 2 mitoses/mm^2), patient age (≥ 55 years), and tumour size stratified by 5 cm tiers to classify tumours into low, intermediate, and high risk groups {788}. This model has been validated for both thoracic and extrathoracic SFTs {788,790, 1074,2596}; a subsequent refinement includes necrosis as a fourth variable, resulting in higher numbers of cases being classified as low-risk {790,2596}.

Inflammatory myofibroblastic tumour

Yamamoto H

Definition

Inflammatory myofibroblastic tumour (IMT) is a distinctive, rarely metastasizing neoplasm composed of myofibroblastic and fibroblastic spindle cells accompanied by an inflammatory infiltrate of plasma cells, lymphocytes, and/or eosinophils.

ICD-O coding

8825/1 Inflammatory myofibroblastic tumour

ICD-11 coding

2B53.Y & XH66Z0 Other specified fibroblastic or myofibroblastic tumour, primary site & Myofibroblastic tumour NOS

Related terminology

Not recommended: plasma cell granuloma; inflammatory pseudotumour; inflammatory myofibrohistiocytic proliferation; omental-mesenteric myxoid hamartoma; inflammatory fibrosarcoma.

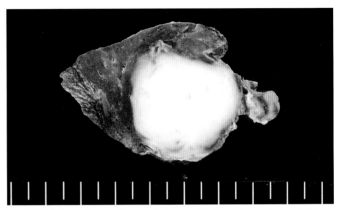

Fig. 1.115 Inflammatory myofibroblastic tumour. The tumour presented as a circumscribed, solid mass in the lung.

Subtype(s)

Epithelioid inflammatory myofibroblastic sarcoma

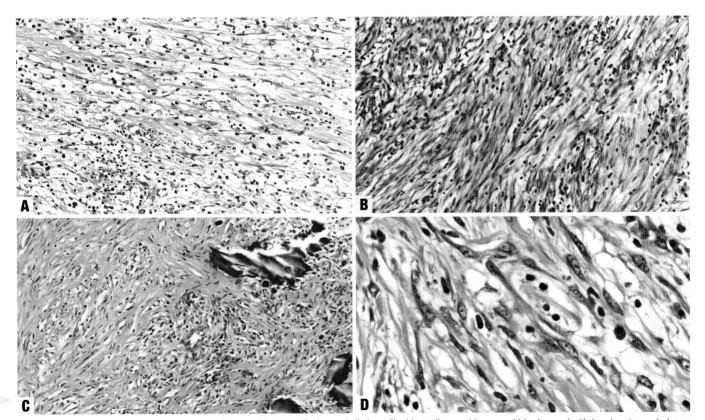

Fig. 1.116 Inflammatory myofibroblastic tumour. **A** The myxoid pattern displays spindled myofibroblasts dispersed in a myxoid background with lymphocytes and plasma cells. **B** The hypercellular pattern shows a fascicular spindle cell proliferation intermingled with inflammatory cells. **C** The hypocellular fibrous pattern is characterized by hyalinized collagenous stroma with sparse spindle cells and lymphoplasmacytic inflammation. Focal calcification is noted. **D** The spindled myofibroblasts show vesicular nuclei, small nucleoli, and eosinophilic cytoplasm.

Localization

IMT shows a wide anatomical distribution, most frequently arising in the abdominal soft tissues, including the mesentery, omentum, retroperitoneum, and pelvis, followed by the lung, mediastinum, head and neck, gastrointestinal tract, and genito-urinary tract (including the bladder and uterus) {631,1167,1588, 3116}. Unusual locations include somatic soft tissues, pancreas, liver, and CNS {631,1167,2570}.

Clinical features

The site of origin determines symptoms {631,1167,1588}. Abdominal tumours may cause gastrointestinal obstruction or bleeding. Pulmonary IMT is sometimes associated with chest pain and dyspnoea {2505}. As many as one third of patients have a clinical syndrome, possibly cytokine-mediated, of fever, malaise, weight loss, and laboratory abnormalities including microcytic hypochromic anaemia, thrombocytosis, polyclonal hypergammaglobulinaemia, elevated ESR, and elevated C-reactive protein {597,631,3042}. Epithelioid inflammatory myofibroblastic sarcoma (EIMS) is predominantly intra-abdominal and associated with a more aggressive course. Radiological imaging studies reveal a lobulated heterogeneous solid mass with or without calcification {1588}.

Epidemiology

IMT primarily affects children and young adults, although the age range extends throughout adulthood {626,631,1167}. There is a slight female predominance.

Etiology

Unknown

Pathogenesis

IMTs are genetically heterogeneous. In 50–60% of cases of IMT in children and young adults, the tumours harbour clonal cytogenetic rearrangements, involving chromosome band 2p23, that fuse the 3′ kinase region of the *ALK* gene with various partner genes, including *TPM3*, *TPM4*, *CLTC*, *CARS*, *ATIC*, *SEC31L1*, *PPFIBP1*, *DCTN1*, *EML4*, *PRKAR1A*, *LMNA*, *TFG*, *FN1*, *HNRNPA1*, and others in a growing list {413,560,769,1220, 1778,3029,3338,1468,1895}. EIMS is often associated with *RANBP2-ALK* or *RRBP1-ALK* gene rearrangements {560,1984, 1804}. IMT with *ALK* genomic rearrangement features activation

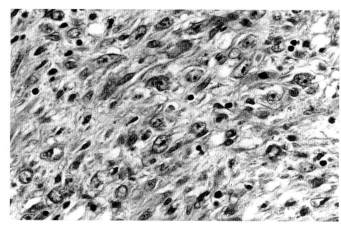

Fig. 1.118 Inflammatory myofibroblastic tumour. Ganglion-like polygonal cells show large rounded nuclei and prominent nucleoli.

and overexpression of the ALK C-terminal kinase region, which is restricted to the neoplastic myofibroblastic component {413, 630,656,1220,1778}.

ROS1 and *NTRK3* gene rearrangements are each found in 5–10% of IMTs; *TFG-ROS1*, *YWHAE-ROS1*, and *ETV6-NTRK3* gene fusions have been reported {1895,1415,62,139,3339}. Very rare cases have *RET* or *PDGFRB* gene rearrangements {139,1895}. In contrast, such rearrangements are uncommon in IMTs diagnosed in adults aged > 40 years {534,1778,3339, 1895,139}.

Macroscopic appearance

IMT is a nodular, circumscribed, or multinodular mass with a tan, whorled, fleshy, or myxoid cut surface and variable haemorrhage, necrosis, and calcification {626,631,1167}. The diameter of the lesion ranges from 1 to 20 cm or more, with a median size of 5–6 cm.

Histopathology

The spindled fibroblastic-myofibroblastic cells and inflammatory cells form three basic histological patterns {626,631, 1167}. The first is a myxoid pattern, which consists of loosely arranged plump or spindled myofibroblasts in an oedematous myxoid background with abundant blood vessels and an infiltrate of plasma cells, lymphocytes, and eosinophils, mimicking

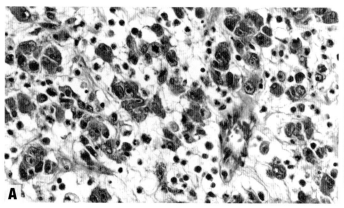

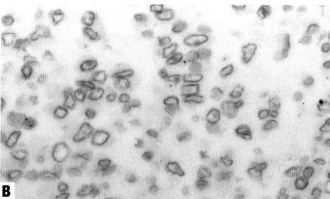

Fig. 1.117 Epithelioid inflammatory myofibroblastic sarcoma with *RANBP2-ALK* rearrangement. **A** Plump polygonal and epithelioid tumour cells with prominent nucleoli are characteristic. The neutrophilic infiltration seen here is often present. **B** Distinctive nuclear membranous immunoreactivity for ALK is seen.

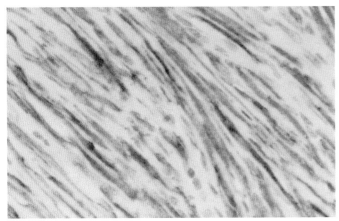

Fig. 1.119 Inflammatory myofibroblastic tumour with *TPM3-ALK* gene fusion. Diffuse cytoplasmic staining for ALK is seen.

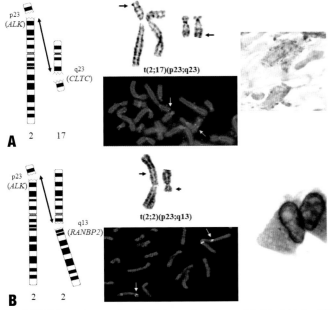

Fig. 1.120 Inflammatory myofibroblastic tumour karyotypes. **A** Left to right: the 2;17 translocation resulting in *CLTC-ALK* fusion (schematic and partial G-banded karyotype) with corresponding *ALK* breakpoint-spanning probe FISH demonstrating a signal split; the white arrow indicates der(2) and the yellow arrow der(17). ALK granular cytoplasmic immunostaining is seen with *CLTC* partnership; *CLTC* encodes a protein component of the cytoplasmic face of intracellular organelles (coated vesicles and coated pits). **B** Left to right: schematic, partial G-banded karyotype and differentially labelled, dual-spanning *RANBP2* and *ALK* FISH illustrating the *RANBP2-ALK* fusion; both chromosome 2 homologues involved in the translocation in this fusion example and juxtaposed orange/green signals indicate fusion (white arrows). Nuclear membrane ALK immunostaining is featured when the *ALK* fusion partner is *RANBP2*, because *RANBP2* encodes a large nucleopore protein localized at the cytoplasmic side of the nuclear pore complex.

granulation tissue or a reactive process. The second is a hypercellular pattern, which is characterized by a compact fascicular spindle cell proliferation with variable myxoid and collagenous stroma and inflammatory infiltrate. The third is a hypocellular fibrous pattern, which features hyalinized collagenous stroma with lower cellularity of spindle cells and a relatively sparse inflammatory infiltrate, mimicking desmoid fibromatosis. Dystrophic calcifications and osseous metaplasia are occasionally

seen. One or more patterns are often seen within a single tumour. Myofibroblasts with vesicular nuclei, 1–3 small nucleoli, and eosinophilic cytoplasm are typical and sometimes show a ganglion-like appearance. Necrosis is uncommon. Mitotic activity varies but is generally low.

EIMS is an aggressive IMT subtype with plump epithelioid or histiocytoid tumour cells with vesicular chromatin, prominent nucleoli, and amphophilic or eosinophilic cytoplasm, often admixed with neutrophils in an abundant myxoid stroma {560,1984}.

By immunohistochemistry, IMT displays variable staining for SMA, MSA, calponin, and desmin. Focal keratin immunoreactivity can be seen in as many as 30% of cases. Immunoreactivity for ALK is detectable in 50–60% of cases and correlates well with the presence of *ALK* gene rearrangement {526,534, 630,656,1167}. Of note, the ALK immunostaining pattern varies depending on the *ALK* fusion partner; for example, *RANBP2-ALK* is associated with a nuclear membranous pattern, *RRBP1-ALK* with a perinuclear accentuated cytoplasmic pattern, and *CLTC-ALK* with a granular cytoplasmic pattern; many other *ALK* fusion variants show a diffuse cytoplasmic pattern (most commonly seen in IMT) {413,1984,1804}. Highly sensitive ALK antibody clones (5A4, D5F3) may improve detection of the ALK protein in IMT {3029,3339}. *ROS1*-rearranged IMT typically shows cytoplasmic expression of ROS1 {3339,1415}.

Cytology

The cytology of IMT consists of bland spindle cells with oval nuclei and small distinct nucleoli in a background of lymphocytes and plasma cells. Atypical ganglion-like polygonal cells can be seen {2956}.

Diagnostic molecular pathology

In addition to immunohistochemical detection of ALK protein, molecular assays for *ALK* may be used to confirm the diagnosis but are generally not required {630}. Exceptional situations such as inversion of *ALK* on the same chromosome arm may lead to a false-negative FISH result {1273}. In ALK-negative cases, immunohistochemistry for ROS1 and/or molecular tests for non-*ALK* gene fusions (e.g. *NTRK3*) may be useful {3339,1895,62, 139}.

Essential and desirable diagnostic criteria

Essential: loose or compact fascicles of spindle cells with a prominent inflammatory infiltrate and a variable fibrous or myxoid stroma; expression of ALK (seen in as many as 60% of cases).
Desirable: ALK or other gene rearrangements (in selected cases).

Staging

Not clinically relevant

Prognosis and prediction

Approximately 25% of extrapulmonary IMTs recur, in part depending on anatomical site and resectability {57,631,1167}. ALK-negative IMTs may have a higher likelihood of metastasis, but ALK immunoreactivity does not appear to correlate with recurrence {626,597,630}. Distant metastases are rare (< 5%) and involve the lungs, brain, liver, and bone. However, reliable prognostic indicators have not been developed for conventional IMT {626,1445}. Intra-abdominal EIMS behaves much more aggressively {560,1984}.

Low-grade myofibroblastic sarcoma

Mentzel TDW

Definition
Low-grade myofibroblastic sarcoma is a rarely metastasizing mesenchymal neoplasm, often having fibromatosis-like features, which tends to arise in the head and neck region.

ICD-O coding
8825/3 Myofibroblastic sarcoma

ICD-11 coding
2B53.Y & XH2668 Other specified fibroblastic or myofibroblastic tumour, primary site & Low-grade myofibroblastic sarcoma

Related terminology
Acceptable: myofibrosarcoma.

Subtype(s)
None

Localization
Low-grade myofibroblastic sarcoma shows a wide anatomical distribution; extremities and the head and neck region, especially the tongue and oral cavity, are preferred locations, whereas the skin and gastrointestinal tract are rarely affected {2083,2177,29,535}. These neoplasms arise predominantly in subcutaneous and deeper soft tissues; dermal presentation is very uncommon {539}. Rare cases involving salivary gland and nasal cavity / paranasal sinuses have been reported {331,1680}.

Clinical features
Most patients report a painless swelling or an enlarging mass. Pain or related symptoms have more rarely been reported. Radiologically, these lesions have a destructive growth pattern.

Epidemiology
Low-grade myofibroblastic sarcoma occurs predominantly in adults, with a slight male predominance; children are more rarely affected {2083,2177,2892}.

Etiology
Unknown

Pathogenesis
Unknown

Macroscopic appearance
Grossly, the tumour is usually a firm mass with pale, fibrous cut surfaces and ill-defined margins {2083}; a minority are well circumscribed with pushing margins {2177}.

Histopathology
Histologically, low-grade myofibroblastic sarcomas are characterized by a diffusely infiltrative growth pattern, and (in deeply located neoplasms) tumour cells often grow between individual skeletal muscle fibres. Most cases are composed of spindle-shaped tumour cells arranged in cellular fascicles or show a storiform growth pattern. Neoplastic cells have ill-defined palely eosinophilic cytoplasm and fusiform nuclei that are either elongated and wavy with evenly distributed chromatin or plumper, more rounded, and vesicular with small nucleoli. Rarely, hypocellular neoplasms with a more prominent collagenous (sometimes hyalinized) stroma have been described. Importantly, neoplastic cells show, at least focally, moderate nuclear atypia with enlarged, hyperchromatic, and irregular nuclei and slightly increased proliferative activity. These neoplasms may contain numerous thin-walled capillaries. The tumours may progress to morphologically higher-grade myofibroblastic sarcomas {2177}.

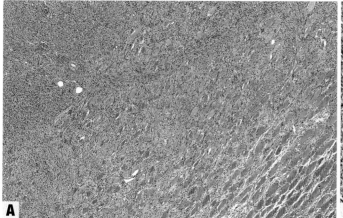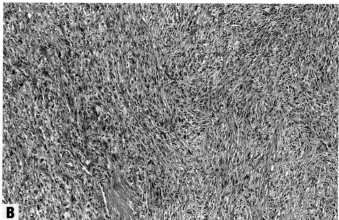

Fig. 1.121 Low-grade myofibroblastic sarcoma. **A** Diffuse infiltration of skeletal muscle by a cellular spindle cell neoplasm. **B** The neoplasm is composed of enlarged spindled tumour cells arranged in cellular bundles and fascicles.

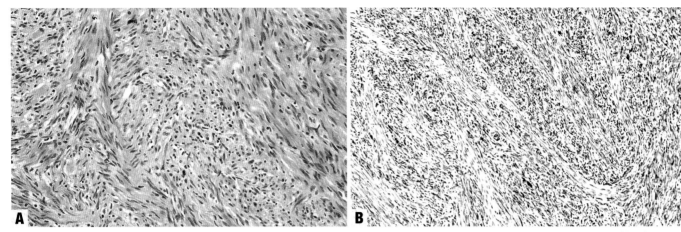

Fig. 1.122 Low-grade myofibroblastic sarcoma. **A** Some tumours contain more-abundant, palely eosinophilic cytoplasm. Note enlarged, hyperchromatic nuclei and scattered mitotic figures. **B** Tumour cells are often positive for desmin.

By immunohistochemistry, neoplastic cells in low-grade myofibroblastic sarcoma show variable positivity for SMA and/or desmin. A subset show nuclear β-catenin staining {480}.

Cytology
Not clinically relevant

Diagnostic molecular pathology
Not clinically relevant

Essential and desirable diagnostic criteria
Essential: diffusely infiltrative growth, often between skeletal muscle fibres; cellular fascicles of spindle cells with pale eosinophilic cytoplasm; at least focally moderate nuclear atypia; variable expression of SMA and/or desmin.

Staging
Not clinically relevant

Prognosis and prediction
Low-grade myofibroblastic sarcoma often recurs locally, but metastases are rare, most often occurring after a prolonged time interval {2083}.

Superficial CD34-positive fibroblastic tumour

Rekhi B
Folpe AL
Yu L

Definition
Superficial CD34-positive fibroblastic tumour is a distinctive low-grade neoplasm of the skin and subcutis, characterized by a fascicular to sheet-like proliferation of spindled cells with abundant, eosinophilic, granular to glassy cytoplasm, marked nuclear pleomorphism, a low mitotic count, diffuse CD34 expression, and frequent aberrant keratin immunoreactivity.

ICD-O coding
8810/1 Superficial CD34-positive fibroblastic tumour

ICD-11 coding
2B53.Y Other specified fibroblastic or myofibroblastic tumour, primary site

Related terminology
Acceptable: PRDM10-rearranged soft tissue tumour.

Subtype(s)
None

Localization
This tumour most frequently occurs in the lower extremities, especially thigh, followed by arm, buttock, shoulder, and (rarely) vulva {497,3212,1747,2601}. Tumour size varies from 1.5 to 10 cm but is usually < 5 cm {497,1747,2910}.

Clinical features
This tumour typically presents as a slow-growing, painless mass of the superficial soft tissues. A long pre-biopsy duration (> 5 years) is often noted {497}.

Epidemiology
Fewer than 40 cases have been reported. Most have occurred in middle-aged adults (median age: 37 years), with a slight male predominance {497,1747}.

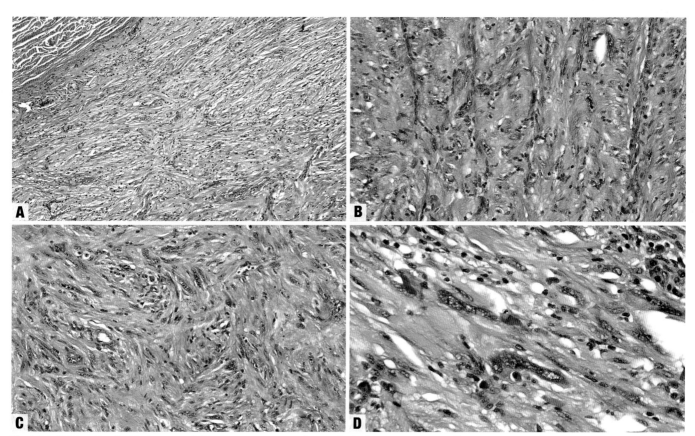

Fig. 1.123 CD34-positive fibroblastic tumour. **A** The tumour presents as a circumscribed subcutaneous mass. **B** The tumour displays a fascicular to sheet-like proliferation of pleomorphic spindle cells with abundant, granular to glassy eosinophilic cytoplasm. **C** Superficial CD34-positive fibroblastic tumour. The tumour shows vague nuclear palisading, nuclear pleomorphism, and a mixed inflammatory infiltrate, including eosinophils. **D** Superficial CD34-positive fibroblastic tumour. The cells show marked nuclear enlargement and pleomorphism, with frequent intranuclear pseudoinclusions; mitotic activity is extremely low.

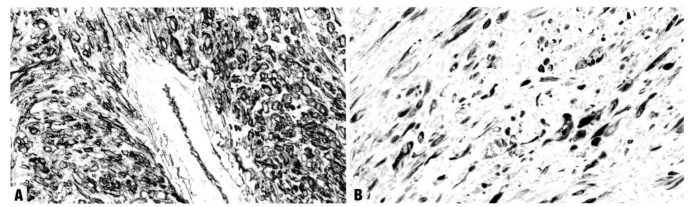

Fig. 1.124 Superficial CD34-positive fibroblastic tumour. **A** Diffuse CD34 expression is invariably present. **B** Patchy keratin expression, most often with the AE1/AE3 clones, is typically present.

Etiology
Unknown

Pathogenesis
PRDM10 rearrangements have been reported in 3 cases previously classified as superficial CD34-positive fibroblastic tumour {2553}.

Macroscopic appearance
The tumours are circumscribed, firm, yellow to tan soft tissue masses with a variably gelatinous appearance {497,1747,2910}.

Histopathology
The lesions grow in a relatively circumscribed, but at least partially infiltrative, fashion and are composed of highly cellular fascicles and sheets of spindled to epithelioid cells with abundant eosinophilic cytoplasm, often having a granular or glassy appearance. Lipidized tumour cells are commonly present. The neoplastic cells show moderate to marked nuclear pleomorphism, often with bizarre, hyperchromatic nuclei containing prominent nucleoli and intranuclear cytoplasmic pseudoinclusions. Despite these alarming nuclear features, mitotic activity is very low and necrosis is rarely seen {497,1747,3212,2601}. A mixed inflammatory cell infiltrate is often present. There is morphological overlap with tumours reported as *PRDM10*-rearranged soft tissue tumours {2553,1390}. By immunohistochemistry, superficial CD34-positive fibroblastic tumours invariably express CD34 and are focally immunoreactive for keratins in close to 70% of cases (most often with the AE1/AE3 clones).

Cytology
Cytology shows cellular smears composed of large, pleomorphic cells with granular to glassy cytoplasm {1844}.

Diagnostic molecular pathology
Not clinically relevant

Essential and desirable diagnostic criteria
Essential: superficial location; large eosinophilic cells with granular to glassy cytoplasm; marked nuclear pleomorphism but a very low mitotic count; diffuse CD34 expression and frequent keratin immunoreactivity.

Staging
Not clinically relevant

Prognosis and prediction
The prognosis for patients with this tumour is excellent, with only a single reported case with lymph node metastasis and no local recurrences in 30 cases with follow-up. All patients with this disease have been reported to be alive and disease-free at the time of last follow-up {497,1747}.

Myxoinflammatory fibroblastic sarcoma

Montgomery EA
Antonescu CR
Folpe AL

Definition

Myxoinflammatory fibroblastic sarcoma (MIFS) is an infiltrative, locally aggressive fibroblastic neoplasm that typically arises in the distal extremities. It is characterized by pleomorphic fibroblastic cells with macronucleoli in a myxohyaline background with a variably prominent inflammatory cell infiltrate.

ICD-O coding

8811/1 Myxoinflammatory fibroblastic sarcoma

ICD-11 coding

2B5F.2 & XH2D15 Sarcoma, not elsewhere classified of other specified sites & Myxoinflammatory fibroblastic sarcoma

Related terminology

Not recommended: inflammatory myxohyaline tumour of the distal extremities with virocyte-like or Reed–Sternberg–like cells; acral myxoinflammatory fibroblastic sarcoma; inflammatory myxoid tumour of the soft parts with bizarre giant cells.

Subtype(s)

None

Localization

MIFS usually affects the acral dorsal extremities, particularly the hands {2179,2063}, but occasional proximal examples have been highlighted {1557} and accounted for about 5% of cases in the largest series to date {1755}. The hand, finger, and wrist account for about 60% of cases, and the foot and ankle for about 20% {1755}.

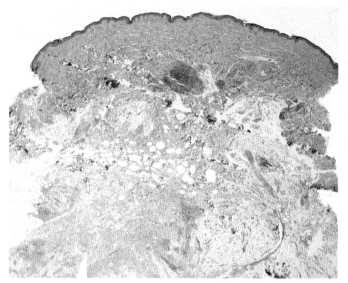

Fig. 1.126 Myxoinflammatory fibroblastic sarcoma. These tumours most commonly arise in the subcutaneous tissue of the distal extremities. In this image, the lesion is seen in the adipose tissue at the bottom of the image. Note the lymphoid aggregate in the deep dermis.

Clinical features

These neoplasms present as solitary painless masses, typically of the distal extremities. Most examples measure about 3 cm, but the size range is wide. On imaging, they are centred in the subcutis (about two thirds) or deeper and typically display infiltration into adjoining tissues such that they mimic infection, tenosynovial giant cell tumour, or ganglion cysts {1712,2249, 3053}.

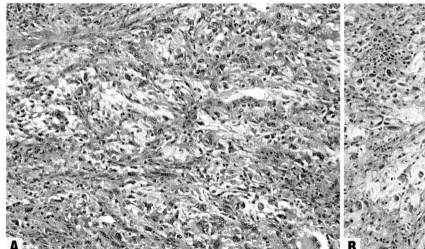
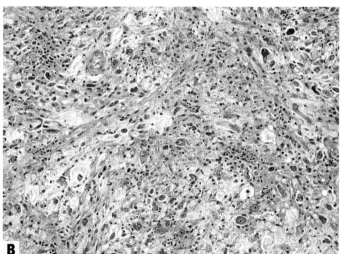

Fig. 1.125 Myxoinflammatory fibroblastic sarcoma. **A** Note the myxoid background, scattered inflammation, and spindle cells in this *BRAF*-mutated case. **B** This example shows haemosiderin and scattered large cells with macronucleoli.

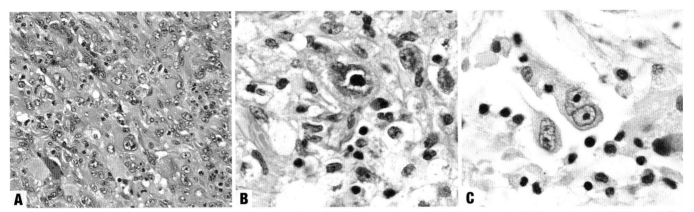

Fig. 1.127 Myxoinflammatory fibroblastic sarcoma. **A** In some examples, the atypical cells are more numerous. Note the macronucleoli. This case showed a *BRAF* fusion. **B** The cell in the centre is reminiscent of a Hodgkin cell. The presence of the eosinophil beneath it and scattered lymphocytes adds to the mimicry. **C** Note the binucleated cell in the centre of the field, with macronucleoli.

Epidemiology

These are rare neoplasms. The reported age range is 4–91 years (median: ~40 years), with no sex predilection {1755,1691,2063, 2179,2107}.

Etiology

Unknown

Pathogenesis

Tumours showing histological overlap with MIFS and haemosiderotic fibrolipomatous tumour (HFLT) have been reported {353,3407,495,1877,144}, suggesting a link between these two tumour types, but this link remains incompletely understood and controversial. MIFSs have also been reported to coexist with pleomorphic hyalinizing angiectatic tumour {353,495,1279}, but the precise classification of these unusual tumours remains the subject of debate.

A complex karyotype including a reciprocal t(1;10)(p22;q24) was initially reported in MIFS {1740}, followed by a report of a reciprocal t(1;10) in a case of HFLT {3279} and a hybrid

MIFS/HFLT with der(10)t(1;10) {892}. The breakpoints in chromosomes 1 and 10 cluster in *TGFBR3* and in or near *OGA* (*MGEA5*), respectively, but do not result in an expressed fusion gene {1279}. The t(1;10) has been detected in most HFLT cases and appears much more common in hybrid HFLT-MIFS tumours than in classic MIFS {2179,144}. Although these findings resulted in the proposal of an initial pathogenetic link between MIFS and HFLT, suggesting that they represent a morphological continuum or pathological spectrum {144}, later studies have questioned this hypothesis, postulating that these two entities are unrelated and that hybrid HFLT-MIFS tumours more likely represent sarcomatous progression in HFLT, rather than true MIFS {2179,3407}. Additionally, one third of MIFSs demonstrate *BRAF*-related fusions, which were not detected in any of the HFLTs tested {1577}. Another common genetic event in both MIFS and HFLT is the presence of a 3p11.1-p12.1 amplicon, including the *VGLL3* gene {1279,144,1577}.

Macroscopic appearance

Tumours are lobulated and variably gelatinous, fleshy, or firm, typically attaining a size of roughly 3 cm.

Histopathology

These tumours are infiltrative and multinodular, being centred in the subcutaneous tissue in most cases. They are characterized histologically by dense inflammation merging with stroma varying from myxoid to hyalinized and containing sheets and small foci of epithelioid and spindled cells. Some lesions contain foamy histiocytes, giant cells, and haemosiderin. The cellularity is quite variable between lesions. Amid the inflammatory background, scattered bizarre cells with large vesicular nuclei and macronucleoli reminiscent of Reed–Sternberg cells or virocytes are present. Many cells show degenerated smudged chromatin. Pseudolipoblasts akin to those encountered in myxofibrosarcoma with cytoplasmic mucopolysaccharide matrix compressing nuclei may be seen. The spindle cells often coalesce at the periphery of myxoid lobules to form a reticular pattern as they merge with myxoid tissue. The inflammatory infiltrate is mixed, consisting of lymphocytes, plasma cells, histiocytes, and eosinophils in varying proportions. Emperipolesis may be present. Despite the cytological atypia, mitotic activity is minimal. Immunohistochemistry is unhelpful {1755,1691,2063,2179}.

Fig. 1.128 Myxoinflammatory fibroblastic sarcoma. Multiple green signals depict the *VGLL3* amplification at 3p12.1; the red signal is the reference probe on 3q12.1-q12.2.

Cytology

Cytological preparations show large epithelioid cells with macronucleoli and lipoblast-like features enmeshed in myxoid stroma with prominent inflammation and spindle cells {3086}.

Diagnostic molecular pathology

Not clinically relevant

Essential and desirable diagnostic criteria

Essential: typical distal extremity location; atypical fibroblastic cells with macronucleoli; variably myxoid and hyalinized matrix with a mixed inflammatory infiltrate.
Desirable: pseudolipoblasts.

Staging

Not clinically relevant

Prognosis and prediction

Local recurrences are common and often repeated. Metastases are rare, occurring in < 1% of cases after multiple recurrences. Initial complete excision is the best predictor of a favourable outcome {1755}.

Infantile fibrosarcoma

Davis JL
Antonescu CR
Bahrami A

Definition

Infantile fibrosarcoma (IFS) is a malignant fibroblastic tumour most commonly occurring in infancy, frequently characterized by an *ETV6-NTRK3* fusion. It is a locally aggressive and rapidly growing tumour that only rarely metastasizes.

ICD-O coding

8814/3 Infantile fibrosarcoma

ICD-11 coding

2B5F.2 & XH7BC6 Sarcoma, not elsewhere classified of other specified sites & Infantile fibrosarcoma

Related terminology

Acceptable: congenital fibrosarcoma; infantile fibrosarcoma-like tumour; cellular congenital mesoblastic nephroma.

Subtype(s)

None

Localization

The most common sites of involvement are the superficial and deep soft tissues of the extremities, followed by the trunk and the head and neck. Less commonly, IFS arises in the abdomen or retroperitoneum {2386,603,628} and rarely in skeletal or visceral locations (e.g. lung, bowel) {2936,2452}. Analogous tumours in the kidney are designated cellular congenital mesoblastic nephroma {1655}.

Clinical features

IFS typically manifests as a localized, rapidly enlarging, painless mass or swelling, or as an exophytic nodule {603}. One third of cases are found at birth {603} and 14% are detected at prenatal ultrasound {2386}. IFS may ulcerate the skin surface and resemble vascular tumours {3345}. Intratumoural haemorrhage in utero or in neonates may lead to anaemia or haemorrhagic shock {869,2760}. Imaging shows a heterogeneously enhancing mass with nonspecific characteristics that sometimes contains haemorrhage {49}.

Epidemiology

More than 75% of cases occur in the first year of life, 15% in the second year, and < 10% in older children {603,2386}. Some of the tumours with alternative kinase fusions have been reported in older children {1573,743}. IFS has a slight male predominance {603,2386}.

Etiology

Unknown

Pathogenesis

IFS is driven by oncogenic activation of kinase signalling, mostly as a result of in-frame fusions upstream of the kinase domains and in rare cases due to complex activating mutations {3258}. Most cases harbour the canonical *ETV6-NTRK3* fusion resulting from t(12;15)(p13;q25), although rare cases involving other partners, such as *EML4-NTRK3*, have been reported {607,743}. In addition, alternative fusions involving other kinases have been reported in a subset of cases, including *NTRK1, NTRK2, BRAF,* and *MET* {743,1573,3258,1039}. *NTRK1* fusion gene partners include *TPM3, LMNA, TPR, SQSTM1,* and *MIR584F1* {1573,743}. *BRAF* fusions and complex deletions have been described, which probably result in the loss of the negative regulatory RAS-binding domain, resulting in constitutive activation of BRAF {1573,3258}. A single case with *TFG-MET* fusion has been reported {1039}. The genetic abnormalities of cellular congenital mesoblastic nephroma share substantial overlap, in keeping with a common pathogenesis {1655,607,3258}. Secretory carcinomas of the breast and salivary gland also harbour the *ETV6-NTRK3* fusion {3079,780,2882}.

Macroscopic appearance

Tumours vary in size but can be quite large (median size: 5–6 cm; range: 1 to > 15 cm) {2915,743}. Grossly, they are typically poorly circumscribed, with infiltrative borders into surrounding structures; some tumours may have a thin pseudocapsule.

Histopathology

Histologically, IFS can display a broad morphological spectrum. Most commonly, it is a cellular neoplasm composed of monomorphic spindled to ovoid cells with scant cytoplasm and

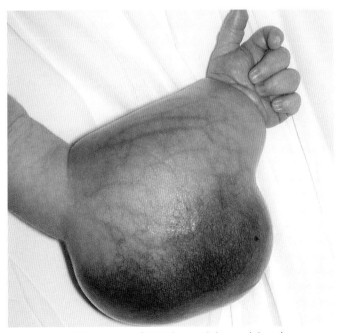

Fig. 1.129 Infantile fibrosarcoma. Clinical photograph. Large soft tissue forearm mass.

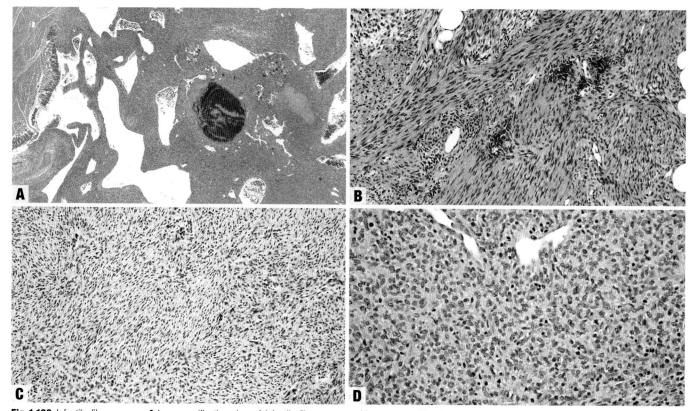

Fig. 1.130 Infantile fibrosarcoma. **A** Low-magnification view of infantile fibrosarcoma with numerous dilated, irregularly branching blood vessels (with *ETV6-NTRK3* fusion). **B** Long intersecting fascicles or herringbone pattern of growth (with *TPR-NTRK1* fusion). **C** Poorly formed fascicular growth pattern (with *LMNA-NTRK1* fusion). **D** Cellular ovoid to round cell pattern (with *ETV6-NTRK3* fusion).

slightly angulated nuclei. The cells may be arranged in randomly oriented compact sheets or in herringbone fascicles. The background stroma can range from collagenous to myxoid. A prominent haemangiopericytoma-like vascular pattern is often present. Tumours with decreased cellularity and prominent collagen resembling fibromatosis or myofibromatosis can also be

seen {624,743}. A rich mixed chronic inflammatory infiltrate may be present. Infiltrative growth into and entrapping adipose tissue, skeletal muscle, and other structures is common. Mitoses range from infrequent to numerous, without prognostic significance; no atypical mitoses are seen. Patchy necrosis may be present. The immunohistochemical profile is nonspecific, with variable expression of SMA, CD34, S100, and desmin {624, 743}. IFSs with NTRK gene rearrangements are often positive by immunohistochemistry using a pan-TRK antibody {1442, 2688}.

Cytology
Not clinically relevant

Diagnostic molecular pathology
ETV6-NTRK3 or other gene fusions/rearrangements can be demonstrated by a variety of molecular approaches {377,158,743}.

Essential and desirable diagnostic criteria
Essential: the majority of patients are aged < 2 years; spindle to primitive ovoid/round cell tumour; often arranged in a fascicular/herringbone pattern; staghorn vasculature and mixed inflammation.
Desirable: *ETV6-NTRK3* fusion or other rearrangements involving *NTRK1*, *BRAF*, and *MET*.

Staging
Not clinically relevant

Fig. 1.131 Infantile fibrosarcoma. Primitive stellate cells in a predominantly myxoid stroma (with *ETV6-NTRK3* fusion).

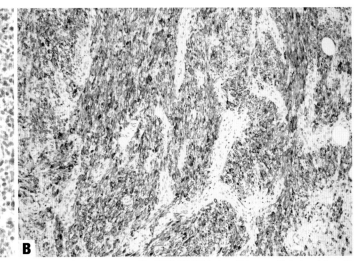

Fig. 1.132 Infantile fibrosarcoma. **A** Immunohistochemistry with pan-TRK antibody. Nuclear expression in a tumour with *ETV6-NTRK3* fusion. **B** Immunohistochemistry with pan-TRK antibody. Cytoplasmic expression in a tumour with *TPM3-NTRK1* fusion.

Prognosis and prediction

IFS is locally aggressive but with relatively infrequent metastases and an overall favourable outcome. The overall 10-year survival rate for IFS with standard treatment regimens (various combinations of surgery and/or standard chemotherapy) is about 90% {603,2915,2386}. Reported local recurrence rates are 25–40%, with recurrence highly associated with incomplete resection {2386,743}. However, for many tumours, complete surgical resection would result in substantial morbidity and is therefore not the ideal management. The rate of metastasis is 8–15% {743,2386,2915}. Rare cases of spontaneous tumour regression have been observed {2707}. The advent of targeted tyrosine kinase inhibitors may alter the prognosis and clinical management of this disease in advanced or intractable disease {1733,862}.

Adult fibrosarcoma

Yoshida A
Folpe AL

Definition
Adult fibrosarcoma is a rare sarcoma composed of relatively monomorphic fibroblastic tumour cells with variable collagen production and often herringbone architecture. It is a diagnosis of exclusion.

ICD-O coding
8810/3 Fibrosarcoma NOS

ICD-11 coding
2B5F.2 & XH4EP1 Sarcoma, not elsewhere classified of other specified sites & Fibrosarcoma NOS

Related terminology
None

Subtype(s)
None

Localization
Adult fibrosarcoma most often involves the deep soft tissues of the extremities, trunk, and head and neck.

Clinical features
Adult fibrosarcoma presents as a mass with or without pain.

Epidemiology
Once considered the most common soft tissue sarcoma in adults {1495}, adult fibrosarcoma has become exceedingly rare, due to changes in diagnostic criteria and advances in ancillary testing {203}. Most cases previously classified as adult fibrosarcoma are currently best classified as another type of spindle cell sarcoma or a specific fibrosarcoma subtype. Strictly defined, adult fibrosarcomas probably account for < 1% of adult soft tissue sarcomas. These tumours most often occur in middle-aged and older adults (median age: 50 years), with a slight male predominance {203}.

Etiology
Some arise in the field of previous irradiation and rarely in association with implanted foreign material {203}.

Pathogenesis
Adult fibrosarcoma has been reported to show multiple numerical and structural chromosomal abnormalities {718,3150,1862}, although older data should be interpreted with caution. A recent report of an *STRN3-NTRK3* fusion in a strictly defined adult fibrosarcoma suggests a possible link to other NTRK-rearranged mesenchymal neoplasms {3344}.

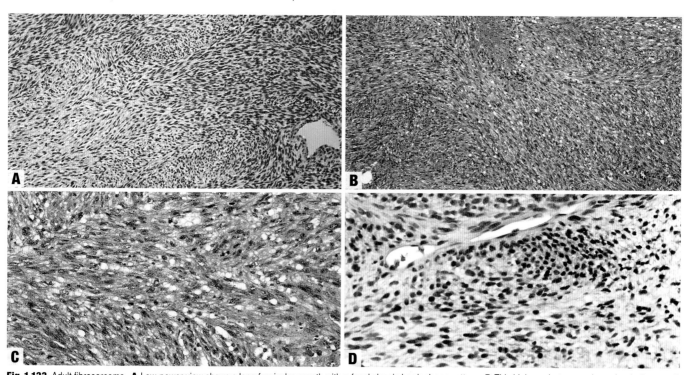

Fig. 1.133 Adult fibrosarcoma. **A** Low-power view shows a long fascicular growth with a focal classic herringbone pattern. **B** This high-grade tumour shows fascicular growth and necrosis. **C** The tumour consists of monomorphic spindle cells with nuclear atypia. **D** Radiation-induced adult fibrosarcoma showing monomorphic nuclear features.

Macroscopic appearance

Adult fibrosarcoma is a circumscribed, firm, white or tan mass. Haemorrhage and necrosis can be seen in high-grade tumours.

Histopathology

Adult fibrosarcoma is composed of relatively monomorphic spindle cells, showing no more than a moderate degree of pleomorphism. The tumour cells are characteristically arranged in long, sweeping fascicles that may be angled in a chevron-like or herringbone pattern. Storiform areas can be focally present. The cells have tapering hyperchromatic nuclei with variably prominent nucleoli and scant cytoplasm. Mitotic activity is almost always present but variable. The stroma has variable collagen, from a delicate intercellular network to paucicellular areas with diffuse or keloid-like sclerosis or hyalinization. Some adult fibrosarcomas may contain relatively bland zones mimicking fibromatosis. By immunohistochemistry, adult fibrosarcomas may occasionally show limited expression of SMA or calponin, representing focal myofibroblastic differentiation. CD34-positive tumours showing fibrosarcoma morphology typically represent fibrosarcomatous dermatofibrosarcoma protuberans or high-risk solitary fibrous tumours.

Cytology

Not clinically relevant

Diagnostic molecular pathology

Not clinically relevant

Essential and desirable diagnostic criteria

Essential: relatively monomorphic spindle cells showing no more than moderate nuclear pleomorphism; fascicular, herringbone architecture with variable collagen production; an immunohistochemical and molecular genetic diagnosis of exclusion.

Staging

Union for International Cancer Control (UICC) or American Joint Committee on Cancer (AJCC) staging would be appropriate.

Prognosis and prediction

More than 80% of strictly defined adult fibrosarcomas are high-grade {203}, with an overall survival rate of < 70% at 2 years and < 55% at 5 years. These sarcomas metastasize to lungs and bone, especially the axial skeleton, and rarely to lymph nodes. It is likely that behaviour is related to grade, tumour size, and depth, although data are limited {203}. The probability of local recurrence relates to completeness of excision.

Myxofibrosarcoma

Huang HY
Mentzel TDW
Shibata T

Definition
Myxofibrosarcoma comprises a spectrum of malignant fibroblastic neoplasms with variably myxoid stroma, pleomorphism, and a distinctive curvilinear vascular pattern.

ICD-O coding
8811/3 Myxofibrosarcoma

ICD-11 coding
2B53.0 Myxofibrosarcoma, primary site

Related terminology
Not recommended: myxoid malignant fibrous histiocytoma.

Subtype(s)
Epithelioid myxofibrosarcoma

Localization
The majority of myxofibrosarcomas arise in the limbs, including the limb girdles (in the lower extremities more commonly than in the upper extremities), whereas they are seen only rarely on the trunk, in the head and neck area, and on the hands and feet. Notably, more than half of cases occur in dermal/subcutaneous tissues, with the remainder involving the underlying fascia and skeletal muscle {2080,1428}. Origin in the retroperitoneum and in the abdominal cavity is extremely uncommon, and most lesions with myxofibrosarcoma-like features in these locations represent dedifferentiated liposarcomas {1427,2873}.

Clinical features
Most patients present with a slowly enlarging and painless mass.

Epidemiology
Myxofibrosarcoma is one of the most common sarcomas of elderly patients, with a slight male predominance. Although the overall age range is wide, these neoplasms mainly affect patients in the sixth to eighth decades of life, whereas they only exceptionally rarely arise in patients aged < 30 years {2080,2731,1798}.

Etiology
Unknown

Pathogenesis
Karyotypes are highly complex, with intratumoural heterogeneity and chromosome numbers in the triploid or tetraploid range in most cases, including even grade 1 neoplasms {2080}. Progression in grade is accompanied by an increase in cytogenetic aberrations. Local recurrences may show more complex cytogenetic aberrations than the primary neoplasms, suggesting tumour progression {3293}.

Recent integrated genomic studies indicate a predominance of somatic copy-number alterations in myxofibrosarcoma, with

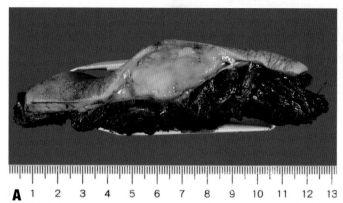

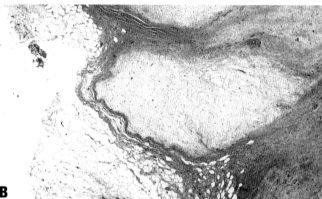

Fig. 1.134 Myxofibrosarcoma. **A** Subcutaneous myxofibrosarcoma. Superficially located, high-grade myxofibrosarcoma with a multinodular growth pattern and a soft, gelatinous, myxoid cut surface. **B** A low-grade myxofibrosarcoma showing multinodular and highly infiltrative growth with a prominent myxoid matrix (shown here) is characterized by the following features: a hypocellular appearance with atypical fibroblastic cells with hyperchromatic, pleomorphic nuclei and elongated, curvilinear blood vessels (shown in Fig. 1.135A) and pseudolipoblasts (shown in Fig. 1.135B).

comparatively lower mutation burdens than many other pleomorphic sarcoma types {224,472,2357}. These include frequent gains of chromosome 5p, where several oncogenes (*TRIO*, *RICTOR*, *SKP2*, and *AMACR*) are variably coamplified and potentially associated with increased grade {1838,1837,1343,2366}. Occurring almost mutually exclusively, genetic aberrations in p53 signalling and the cell-cycle G1/S checkpoint collectively play a central pathogenetic role in half of myxofibrosarcomas; *TP53* (46%; most frequently mutated), *RB1* (18%), and *CDKN2A/CDKN2B* (16%) tumour suppressor gene mutations are more common than *CDK6*, *CCND1*, and *MDM2* amplifications {2357}. Components of driver regulomic pathways also harbour recurrently altered targets, such as missense mutation and amplification of *NTRK1* and loss-of-function mutations and homozygous deletion of *NF1* in the RTK/RAS/MAPK pathway and amplification of *VGLL3* in the Hippo pathway {224,472,2357}, as well as amplifications of *TRIO* and *RICTOR* that activate the RAC/PAK and AKT/mTOR pathways, respectively {1343,2366}.

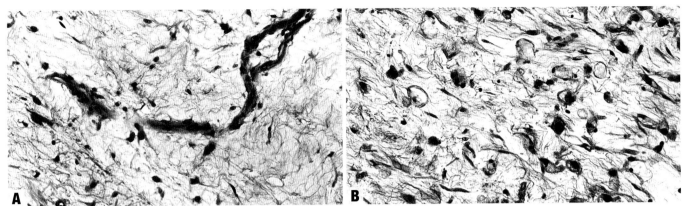

Fig. 1.135 Myxofibrosarcoma, low-grade. A low-grade myxofibrosarcoma showing multinodular and highly infiltrative growth with a prominent myxoid matrix (shown in Fig. 1.134B) is characterized by the following features: a hypocellular appearance with atypical fibroblastic cells with hyperchromatic, pleomorphic nuclei and elongated, curvilinear blood vessels (**A**) and pseudolipoblasts (**B**).

Macroscopic appearance

Superficially located neoplasms typically consist of multiple, variably gelatinous or firmer nodules, whereas deep-seated neoplasms often form a single mass with an infiltrative margin. In high-grade lesions, areas of tumour necrosis are often found.

Histopathology

Myxofibrosarcoma shows a broad spectrum of cellularity, pleomorphism, and proliferative activity; however, all cases share distinct morphological features, particularly multinodular growth with incomplete fibrous septa and myxoid stroma. Subcutaneous examples commonly have very infiltrative margins, often extending beyond what is detected clinically {2080,1428}. The low-grade end of the morphological spectrum is characterized by hypocellular neoplasms composed of only a few, non-cohesive, plump spindled or stellate tumour cells with ill-defined, slightly eosinophilic cytoplasm and atypical, enlarged, hyperchromatic nuclei. Mitotic figures are infrequent in low-grade lesions. A characteristic finding is the presence of prominent elongated, curvilinear, thin-walled blood vessels with a perivascular condensation of tumour cells and/or inflammatory cells (mainly lymphocytes and plasma cells). Frequently, so-called pseudolipoblasts containing cytoplasmic mucin are noted in the form of vacuolated neoplastic fibroblastic cells. In contrast, high-grade neoplasms are composed partly of solid sheets and cellular fascicles of spindled and pleomorphic tumour cells with numerous, often atypical mitoses, areas of haemorrhage, and necrosis. In many cases, bizarre, multinucleated giant cells with abundant eosinophilic cytoplasm (resembling myoid cells) and irregularly shaped nuclei are noted. However, high-grade lesions also focally show features of a lower-grade neoplasm, with a prominent myxoid matrix and numerous elongated capillaries. The intermediate-grade lesions are more cellular and pleomorphic relative to purely low-grade neoplasms, but they lack well-developed solid areas, pronounced cellular pleomorphism, and necrosis.

The rare epithelioid subtype of myxofibrosarcoma is composed predominantly of atypical epithelioid tumour cells with abundant eosinophilic cytoplasm and round vesicular nuclei arranged in small cohesive clusters in the myxoid areas or forming sheets in the hypercellular areas, mimicking metastatic

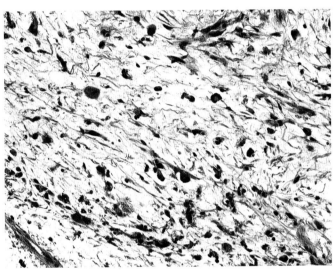

Fig. 1.136 Myxofibrosarcoma, intermediate-grade. Intermediate-grade myxofibrosarcomas retain myxoid stroma and the characteristic vascular pattern, but they are more cellular and pleomorphic than low-grade lesions.

carcinoma or melanoma {2250}. By immunohistochemistry, focal SMA and/or CD34 reactivity is occasionally seen in myxofibrosarcoma, whereas desmin and S100 are negative.

Cytology
Not clinically relevant

Diagnostic molecular pathology
Not clinically relevant

Essential and desirable diagnostic criteria
Essential: multinodular architecture with infiltrative margins; myxoid stroma; variably prominent pleomorphic cells; distinctive curvilinear vessels; hypercellular areas in higher-grade tumours.

Staging
The Union for International Cancer Control (UICC) or American Joint Committee on Cancer (AJCC) TNM system is applicable.

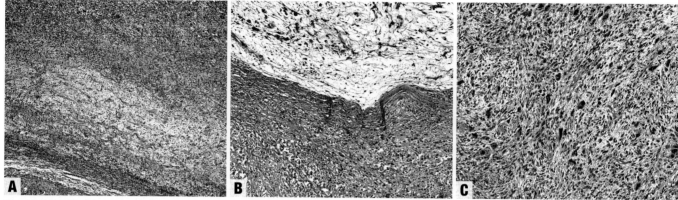

Fig. 1.137 Myxofibrosarcoma, high-grade. **A** A component of the tumour with myxoid stroma and the typical vasculature is required to differentiate high-grade myxofibrosarcoma from undifferentiated pleomorphic sarcoma. **B** A high-grade solid component resembling undifferentiated pleomorphic sarcoma is seen (bottom), juxtaposed to a myxoid area exhibiting typical features of myxofibrosarcoma (top). **C** Frequent pleomorphic giant cells with eosinophilic cytoplasm are present in the high-grade component, mimicking high-grade undifferentiated pleomorphic sarcoma.

Prognosis and prediction

Local, often repeated recurrences, unrelated to histological grade, occur in 30–40% of cases, usually as a result of inadequate surgery, sometimes even in experienced hands.

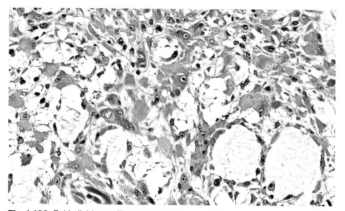

Fig. 1.138 Epithelioid myxofibrosarcoma, high-grade. Note the large, somewhat discohesive epithelioid cells with copious eosinophilic cytoplasm.

Metastases and tumour-related mortality are closely related to tumour grade. The overall 5-year mortality rate is 30–35%. Although none of the low-grade neoplasms metastasize, high-grade tumours develop metastases in 20–35% of cases. In addition to pulmonary and osseous metastases, lymph node metastases are sometimes seen {1428,2731,1798}. Local recurrence within 12 months increases tumour-associated mortality {2080}. Given the propensity for relentless local recurrence associated with highly infiltrative growth, aggressive surgery combined with radiotherapy is advised for myxofibrosarcoma in order to achieve improved local control, which may translate into survival benefits {375}. Compared with other high-grade pleomorphic sarcomas of somatic soft tissue, intermediate-grade and high-grade myxofibrosarcomas have a lower metastatic rate {1428,2731,1798}. Tumour size, morphological grade (inversely related to the percentage of the myxoid component), and surgical margins are significant predictors of survival {2731, 1798}. The epithelioid subtype of myxofibrosarcoma behaves more aggressively, with an increased risk of metastasis (> 50%) {2250}.

Low-grade fibromyxoid sarcoma

Doyle LA
Mertens F

Definition

Low-grade fibromyxoid sarcoma is a malignant fibroblastic neoplasm characterized by alternating collagenous and myxoid areas, deceptively bland spindle cells with a whorling growth pattern, and arcades of small blood vessels. These tumours consistently have either *FUS-CREB3L2* or *FUS-CREB3L1* gene fusions.

ICD-O coding

8840/3 Low-grade fibromyxoid sarcoma

ICD-11 coding

2B5F.2 & XH4V76 Sarcoma, not elsewhere classified of other specified sites & Low-grade fibromyxoid sarcoma

Related terminology

Not recommended: hyalinizing spindle cell tumour with giant rosettes.

Subtype(s)

None

Localization

The most common sites of involvement are the proximal extremities and trunk, usually subfascial in depth {945,1245,2602}. Less common locations include central body sites (abdominal cavity, retroperitoneum, mediastinum) and superficial soft tissues, with the latter being affected relatively more commonly in children {1510,1776,3121,323}. Origin at other anatomical sites is rare.

Clinical features

Presentation is typically with a painless mass. In many cases, the mass has reportedly been present for > 5 years.

Epidemiology

Although relatively rare among sarcomas, the true incidence of low-grade fibromyxoid sarcoma may have been underestimated before the availability of ancillary diagnostic markers and due to its propensity to mimic other soft tissue neoplasms histologically. There is a slight male predilection, and tumours typically arise in young adults, but the overall age range is wide, and as

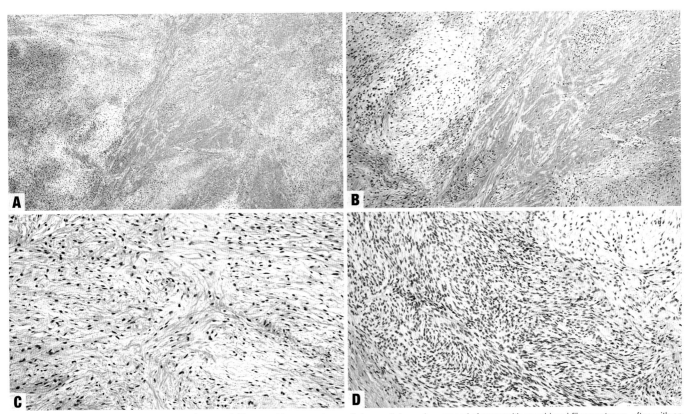

Fig. 1.139 Low-grade fibromyxoid sarcoma. **A** Low-grade fibromyxoid sarcoma is usually hypocellular and composed of areas with myxoid and fibrous stroma, often with an abrupt transition between the two areas. **B** Higher power showing the distinct fibrous and myxoid areas. **C** The tumour cells are spindled and cytologically bland and grow in short fascicles or in a storiform pattern. **D** Areas of hypercellularity.

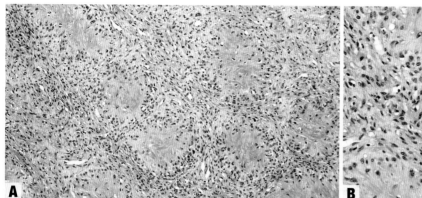
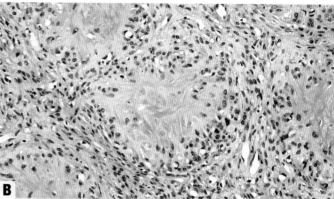

Fig. 1.140 Low-grade fibromyxoid sarcoma. **A** An example with giant collagen rosettes. **B** The tumour cells surround nodules of hyaline collagen.

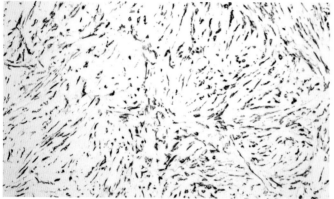

Fig. 1.141 Low-grade fibromyxoid sarcoma. Diffuse strong cytoplasmic expression of MUC4.

many as 20% of cases occur in patients aged < 18 years {323, 945,1055,1245,1189}.

Etiology
Unknown

Pathogenesis
The cytogenetic hallmark of low-grade fibromyxoid sarcoma is the t(7;16)(q33;p11), which is present, often as the sole change, in two thirds of cases. Another 25% show supernumerary ring chromosomes {2592,2426,2094}. Both aberrations result in fusion of the 5′ part of the FUS gene in 16p11 with the 3′ part of CREB3L2 in 7q33; a chimeric FUS-CREB3L2 transcript is seen in > 90% of cases {2094,2018,1245,2170}. Rare cases have one of the fusion variants FUS-CREB3L1 or EWSR1-CREB3L1 {2094,1770,2684}. Apart from recurrent microdeletions in association with the t(7;16) chromosomal breakpoints and gain of 7q in cases with ring chromosomes, no recurrent genomic imbalances or single-nucleotide variants have been found in low-grade fibromyxoid sarcoma {2170,152}. The chimeric FUS-CREB3L2 protein functions as an aberrant transcription factor, causing deregulated expression of CREB3L2 target genes {2170}. Many of these target genes, such as CD24 and MUC4, are shared with sclerosing epithelioid fibrosarcoma, with which low-grade fibromyxoid sarcoma overlaps with regard to underlying gene fusions but differs with regard to additional genomic imbalances {152}.

Macroscopic appearance
Grossly, low-grade fibromyxoid sarcomas are well-circumscribed, fibrous, and often focally mucoid. Tumour size ranges from 1 to > 20 cm in greatest dimension.

Histopathology
Low-grade fibromyxoid sarcoma is composed of collagenous hypocellular areas and more-cellular myxoid nodules. An abrupt transition between these two areas is typical. The tumour cells are bland, spindled, and sometimes plump, and they grow in short fascicles or in a whorling pattern. Mitotic activity is generally inconspicuous. Arcades of small vessels and arteriole-sized vessels with perivascular sclerosis are seen. Occasionally, the vessels have a haemangiopericytoma-like pattern {852}. Approximately 30% of cases contain collagen rosettes – a central core of hyalinized collagen surrounded by a cuff of epithelioid tumour cells {1055,1743}. In some cases, areas of sclerosing epithelioid fibrosarcoma are present, reflecting the overlap between these two entities {852,945,1245,2602,3240}. Unusual features (< 10% of cases) include the presence of focal pleomorphism or nuclear atypia, hypercellularity, epithelioid or round cell features, and heterotopic ossification {852,945,1245}. By immunohistochemistry, tumour cells show strong, diffuse cytoplasmic expression of MUC4, an epithelial glycoprotein, in approximately 99% of cases {852}. MUC4 is highly sensitive and specific for low-grade fibromyxoid sarcoma and sclerosing epithelioid fibrosarcoma among fibroblastic and neural tumours. Expression of EMA is present in 80% of cases and focal expression of SMA in approximately 30% {852,1245,1055}.

Cytology
Not clinically relevant

Diagnostic molecular pathology
If MUC4 is negative or not available to confirm the diagnosis, identification of FUS-CREB3L2 (or other rare variants) offers molecular genetic support for the diagnosis.

Essential and desirable diagnostic criteria
Essential: alternating fibrous and myxoid areas; bland spindle cells in a whorled or short fascicular growth pattern; diffuse strong MUC4 expression (in nearly all cases).
Desirable: FUS gene rearrangement (in selected cases).

Staging

American Joint Committee on Cancer (AJCC) eighth-edition staging is appropriate

Prognosis and prediction

Although low-grade fibromyxoid sarcoma shows low rates of recurrence and metastasis in the first 5 years after excision of the primary tumour (10% and 5%, respectively), rates are much higher with long-term follow-up {323,944,943,945,1055,1189, 1245}. A large study with long follow-up showed recurrences, metastases, and death from disease in 64%, 45%, and 42% of patients, respectively {945}. Metastases occurred as long as 45 years after primary excision (median: 5 years), and the median interval to tumour-related death was 15 years {945}. The most common metastatic sites are lung and pleura. Histological features generally do not correlate with clinical behaviour {945,1055}, although tumours with areas of sclerosing epithelioid fibrosarcoma or round cell morphology tend to pursue a more aggressive clinical course {945}, similar to that expected for sclerosing epithelioid fibrosarcoma.

Sclerosing epithelioid fibrosarcoma

Doyle LA
Mertens F

Definition
Sclerosing epithelioid fibrosarcoma is a rare malignant fibroblastic neoplasm characterized by epithelioid fibroblasts arranged in cords and nests and embedded in a dense sclerotic hyalinized stroma. A subset of sclerosing epithelioid fibrosarcomas are related morphologically and molecularly to low-grade fibromyxoid sarcoma.

ICD-O coding
8840/3 Sclerosing epithelioid fibrosarcoma

ICD-11 coding
2B5F.2 & XH4BT2 Sarcoma, not elsewhere classified of other specified sites & Sclerosing epithelioid fibrosarcoma

Related terminology
None

Subtype(s)
None

Localization
Tumours are deep-seated and arise most often in the upper or lower extremities or limb girdle, followed by the trunk and the head and neck {136,2065,1042}. Rarely, tumours arise in the pelvis, retroperitoneum, viscera, or bone {3251,3302,161}.

Clinical features
Most patients present with a mass of variable duration, with one third reporting recent enlargement or pain {2065}.

Epidemiology
Sclerosing epithelioid fibrosarcoma usually arises in middle-aged and elderly adults, with an equal sex distribution {2065}.

Etiology
Unknown

Pathogenesis
Sclerosing epithelioid fibrosarcoma usually displays a near-diploid karyotype with multiple chromosomal rearrangements. Tumours consistently harbour translocations resulting in gene fusions, the most frequent (> 60%) of which is *EWSR1-CREB3L1* {855,153,2952,2544,850}. In rare cases, *EWSR1* is exchanged for *FUS* or *PAX5* and/or *CREB3L1* for *CREB3L2*, *CREB3L3*, or *CREM* {809,152}. The most common of these variant fusion partners is *FUS*, which is involved in 10% of cases with pure sclerosing epithelioid fibrosarcoma morphology {1245,3240,2544}. Furthermore, most so-called hybrid sclerosing epithelioid fibrosarcomas / low-grade fibromyxoid sarcomas display a *FUS-CREB3L2* chimera, identical to that seen in most low-grade fibromyxoid sarcomas. Sclerosing epithelioid fibrosarcoma and

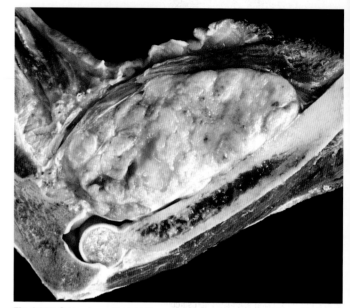

Fig. 1.142 Sclerosing epithelioid fibrosarcoma. Deep, large sclerosing epithelioid fibrosarcoma of the upper arm.

low-grade fibromyxoid sarcoma also have overlapping gene expression profiles, for example, with high expression of MUC4 and CD24 in both tumours {2170,152}. In contrast to low-grade fibromyxoid sarcoma, however, both pure and hybrid sclerosing epithelioid fibrosarcoma cases typically have complex genomic profiles, including deletions / copy-neutral loss of heterozygosity at chromosome arm 11p, loss of chromosome 22, and intragenic deletions of the *DMD* gene {152}. No recurrent single-nucleotide variant has been detected {152}. A small subset of sclerosing epithelioid fibrosarcomas do not have MUC4 expression or harbour any of the above fusion genes; little is known about the molecular pathogenesis of this group.

Macroscopic appearance
Sclerosing epithelioid fibrosarcoma is usually well circumscribed, is lobular or multilobulated, and involves deep musculature and fascia. Periosteal adherence is common, and there is occasionally erosion of underlying bone. The cut surface is firm and white. Areas of calcification may be present. Most tumours are < 10 cm, but occasional cases measure > 20 cm {136,2065}.

Histopathology
The margins of sclerosing epithelioid fibrosarcoma are typically infiltrative into muscle, fascia, or periosteum. A characteristic feature is a prominent hyalinized sclerotic collagenous stroma, within which relatively bland and monomorphic epithelioid cells are arranged in cords, nests, or occasionally sheets. Some tumours contain more cellular fascicular areas. Pseudoalveolar

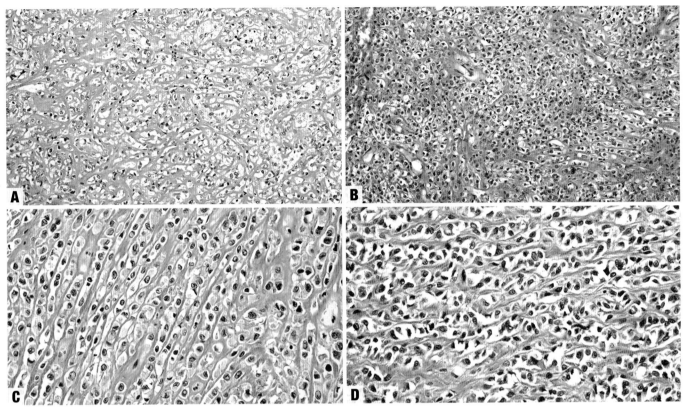

Fig. 1.143 Sclerosing epithelioid fibrosarcoma. **A** Low power shows small nests and cords of epithelioid cells in a dense sclerotic stroma. **B** Sclerosing epithelioid fibrosarcoma with areas of solid growth and less-dense stroma. **C** Classic growth pattern of sclerosing epithelioid fibrosarcoma. This image shows cords and strands of epithelioid cells with pale cytoplasm and round to oval nuclei. **D** Classic growth pattern of sclerosing epithelioid fibrosarcoma. This image shows epithelioid cells arranged in trabeculae with a pseudoalveolar pattern.

or acinar growth patterns are occasionally seen. Hypocellular areas with myxoid or fibrous stroma are common. The tumour cells usually have clear cytoplasm and inconspicuous nucleoli.

Unusual features include marked pleomorphism, necrosis, prominent mitotic activity, and haemangiopericytoma-like vessels {136,2065,951,855}. Calcifications or chondro-osseous differentiation may be seen. Areas of conventional low-grade fibromyxoid sarcoma may be present {2544,855}. Rarely, the sclerotic stroma is absent in large areas of the tumour in either sclerosing epithelioid fibrosarcoma or low-grade fibromyxoid

sarcoma, making recognition difficult {2551,945}. Clues to the diagnosis in such cases include the relatively monomorphic appearance of the tumour cells and the presence of MUC4 expression in the absence of keratin expression, which would be unusual for carcinoma.

MUC4 expression is present in 80–90% of cases and is strong, diffuse, and cytoplasmic {855}. Expression of EMA and SMA is present in approximately 40% of cases. Keratins are typically negative, which is helpful in the differential diagnosis with carcinoma {136,1042}.

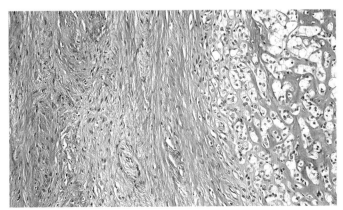

Fig. 1.144 Sclerosing epithelioid fibrosarcoma. Sclerosing epithelioid fibrosarcoma showing abrupt transition to areas of low-grade fibromyxoid sarcoma.

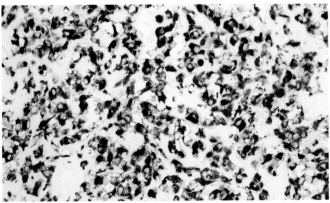

Fig. 1.145 Sclerosing epithelioid fibrosarcoma. Diffuse strong cytoplasmic expression of MUC4 in sclerosing epithelioid fibrosarcoma.

Cytology
Not clinically relevant

Diagnostic molecular pathology
Demonstration of *EWSR1-CREB3L1* or other rearrangements can help confirm the diagnosis. For cases with characteristic morphology and MUC4 expression, additional molecular studies are not needed.

Essential and desirable diagnostic criteria
Essential: epithelioid cells arranged in cords, nests, or trabeculae and embedded in a dense sclerotic hyalinized stroma; diffuse strong MUC4 expression (in most cases); keratin-negative.
Desirable: *EWSR1-CREB3L1* or other rearrangements (in selected cases).

Staging
Union for International Cancer Control (UICC) or American Joint Committee on Cancer (AJCC) staging is appropriate.

Prognosis and prediction
Sclerosing epithelioid fibrosarcoma pursues a more aggressive clinical course than the related low-grade fibromyxoid sarcoma, with recurrences (often multiple) in about 50% of cases. Metastases are common, occurring in 40–50% of cases to lung, pleura, bone, and brain. Poor prognostic features include large tumour size and proximal location {136,2065}. Whether sclerosing epithelioid fibrosarcoma that arises in the context of low-grade fibromyxoid sarcoma has the same prognosis has not yet been established.

Tenosynovial giant cell tumour

de Saint Aubain Somerhausen N
van de Rijn M

Definition

The term "tenosynovial giant cell tumour" encompasses a group of lesions most often arising from the synovium of joints, bursae, and tendon sheaths and showing synovial differentiation. The very uncommon malignant tenosynovial giant cell tumour is defined by the coexistence of a benign tenosynovial giant cell tumour with overtly malignant areas or by recurrence of a typical giant cell tumour as a sarcoma.

ICD-O coding

9252/0 Tenosynovial giant cell tumour NOS

ICD-11 coding

2F7Z & XH0HZ1 Neoplasms of uncertain behaviour of unspecified site & Tenosynovial giant cell tumour NOS

2F7Z & XH6911 Neoplasms of uncertain behaviour of unspecified site & Tenosynovial giant cell tumour, localized

2F7Z & XH52J9 Neoplasms of uncertain behaviour of unspecified site & Tenosynovial giant cell tumour, diffuse

2D4Y & XH5AQ9 Other specified malignant neoplasms of ill-defined or unspecified primary sites & Malignant tenosynovial giant cell tumour

Related terminology

Acceptable: giant cell tumour of tendon sheath.
Not recommended: pigmented villonodular synovitis.

Subtype(s)

Tenosynovial giant cell tumour, diffuse; malignant tenosynovial giant cell tumour

Localization

Localized giant cell tumours occur predominantly in the hand. Approximately 85% of the tumours occur in the fingers, in close proximity to the synovium of the tendon sheath or interphalangeal joint. The lesions may rarely erode bone or involve the skin. Other sites include the wrist, ankle, foot, knee, and rarely the elbow and hip. Rarely, localized lesions may be found in large joints {2173,2005,3138}. Intra-articular diffuse-type giant cell

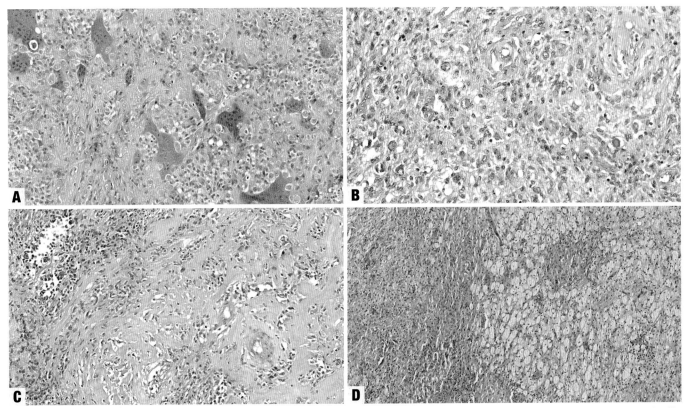

Fig. 1.146 Tenosynovial giant cell tumour, localized type. **A** Tumours are composed of an admixture of small histiocyte-like cells, larger epithelioid cells, and osteoclast-like giant cells. **B** The cytoplasm of larger mononuclear cells often contains a peripheral rim of haemosiderin. **C** The stroma shows variable degrees of hyalinization. **D** Collections of foamy histiocytes are common.

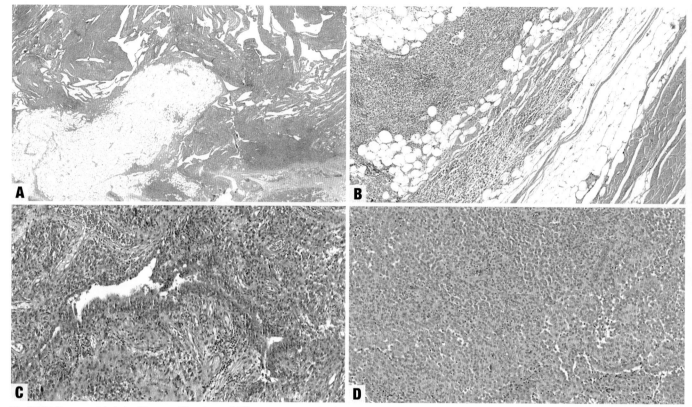

Fig. 1.147 Tenosynovial giant cell tumour, diffuse type. **A** Villous appearance of an intra-articular tumour. **B** Purely extra-articular tumour infiltrating muscular and adipose tissue. **C** Pseudosynovial clefts are common. **D** Osteoclast-like giant cells may be absent or extremely rare in the diffuse type.

tumours most commonly affect the knee (75% of cases), followed by the hip (15%), ankle, elbow, and shoulder {2787,2399, 3323,2005}. Rare cases are reported in the temporomandibular and spinal facet joints {481}. Extra-articular tumours most commonly involve the knee region, thigh, and foot. Uncommon locations include the finger, wrist, groin, elbow, and toe. Most extra-articular tumours are located in periarticular soft tissues, but these lesions can be purely intramuscular or subcutaneous {2904}. Most malignant tenosynovial giant cell tumours involve the lower limbs, with a strong predilection for the knee. Other locations include the hip, ankle, fingers, wrist, and pelvic area {69,2243,297,1839}.

Clinical features

These tumours are usually divided according to their site (intra- or extra-articular) and growth pattern (localized or diffuse) into two main subtypes, which differ in their clinical features and biological behaviour but appear to share a common pathogenesis. Localized-type giant cell tumours present as a painless mass that develops gradually over a long period; a preoperative duration of several years is often mentioned. Diffuse-type giant cell tumours are associated with pain, tenderness, swelling, or limitation of motion. Haemorrhagic joint effusions are common. The symptoms are usually of relatively long duration (often several years) {2904,2459,2399}. Repeated local recurrences can be destructive, leading to major functional loss {2629}. Radiographically, most tumours present as ill-defined periarticular masses, frequently associated with degenerative joint disease and cystic lesions in the adjacent bone (often on both sides of

the joint). On MRI, giant cell tumours show decreased signal intensity in both T1- and T2-weighted images, with artefacts from haemosiderin deposition {2224,1921}. Malignant tenosynovial giant cell tumours can arise de novo or occur after multiple recurrences of a conventional tenosynovial giant cell tumour {2004,69,2243,297,1839}.

Epidemiology

The estimated incidence rates in digits, localized-extremity, and diffuse tenosynovial giant cell tumours are 29, 10, and 4 cases per 1 million person-years, respectively {2005}. The localized form is more common than the diffuse form of tenosynovial giant cell tumour. Tumours may occur at any age, but they usually occur in patients aged 30–50 years, with a female predominance (M:F ratio: 0.5:1) {15,2005,3138}. The diffuse type usually affects young adults (< 40 years of age). There is a slight female predominance {2904,2399,2231}. Malignant tenosynovial giant cell tumour is exceedingly uncommon, with only 50 reported cases. Most patients are adults aged 50–60 years {69,2243, 297,1839}.

Etiology
Unknown

Pathogenesis
Cytogenetic studies have demonstrated relatively simple structural changes that most often involve a translocation of the *CSF1* gene, encoding colony stimulating factor 1 (CSF1). Cells with this translocation synthesize large amounts of the CSF1 protein.

Within tumours that have this translocation, only a small subset of cells actually harbour the translocation, with the majority of the cells that make up the tumour mass consisting of macrophages that are apparently there as a result of the high CSF1 levels {693,3277,2003}.

Macroscopic appearance
Grossly, most tenosynovial giant cell tumours of localized type are small (0.5–4 cm), although lesions of greater size may be found in large joints. Tumours are well circumscribed and typically lobulated and white to grey with yellowish and brown areas. Diffuse-type tenosynovial giant cell tumours are usually large (often > 5 cm), firm, or sponge-like. The villous pattern is usually present in intra-articular tumours, whereas extra-articular tumours have a multinodular appearance and a variegated colour, with alternation of white, yellowish, and brownish areas {2224}. Malignant tenosynovial giant cell tumours are usually large, fleshy, and poorly circumscribed, with areas of haemorrhage and necrosis {1839,69}.

Histopathology
The microscopic appearance of tenosynovial giant cell tumours is variable, depending on the proportions of mononuclear cells, multinucleated giant cells, foamy macrophages, inflammatory cells, and haemosiderin, as well as the degree of collagenization of the stroma. Two principal cell types are identified within the mononuclear component: small histiocyte-like cells, with pale cytoplasm and round or reniform nuclei, and larger epithelioid cells, with amphophilic cytoplasm and rounded vesicular nuclei. These larger cells often contain a peripheral rim of haemosiderin granules. Most tumours contain a majority of small histiocyte-like cells, but larger cells may predominate. In both types, mitotic activity may be brisk. Necrosis can be present. Chondroid metaplasia can be seen in tenosynovial giant cell tumours of the temporomandibular joint {2346,1383}.

Localized-type tenosynovial giant cell tumours are lobulated and well circumscribed. Osteoclast-like giant cells are usually readily apparent, but they may be inconspicuous in some tumours. Xanthoma cells are frequent, tend to aggregate locally near the periphery of nodules, and may be associated with cholesterol clefts. Haemosiderin deposits are virtually always identified. The stroma shows variable degrees of hyalinization {2173,1543,3138}.

Diffuse-type tenosynovial giant cell tumours are infiltrative and grow as diffuse, expansile sheets. Osteoclast-like giant cells are less common in the diffuse form than in the localized form, and they may be absent or extremely rare in as many as 20% of cases. Cleft-like spaces are common and appear either as artefactual tears or as synovial-lined spaces. Blood-filled pseudoalveolar spaces are seen in approximately 10% of cases {2904,3138,2224}.

Most malignant tenosynovial giant cell tumours are composed of sheets and nodules of enlarged mononuclear cells. These neoplasms tend to show significantly increased mitotic count, including atypical mitoses, necrosis, enlarged nuclei with nucleoli, spindling of mononucleated cells, and myxoid changes. Less commonly, these tumours contain areas resembling undifferentiated pleomorphic sarcoma or myxofibrosarcoma {69,2243,297,1839}.

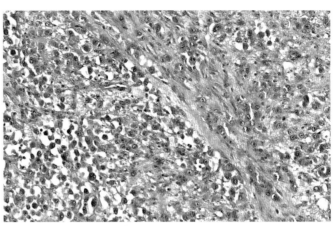
Fig. 1.148 Malignant tenosynovial giant cell tumour. Sheets of large mononuclear cells, with enlarged nuclei and increased mitotic activity.

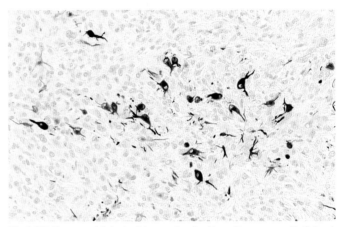
Fig. 1.149 Tenosynovial giant cell tumour, localized type. Some cases of both localized and diffuse types contain numerous desmin-positive mononuclear cells, often with dendritic processes.

The larger mononuclear cells express clusterin, and in 45–80% of cases a small subset of these cells stain for desmin, which highlights their dendritic processes. The smaller histiocyte-like cells are positive for CD68, CD163, and CD45. Multinucleated giant cells display an osteoclastic phenotype {354, 2342}.

Cytology
The presence of large mononuclear cells with eccentric nuclei, finely granulated cytoplasm, and a cytoplasmic rim of haemosiderin is distinctive {3400}.

Diagnostic molecular pathology
Not clinically relevant

Essential and desirable diagnostic criteria
Essential: intra- or extra-articular location; varying proportions of small histiocytic cells, large amphophilic cells, foam cells, multinucleated giant cells.
Desirable: demonstration of *CSF1* rearrangement (selected cases).

Staging

Not clinically relevant

Prognosis and prediction

Tenosynovial giant cell tumour of localized type is a benign lesion with a capacity for local recurrence. Although 4–30% of cases recur, these recurrences are usually non-destructive and are controlled by surgical re-excision {2005,3138,2173,1543}. Recurrences are more common in diffuse-type tumours, and repeated recurrences may severely compromise joint function. The recurrence rate has been estimated at 40–60% {2004}. In addition, rare cases with benign histology may develop metastatic disease (in the lungs or lymph nodes) {2005,2904,2399, 2459}. Malignant tenosynovial giant cell tumour is an aggressive neoplasm, with substantial mortality (roughly one third of cases). Approximately 50% of cases metastasize to lymph nodes (inguinal and pelvic) and the lungs {69,2243,297,1839}. Surgery is the mainstay of the treatment of tenosynovial tumours. Molecular targeted therapy targeting the CSF1/CSF1R pathway has shown promising results for unresectable or metastasizing tumours {339,510,511}.

Deep fibrous histiocytoma

Jo VY

Definition
Deep fibrous histiocytoma is a morphologically benign fibrous histiocytoma that arises entirely within subcutaneous or deep soft tissue and that may occasionally metastasize.

ICD-O coding
8831/0 Deep benign fibrous histiocytoma

ICD-11 coding
2F7C & XH5DP4 Neoplasms of uncertain behaviour of connective or other soft tissue & Deep benign fibrous histiocytoma
2F23.0 Dermatofibroma

Related terminology
None

Subtype(s)
None

Localization
The most common site is the extremities, representing more than half of cases, followed by the head and neck region. Most deep fibrous histiocytomas are subcutaneous, but nearly 10% arise in visceral soft tissue (e.g. retroperitoneum, mediastinum, pelvis) {1015,1165}. Intramuscular tumours are uncommon, and tumours arising in visceral organs are exceedingly rare {2709}.

Clinical features
Most lesions present as a painless, slowly enlarging mass {1165}.

Epidemiology
Deep-seated fibrous histiocytomas are rare, accounting for < 1% of fibrohistiocytic tumours {1015}. Patients are affected over a wide age range (6–84 years; median age: 37 years). There is a slight predominance in males.

Etiology
Unknown

Pathogenesis
Rearrangements involving either *PRKCB* or *PRKCD* (members of the gene family encoding PKC) have been identified in all morphological subtypes of benign fibrous histiocytoma, including deep fibrous histiocytoma {2521,3223}. Known fusion partners are genes encoding membrane-associated proteins (*PDPN*, *CD63*, and *LAMTOR1*), resulting in chimeric proteins localizing the catalytic domain of PKC to the cell membrane {2521}.

Macroscopic appearance
These tumours form well-circumscribed nodules, with a median size of 2.5 cm for subcutaneous lesions. Subcutaneous tumours may be observed intraoperatively to be attached to fascia or tendon. Deep-seated lesions may be larger {1165}.

Histopathology
Unlike their cutaneous counterparts, deep fibrous histiocytomas are well circumscribed. The lesions are more cellular than typical cutaneous fibrous histiocytomas, but they share a storiform architecture. A minority of tumours have a predominantly short fascicular pattern – similar to that seen in cellular fibrous histiocytoma in skin – with only focal storiform areas. A branching,

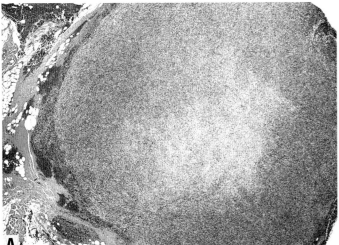 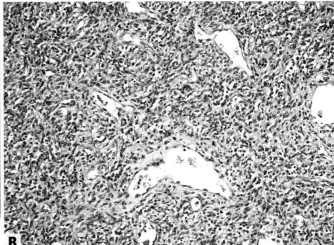

Fig. 1.150 Deep fibrous histiocytoma. **A** Tumours often arise in the subcutis and are well circumscribed, often with a fibrous pseudocapsule. **B** Thin-walled branching (haemangiopericytoma-like) vessels are common.

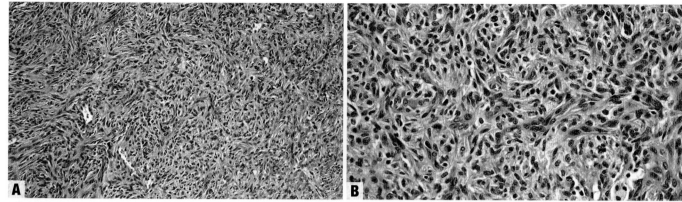

Fig. 1.151 Deep fibrous histiocytoma. **A** Monomorphic storiform pattern is typical. **B** Tumour cells are generally uniform, with less cytological pleomorphism than their dermal counterparts.

haemangiopericytoma-like vascular pattern is common, which may cause confusion with solitary fibrous tumour, particularly when CD34 is expressed. Generally, deep fibrous histiocytoma can be distinguished by its uniform cellularity and storiform architecture. The tumour cells are spindled, with plump, ovoid to elongated vesicular nuclei and indistinct, palely eosinophilic cytoplasm. Nearly half of all deep fibrous histiocytomas are cytologically monomorphic, lacking the foamy histiocytes and giant cells that are often seen in cutaneous lesions. Stromal hyalinization is relatively common; less frequent findings include haemorrhage, myxoid change, cystic degeneration, central infarction, and a peripheral lymphoid infiltrate. There is generally no nuclear pleomorphism or hyperchromasia, although rare examples of atypical deep fibrous histiocytoma (akin to atypical cutaneous fibrous histiocytoma) have been reported {1165}. Tumour necrosis is rare.

CD34 positivity is far more common in deep fibrous histiocytomas than in those in the skin, with 40% of the former expressing this marker, sometimes diffusely {1165}. Such examples may be difficult to distinguish from solitary fibrous tumour; however, deep fibrous histiocytomas are negative for STAT6 {3371,854}. A similar number of cases express SMA, usually focally.

Cytology
Not clinically relevant

Diagnostic molecular pathology
Not clinically relevant

Essential and desirable diagnostic criteria
Essential: well-circumscribed lesion located in subcutaneous or deep/visceral tissue; mixed fascicular and storiform growth pattern; monomorphic population of spindled or histiocytoid cells; branching vessels.

Staging
Not clinically relevant

Prognosis and prediction
Deep fibrous histiocytomas recur locally in approximately 20% of cases, usually if incompletely or marginally excised {1015, 1165}. Metastasis is rare, reported to occur in 5% of cases in a series of 69 cases {1165}, possibly reflecting referral bias.

Plexiform fibrohistiocytic tumour

Brenn T

Definition
Plexiform fibrohistiocytic tumour is a rare dermal and subcutaneous neoplasm showing plexiform architecture and biphasic morphology, composed of nodules of histiocytoid cells and bundles of myofibroblastic spindle cells.

ICD-O coding
8835/1 Plexiform fibrohistiocytic tumour

ICD-11 coding
2F7C & XH4GL1 Neoplasms of uncertain behaviour of connective or other soft tissue & Plexiform fibrohistiocytic tumour

Related terminology
None

Subtype(s)
None

Localization
There is a strong predilection for the upper limbs followed by the lower limbs. The trunk and the head and neck area are less often affected {2186,920,1397}.

Clinical features
The tumours present as slow-growing, ill-defined plaques and nodules, typically measuring 1–3 cm in diameter {920}.

Epidemiology
The age range is wide, but children and young adults are typically affected, with a median age of 14.5–20 years and an equal sex distribution {2186,920,1397,2610}.

Etiology
Unknown

Pathogenesis
Unknown

Macroscopic appearance
These tumours form a nondescript mass at the dermal–subcutaneous junction, usually < 3 cm in size.

Histopathology
Plexiform fibrohistiocytic tumours are centred at the dermal–subcutaneous junction. They show an infiltrative architecture with overall plexiform outlines and may extend into skeletal muscle. The tumours are composed of small nodules of histiocytoid cells and osteoclast-like multinucleated giant cells, surrounded by fascicles of spindle cells in varying proportions. There may

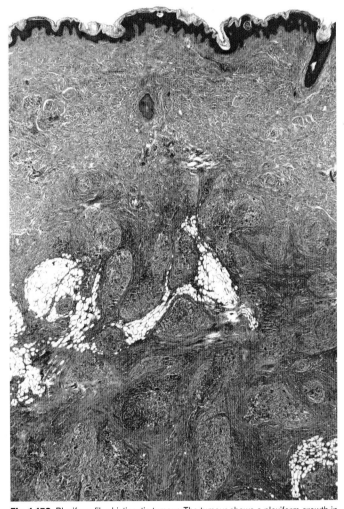

Fig. 1.152 Plexiform fibrohistiocytic tumour. The tumour shows a plexiform growth in deep dermis and subcutaneous adipose tissue.

be haemorrhage, haemosiderin deposition, and a chronic inflammatory infiltrate. Lymphovascular invasion can rarely be seen. Additional rare findings include myxoid or hyalinized stromal changes and metaplastic bone formation. By immunohistochemistry, the spindle cells express SMA {1065}.

Cytology
Not clinically relevant

Diagnostic molecular pathology
Not clinically relevant

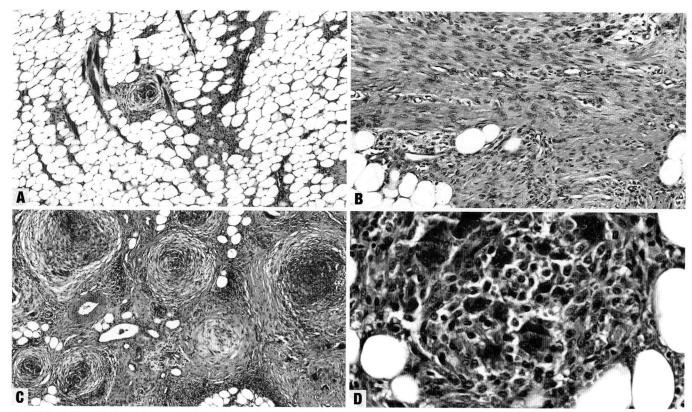

Fig. 1.153 Plexiform fibrohistiocytic tumour. **A** Note the infiltrative tumour growth within subcutaneous adipose tissue and extension into skeletal muscle. **B** Bland-appearing spindle cells are arranged in intersecting fascicles. **C** The distinctive nodules are distributed within adipose tissue in a plexiform distribution. **D** The nodules are composed of bland and uniform epithelioid cells with admixed osteoclast-like multinucleated giant cells.

Essential and desirable diagnostic criteria

Essential: plexiform architecture; involvement of dermis and/or subcutaneous adipose tissue; nodules composed of histiocytoid epithelioid cells and osteoclast-like giant cells; fascicles of myofibroblastic spindle cells.

Staging

Not clinically relevant

Prognosis and prediction

Plexiform fibrohistiocytic tumour is associated with a risk for local recurrence ranging from 12.5% to 37.5% and rare lymph node metastasis {2186,920,1397,2610}. Distant metastasis to the lung is exceptional {2725,2610}.

Giant cell tumour of soft tissue

Oliveira AM
Lee JC

Definition
Giant cell tumour of soft tissue is morphologically similar to but genetically unrelated to giant cell tumour of bone.

ICD-O coding
9251/1 Giant cell tumour of soft parts NOS

ICD-11 coding
2F7C & XH81M1 Neoplasms of uncertain behaviour of connective or other soft tissue & Giant cell tumour of soft parts NOS

Related terminology
Not recommended: giant cell tumour of low malignant potential.

Subtype(s)
None

Localization
Giant cell tumour of soft tissue usually occurs in superficial soft tissues of the upper and lower extremities (70% of tumours). Affected less frequently are the trunk (20%) and head and neck (7%) regions {1058,2345,2372,2488,2643}. Occasional cases have been reported in other anatomical locations {1176,2158, 1645}.

Clinical features
The tumours usually present as painless growing masses {2345, 2372}, with an average duration of 6 months {2372}. Peripheral mineralization is common.

Epidemiology
Giant cell tumour of soft tissue occurs predominantly in the fifth decade of life, but it can affect patients ranging in age from 5 to 89 years. Giant cell tumour of soft tissue shows no apparent difference in incidence with regard to sex or ethnicity {1058, 2345,2372}.

Etiology
Unknown

Pathogenesis
Giant cell tumour of soft tissue lacks the mutations of the *H3-3A* (*H3F3A*) gene that are present in the vast majority of giant cell tumours of bone, suggesting a different pathogenesis {1805, 1961}.

Macroscopic appearance
Tumours range in size from 0.7 to 10 cm (mean: 3 cm) {1058, 2345,2372}. Subcutaneous adipose tissue or dermis is involved in 70% of tumours; 30% are situated deep to superficial fascia. Giant cell tumour of soft tissue is a well-circumscribed, mostly solid, nodular mass with a fleshy, reddish-brown or grey cut surface. Gritty regions of mineralized bone are frequently present at the periphery {2345}.

Histopathology
Giant cell tumour of soft tissue displays a multinodular architecture (85%). Cellular nodules are separated by fibrous septa of varying thickness, containing haemosiderin-laden macrophages {2345}. The nodules are composed of a mixture of round to oval mononuclear cells and osteoclast-like multinucleated giant cells, with both cell types immersed in a richly

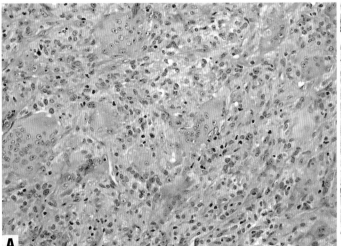 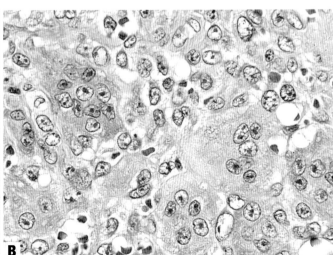

Fig. 1.154 Giant cell tumour of soft tissue. **A** Giant cell tumour of soft tissue is composed of nodules of osteoclast-like multinucleated giant cells intermixed with ovoid mononuclear cells. **B** The cellular nodules contain a mixture of round/oval mononuclear and multinucleated osteoclast-like giant cells.

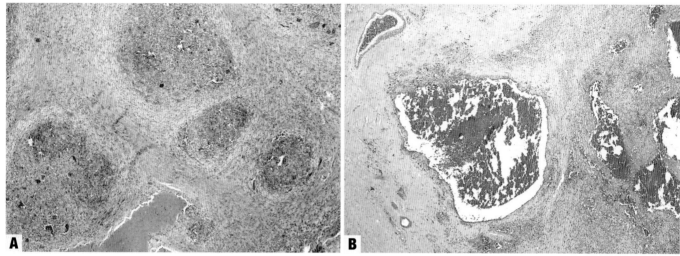

Fig. 1.155 Giant cell tumour of soft tissue. **A** Giant cell tumour of soft tissue shows a characteristic multinodular architecture where clusters of osteoclast-like multinucleated giant cells are often separated by fibrous septa. Metaplastic bone formation is also commonly observed (bottom). **B** Aneurysmal bone cyst–like changes can occur in giant cell tumour of soft tissue.

vascularized stroma. Mitotic activity is readily seen in giant cell tumour of soft tissue {1058,2345,2372}. Nuclear pleomorphism and bizarre giant cells are absent, and necrosis is rarely found {1058,2345,2372}. Metaplastic bone formation is present in approximately 50% of tumours, most often in the form of a peripheral shell of woven bone. Aneurysmal bone cyst–like changes may be seen. Vascular invasion is identified in about 30% of tumours {1058,2372}. Additional histological features include stromal haemorrhage (50%) and regressive changes in the form of marked stromal fibrosis and clusters of foamy macrophages (70%). Immunohistochemistry is not helpful.

Cytology
Not clinically relevant

Diagnostic molecular pathology
Not clinically relevant

Essential and desirable diagnostic criteria
Essential: multinodular superficial soft tissue neoplasm; histiocytoid mononuclear cell population with osteoclastic giant cells; haemosiderin deposition and metaplastic bone formation are commonly observed.

Staging
Not clinically relevant

Prognosis and prediction
Giant cell tumour of soft tissue is associated with a local recurrence rate of 12%, with very rare metastasis {1058,2345,2372}.

Synovial haemangioma

Calonje JE

Definition
Synovial haemangioma is a benign proliferation of blood vessels arising in a synovium-lined surface, including the intra-articular space or a bursa. Similar lesions occurring within the tendon sheath do not fall into this category.

ICD-O coding
9120/0 Haemangioma NOS

ICD-11 coding
2E81.0Y Other specified neoplastic haemangioma

Related terminology
None

Subtype(s)
None

Localization
The most common site is the knee, followed much less commonly by the elbow and hand. Involvement of hip or other joints is exceptional {784}.

Clinical features
The tumour presents as a slow-growing lesion, often associated with swelling and joint effusion {807}. Recurrent haemarthrosis has been reported {490,1864} and recurrent pain is a frequent symptom. Delayed diagnosis causes osteoarthritic damage. In about one third of cases, the lesion is painless. Rarely, destructive growth may be seen {3142}, exceptionally with extra-articular extension, bone involvement, and pathological fracture of bone {5,1399}. MRI is the best radiological technique for diagnosis and for determining the extent of involvement.

Epidemiology
Synovial haemangioma is very rare. Most patients are children or adolescents, and males are affected more commonly than females {807,2217}.

Etiology
Unknown

Pathogenesis
Unknown

Macroscopic appearance
Numerous congested, variably dilated vessels of different calibre can be seen, and the tumour can be fairly circumscribed or diffuse.

Histopathology
The tumour is composed of numerous congested, variably dilated vessels of different calibre, with either a fairly circumscribed or

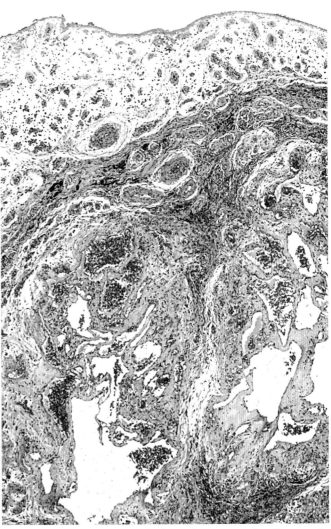

Fig. 1.156 Synovial haemangioma. A mixture of cavernous and capillary vascular channels underlies the synovium.

a diffuse growth pattern. It often has the appearance of a cavernous haemangioma with multiple dilated thin-walled vascular channels; a smaller percentage of cases have the appearance of either a capillary or an arteriovenous haemangioma. The vascular channels are located beneath the synovial membrane and are surrounded by myxoid or fibrotic stroma. Haemosiderin deposition in lining synoviocytes and in histiocytes can be prominent. Villous hyperplasia of the synovium is present in some cases.

Cytology
Not clinically relevant

Diagnostic molecular pathology
Not clinically relevant

Essential and desirable diagnostic criteria

Essential: a tumour composed of numerous congested, variably dilated vessels of different calibre; origin from a synovium-lined space.

Staging

Not clinically relevant

Prognosis and prediction

Small lesions are usually easy to remove completely by synovectomy with no risk of local recurrence {2217}. When more-diffuse involvement of the joint is present, complete excision can be difficult to achieve and may predispose to recurrence.

Intramuscular angioma

Calonje JE

Definition
Intramuscular angioma is a proliferation of benign vascular channels within skeletal muscle, associated in most instances with variable amounts of mature adipose tissue.

ICD-O coding
9132/0 Intramuscular haemangioma

ICD-11 coding
2E81.0Y & XH0553 Other specified neoplastic haemangioma & Intramuscular haemangioma

Related terminology
Acceptable: intramuscular haemangioma.
Not recommended: intramuscular-infiltrating angiolipoma.

Subtype(s)
None

Localization
Intramuscular angioma most commonly affects the lower limbs, particularly the thigh and calf, followed by the head and neck, upper limbs, and trunk. Cases can present rarely in the mediastinum and retroperitoneum and exceptionally within cardiac muscle {2913}.

Clinical features
Typical presentation is of a slow-growing mass that is often painful, particularly after exercise. Pain is mainly present in tumours located in the limbs. Giant lesions may exceptionally induce osteolysis {2015}. Radiological examination often reveals the presence of calcification due to phleboliths or metaplastic ossification. MRI is the most important radiological technique to establish the diagnosis {2216}.

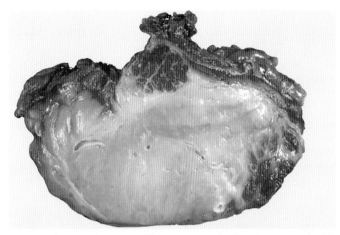

Fig. 1.157 Intramuscular angioma. This lesion was excised from the rectus abdominis muscle of a young woman. Note the poorly circumscribed margins and prominent fatty stroma.

Epidemiology
Although relatively uncommon, intramuscular angioma is one of the most frequent deep-seated soft tissue tumours. The age range is wide, but adolescents and young adults are most commonly affected (as many as 90% of cases) {78,254,983}, with equal sex distribution. Lesions have often been present for many years and it is therefore likely that many examples are congenital.

Etiology
Unknown

Pathogenesis
Unknown

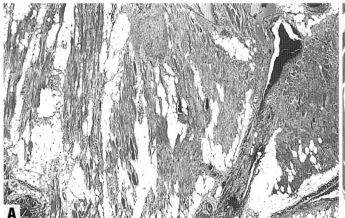 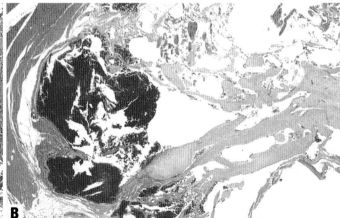

Fig. 1.158 Intramuscular angioma. **A** Extensive replacement of the muscle by dilated vascular channels with focal thrombosis. There is a prominent adipocytic component. **B** Predominance of cavernous-like vascular spaces.

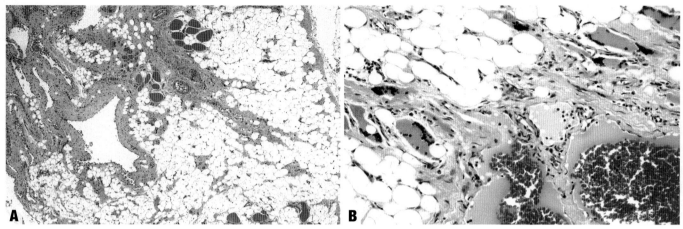

Fig. 1.159 Intramuscular angioma. **A** Extensive adipocytic component with muscle atrophy. **B** Entrapped muscle fibres with hyperchromatic, reactive nuclei.

Macroscopic appearance
Tumours are often large and there is diffuse infiltration of the involved muscle. Variably sized vascular channels with thrombosis and haemorrhage are usually readily seen. The appearance of the tumour can be solid and yellowish as a result of the presence of adipose tissue. Lesions also appear solid when capillaries predominate.

Histopathology
Intramuscular angiomas are mostly composed of mixed vessel types, including lymphatics {78}, large thick-walled veins, a mixture of cavernous-like vascular spaces and capillaries, or a prominent arteriovenous component. Tumours purely composed of capillaries are more common in the head and neck area, and those with a predominant cavernous lymphatic component are seen mainly on the trunk, proximal upper limb, and head. Variable amounts of mature adipose tissue are almost always present and may be very prominent. This explains why intramuscular angioma was sometimes inappropriately known in the past as deep or infiltrating angiolipoma {1867}. Atrophy of muscle fibres because of tumour infiltration often results in degenerative/reactive sarcolemmal changes with hyperchromatic nuclei. Perineural involvement may be present.

Cytology
Not clinically relevant

Diagnostic molecular pathology
Not clinically relevant

Essential and desirable diagnostic criteria
Essential: mass composed of mixed vessel types including lymphatics; situated within muscle and often presents with pain (worse on exercise).

Staging
Not clinically relevant

Prognosis and prediction
The rate of local recurrence is high (30–50%) and wide local excision is therefore recommended. Local recurrence seems to be determined only by size of the tumour and excision margins {263}.

Arteriovenous malformation/haemangioma

Calonje JE

Definition
Arteriovenous malformation/haemangioma (AVM/H) is a fast-flow, mostly congenital vascular anomaly characterized by the presence of arteriovenous shunts. There are two distinctive forms: deep-seated and cutaneous (cirsoid aneurysm or acral arteriovenous tumour). Most cases of extracranial AVM/H harbour *MAP2K1* mutations, resulting in upregulated MAP2K1 (MEK1) activity. When these lesions involve multiple tissue planes, they are termed angiomatosis.

ICD-O coding
9123/0 Arteriovenous haemangioma

ICD-11 coding
LA90.3Y Other specified peripheral arteriovenous malformations

Related terminology
None

Subtype(s)
None

Localization
AVM/H affects predominantly the head and neck (including the brain), followed by the limbs. Internal organs, including the lungs and uterus, may be involved {732}.

Clinical features
Angiography is an essential tool to confirm the diagnosis and establish the extent of disease. Lesions are often associated with a variable degree of arteriovenous shunting, and this can be severe enough to induce limb hypertrophy, heart failure, and consumption coagulopathy (Kasabach–Merritt syndrome). Pain is also a frequent symptom, and superficial cutaneous changes mimicking Kaposi sarcoma clinically and histologically can be seen (pseudo-Kaposi sarcoma or acroangiodermatitis) {2967}. The presence of shunting can be confirmed clinically by auscultation. AVM/H should not be confused with juvenile, cutaneous (cellular) haemangiomas because they do not usually regress spontaneously. Spontaneous regression of AVM/H is exceptional {2786}.

Epidemiology
Deep-seated AVM/H is uncommon and affects children and young adults. AVM/H represents about 14.3% of all vascular anomalies in children {1216}. Although a large proportion of lesions (particularly those that are deep-seated) are congenital, acquired lesions are increasingly being recognized {1942}.

Etiology
Unknown

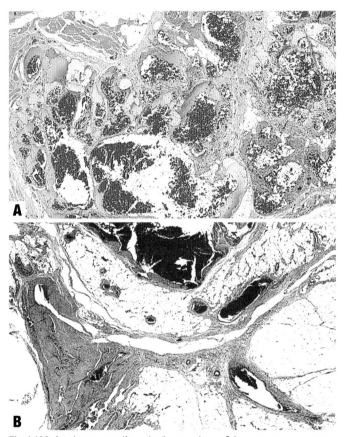

Fig. 1.160 Arteriovenous malformation/haemangioma. **A** In some cases, cavernous vascular spaces predominate. **B** There is extensive infiltration of the subcutaneous tissue by large vessels.

Pathogenesis
Unknown

Macroscopic appearance
Tumours are ill defined and contain variable numbers of small and large blood vessels, many of which are dilated.

Histopathology
This diagnosis always requires clinicopathological and radiological correlation. AVM/H is characterized by large numbers of vessels of different sizes, including veins and arteries, with the former largely outnumbering the latter. Areas resembling a cavernous or capillary haemangioma are frequent, as are thrombosis and calcification. Lymphatic vessels may be present. Recognition of arteriovenous shunts is difficult and requires examination of numerous serial sections. Fibrointimal thickening in veins is a useful diagnostic clue. Elastic stains are helpful in distinguishing between arteries and veins. True arteriovenous shunts are sometimes impossible to demonstrate in superficial

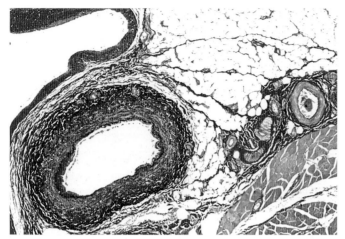

Fig. 1.161 Arteriovenous malformation/haemangioma. An elastic stain (elastic Van Gieson) is useful to determine the type of vessels involved.

lesions. Some malformations may be purely venous (see *Venous haemangioma*, p. 149).

Negative staining for GLUT1 may facilitate distinction from juvenile haemangioma {2327}. WT1 protein, a marker that is usually positive in haemangiomas, tends to be negative or focally positive in other vascular malformations {55}. However, this marker has recently been reported to be positive in AVM/H {3101}.

Cytology
Not clinically relevant

Diagnostic molecular pathology
Not clinically relevant

Essential and desirable diagnostic criteria
Essential: radiological (angiographic) or auscultatory evidence of an arteriovenous shunt within an ill-defined vascular lesion.
Desirable: histology showing vessels of different sizes, including both arteries and veins; fibrointimal thickening in veins.

Staging
Not clinically relevant

Prognosis and prediction
Treatment is sometimes difficult because of the extent of tumour involvement, which must be determined by angiographic examination. Local recurrence is common because of difficulty in achieving complete excision.

Venous haemangioma

Calonje JE

Definition
Venous haemangioma is composed of veins of variable size, often having thick muscular walls. Intramuscular angiomas and angiomatosis, which are described separately, can be composed almost exclusively of veins but are usually intermixed with other vessel types.

ICD-O coding
9122/0 Venous haemangioma

ICD-11 coding
2E81.0Y Other specified neoplastic haemangioma

Related terminology
None

Subtype(s)
None

Localization
Tumours present in the subcutaneous or deeper soft tissues and are commonly located in the limbs. Rarely, lesions have been described elsewhere, including the mandibular division of the trigeminal nerve {2048}, the orbit {1704}, the superior sulcus of the lung {3379}, the mediastinum {1369}, the retroperitoneum {1660}, the breast {1634}, the brain {1251}, and the parapharyngeal space {578}.

Clinical features
Venous haemangioma often presents as a longstanding slow-growing tumour. Radiological examination often shows the presence of calcification due to phleboliths.

Epidemiology
Venous haemangioma is rare and data are limited, but these lesions occur mainly in adults.

Etiology
The clinical evolution and clinicopathological features suggest that these lesions represent vascular malformations.

Pathogenesis
Unknown

Macroscopic appearance
Venous haemangioma is ill defined and consists of dilated congested vascular spaces with areas of haemorrhage.

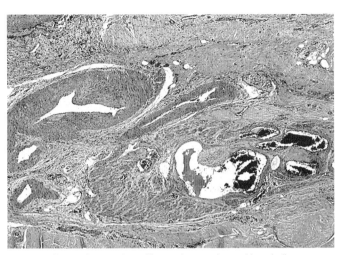

Fig. 1.162 Venous haemangioma. Venous haemangioma with typically numerous prominent thick-walled veins.

Histopathology
Venous haemangioma typically consists of large thick-walled muscular vessels, which are variably dilated and commonly display thrombosis, with occasional formation of phleboliths. Widely dilated vessels can show attenuation of their walls, mimicking a cavernous haemangioma. Elastic stains reveal the absence of an internal elastic lamina. This aids in the distinction from an arteriovenous haemangioma.

Cytology
Not clinically relevant

Diagnostic molecular pathology
Not clinically relevant

Essential and desirable diagnostic criteria
Essential: ill-defined lesion with thick-walled muscular vessels, variable dilation, and area of thrombosis; absence of internal elastic lamina.
Desirable: longstanding, slow-growing tumour, often with calcifications (phleboliths).

Staging
Not clinically relevant

Prognosis and prediction
Deep-seated tumours are difficult to excise and can recur locally, but subcutaneous tumours do not usually recur.

Anastomosing haemangioma

Montgomery EA
Umetsu SE

Definition
Anastomosing haemangioma is a benign vascular neoplasm that is poorly marginated and consists of thin-walled anastomosing vessels lined by a monolayer of endothelial cells with somewhat protuberant nuclei.

ICD-O coding
9120/0 Haemangioma NOS

ICD-11 coding
2E81.0Z Neoplastic haemangioma, unspecified

Related terminology
None

Subtype(s)
None

Localization
Anastomosing haemangioma was initially reported in the male genital tract {2176}, and the most common site is the kidney and retroperitoneal adipose tissue {2383,435}, but this type of haemangioma has been reported in multiple sites, including the female genital tract {1702,871}, gastrointestinal tract and liver {1551,1865}, soft tissue {1539}, and skin {3095}.

Clinical features
Because many cases arise in the viscera, they may be incidental findings on imaging studies, although some patients with renal lesions present with haematuria {2176}; patients with superficial examples present with palpable masses or with pain {1539}. Colorectal lesions can manifest as polyps {1865}, and hepatic lesions often present during the evaluation of another process {1865,1154,1551}. Imaging studies often show a well-marginated

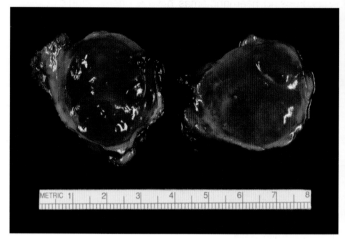

Fig. 1.163 Anastomosing haemangioma. The lesion is well marginated, which is generally the case.

lesion that is mildly hyperdense with heterogeneous attenuation that is inconclusive for malignancy {2383,1539}. Multifocality has been documented {3}. Most lesions are 1–2 cm, but larger examples (as large as 7.5 cm in soft tissue {1539}) are known. Hepatic examples can not only appear infiltrative but can also be as large as 16 cm {1154,3217}.

Epidemiology
Patients are predominantly adults (mean age in the initial series: ~60 years {2176}), but lesions in the paediatric age group have been reported {454}. There does not appear to be a sex predilection overall.

Etiology
Unknown

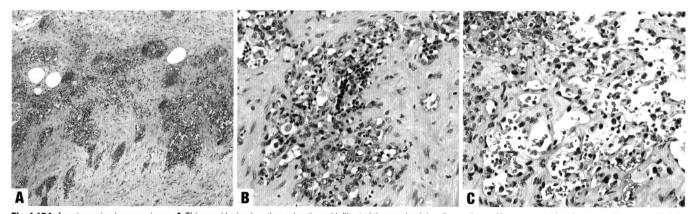

Fig. 1.164 Anastomosing haemangioma. **A** This renal lesion is rather sclerotic and infiltrated the renal pelvic adipose tissue. However, note that the tumour is arranged in lobules. **B** The lesion is composed of vascular spaces that are cuffed by supporting cells. Note the extramedullary haematopoiesis (erythropoiesis) in the upper-central part of the image. **C** Note the anastomosing growth pattern and tiny hobnail endothelial cells.

Pathogenesis

The vast majority of cases contain an activating hotspot mutation in *GNAQ* or *GNA14*; similar mutations have been identified in hepatic small vessel neoplasms {243,242,1551}. No other molecular alterations have been identified.

Macroscopic appearance

Anastomosing haemangiomas have a haemorrhagic, mahogany-coloured, spongy appearance.

Histopathology

These lesions have a loosely lobulated architecture at low magnification and can be associated with a medium-calibre vessel. There is often focal infiltration into adjoining tissue. The neoplasms consist of anastomosing sinusoidal capillary-sized vessels with scattered hobnail endothelial cells {1748}. There may be a lymphocytic infiltrate. Mitoses are absent or rare. Mild cytological atypia can be present, but no multilayering of endothelial cells is seen. Vascular thrombi are typical, and zones of central sclerosis with focal necrosis are common. Extramedullary haematopoiesis can be a prominent feature, and some examples have striking hyaline globules. Immunohistochemistry shows labelling with CD34, CD31, and ERG in the endothelial cells.

Cytology

Not clinically relevant

Diagnostic molecular pathology

Not clinically relevant

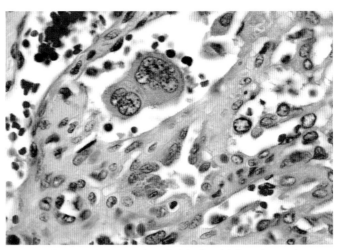

Fig. 1.165 Anastomosing haemangioma. Both hyaline globules and a megakaryocyte are seen.

Essential and desirable diagnostic criteria

Essential: anastomosing vessels lined by hobnail endothelial cells.

Desirable: hyaline globules and extramedullary haematopoiesis are common.

Staging

Not clinically relevant

Prognosis and prediction

Anastomosing haemangiomas, even when multicentric or infiltrative, are benign.

Epithelioid haemangioma

Bovée JVMG
Huang SC
Wang J

Definition

Epithelioid haemangioma is a benign vascular neoplasm composed of well-formed blood vessels lined by plump, epithelioid (histiocytoid) endothelial cells, with abundant eosinophilic cytoplasm and a variable eosinophilic infiltrate. As many as half of the cases show recurrent gene fusions in the *FOS* and *FOSB* genes.

ICD-O coding

9125/0 Epithelioid haemangioma

ICD-11 coding

2E81.0Y & XH10T4 Other specified neoplastic haemangioma & Epithelioid haemangioma

Related terminology

Not recommended: angiolymphoid hyperplasia with eosinophilia; histiocytoid haemangioma.

Subtype(s)

Cellular epithelioid haemangioma; atypical epithelioid haemangioma

Localization

Cutaneous and soft tissue lesions are most commonly located in the head and neck region, especially the forehead, preauricular region, and scalp, followed by the distal extremities and trunk {2380,1432}. The penis is uncommonly involved {1001}. Visceral occurrences are exceedingly rare {2188}. Some arise in large vessels.

Clinical features

The most common presentation is a single cutaneous erythematous-violaceous papule or angiomatoid nodule, asymptomatic or slightly painful. Approximately 10–20% of patients present with multiple (sometimes numerous) lesions, usually within the same anatomical region {1883}.

Epidemiology

Epithelioid haemangioma occurs over a wide age range, with peak incidence in the fourth decade of life and no sex predilection {1432}.

Etiology

Unknown

Pathogenesis

Epithelioid haemangioma is characterized by recurrent fusion genes involving the *FOS* or *FOSB* gene in as many as half of the cases. The fusion-positive tumours are more often in the extremities/trunk, non-cutaneous, and of the cellular/atypical subtypes {1432}. The gene partners for *FOS* are variable, including *LMNA*, *MBNL1*, *VIM*, and lincRNA {3162,1432}, whereas *FOSB* is often fused to *ZFP36* or very rarely to *WWTR1* or *ACTB* {128,36}. Dysregulation of the FOS family of transcription factors through chromosomal translocation is the key event. The FOS family includes FOS, FOSB, FOSL1, and FOSL2, which encode leucine zipper proteins that can dimerize with proteins of the JUN family, thereby forming the transcription factor complex AP-1. FOS proteins regulate cell proliferation, differentiation, angiogenesis, and survival. In the FOS fusions, the various fusion partners are at the C-terminal end of the protein and cause loss of the transactivating domain {3162}. The C-terminal part is essential for fast, ubiquitin-independent FOS degradation via the 20S proteasome. Loss of the C-terminal part prevents the normal rapid degradation of FOS, resulting in prolonged FOS activation {3163}. The FOSB fusions occur at the N-terminal part of the protein and are most likely activating promoter-swap events causing upregulation of FOSB {3177}. Recent data suggest that cutaneous epithelioid

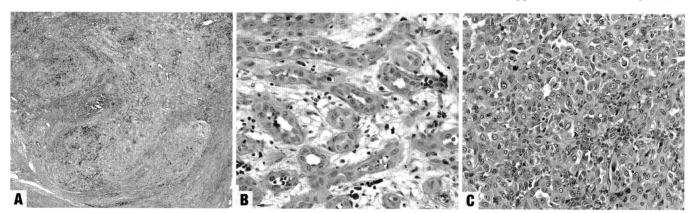

Fig. 1.166 Epithelioid haemangioma. **A** Epithelioid haemangioma shows a multilobular growth pattern. **B** High-power view details the endothelial cells, which have glassy and eosinophilic cytoplasm and central enlarged nuclei with prominent nucleoli. **C** Exuberant or cellular examples of epithelioid haemangioma exhibit high cellularity and sheet-like areas with inconspicuous or slit-like vascular lumina and scant intervening stroma. These lesions usually have a conventional vasoformative pattern and peripheral maturation.

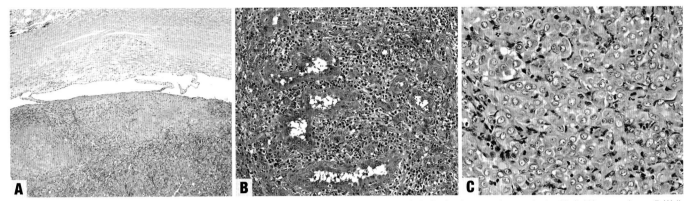

Fig. 1.167 Epithelioid haemangioma. **A** Histological variations: this lesion is confined within a large vein, indicating intravascular growth of epithelioid haemangioma. **B** Well-formed vessels with abundant eosinophilic infiltration in angiolymphoid hyperplasia with eosinophilia–type epithelioid haemangioma. **C** Compact proliferation of epithelioid endothelial cells in an exuberant example of penile epithelioid haemangioma.

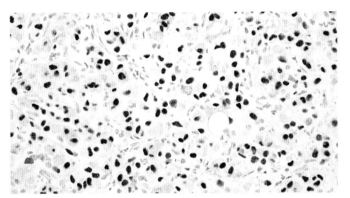

Fig. 1.168 Epithelioid haemangioma. There is strong nuclear staining for FOSB in this cellular example of epithelioid haemangioma.

haemangioma (angiolymphoid hyperplasia with eosinophilia type) may be non-neoplastic, lacking abnormalities in the *FOS* or *FOSB* gene {1432}.

Macroscopic appearance
Superficial epithelioid haemangiomas are usually 0.5–2.0 cm in size, only rarely exceeding 5 cm {2380}. Most have a nonspecific nodular appearance.

Histopathology
Epithelioid haemangioma typically exhibits a proliferation of well-formed small blood vessels lined by plump and epithelioid endothelial cells with abundant eosinophilic cytoplasm and enlarged round nuclei. The tumour is typically well demarcated and has a distinctive lobulated growth at low power. Moreover, it shows increased maturation of the vascular lumina at the periphery of the lesion. These vessels are lined by a monolayered endothelium and an intact pericytic layer in a loose stroma. The endothelial cells may show intracytoplasmic vacuoles (so-called blister cells). Tumour cells have vesicular or fine chromatin, with only mild cytological atypia and mostly low mitotic activity. The stromal component is often oedematous, and the tumour may show haemorrhagic changes within the solid component. A subset of cases may display centrifugal growth around a central small artery and evenly complete intravascular growth. Marked lymphoplasmacytic infiltrates, prominent lymphoid follicles, and abundant eosinophils are not uncommon,

especially for head and neck cases. Dermal cases usually have less demarcation, more well-canalized lumina, and less plump endothelial cells. A subset of cases, referred to as atypical epithelioid haemangiomas, can display more-solid growth, exuberant and compact proliferation with increased cellularity, nuclear pleomorphism with sheet-like appearance with inconspicuous or slit-like spaces and little intervening stroma, and necrosis {128}. These cases more often have *FOSB* fusions and are more often localized in the penis, with more infiltrative growth.

Tumour cells express the endothelial markers CD31, FLI1, and ERG, and CD34 is expressed to a lesser extent. Many cases are also positive for keratin and EMA {2343,3190}. SMA highlights the pericytic lining and therefore the vasoformative architecture. FOSB was shown to be positive in 54% of epithelioid haemangiomas {1440}. The angiolymphoid hyperplasia with eosinophilia subtype is also positive for FOSB, although gene fusions are absent {1440,2387,3162,1432}.

Cytology
Not clinically relevant

Diagnostic molecular pathology
Rearrangement of the *FOS* or *FOSB* gene can be detected by molecular methods if required {1440,2387}.

Essential and desirable diagnostic criteria
Essential: lobular architecture with vasoformation; lining endothelial cells are epithelioid, with eosinophilic cytoplasm and enlarged round nuclei; loose haemorrhagic stroma, often with eosinophils.
Desirable: demonstration of *FOS/FOSB* rearrangements or expression may be helpful in selected cases.

Staging
Not clinically relevant

Prognosis and prediction
As many as one third of patients experience local recurrence, related to incomplete excision or multicentricity. Most of the recurrences are indolent and can be cured by re-excision, although very rare recurrences can be locally aggressive. Rare lymph node metastasis may occur. To date, no patients have developed distant metastases.

Lymphangioma and lymphangiomatosis

Thway K
Doyle LA

Definition

Lymphangioma is a benign vascular lesion composed of a localized collection of dilated lymphatic channels. Lymphangiomatosis is multicentric or extensively infiltrating lymphangioma, and it typically involves multiple tissue planes or more than one organ.

ICD-O coding

9170/0 Lymphangioma NOS
9173/0 Cystic lymphangioma

ICD-11 coding

LA90.12 & XH9MR8 Lymphatic malformations of certain specified sites & Lymphangioma
2E81.10 Disseminated lymphangiomatosis

Related terminology

Acceptable: cystic hygroma; lymphatic malformation; lymphangioma circumscriptum; cavernous lymphangioma; intra-abdominal cystic lymphangioma; haemangiolymphangioma.

Subtype(s)

Lymphangiomatosis

Localization

Lymphangiomas may be superficial or deep, or they may involve both superficial and deep tissue planes. Superficial lesions are often referred to as lymphangioma circumscriptum, and deep lesions as cavernous lymphangioma {3280,2469,1013}. Most cases of superficial lymphangioma / lymphangioma circumscriptum arise on the skin of proximal extremities and limb girdles. Cavernous lymphangiomas most commonly involve the head and neck, followed by the extremities, axilla, groin, and abdominal sites, including the gastrointestinal tract, mesentery, and retroperitoneum {83,1409}. Cystic hygroma (cystic lymphangioma) presents as a large mass in the neck, axilla, or groin of infants. Lymphangiomatosis can involve either a single anatomical structure/organ or multiple structures (e.g. skeletal muscle, liver, spleen, lungs, and bones) {1184,2783,87}.

Clinical features

Superficial lymphangioma appears as pale or pink vesicles involving skin. Deeper lesions may present as circumscribed, soft, and fluctuant painless swellings. Deep lesions may displace surrounding organs at mediastinal sites (compression of trachea and oesophagus) or intra-abdominal sites (intestinal obstruction).

Epidemiology

Lymphangiomas are common paediatric lesions, presenting most often at birth or during early life {83}. Some are identified in the context of Turner syndrome or other malformative

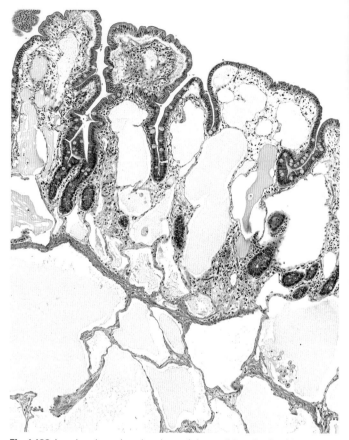

Fig. 1.169 Lymphangioma. Lymphangioma of the small intestine involving mucosa and submucosa. The lymphatic channels are dilated and lined by inconspicuous endothelium, and they contain lymphatic fluid and occasional lipid-laden macrophages.

syndromes {264,453,569}. Head and neck lymphangiomas represent the most frequent subtype. Although lymphangiomas primarily occur in children and young adults, there is a wide age range including older adults, particularly for mesenteric lesions {3030,2624,2199}, and an overall slight male predominance.

Etiology

Early or congenital lesions favour developmental malformations, with genetic abnormalities playing an additional role {3288}. Somatic mutations in *PIK3CA* have been reported to be involved {1912}.

Pathogenesis

Lymphangiomas are thought to arise from abnormal lymphatic system development. *PIK3CA* and other mutations are likely to drive this process through endothelial growth receptor pathways {1912,3024}.

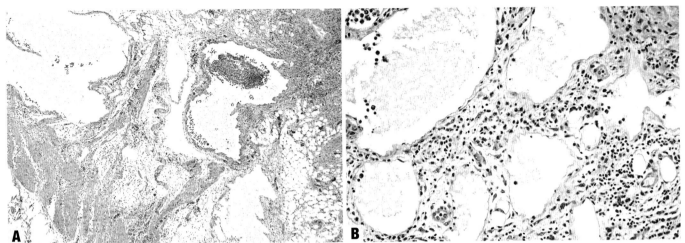

Fig. 1.170 Lymphangioma of the mesentery. **A** Present within the bowel muscularis propria, this lymphangioma shows well-formed, dilated lymphatic channels that contain lymphocytes and are lined by flattened endothelial cells lacking any atypia. **B** Showing multiple, markedly ectatic lymphatic channels containing lymph and lined by small bland endothelial cells.

Macroscopic appearance

Lymphangiomas are multicystic and spongy, with cavities containing watery/milky chylous fluid.

Histopathology

Cutaneous lesions consist of dilated thin-walled lymphatics in superficial dermis that connect with thick-walled, often muscular, lymphatic channels in deep dermis, often with overlying epidermal hyperplasia. Cavernous lymphangiomas contain variably sized thin-walled, dilated lymphatic vessels lined by flattened endothelium, frequently surrounded by lymphocytic aggregates. Lumina may be empty or may contain proteinaceous fluid, lymphocytes, and sometimes erythrocytes. Larger vessels can be surrounded by a smooth muscle layer, and longstanding lesions may show interstitial fibrosis and stromal inflammation. Stromal mast cells and haemosiderin deposition are common. Xanthogranulomatous inflammation with florid cellular reactive myofibroblastic proliferations can obscure the underlying lymphatic abnormality, particularly in mesenteric or retroperitoneal lesions {1409}. In lymphangiomatosis, the vessels are similarly thin-walled and variably dilated, but they usually also show an anastomosing growth pattern and may dissect around normal structures. The endothelium expresses podoplanin (D2-40) and PROX1 {2138}, as well as CD31 (consistently) and CD34 (variably) {1409}. SMA is positive in smooth muscle cells surrounding the cysts.

Cytology

Not clinically relevant

Diagnostic molecular pathology

Not clinically relevant

Essential and desirable diagnostic criteria

Essential: tumour composed of thin-walled vascular spaces.
Desirable: immunohistochemical expression of CD31 and D2-40, with variable CD34 expression.

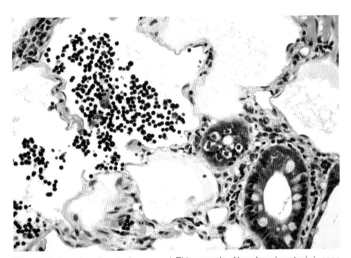

Fig. 1.171 Lymphangiomatosis, mucosal. This example of lymphangiomatosis is seen within bowel mucosa. The ectatic lymphatic channels are lined by small, almost imperceptible spindle cells and contain prominent cloudy lymph as well as numerous lymphocytes.

Staging

Not clinically relevant

Prognosis and prediction

Lymphangiomas are benign, but because of their propensity for involvement of deeper tissue planes, recurrences occur in as many as 20% of patients after removal of apparently superficial lesions {1290,83}. In general, the recurrence rate varies depending on lesion size and depth. However, lymphangiomatosis has a much higher recurrence rate, and diffuse lymphangiomatosis with visceral involvement can be fatal.

Tufted angioma and kaposiform haemangioendothelioma

North PE

Definition
Kaposiform haemangioendothelioma (KHE) is a rare, often deep-seated, vascular neoplasm usually presenting in children, characterized by lobular infiltrates of capillaries and spindled endothelial cells associated with lymphatic vessels. Tufted angioma (TA), a more superficial lesion, is otherwise essentially identical to KHE. Together, KHE and TA are responsible for virtually all instances of the platelet-trapping syndrome Kasabach–Merritt phenomenon (KMP).

ICD-O coding
9161/0 Acquired tufted haemangioma
9130/1 Kaposiform haemangioendothelioma

ICD-11 coding
2F2Y & XH6PA4 Other specified benign cutaneous neoplasms & Kaposiform haemangioendothelioma

Related terminology
Not recommended: Kaposi-like infantile haemangioendothelioma; haemangioma with Kaposi-like features; angioblastoma of Nakagawa.

Subtype(s)
None

Localization
TA and KHE most commonly affect the skin and deep soft tissues of the extremities, head and neck, trunk, and retroperitoneum;

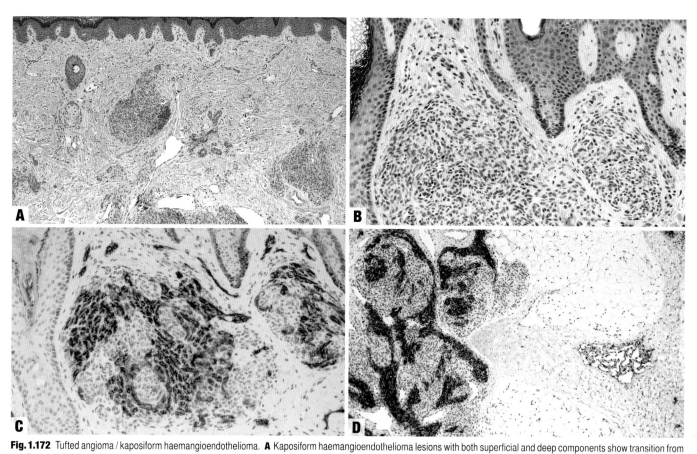

Fig. 1.172 Tufted angioma / kaposiform haemangioendothelioma. **A** Kaposiform haemangioendothelioma lesions with both superficial and deep components show transition from smaller superficial tumour nodules with subtle endothelial spindling (tufted angioma pattern) to deeper coalescent nodules with more prominent spindling and platelet-trapping (classic kaposiform haemangioendothelioma pattern). **B** This lesion shows the typical superficial (tufted angioma) pattern. Higher magnification reveals pinpoint lumina and relatively subtle endothelial cell spindling without nuclear pleomorphism. Mitotic activity is very low. **C** This lesion with a superficial (tufted angioma) pattern shows focal strong positivity for podoplanin within tumour nodules, sharply sparing other areas within the same nodule. A matching pattern of positivity is seen for other lymphatic endothelial markers, including PROX1 and LYVE1, as well as for CD34 (which is normally expressed preferentially in blood vascular endothelial cells). **D** Within tumour nodules of kaposiform haemangioendothelioma, an alternating pattern of strong positivity and negativity for podoplanin is striking. Note the presence of abnormal lymphatic vasculature in adjacent stroma, a common finding.

less commonly, the mediastinum, spleen, bone, and testis are affected {1922,3410,908,3291,2325,663}.

Clinical features
Cutaneous forms are violaceous, infiltrative patches/plaques that may develop nodularity. Deeper soft tissue lesions are bulging indurated masses. Congenital/early infantile cases, especially when large, commonly present with profound thrombocytopenia (KMP) {1922}. MRI shows an ill-defined, diffusely enhancing T2-hyperintense mass involving multiple tissue layers.

Epidemiology
Most cases present in children aged < 5 years; some are congenital. Congenital/early infantile tumours cause most KMP cases. Rare cases present in older children and adults, without KMP {2087,657,663}. There is no sex or racial predilection.

Etiology
Unknown

Pathogenesis
Somatic activating *GNA14* mutations have been reported in 2 cases {1860}. KMP can be attributed to histologically observed platelet-trapping within tumoural vascular beds, because podoplanin is the natural ligand of CLEC2, a platelet-bound receptor {3007}. Platelet transfusions may worsen KMP by stimulating vascular proliferation by intratumoural platelet activation {13}. A self-sustaining cycle of platelet-trapping and tumour growth may drive tumour progression and KMP development.

Macroscopic appearance
Macroscopically, TA and KHE appear as multiple grey to red infiltrative nodules, encased in fibrous tissue.

Histopathology
Classic KHEs are composed of ill-defined, coalescing nodules of spindled endothelial cells forming elongated slit-like lumina containing erythrocytes, curving around epithelioid nodules enriched in pericytes surrounding platelet-rich microthrombi.

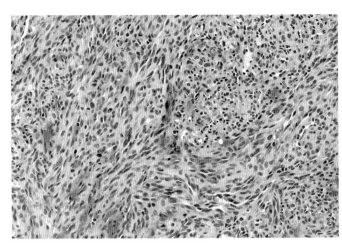

Fig. 1.174 Kaposiform haemangioendothelioma, classic pattern. Classic histological manifestations of kaposiform haemangioendothelioma, such as prominent endothelial spindling and numerous platelet-rich microthrombi, are best developed in larger, more deeply seated lesions, as shown in this example from the lateral neck of an 8-day-old girl. Platelet-trapping within compressed spaces is highlighted by CD61 immunostaining (not shown) and is the presumed histological correlate of Kasabach–Merritt phenomenon. Note the presence of abnormal lymphatic vasculature in adjacent stroma, a common finding.

Mitoses are infrequent. Variably prominent areas show more typical capillary formation. Dilated crescentic lymphatic vessels surround and intermingle with nodules, most prominently at peripheral margins. Peripheral fibrosis is common around endothelial cell nodules. Perineural invasion may be present. Residua after medical treatment or spontaneous regression are sclerotic versions of the original. Spindled endothelial cells of KHE are positive for CD31, CD34, and ERG, as well as strongly positive for the lymphatic markers podoplanin, LYVE1, and PROX1 {2324,1787}. TAs are less extensively positive for lymphatic markers, seemingly correlated with reduced endothelial spindling {1787}. Expression of the infantile haemangioma–associated marker GLUT1 is absent in KHE/TA {2327, 2326,1922}. CD31/CD61 immunostaining highlights platelet-rich microthrombi.

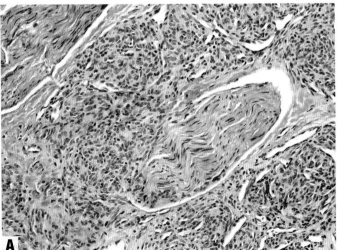
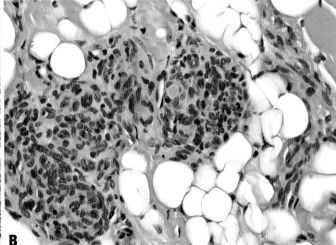

Fig. 1.173 Tufted angioma / kaposiform haemangioendothelioma. **A** A lesion from the knee in a 5-month-old girl. This kaposiform haemangioendothelioma shows solid growth composed of nests of ovoid cells, forming slit-like lumina. Perineurial invasion is present. **B** This lesion from the buttock of a 5-year-old girl shows tightly packed lobules of capillaries involving subcutis.

Cytology
Not clinically relevant

Diagnostic molecular pathology
Not clinically relevant

Essential and desirable diagnostic criteria
Essential: superficial dermal lesions (TA pattern): discrete lobules of capillaries in cannonball pattern within dermal collagen; deeper lesions (KHE pattern): ill-defined, coalescing nodules composed of fascicles of plump spindled endothelial cells that form slit-like lumina that contain erythrocytes – a prominent component of dilated lymphatic vessels is seen at the periphery and in surrounding fibrotic stroma; the spindled cells are positive for CD31, ERG, CD34, and lymphatic markers (podoplanin, LYVE1, PROX1).

Staging
Not clinically relevant

Prognosis and prediction
Untreated lesions may partially undergo fibrosis and regress, but they invariably recur. Large lesions are associated with high mortality due to thrombocytopenia or tumour infiltration. Wide local excision, when feasible, can be curative. Medical therapies (e.g. vincristine and steroids) are the first line for high-risk patients with KMP; mTOR inhibition (e.g. sirolimus) is also promising {13,14}. No distant metastases have been reported; lymph node involvement is rarely seen {1922,1736}. This may represent multifocal lymphatic chain involvement rather than true metastasis.

Retiform haemangioendothelioma

Calonje JE

Definition
Retiform haemangioendothelioma is a locally aggressive, rarely metastasizing vascular lesion, characterized by distinctive arborizing blood vessels lined by endothelial cells with characteristic hobnail morphology.

ICD-O coding
9136/1 Retiform haemangioendothelioma

ICD-11 coding
2B56.1 & XH64U8 Angiosarcoma of skin & Retiform haemangioendothelioma

Related terminology
Acceptable: hobnail haemangioendothelioma.

Subtype(s)
None

Localization
The tumour involves predominantly the skin and subcutaneous tissue and is most commonly found in the distal extremities, particularly the lower limb.

Clinical features
Retiform haemangioendothelioma presents as a red/bluish slow-growing plaque or nodule, usually < 3 cm in maximum dimension. A case with multiple lesions has been described {868}. Exceptional cases occur in the setting of previous radiotherapy {462} or pre-existing lymphoedema {462} (including Milroy disease {173}), as well as in association with a cystic lymphangioma {65}.

Epidemiology
Retiform haemangioendothelioma is uncommon. Since its original description in 1994, only about 40 cases have been reported {65,462,1090,2092,3036}. The age range is wide, but this lesion usually affects young adults or children; males and females are affected equally frequently.

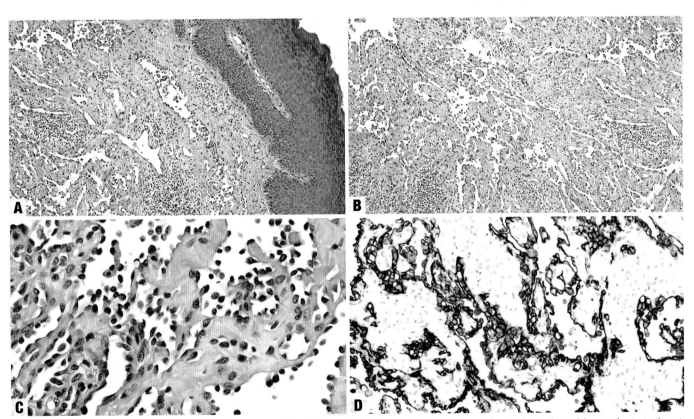

Fig. 1.175 Retiform haemangioendothelioma. **A** A cutaneous example showing an infiltrative growth of well-formed elongated vessels reminiscent of rete testis pattern. **B** Branching vessels within a sclerotic stroma with associated lymphocytic infiltrate. Dabska-like intravascular papillary structures are present. **C** High-power view showing vascular structures lined by monomorphic hobnail endothelial cells, lacking nuclear pleomorphism or increased mitotic activity. **D** Diffuse podoplanin expression, confirming lymphatic endothelial phenotype.

Etiology
Unknown

Pathogenesis
Unknown

Macroscopic appearance
Macroscopic examination reveals diffuse, sometimes discoloured induration of the dermis, with frequent involvement of the underlying subcutaneous tissue.

Histopathology
Scanning magnification reveals characteristic elongated and narrow arborizing vascular channels with a striking resemblance to normal rete testis. Although this pattern is usually readily apparent, if the vascular channels are small or collapsed, then the retiform architecture may be difficult to recognize. Monomorphic hyperchromatic endothelial cells with prominent protuberant nuclei having a characteristic tombstone or hobnail appearance line the blood vessels. These cells have scant cytoplasm, which seems to blend with the underlying stroma. Pleomorphism is absent and mitotic figures are rare. A prominent stromal and often intravascular lymphocytic infiltrate is present in about half of the cases. The stroma surrounding the tumour tends to be sclerotic. Focal solid areas composed of sheets of endothelial cells are often identified. Vacuolated cells are uncommonly seen. Monomorphic endothelial spindle-shaped cells are also a rare feature and were described in a case of metastatic disease in a lymph node {462}. In some cases, there are intravascular papillae with hyaline collagenous cores similar to those seen in papillary intralymphatic angioendothelioma {65}. Retiform haemangioendothelioma can be one of the components of a composite haemangioendothelioma. The neoplastic cells in retiform haemangioendothelioma stain for vascular markers, including CD31, CD34, and ERG. Staining for CD34 is often stronger than for other vascular markers. Although the lymphatic marker PROX1 is positive in retiform haemangioendothelioma, other lymphatic markers, including podoplanin (D2-40) and the less specific VEGFR3, are usually (but not always) negative {900,2138,2453}. These lesions are negative for HHV8.

Cytology
Not clinically relevant

Diagnostic molecular pathology
Not clinically relevant

Essential and desirable diagnostic criteria
Essential: arborizing branching vascular channels; bland endothelial cells with hobnail morphology and no or very low mitotic activity.

Staging
Not clinically relevant

Prognosis and prediction
Multiple local recurrences (occurring in as many as 60% of cases), often over many years, are the rule, unless wide local excision is performed {462}. Very rarely, lymph node or locoregional soft tissue metastasis may occur {307,462,2092}. To date, no patients have developed distant metastases or died from this disease.

Papillary intralymphatic angioendothelioma

Fanburg-Smith JC

Definition
Papillary intralymphatic angioendothelioma (PILA) is an uncommon, rarely metastasizing, superficial lymphatic vascular tumour, showing tufting and hobnail endothelial proliferations within lymphatic channel lumina, in a background of lymphatic vascular proliferation or lymphangioma.

ICD-O coding
9135/1 Papillary intralymphatic angioendothelioma

ICD-11 coding
2F72.Y & XH4SY7 Other specified neoplasms of uncertain behaviour of skin & Endovascular papillary angioendothelioma

Related terminology
Not recommended: Dabska tumour; endovascular papillary angioendothelioma; hobnail haemangioendothelioma.

Subtype(s)
None

Localization
Most PILAs involve the proximal extremities, especially the buttock or thigh {967}, and less commonly the distal extremities or trunk, head and neck, intra-abdominal sites, or parenchymal sites (including testis) {2792}. Intraosseous locations are rarely reported {967,2028,1836,1112}.

Clinical features
There is a slight female predilection (M:F ratio: ~0.7:1). PILA presents as a slow-growing asymptomatic cutaneous induration, plaque, or rarely nodule, often with unremarkable overlying skin. Radiology data are scant; intraosseous tumours are lytic and destructive and may be multifocal {1836,1112}.

Epidemiology
PILA is exceedingly rare, with < 50 reported cases {699,967}.

Etiology
Unknown

Pathogenesis
Unknown

Macroscopic appearance
Tumours are ill defined and usually involve dermis and subcutaneous tissue {967}. Grossly, greyish-white to pink streaks or cystic change in otherwise normal dermis and subcutis may be present, without haemorrhage or necrosis. Tumour size ranges from 1 to > 40 cm (mean: 7 cm) {967}.

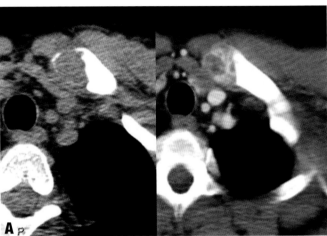

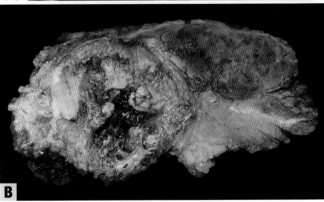

Fig. 1.176 Papillary intralymphatic angioendothelioma. **A** This is a rare intraosseous papillary intralymphatic angioendothelioma of the clavicle that is a lytic destructive lesion, seen here on radiological CT without contrast (**left**) and with contrast (**right**). **B** This is a gross photograph of the same lesion. Notice the extensive vascular proliferation of clavicle and the extension into soft tissue around the bone.

Histopathology
PILA is an extensive, poorly delineated dermal and/or subcutaneous proliferation of lymphatic channels. A cavernous lymphangioma is often present nearby. The cavernous or slit-like lymphatic vascular channels are lined by columnar, matchstick-like, or hobnail endothelial cells. In addition, variable proliferations of intraluminal papillary tufts are noted, with hyaline cores and intermixed intraluminal lymphocytes with proteinaceous fluid. The lesional cells have eosinophilic cytoplasm and round uniform nuclei with indistinct nucleoli; they lack cytological atypia and mitoses {967}. Tumour cells express pan-endothelial markers, such as CD31, ERG, and less often CD34, as well as lymphatic endothelial markers, such as podoplanin, VEGFR3, and PROX1 {967,2138,2792}.

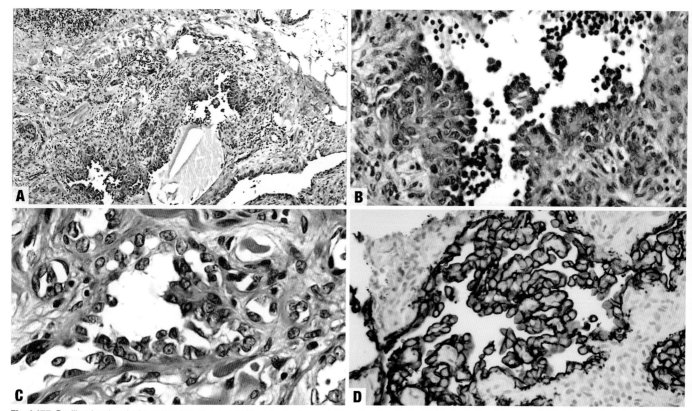

Fig. 1.177 Papillary intralymphatic angioendothelioma. **A,B** There is a background of lymphangiomatosis with intraluminal proteinaceous fluid and stromal lymphocytes. **C** This image shows the intraluminal proliferation of hobnail or matchstick-like columnar endothelial cells. **D** The cells are immunopositive for VEGFR3.

Cytology
Not clinically relevant

Diagnostic molecular pathology
Not clinically relevant

Essential and desirable diagnostic criteria
Essential: extensive infiltration of lymphatic vessels with stromal and intraluminal lymphocytes and proteinaceous fluid; intralymphatic, intraluminal hobnail proliferation of polarized matchstick-like columnar endothelial cells; expression of pan-endothelial and lymphatic markers.

Staging
Not clinically relevant

Prognosis and prediction
Most patients have excellent prognosis after complete excision {967}. Very rarely, lymph node metastases and death from disease occur {699}.

Composite haemangioendothelioma

Rubin BP
Folpe AL

Definition
Classic composite haemangioendothelioma (CHE) is a locally aggressive, rarely metastasizing vascular neoplasm, containing an admixture of histologically distinct components. An aggressive form showing neuroendocrine marker expression has also been described.

ICD-O coding
9136/1 Composite haemangioendothelioma

ICD-11 coding
2F72.Y & XH8D24 Other specified neoplasms of uncertain behaviour of skin & Composite haemangioendothelioma

Related terminology
None

Subtype(s)
Neuroendocrine composite haemangioendothelioma

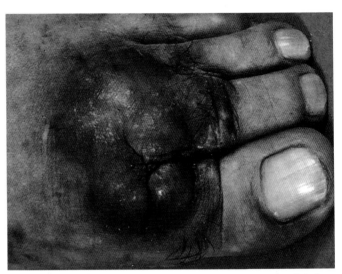

Fig. 1.178 Composite haemangioendothelioma. Composite haemangioendothelioma presenting as a bluish-purple multinodular mass.

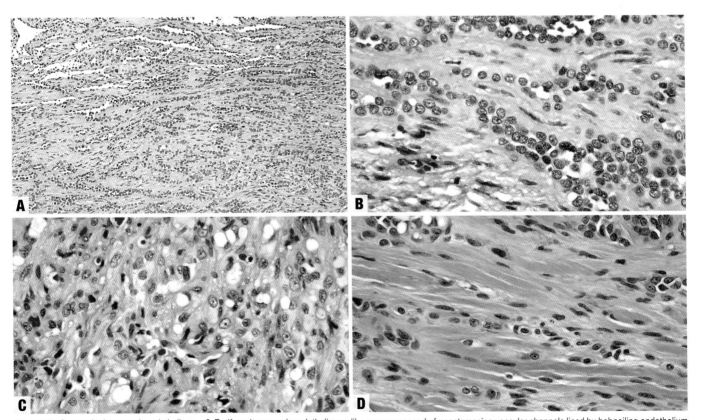

Fig. 1.179 Composite haemangioendothelioma. **A** Retiform haemangioendothelioma–like area composed of anastomosing vascular channels lined by hobnailing endothelium with an appearance reminiscent of rete testis. **B** Uniform hobnail endothelial cells with round nuclei and fine chromatin lining the vascular spaces. **C** Epithelioid haemangioendothelioma–like area composed of sheets of epithelioid cells with occasionally prominent cytoplasmic vacuolization. **D** Epithelioid haemangioendothelioma–like component composed of cords and nests of epithelioid cells in a hyalinized stroma.

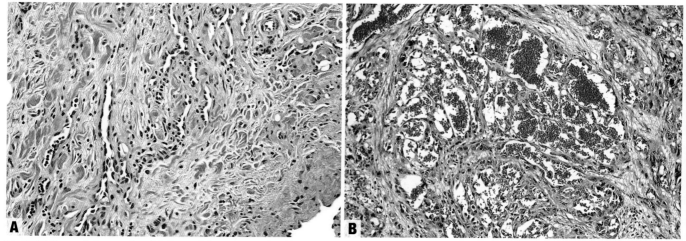

Fig. 1.180 Composite haemangioendothelioma. **A** An area suggestive of low-grade angiosarcoma composed of irregular vascular structures with a dissecting/infiltrative growth pattern. **B** Haemangioma-like area with dilated vascular spaces lined by flat, unremarkable endothelium. Other components of this lesion were epithelioid haemangioendothelioma–like, retiform haemangioendothelioma–like, and epithelioid angiosarcoma–like.

Localization
Most cases occur on the distal extremities, especially the hands and feet or the head and neck. Multiple other sites have been affected {2260,2615,2824,2496,1092}.

Clinical features
Several patients with CHE had a history of lymphoedema. Lesions are usually longstanding (for as long as several decades) and have a reddish-blue, variably nodular appearance.

Epidemiology
CHE is a rare neoplasm {2496,2824}. There is a slight female predominance and the majority of cases occur in adults, with a median age of 42.5 years. Rare cases may occur in childhood.

Etiology
Rare cases have arisen in the setting of chronic lymphoedema and after irradiation {2260,2615,2824,2496,1092}.

Pathogenesis
PTBP1-MAML2 and *EPC1-PCH2* gene fusions have been identified in single cases of neuroendocrine CHE {2496}.

Macroscopic appearance
CHE presents as an infiltrative, uninodular or multinodular mass (individual nodules measure 0.4–30 cm; median: 3.2 cm) or as an area of ill-defined swelling. Some of the lesions are associated with reddish-purple skin discolouration, suggestive of a vascular neoplasm.

Histopathology
CHE is a poorly circumscribed, infiltrative lesion that is typically centred in the dermis and subcutis, although occasional cases are deep-seated or involve viscera. It comprises a complex admixture of histologically benign and malignant vascular components that vary greatly in their relative proportions. These lesions are unified by a similar admixture of the different components, which include epithelioid haemangioendothelioma, retiform haemangioendothelioma, spindle cell haemangioma,

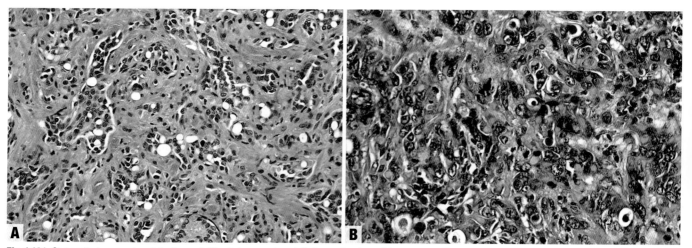

Fig. 1.181 Composite haemangioendothelioma. **A** Classic haemangioendothelioma showing solid nests or papillary growth pattern. **B** This composite haemangioendothelioma had an area composed of sheets of malignant-appearing epithelioid cells with high mitotic activity, overall with an epithelioid angiosarcoma–like appearance.

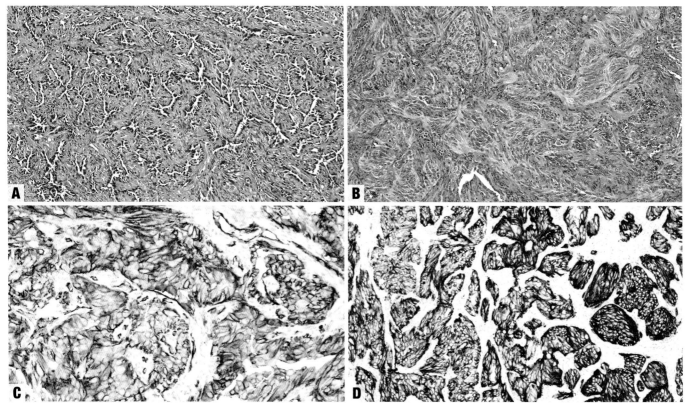

Fig. 1.182 Neuroendocrine composite haemangioendothelioma (CHE). **A** Retiform haemangioendothelioma–like area from a neuroendocrine CHE composed of anastomosing vessels lined by hobnailing endothelium with an appearance reminiscent of rete testis. **B** Nests of epithelioid cells characteristic of neuroendocrine CHE. **C** Neuroendocrine CHE showing diffuse and strong immunoreactivity for CD31. **D** Neuroendocrine CHE exhibiting diffuse and strong immunoreactivity for synaptophysin.

angiosarcoma-like areas, and benign vascular lesions (lymphangioma, angiomatosis, vascular malformation, and cavernous haemangioma). Not all cases contain every component. Vacuolated, pseudolipoblastic endothelial cells are frequently present. The angiosarcoma-like areas are usually characterized by a low-grade angiosarcomatous appearance, composed of complex dissecting vascular channels with subtle endothelial atypia and relatively few mitotic figures. However, there is a single convincing reported case containing foci resembling high-grade epithelioid angiosarcoma {1821}. Neuroendocrine CHE is characterized by a distinctive admixture of retiform haemangioendothelioma–like areas, epithelioid haemangioendothelioma–like areas, and a component with a striking nested appearance, as well as by expression of neuroendocrine markers (most often synaptophysin). CHEs are more generally consistently positive for CD31, ERG, and FLI1. About half of cases are positive for CD34 and D2-40; they are negative for CAMTA1 {2260,2615, 2824,2496,1092}.

Cytology
Not clinically relevant

Diagnostic molecular pathology
Not clinically relevant

Essential and desirable diagnostic criteria
Essential: minimal criteria for CHE include the presence of at least two morphologically distinct vascular tumour elements, most often closely resembling retiform haemangioendothelioma and epithelioid haemangioendothelioma; cases arising in pre-existing (lymphatic) vascular malformations must show at least two additional, discrete endothelial tumour components; CHEs showing foci resembling high-grade angiosarcoma are exceptionally rare, and this diagnosis should be made only after conventional angiosarcoma is rigorously excluded on clinical and morphological grounds.

Staging
Not clinically relevant

Prognosis and prediction
The behaviour of CHE in general appears to be much less aggressive than that of conventional angiosarcoma {2260, 1092}. Several lesions recurred locally between 4 months and 10 years after excision of the primary mass, often with multiple recurrences. There is potential for lymph node metastasis. Neuroendocrine CHE appears to be considerably more aggressive, with distant metastases to bone, lung, liver, or brain reported in half of patients {2496}.

Kaposi sarcoma

Thway K
Doyle LA
Grayson W
Mentzel TDW

Definition

Kaposi sarcoma (KS) is a locally aggressive endothelial proliferation that usually presents with cutaneous lesions in the form of multiple patches, plaques, or nodules, but it may also involve mucosal sites, lymph nodes, and visceral organs. KS is uniformly associated with HHV8 infection, and it represents an example of virus-induced vascular proliferation.

ICD-O coding

9140/3 Kaposi sarcoma

ICD-11 coding

2B57.Z & XH36A5 Kaposi sarcoma of unspecified primary site & Kaposi sarcoma

Related terminology

Not recommended: idiopathic multiple pigmented sarcoma of skin; angiosarcoma multiplex; granuloma multiplex haemorrhagicum.

Subtype(s)

Classic indolent Kaposi sarcoma; endemic African Kaposi sarcoma; AIDS-associated Kaposi sarcoma; iatrogenic Kaposi sarcoma

Localization

The most typical site of involvement is the skin. Mucosal membranes, lymph nodes, and visceral organs can be affected, sometimes without skin involvement. Brain and bone involvement are rare, even in disseminated disease.

Clinical features

Classic KS is characterized by reddish-purple/dark-brown macules, plaques, and nodules that can ulcerate, are particularly frequent in distal extremities, and may be accompanied by lymphoedema. It is usually indolent, with nodal and visceral involvement occurring rarely. Endemic KS may be localized to skin and has a protracted course; a lymphadenopathic form in children is rapidly progressive and highly lethal. Untreated AIDS-associated KS is the most aggressive type. In skin, lesions are most common on the face, genitals, and lower extremities; oral mucosa, lymph nodes, gastrointestinal tract (the most common extracutaneous site), and lungs are frequently involved. Nodal and visceral disease can occur without mucocutaneous lesions. KS can develop at any stage of HIV infection, but it is more frequent in advanced immunosuppression {1832,271,1796}. Iatrogenic KS is relatively uncommon, developing months to years after solid-organ transplantation or immunosuppressive treatment {3097,2566}; it may resolve upon immunosuppressant withdrawal, although its course is unpredictable. Whereas skin lesions and lymphadenopathy are obvious disease signs, visceral organ involvement may be silent or symptomatic, depending on the lesion site and extent.

Epidemiology

Four clinical and epidemiological forms are recognized. Classic indolent KS predominantly occurs in elderly men of Mediterranean, eastern European, or Ashkenazi Jewish descent. Endemic African KS occurs in non–HIV-infected middle-aged adults and children in equatorial Africa. AIDS-associated KS, the most aggressive form when untreated, is found in HIV-1–infected individuals (most frequently in men who have sex with

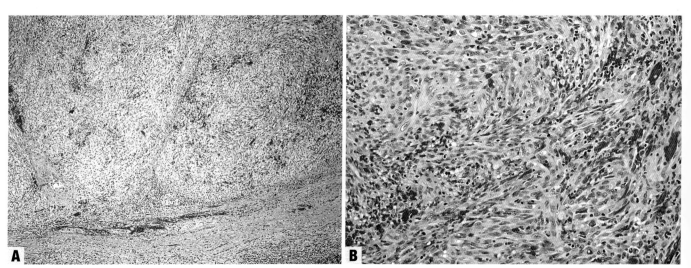

Fig. 1.183 Nodular-stage Kaposi sarcoma. **A** This example shows a cellular proliferation comprising fascicles of spindle cells, with prominent surrounding haemorrhage. Numerous small slit-like spaces containing erythrocytes are discernible, even at low power, with small numbers of ectatic vessels. **B** At higher power, the cells are uniform and contain minimally atypical elongated spindled vesicular nuclei.

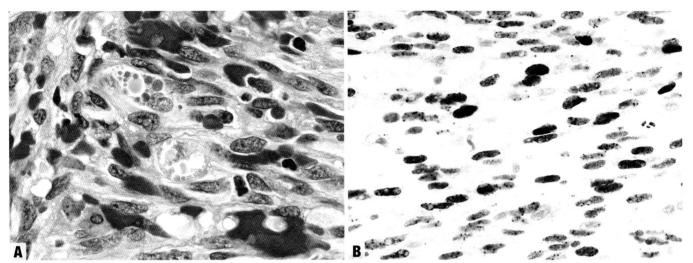

Fig. 1.184 Kaposi sarcoma. **A** Hyaline globules, which can be intracellular or extracellular, are scattered within this lesion. **B** This example of nodular Kaposi sarcoma shows strong nuclear expression of HHV8 in spindle cells.

men); its incidence has been reduced with the advent of highly active antiretroviral therapy (HAART) {1171,317}. Iatrogenic KS arises in solid-organ transplant recipients treated with immunosuppressive therapy and in patients treated with immunosuppressive agents, notably corticosteroids.

Etiology

HHV8 (KS-associated herpesvirus), found in KS endothelial cells in all disease forms, is a DNA virus encoding a latent nuclear antigen, the product of the viral gene *ORF73* {540, 2184}. Sequencing shows linkage of HHV8 genetic variants with specific populations {3088}. HHV8 is mainly sexually transmitted. HHV8 DNA is detected in all KS forms (> 95% of AIDS-related and non-related KS) {370,1793,121}. Antibodies against HHV8 nuclear antigens appear before clinical KS {1115} and can be detected in peripheral blood. Not all HHV8 infections lead to pathological manifestations, and most primary infections are asymptomatic {829}.

Pathogenesis

There is serological correlation between HHV8 infection and KS. Not all seropositive individuals have KS; infection is required but not sufficient for disease induction, which results from a complex interplay of genetic, immunological, and environmental factors {911,2735}. Comparative genomic hybridization analyses show recurrent 11q13 involvement, including of *FGF4* and *FGF3* target genes. Y chromosome loss appears recurrent in early disease, whereas additional changes of chromosomes 16, 17, 21, X, and Y appear during tumour growth {1648,2555}. *KRAS* and *TP53* alterations are reported {2279,2795,593} in addition to aberrant expression of genes related to neoangiogenesis and proliferation that may impact endothelial cell transformation by HHV8 (KS-associated herpesvirus) {2203,2567,1845}. Both viral and cellular DNA-encoded microRNAs have been shown to play an important role in pathogenesis {1114,2727}.

Macroscopic appearance

Skin lesions (patches, plaques, nodules) range from small to several centimetres. Involvement of mucosa, soft tissues, lymph

nodes, and visceral organs presents as variably sized haemorrhagic nodules that can coalesce.

Histopathology

All four KS types show identical histological features. Early skin lesions show subtle vascular proliferation {2693}. In the patch stage, vascular spaces are increased in number, dissecting collagen fibres in the upper reticular dermis. Lining endothelial cells are flattened or oval, with no or minimal atypia. Pre-existing vessels may protrude into lumina of new vessels. Ovoid/spindle endothelial cell proliferations surround pre-existing vessels, and admixed lymphoplasmacytic infiltrates, extravasated erythrocytes, and haemosiderin deposits are common. Rarely, lesions resemble lymphangioma or haemangioma, causing diagnostic confusion {2574,3353,662}. The papillary dermis is uninvolved in early stages. In the plaque stage, all patch-stage characteristics are exaggerated, and angioproliferation is extensive, with jagged vascular spaces. The inflammatory infiltrate is denser, with extravascular erythrocytes and siderophages, as well as frequent intracellular or extracellular hyaline globules. The nodular stage comprises circumscribed, cellular nodules of spindle cell fascicles with minimal atypia, hyaline globules, and numerous slit-like spaces containing erythrocytes, with peripheral ectatic vessels. Rare histological subtypes include anaplastic KS, which is clinically aggressive with increased metastatic potential {1454,3381}, and intravascular KS {1915}.

In nodal disease, KS may be unifocal or multifocal and may entirely efface nodes. Early lesions may be subtle, showing only increased numbers of vascular channels with sinusoidal plasma cell infiltrates {1900}. In viscera, lesions tend to respect organ architecture and spread along native structures, such as pre-existing vessels, bronchi, and liver portal areas, before involving surrounding parenchyma {956}.

Both lining endothelial cells of vessels and spindled tumour cells express endothelial markers, including CD31, CD34, and ERG, and lymphatic markers such as podoplanin (D2-40), and they show almost invariable nuclear expression of HHV8.

Cytology
Not clinically relevant

Diagnostic molecular pathology
PCR and in situ hybridization show HHV8 in the flat endothelial cells lining vascular spaces and in spindle cells {369}.

Essential and desirable diagnostic criteria
Essential: proliferation of small slit-like vessels lined by mildly atypical cells and surrounded by bland spindle cells; extravasated erythrocytes and lymphoplasmacytic patchy infiltrates in the early stage.
Desirable: nuclear HHV8 expression (by immunohistochemistry).

Staging
Not clinically relevant

Prognosis and prediction
Disease evolution depends on the epidemiological–clinical type and extent. Degree of immunosuppression at diagnosis is the most important survival determinant, but this is modified by treatment (including surgery, radiotherapy, and chemotherapy). Immunosuppression withdrawal can sometimes cause disease resolution. Combined HAART and systemic chemotherapy improves morbidity and mortality {1992}. Patients with widespread visceral involvement are commonly poorly responsive to treatment.

Pseudomyogenic haemangioendothelioma

Hornick JL
Agaram NP
Bovée JVMG

Definition

Pseudomyogenic haemangioendothelioma is a rarely metastasizing endothelial neoplasm that occurs more frequently in young adult males. It often presents as multiple discontiguous nodules in different tissue planes and histologically mimics a myoid tumour or epithelioid sarcoma.

ICD-O coding

9138/1 Pseudomyogenic (epithelioid sarcoma–like) haemangioendothelioma

ICD-11 coding

2E81.0Z & XH26F6 Neoplastic haemangioma, unspecified & Pseudomyogenic (epithelioid sarcoma–like) haemangioendothelioma

Related terminology

Acceptable: epithelioid sarcoma–like haemangioendothelioma.

Subtype(s)

None

Localization

Pseudomyogenic haemangioendothelioma usually arises on the lower limbs (55% of cases); the upper limbs and trunk are less commonly affected (20% each); tumours rarely occur on the head or neck (5%) {322,2156,1412,97}.

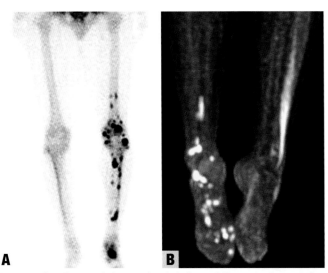

Fig. 1.185 Pseudomyogenic haemangioendothelioma. **A** Bone scan from a patient with pseudomyogenic haemangioendothelioma showing multiple lesions involving the tibia and ankle. **B** FDG PET from a patient with pseudomyogenic haemangioendothelioma showing multiple lesions in the foot.

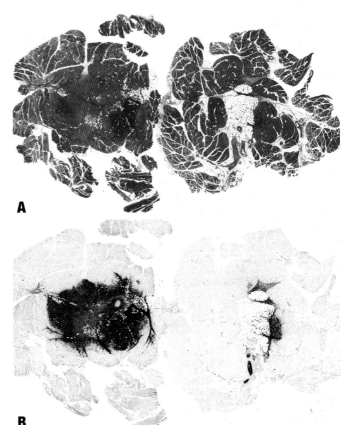

Fig. 1.186 Pseudomyogenic haemangioendothelioma. **A** Scanning image from a multifocal intramuscular pseudomyogenic haemangioendothelioma of the lower leg. **B** Immunohistochemistry for FOSB is strongly positive in tumour cells and highlights the multifocality.

Clinical features

About half of affected patients present with painless and half with painful nodules. In approximately 60% of patients, this disease is multifocal, often involving multiple tissue planes {1412}. Most patients (75%) present with cutaneous and subcutaneous nodules. About 50% of affected patients have intramuscular lesions, and 20% of patients have lytic bone lesions {322,2156, 1412,97}. Some patients have intraosseous lesions without soft tissue involvement {1474}. By PET, the tumours in most patients are highly avid for FDG; this technique can be used to visualize clinically occult deep lesions in patients who present with cutaneous nodules {1412}.

Epidemiology

Pseudomyogenic haemangioendothelioma is rare. There is a marked male predominance (M:F ratio: 3.5:1), with peak incidence in young adults (mean age: 30 years) {1412}. Only 20% of patients are aged > 40 years at presentation.

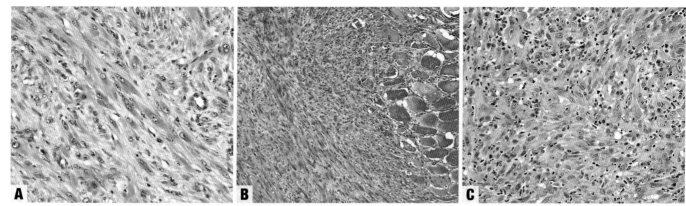

Fig. 1.187 Pseudomyogenic haemangioendothelioma. **A** Some tumour cells with brightly eosinophilic cytoplasm resemble rhabdomyoblasts. **B** The tumour shows infiltrative margins into adjacent skeletal muscle. **C** Prominent stromal neutrophils can be seen in this example. Note the scattered tumour cells with a more epithelioid appearance.

Etiology
Unknown

Pathogenesis
Pseudomyogenic haemangioendothelioma was initially described as being caused by a balanced translocation t(7;19) (q22;q13), resulting in the fusion of *SERPINE1* to *FOSB* {3105, 3224}. Recently, an alternative *ACTB-FOSB* gene fusion was identified in half of the cases {36}. These fusions lead to upregulation of FOSB, probably by a promoter-swapping mechanism, because most of the *FOSB* gene is retained in the fusion (fused at exon 2). *SERPINE1* (fusion occurs in non-coding exon 1) is normally highly expressed in vascular cells {3224}, and *ACTB* (fused at exon 3) is a ubiquitously expressed gene {36}. FOSB is a member of the FOS family of transcription factors, which encode leucine zipper proteins that can dimerize with proteins of the JUN family, thereby forming the transcription factor complex AP-1, regulating cell proliferation, differentiation, angiogenesis, and survival. Upregulation of FOSB causes activation of the AP-1 complex. Overexpression of the retained part of FOSB in endothelial cells affects angiogenesis in vitro, with the retained part acting as an active transcription factor capable of regulating its own transcription {3164}. The clinicopathological features and behaviour do not differ between pseudomyogenic haemangioendotheliomas with *SERPINE1-FOSB* and *ACTB-FOSB* fusions, although tumours with the *ACTB* variant more often present as solitary lesions {36}.

Macroscopic appearance
Grossly, margins are ill defined and the cut surface is firm and grey or white. Most tumour nodules are 1–2.5 cm in greatest dimension; only 10% of tumours are > 3 cm in size {1412}.

Histopathology
The tumour is composed of sheets and loose fascicles of plump spindle cells with abundant, brightly eosinophilic cytoplasm, sometimes mimicking rhabdomyoblasts {1412}. A minor component of cells with epithelioid cytomorphology is often present; but sometimes epithelioid cells predominate {2156}. Intraosseous lesions are often dominated by epithelioid cells with marked cytoplasmic eosinophilia, associated with reactive woven bone, haemorrhage, and osteoclast-like giant cells {1474}. The tumour cells contain vesicular nuclei with generally small nucleoli. The degree of nuclear atypia is usually mild, and mitotic activity is scarce. About 10% of tumours show notable pleomorphism or large nucleoli {1412}. Occasional tumours contain focally myxoid stroma. About 50% of cases contain prominent stromal neutrophils. The tumours show infiltrative margins.

By immunohistochemistry, these tumours show diffuse expression of keratins (with AE1/AE3 but not MNF116) and the endothelial transcription factors FLI1 and ERG {2156,1412}. About 50% of cases are positive for CD31. Focal expression of SMA is observed in one third of tumours. Nuclear staining for FOSB is a consistent finding {2976,1440}.

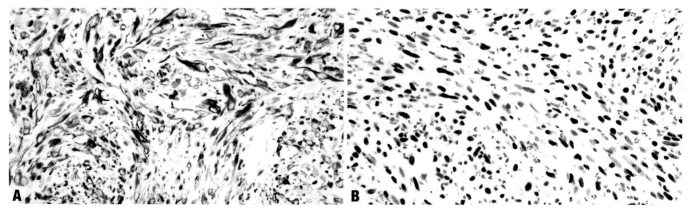

Fig. 1.188 Pseudomyogenic haemangioendothelioma. **A** Diffuse expression of keratin AE1/AE3. **B** Strong nuclear staining for the endothelial transcription factor ERG.

Cytology
Not clinically relevant

Diagnostic molecular pathology
Detection of *FOSB* rearrangement can be helpful for diagnosis.

Essential and desirable diagnostic criteria
Essential: plump spindle or more rarely epithelioid cell morphology with vesicular chromatin and eosinophilic cytoplasm; fascicular or sheet-like growth pattern; expression of ERG, FOSB, and keratins (AE1/AE3).
Desirable: demonstration of *FOSB* gene rearrangement (in selected cases).

Staging
Not clinically relevant

Prognosis and prediction
Approximately 60% of patients with this tumour type experience local recurrences (often multiple) or develop additional nodules in the same anatomical region {1412}. The interval between excision of the primary tumour and recurrence is usually short, within 1–2 years. The relationship between margin status and recurrence has not been established. Regional lymph node and distant metastases are uncommon (< 5%), most often occurring years or decades after presentation, rarely within a short interval {1412}. Metastatic sites may include lungs, bones, and soft tissues. Histological features do not predict metastasis.

Epithelioid haemangioendothelioma

Rubin BP
Deyrup AT
Doyle LA

Definition
Epithelioid haemangioendothelioma is a malignant vascular neoplasm composed of epithelioid endothelial cells within a distinctive myxohyaline stroma; most cases are characterized by the presence of a *WWTR1-CAMTA1* gene fusion. A small subset of tumours show distinct morphology, with well-formed vessels lined by epithelioid endothelial cells with abundant eosinophilic cytoplasm, and are characterized by a *YAP1-TFE3* fusion.

ICD-O coding
9133/3 Epithelioid haemangioendothelioma NOS

ICD-11 coding
2B5Y & XH9GF8 Other specified malignant mesenchymal neoplasms & Epithelioid haemangioendothelioma

Related terminology
Not recommended: malignant epithelioid haemangioendothelioma.

Subtype(s)
Epithelioid haemangioendothelioma with *WWTR1-CAMTA1* fusion; epithelioid haemangioendothelioma with *YAP1-TFE3* fusion

Localization
Epithelioid haemangioendothelioma most commonly involves somatic soft tissue, lung, and liver, but any site or organ can be affected. Skin and soft tissue lesions are usually solitary {3268, 2559,2076}, whereas visceral and bone lesions are often multifocal and may be metastatic at presentation {1480,1948,300, 3115,1650}. Within soft tissues, tumours are more often deep rather than superficial {2076}.

Clinical features
Presenting symptoms depend on the anatomical site of involvement. In soft tissues, epithelioid haemangioendothelioma usually presents as a painful mass. Those arising from large vessels can result in other symptoms of vascular occlusion, such as oedema and thrombophlebitis. For liver lesions, please see the 2019 *Digestive system tumours* volume {3282}.

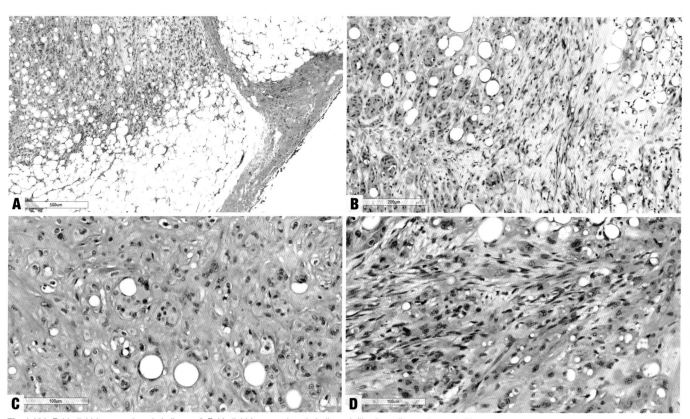

Fig. 1.189 Epithelioid haemangioendothelioma. **A** Epithelioid haemangioendothelioma infiltrating adipose tissue. **B** The lesional cells in this example range from nests of epithelioid cells to more spindled cells focally. Note the fibromyxoid matrix. **C** Typical appearance, with nests and cords of epithelioid cells set in a sclerotic matrix. **D** Epithelioid haemangioendothelioma with a more spindled appearance than is typical.

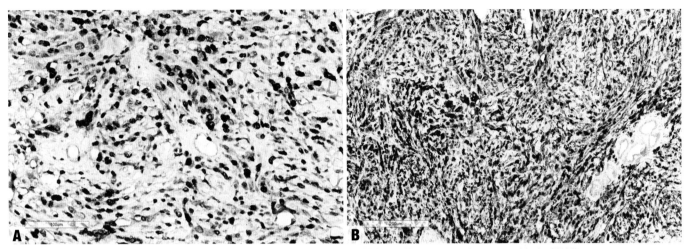

Fig. 1.190 Epithelioid haemangioendothelioma. **A** Diffuse and strong immunoreactivity for ERG. **B** Diffuse and strong immunoreactivity for CAMTA1.

Epidemiology

Epithelioid haemangioendothelioma shows a wide age distribution, but it usually arises in adults and is rare in children {813}. There is a slight female predominance for visceral lesions {813, 2076,3269}. Patients with *YAP1-TFE3* fusion tumours tend to be younger than those with a *WWTR1-CAMTA1* fusion {133}.

Etiology
Unknown

Pathogenesis

Epithelioid haemangioendothelioma is characterized by a t(1;3)(p36;q23-q25) resulting in a *WWTR1-CAMTA1* fusion in > 90% of cases {932,2073,3041}. The translocation is present in tumours across all anatomical sites and clinical behaviours. The WWTR1 (TAZ) protein is one of two end effectors of the Hippo pathway, a highly conserved tumour suppressive signal transduction pathway {1310}. One of the major roles of the Hippo pathway is to phosphorylate WWTR1 (TAZ) and YAP1 (encoded

by *YAP1*), resulting in cytoplasmic sequestration and degradation. WWTR1 (TAZ) and YAP1 are transcription factors that promote a pro-oncogenic transcriptional programme. Fusion of WWTR1 (TAZ) to CAMTA1 results in dysregulation of the Hippo pathway, such that WWTR1-CAMTA1 resides constitutively in the nucleus, driving oncogenic transformation {3040}.

The monoclonal origin of multifocal epithelioid haemangioendotheliomas has also been established using *WWTR1-CAMTA1* breakpoint analysis. This indicates that multiple lesions arise from local or metastatic spread from a single primary as opposed to multiple independent primaries {929}.

A separate translocation event, *YAP1-TFE3*, has been identified in a subset of epithelioid haemangioendotheliomas with distinct morphological features {133}. YAP1, similar to WWTR1 (TAZ), is a downstream transcriptional regulator of the Hippo pathway, and there is substantial sequence homology between the two proteins. TFE3, a well-known oncogenic transcription factor involved in other soft tissue tumour translocations, is upregulated in these lesions as a result of this fusion.

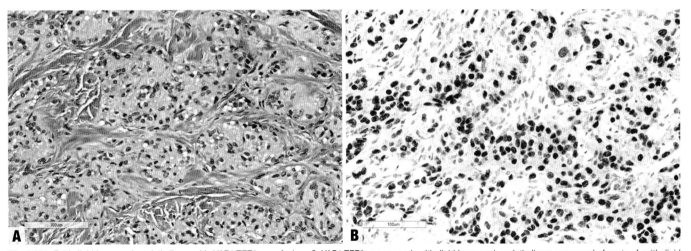

Fig. 1.191 Epithelioid haemangioendothelioma with *YAP1-TFE3* gene fusion. **A** *YAP1-TFE3*–rearranged epithelioid haemangioendothelioma composed of nests of epithelioid cells infiltrating fibrous tissue. Note the focal cytoplasmic vacuolization. **B** Diffuse and strong immunoreactivity for TFE3.

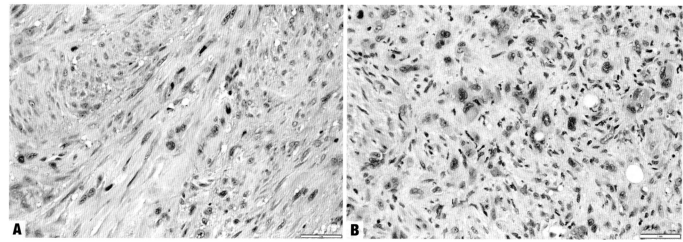

Fig. 1.192 Epithelioid haemangioendothelioma. **A** Epithelioid haemangioendothelioma with spindle/sarcomatous features and increased nuclear pleomorphism. **B** Epithelioid haemangioendothelioma with malignant histological features and increased nuclear pleomorphism.

Macroscopic appearance

Tumours in visceral or deep soft tissue locations are usually larger than superficial ones, and they may measure > 10 cm. The cut surface is typically white and firm. For soft tissue tumours that arise from a small to medium-sized vein (as many as 50%) {3268, 2076}, origin from a vessel can be grossly identifiable, usually as a firm, tan-tinged mass circumscribed by the vessel wall.

Histopathology

Angiocentric tumours expand the vessel wall, obliterate the lumen, and spread centrifugally into surrounding tissue, where they induce a sclerotic response. Infiltrative growth into adjacent skeletal muscle or fat may be seen. Epithelioid haemangioendothelioma is characterized by cords and nests of epithelioid cells in a myxohyaline stroma. Tumour cells have moderate amounts of eosinophilic cytoplasm and round nuclei with inconspicuous nucleoli. Intracytoplasmic vacuoles are sometimes present and may contain erythrocytes. In most cases there is only minimal atypia and mitotic count is very low. The stroma is variably myxoid and hyaline; in some cases, hyaline stroma may obscure the tumour cells. Cystic degeneration, haemorrhage, sclerosis, and metaplastic ossification may be present {2076,3002}.

Epithelioid haemangioendothelioma with *YAP1-TFE3* fusion shows distinctive histological features. The tumour cells usually have brightly eosinophilic cytoplasm and are more likely to show solid growth and often form vascular spaces; the latter feature is generally not seen in the classic form of epithelioid haemangioendothelioma {133}.

A small subset (< 10%) of epithelioid haemangioendotheliomas have atypical histological features, including nuclear pleomorphism, increased mitotic activity, solid sheet-like growth, and necrosis {813,2076}. In some cases, these tumours may resemble epithelioid angiosarcoma. In such cases, the presence of areas of conventional epithelioid haemangioendothelioma or nuclear CAMTA1 expression supports the diagnosis. This latter group of lesions is often associated with more aggressive behaviour.

The tumour cells of epithelioid haemangioendothelioma express the endothelial markers CD34, CD31, podoplanin (D2-40), FLI1, and ERG; however, there may be substantial variability in the degree of staining for a given marker {1046,

2670,2140}. Epithelial antigens are expressed in as many as 40% of cases (CK7, CK8, CK18, pan-keratin), but expression of EMA is unusual {2076,2121}. SMA expression is present in approximately 50% of cases {2076}. Epithelioid haemangioendothelioma with *WWTR1-CAMTA1* typically shows diffuse strong nuclear expression of CAMTA1, which is a surrogate for the WWTR1-CAMTA1 fusion protein {849}. Tumours with *YAP1-TFE3* fusion show diffuse nuclear TFE3 expression {133}; however, TFE3 is less specific in this regard, because expression can be seen in tumours with *WWTR1-CAMTA1* fusion {849,1041}.

Cytology
Not clinically relevant

Diagnostic molecular pathology
Identification of the *WWTR1-CAMTA1* or *YAP1-TFE3* fusion transcripts helps distinguish epithelioid haemangioendothelioma from other tumours.

Essential and desirable diagnostic criteria
Essential: classic epithelioid haemangioendothelioma is composed of cords or nests of epithelioid cells with cytoplasmic vacuolization within a myxochondroid or hyaline stroma; epithelioid haemangioendothelioma with *YAP1-TFE3* fusion shows either solid growth or well-formed vascular channels lined by epithelioid endothelial cells with moderate nuclear atypia and abundant pale cytoplasm.
Desirable (in selected cases): CAMTA1 expression by immunohistochemistry and/or *WWTR1-CAMTA1* fusion; TFE3 overexpression by immunohistochemistry and/or *TFE3* gene rearrangement (*YAP1-TFE3* gene fusion).

Staging
Epithelioid haemangioendothelioma of somatic soft tissue should be staged according to the American Joint Committee on Cancer (AJCC) eighth-edition TNM staging system for soft tissue sarcoma of the trunk and extremities. For tumours occurring within the abdominal and thoracic cavities, AJCC eighth-edition staging is not applicable. Instead, it is recommended that the size of the largest lesion is recorded if possible.

Prognosis and prediction

The prognosis differs depending on anatomical site. Epithelioid haemangioendotheliomas of soft tissues can be indolent; however, approximately 21% will metastasize and pursue an aggressive clinical course, with death in approximately 17% of patients {3268,2076,813,932,1041}. Risk stratification into high-risk and low-risk groups based on a combination of mitotic activity (> 3 mitoses per 10 mm^2; > 3 mitoses per 50 high-power fields, assuming a field diameter of 0.5 mm and an area of 0.2 mm^2) and tumour size (> 3 cm) has shown a worse prognosis for patients with both features (5-year disease-specific survival rate: 59%) compared with patients with neither feature (5-year disease-specific survival rate: 100%) {813}. Severe cytological atypia, spindled morphology, and the presence of necrosis have not been shown to be indicative of aggressive behaviour in epithelioid haemangioendothelioma of soft tissue, and even tumours with bland morphological features can metastasize {813,2076}. However, in the recently identified *YAP1-TFE3* subset of cases, metastatic rate may be higher, with metastases reported in 3 of 6 cases in the original study {133}. Epithelioid haemangioendothelioma arising in lung or bone has a worse prognosis than soft tissue tumours, and patients often present with metastatic disease {2839,108,1948,1769}. By contrast, cutaneous epithelioid haemangioendothelioma has an excellent prognosis {2076,2559}.

Angiosarcoma

Thway K
Billings SD

Definition
Angiosarcoma is a malignant vascular neoplasm that variably recapitulates the morphological, immunohistochemical features of endothelial cells.

ICD-O coding
9120/3 Angiosarcoma

ICD-11 coding
2B56.Y & XH6264 Angiosarcoma, other specified primary site & Haemangiosarcoma

Related terminology
Not recommended: haemangiosarcoma; lymphangiosarcoma; malignant haemangioendothelioma; malignant angioendothelioma.

Subtype(s)
None

Localization
More than 50% of cases arise in cutaneous sites, with the remainder occurring within deep soft tissues, breast, bone, or viscera. Soft tissue angiosarcomas most frequently arise within deep muscles of the lower extremities, followed by retroperitoneum, trunk, and head and neck {2064}. In children, there is a propensity for occurrence in the mediastinum {812}. Angiosarcomas rarely arise within a pre-existing vessel {1419}.

Clinical features
Soft tissue angiosarcomas present as poorly defined, rapidly growing, often painful masses, occasionally associated with acute haemorrhage. Approximately one third of patients have other symptoms, such as anaemia, coagulopathy, and persistent haematoma {2064}.

Epidemiology
Angiosarcoma accounts for approximately 2–4% of soft tissue sarcomas {2665,3089}. There is a male predominance, with peak incidence in the seventh decade of life, and a wide age range, although it is very rare in children {812,2812}.

Etiology
The etiology is unknown in most cases, although a minority arise after radiation exposure or longstanding lymphoedema. Smaller numbers occur in association with implanted foreign material (including synthetic grafts), in the vicinity of arteriovenous fistulas, in a pre-existing haemangioma / vascular malformation, in regions of prior trauma or surgery, in certain syndromes (e.g. neurofibromatosis and Maffucci syndrome), and rarely as heterologous components of other neoplasms (e.g. in benign or malignant nerve sheath tumours) {1524,3257,2084,2666}.

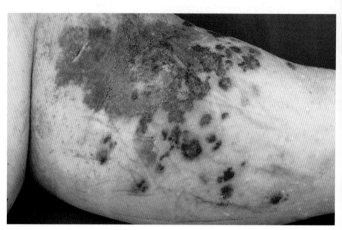

Fig. 1.193 Angiosarcoma. This tumour, present on the lower extremity, is composed of markedly haemorrhagic, purple to bluish-black coalescing macules and papules.

Pathogenesis
Angiosarcomas are genetically heterogeneous. Most harbour complex karyotypes, without recurrent chromosomal changes {1243,3191}. Unlike other sarcomas with complex genomics, angiosarcomas show low levels of alterations in *TP53* and PIK3CA/AKT/mTOR pathways {1488,124}. Genes related to angiogenesis and vascular-specific receptor tyrosine kinases (including *TIE1*, *TEK*, *KDR* [*VEGFR2*], and *FLT4* [*VEGFR3*]) are usually upregulated compared with other sarcomas {142,1483}. A subset of cases, typically in younger patients, are associated with *CIC* gene abnormalities and inferior disease-free survival {1433}. About 40% harbour recurrent somatic mutations involving angiogenic signalling pathways (e.g. in *KDR*, *PTPRB*, and *PLCG1*), and rare mutations occur in RAS genes, *PIK3CA*, *TP53*, *FLT4*, and *TIE1* {142,1488,258}.

High-level *MYC* gene amplifications (at 8q24) occur in almost all postirradiation and chronic lymphoedema-associated angiosarcomas, and rarely in primary angiosarcomas {1255,1973,1658,987}; 25% of secondary angiosarcomas are associated with *FLT4* (*VEGFR3*) coamplification at 5q35 {1255}. *PLCG1* and *KDR* mutations occur in subsets of both primary and secondary angiosarcomas, particularly in breast and bone/visceral sites, regardless of *MYC* status {1433}. *KDR* and *PLCG1* mutations are mutually exclusive, with both genes involved in the angiogenesis signalling pathway. *FLT4*-amplified angiosarcomas lack *PLCG1* or *KDR* mutations, occur predominantly in *MYC*-amplified tumours, and are associated with a poor prognosis {1433}.

Macroscopic appearance
Angiosarcomas are typically haemorrhagic, diffuse or multinodular masses of variable size (1–15 cm in diameter; median: 5 cm) {2064}. They can be relatively well demarcated or ill defined. Better-differentiated tumours often have a haemorrhagic, spongy appearance, whereas more poorly differentiated

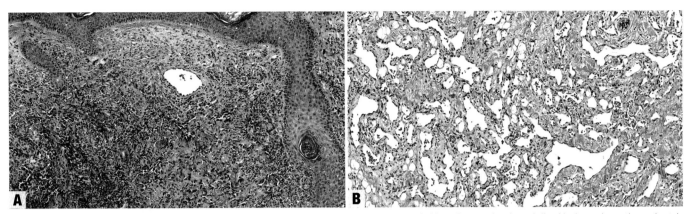

Fig. 1.194 Angiosarcoma. **A** Cutaneous angiosarcoma. The dermis contains ill-defined tumour composed of irregular vascular channels lined by hyperchromatic, moderately atypical vascular endothelial cells. There is a marked surrounding chronic inflammatory infiltrate that makes the tumour difficult to discern. **B** Well-differentiated angiosarcoma. This lesion shows well-formed (although angulated and irregular) vascular spaces lined by mildly atypical flattened endothelial cells.

neoplasms are more solid and fleshy, with firm, greyish-white tissue with focal necrosis or areas of haemorrhage with cystic degeneration.

Histopathology

Angiosarcomas typically have ill-defined margins, and they vary in their degree of cytological atypia and architectural differentiation. They range from well-formed, anastomosing vessels to solid sheets of high-grade epithelioid or spindled cells without clear vasoformation. Tumours often show a mixture of these two patterns. Most show high-grade morphology, with anastomosing vascular channels or more-solid areas, variable nuclear atypia, mitotic activity (most prominent in more-solid areas) and coagulative necrosis. Sometimes atypia is mild and focal, with cells resembling normal vascular endothelium. Marked pleomorphism is rare. Vasoformative areas are composed of ramifying channels lined by atypical spindle or epithelioid cells, with variable endothelial multilayering, intraluminal budding, hobnailing, or papillary-like projections. The vascular channels may be poorly formed, with complex dissecting patterns within fibroadipose tissue, or they may be compressed, with only subtle cleft-like spaces. Solid areas typically comprise cellular sheets of spindled to

epithelioid cells with abundant eosinophilic to amphophilic cytoplasm, large vesicular nuclei, and prominent nucleoli. There may be associated blood lakes or extensive haemorrhage and organizing haematoma that obscures much of the neoplasm, making recognition difficult. More rarely, tumours appear morphologically low-grade, with well-formed vascular channels lined by minimally atypical spindled cells. Epithelioid angiosarcomas typically have a solid architecture, with diffuse, sheet-like patterns of large, atypical epithelioid or polygonal cells with ovoid vesicular nuclei, prominent large central nucleoli, and abundant cytoplasm. Vasoformation is often focal {1020}.

Angiosarcomas typically show membranous CD31 and nuclear ERG positivity, with variable expression of CD34 and factor VIII–related antigen (now rarely used) {2129,2140,1046}. An outer layer of SMA-positive pericytes is usually absent. Keratin and EMA expression may be seen, particularly in epithelioid subtypes, and this can lead to misdiagnosis as carcinoma {56,1020}. Irradiation- and lymphoedema-associated angiosarcomas are frequently strongly positive for MYC.

Cytology

Not clinically relevant

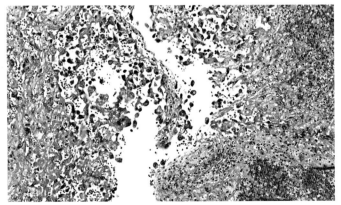

Fig. 1.195 Angiosarcoma with thrombus. This tumour is present amid extensive organizing haemorrhage and thrombus. Sometimes this can be so extensive that it obscures much of the neoplasm.

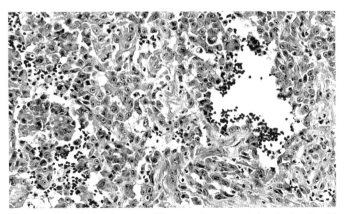

Fig. 1.196 Epithelioid angiosarcoma. The tumour is composed of predominantly solid distributions of moderately atypical, large epithelioid cells with ovoid vesicular nuclei and prominent nuclei.

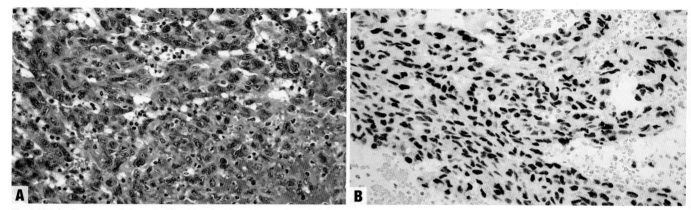

Fig. 1.197 Angiosarcoma. **A** A poorly differentiated angiosarcoma composed of sheets of epithelioid and spindle cells with amphophilic cytoplasm. **B** Nuclear immunoreactivity for ERG, the most sensitive and specific endothelial marker. In the absence of a vasoformative component, confirmation of endothelial differentiation by immunohistochemistry is critical.

Diagnostic molecular pathology

Demonstration of *MYC* amplification may be helpful, although only in the setting of irradiation- or lymphoedema-associated angiosarcoma {987,2091,1255}.

Essential and desirable diagnostic criteria

Essential: vasoformative or sheet-like growth; multilayering of endothelial cells; nuclear atypia, increased mitoses, necrosis; CD31 and ERG expression by immunohistochemistry.

Staging

Staging of angiosarcoma is not recommended, because its typically aggressive natural history is not consistent with soft tissue staging systems.

Prognosis and prediction

Angiosarcomas of soft tissue are highly aggressive. More than half of patients die of disease within 1 year {2064}, with a local recurrence rate of 20% and distant metastases in approximately half {2064}. The most frequent site of distant metastasis is the lungs, followed by the lymph nodes, soft tissues, bone, liver, and other sites (including the brain) {2064,324}. Older patient age, retroperitoneal location, and large size are associated with poor outcome {2064,975,1735}. Factors such as epithelioid change, necrosis, and margin status, which have been shown to be prognostically significant for angiosarcomas in general, require specific validation for angiosarcomas of soft tissue {1735,975}. Standard sarcoma grading systems have been applied to angiosarcoma, although the correlation between histological grade and prognosis has been debated {2194,1395}, and well-differentiated tumours often behave aggressively.

Glomus tumour

Specht K
Antonescu CR

Definition
Glomus tumour is a mesenchymal neoplasm composed of cells resembling the perivascular modified smooth muscle cells of the normal glomus body.

ICD-O coding
8711/0 Glomus tumour NOS

ICD-11 coding
2E81.0Y & XH47J2 Other specified neoplastic haemangioma & Glomus tumour NOS
2E81.0Y & XH21E6 Other specified neoplastic haemangioma & Glomus tumour, malignant

Related terminology
Acceptable: glomangioma; glomangiomyoma; glomuvenous malformation; glomangiosarcoma.

Subtype(s)
Glomangioma; glomangiomyoma; glomangiomatosis; glomus tumour of uncertain malignant potential; glomus tumour, malignant

Localization
The vast majority occur in the distal extremities, particularly the subungual region, the hand, the wrist, and the foot {1050, 2854,2949}. Rare tumours have been reported in almost every location, including gastrointestinal tract {2132}, genitourinary system {2002,2708,2844,2874}, mediastinum {1372}, nerve {460}, bone {2679}, and lung {1103}. Glomus tumours often occur in skin or superficial soft tissues, although occasional cases occur in deep soft tissue or viscera. An unusually large number occur in the stomach {2132}. Malignant glomus tumours are usually deeply situated but may be cutaneous {609,1050,1917}.

Clinical features
Cutaneous glomus tumours are typically small (< 1 cm), reddish-blue nodules often associated with a long history of pain, particularly with exposure to cold or minor tactile stimulation. Deep-seated or visceral glomus tumours present as a nonspecific mass. The vascular tumours in blue rubber bleb naevus syndrome are commonly glomuvenous malformations (also known as glomangiomas).

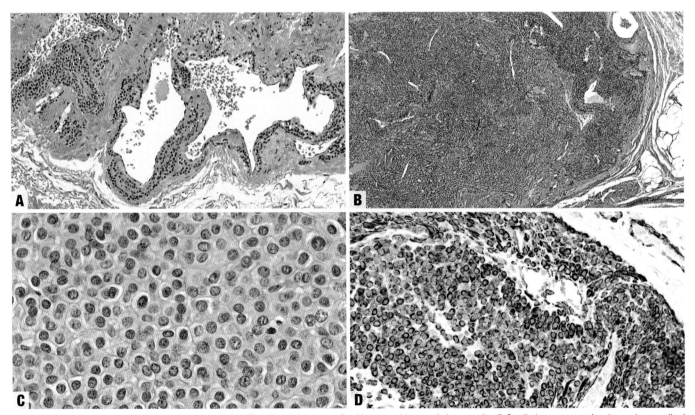

Fig. 1.198 Glomus tumour. **A** Glomangioma, composed of dilated vascular spaces lined by several layers of glomus cells. **B** Small glomus tumour forming a circumscribed mass. **C** Glomus tumour, solid type, consisting of round, uniform cells with well-defined cell margins. **D** The tumour cells are strongly positive for SMA.

Soft tissue tumours   179

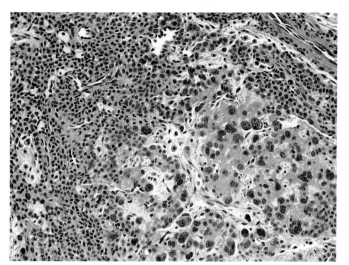

Fig. 1.199 Symplastic glomus tumour. Areas of prominent nuclear atypia but without mitotic activity.

Epidemiology

Glomus tumours are rare, accounting for < 2% of soft tissue tumours {2854}. Multiple lesions may be seen in 10% of patients. They can occur at any age, but most are diagnosed in young adults. Glomus tumours have no sex predilection, except for subungual lesions, which are far more common in women {3028,3159}. Malignant glomus tumours are rare {1050,1585, 1917,2206}.

Etiology

The syndrome of multiple familial glomus tumours (glomuvenous malformations) shows autosomal dominant inheritance {1298, 2021} and is caused by inactivating mutations in the glomulin gene (*GLMN*), which is predominantly expressed in vascular smooth muscle cells {367,433,2038}. Another genetic mechanism, demonstrated in about 70% of familial multiple glomus tumours, is the uniparental disomy, further supporting a somatic second-hit model {105}. An association between digital glomus tumours and neurofibromatosis type 1 has been reported, with frequent involvement of multiple digits {405,803,2748,2948}.

Biallelic *NF1* inactivation underlies the pathogenesis of neurofibromatosis type 1–associated glomus tumours {405}.

Pathogenesis

Sporadic benign and malignant glomus tumours of soft tissue or visceral origin harbour recurrent NOTCH gene family rearrangements, with *MIR143-NOTCH1/2/3* fusion genes in more than half of cases {2206}. Of note, all malignant glomus tumours tested in that study showed the presence of *NOTCH2* gene rearrangements. In contrast, NOTCH gene rearrangements have only rarely been detected in other tumours of pericytic origin. In addition, a small subset of sporadic glomus tumours show oncogenic *BRAF* and *KRAS* mutations {530}, and *BRAF* mutations have been associated with malignant histology {1585,715}.

Macroscopic appearance

Glomus tumours typically form circumscribed, ovoid or round nodules with a solid or cystic and often haemorrhagic surface on sectioning.

Histopathology

Glomus cells are small, uniform, and rounded, with a centrally placed round nucleus, amphophilic to lightly eosinophilic cytoplasm, and sharply defined cell borders. Occasionally, cases show oncocytic or epithelioid change {2548,2887}. Solid glomus tumours account for approximately 75% of cases and are composed of nests of glomus cells surrounding capillary-sized vessels. Glomuvenous malformations (also known as glomangiomas) are most common in patients with multiple or familial lesions, account for approximately 20% of cases, and are characterized by cavernous haemangioma–like vascular structures surrounded by small clusters of glomus cells. Glomangiomyomas show transition from typical glomus cells to elongated cells resembling mature smooth muscle. In some glomus tumours, a branching, haemangiopericytoma-like vasculature is present (glomangiopericytoma) {1207}. Glomangiomatosis is an extremely rare subtype of glomus tumour with an overall architectural resemblance to a diffuse vascular malformation (so-called angiomatosis), but containing nests of glomus cells investing vessel walls {1050,1511,2441,3403}. Symplastic

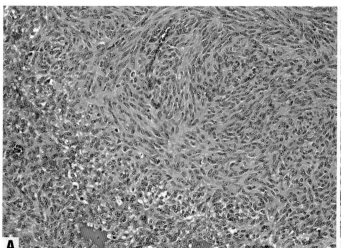

Fig. 1.200 Malignant glomus tumour. **A** Spindle cell type. **B** Round cell type, with mitotic activity.

glomus tumours show striking nuclear atypia in the absence of any other features indicative of malignancy (e.g. large size, deep location, mitotic activity, necrosis) {174,586,1050,1564}.

The diagnosis of malignant glomus tumour should be reserved for tumours showing either marked nuclear atypia (with any level of mitotic activity) or atypical mitotic figures {1050}. A component of pre-existing benign-appearing glomus tumour is often present. There are two types of malignant glomus tumour: one resembling a leiomyosarcoma or fibrosarcoma and the other resembling a primitive round cell tumour. Immunohistochemical demonstration of SMA and pericellular collagen IV is required for this diagnosis in the absence of a clear-cut benign precursor. Glomus tumours not fulfilling the criteria for malignancy but having at least one atypical feature other than nuclear pleomorphism are designated as being of uncertain malignant potential. Although glomus tumours of > 2 cm in size and deep location were previously considered malignant, subsequent experience suggests that these have uncertain malignant potential. An infiltrative growth pattern, high cellularity, and spindled morphology are also features significantly more common in malignant glomus tumours and glomus tumours of uncertain malignant potential {1585}.

Glomus tumours of all types typically express SMA and MSA and have abundant pericellular production of collagen IV. Staining for h-caldesmon is also positive, whereas CD34 expression is focal or absent {1050,2209}. BRAF p.Val600Glu expression is seen in the *BRAF*-mutated molecular subset.

Cytology
Not clinically relevant

Diagnostic molecular pathology
Detection of NOTCH gene rearrangements and/or *BRAF* mutations by various molecular strategies can be helpful, especially in malignant examples. *BRAF* p.Val600Glu mutations have been detected in 6% of glomus tumours, all either malignant or of uncertain malignant potential. BRAF is a potential therapeutic target in patients with progressive disease {1585,696}.

Essential and desirable diagnostic criteria
Essential: monomorphic round to epithelioid cells with centrally placed, round nuclei and well-defined cell borders, arranged in perivascular nests; malignant glomus tumours usually may be recognized by an adjacent benign component and show either a spindle or round cell sarcomatous phenotype; in malignant examples lacking a benign component, immunohistochemistry and/or molecular diagnosis is required for definitive diagnosis.

Desirable: immunohistochemical expression of SMAs, h-caldesmon, and collagen IV; NOTCH gene rearrangements are commonly present in malignant cases.

Staging
Not clinically relevant

Prognosis and prediction
Typical glomus tumours, glomuvenous malformations, and symplastic glomus tumours are benign. Malignant glomus tumours are aggressive, with metastases and death from disease in as many as 40% of patients. Some large, visceral glomus tumours without other atypical features (uncertain malignant potential) have behaved aggressively. The natural history of histologically malignant glomus tumours in the skin may be favourable, although more data are needed {1917}.

Myopericytoma, including myofibroma

Mentzel TDW
Agaram NP

Definition
Myopericytoma is a distinctive perivascular myoid neoplasm that forms a morphological spectrum with myofibroma. Rarely, myopericytomas show malignant features.

ICD-O coding
8824/0 Myopericytoma

ICD-11 coding
2E84.Y & XH0953 Benign fibrogenic or myofibrogenic tumour of other specified sites & Myofibroma

Related terminology
Not recommended: infantile haemangiopericytoma.

Subtype(s)
Myofibromatosis; myofibroma; infantile myofibromatosis

Localization
Myopericytoma generally arises in the dermis or subcutis, and it only rarely involves deep soft tissue. The distal extremities are most commonly involved, followed by the proximal extremities, neck, trunk, and oral cavity {736,1461}. Very rarely, these neoplasms arise in visceral locations and intracranial sites {1772,2673}. The majority of solitary myofibromas arise in the skin and subcutis of the extremities, head and neck, and trunk {253,604}. Infants with myofibromatosis may have involvement of visceral locations, including the liver, heart, gastrointestinal tract, brain, and bone {604}.

Clinical features
Myopericytoma usually presents as a painless, slow-growing, superficially located nodule, which can be present for years. Most cases arise as a solitary lesion, but multiple lesions involving a particular anatomical region or different regions are sometimes seen {2081,1207,3322}. Myofibromas may present as solitary or multicentric lesions (myofibromatosis). Lesions arising congenitally or in the first years of life may involve viscera or bone {2081}.

Epidemiology
Myopericytoma may occur at any age; however, most cases are seen in adults {2081}. Myofibroma may be present at birth, appear in the first 2 years of life, or arise in adults with a male predominance.

Etiology
A subset of solitary and multiple (non-visceral) forms of infantile myofibromatosis are familial, following an autosomal dominant mode of inheritance with variable penetrance and expressivity {1464,2717,2891}. However, some reports have suggested instead an autosomal recessive inheritance {2247}. An association between myopericytoma and EBV has been reported in patients with AIDS {1771}.

Pathogenesis
Mutations in the *PDGFRB* gene appear to represent a common pathogenesis for myopericytoma, myopericytomatosis, and myofibroma {1441,24}. Germline mutations in the *PDGFRB* gene have been shown to underlie familial, autosomal dominant infantile myofibromatosis {573,1988}. Germline mutation in *NOTCH3*, a gene implicated in the pathogenesis of some glomus tumours {2206}, has also been reported in a familial myofibromatosis kindred {1988}. Cellular/atypical myofibromas are associated with *SRF-RELA* gene fusions {138}.

Macroscopic appearance
In superficial locations, myopericytoma tends to be well circumscribed, with nodules measuring < 2 cm in diameter; larger neoplasms may be seen in deep soft tissues {2081}.

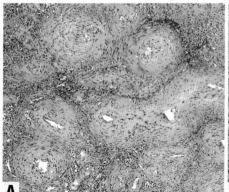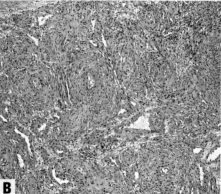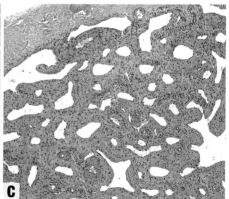

Fig. 1.201 Myopericytoma. **A** The so-called classic, solid type of myopericytoma with thick-walled vessels surrounded concentrically by plump spindled tumour cells. **B** A concentric, perivascular growth of plump spindled, myoid tumour cells is characteristic. **C** Numerous thin-walled branching vessels and a perivascular growth of myoid tumour cells are seen in the haemangiopericytoma type of myopericytoma.

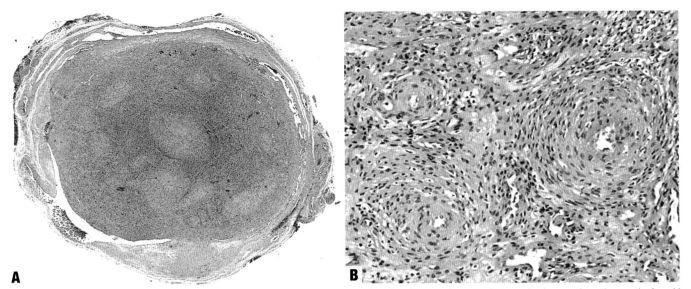

Fig. 1.202 Myopericytoma. **A** An example of intravascular myopericytoma. **B** High-power view of an intravascular myopericytoma showing a perivascular growth of myoid tumour cells.

Histopathology

Myopericytomas are unencapsulated, usually well-circumscribed, nodular or lobular lesions composed of cytologically bland, oval to spindle-shaped, myoid tumour cells with characteristic multi-layered, concentric growth around numerous small vessels. The tumours show variable cellularity, ranging from cellular and solid-appearing to hypocellular and collagenous/myxoid. Lesional blood vessels tend to be numerous and variable in size; branching, haemangiopericytoma-like vessels may be present. Blood vessels outside of the tumour mass may show a similar concentric perivascular proliferation of myoid, spindled cells {2081}. In some cases, a more prominent fascicular or whorled arrangement of neoplastic cells resembling myofibroma or angioleiomyoma is present {857,2017}. Intravascular myopericytomas have been reported {2081,2044}. Some myopericytomas have glomus-like features (glomangiopericytoma) {1207}. Rarely, myopericytomas may show degenerative features, including symplastic nuclear atypia, stromal hyalinization, and cystic change {2081}. A very unusual process of diffuse dermal and subcutaneous involvement by numerous microscopic myopericytomatous nodules has been

reported under the term "myopericytomatosis" {1441}. Rare malignant myopericytomas occur mainly in the deep soft tissues, as infiltrating neoplasms showing marked nuclear atypia and a high mitotic count, in addition to features more typical of myopericytoma {2046}. By immunohistochemistry, myopericytomas express SMAs and h-caldesmon, and they are at most only focally positive for desmin and/or CD34.

Solitary myofibromas are nodular, well-circumscribed neoplasms characterized by a distinctive biphasic growth pattern. Classically, the centre of the lesion is composed of immature-appearing, plump, spindled tumour cells associated with a haemangiopericytoma-like branching vasculature, whereas the periphery of the lesion consists of nodules and fascicles of variably hyalinized, myoid, or even chondroid-appearing cells. This pattern of zonation may be more haphazard or even reversed in older children and adults {253}. Mitotic figures are variable in number and, especially in the immature-appearing tumour areas, may be numerous. The cellular zones of myofibroma may undergo necrosis and calcification. Particularly in infants, myofibromas may be composed almost entirely of these more primitive, cellular

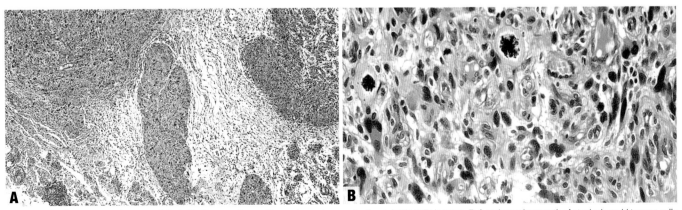

Fig. 1.203 Malignant myopericytoma. **A** An infiltrating neoplasm with a perivascular growth of neoplastic cells is seen. **B** A perivascular growth of atypical myoid tumour cells and numerous mitoses, including atypical mitotic figures, is present.

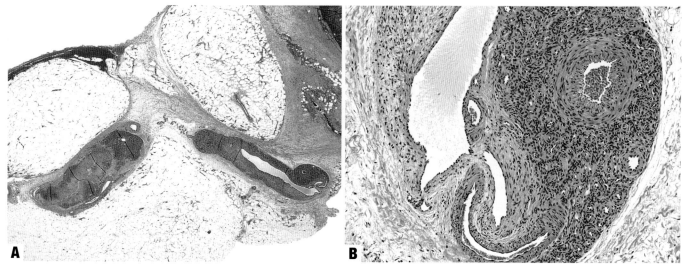

Fig. 1.204 Myopericytomatosis. **A** Numerous small nodular aggregates with features of myopericytoma are seen. **B** An intramural growth is noted.

zones; such cases were historically labelled infantile haemangiopericytoma {2079}. The morphological features of the cellular zones of myofibroma share some features with myopericytoma, suggesting that these are related entities. Intravascular extension is commonly seen and does not imply malignancy. Immunohistochemically, both components of myofibroma express SMAs and are usually negative for desmin and h-caldesmon.

Rare myofibromas/myopericytomas show atypical features, in particular high cellularity, a predominantly fascicular pattern with inapparent myoid nodules, infiltrative growth, and perineurial invasion; proper classification of such lesions usually requires identification of small foci of more-typical myofibroma {1871}. Despite the dense cellularity and variable mitotic activity, these lesions lack nuclear pleomorphism or necrosis {138}. In contrast with classic myofibromas, these tumours often show coexpression of SMA and desmin.

Cytology
Not clinically relevant

Diagnostic molecular pathology
SRF and *RELA* gene rearrangements in cellular/atypical myofibromas can be identified by molecular studies {138}.

Essential and desirable diagnostic criteria
Essential: myopericytoma: bland, myoid-appearing spindled cells growing in a concentric pattern around numerous small vessels; myofibroma: biphasic growth pattern, with primitive cellular zones often showing necrosis, calcification, and mitotic activity, surrounded by hyalinized nodules of myoid spindled cells; cellular/atypical myofibroma/myopericytoma: predominant cellular spindle cell growth pattern lacking nuclear pleomorphism, often with coexpression of SMA and desmin.

Desirable (in selected cases): PDGFRB mutations in myopericytoma and myofibroma; *SRF-RELA* gene fusions in cellular/atypical myofibroma.

Staging
Not clinically relevant

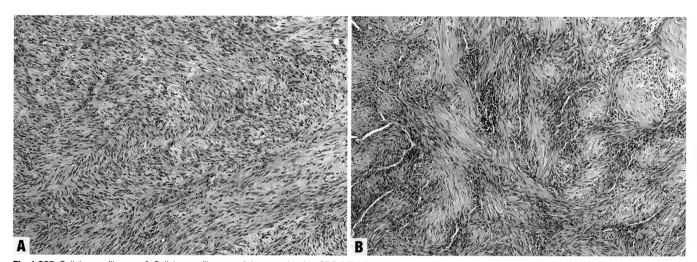

Fig. 1.205 Cellular myofibroma. **A** Cellular myofibromas of the type showing *SRF-RELA* fusions may consist largely of intersecting fascicles of spindled cells, simulating a spindle cell sarcoma. **B** Identification of more-typical areas of myofibroma, showing hyalinized nodules, is key to their distinction from various spindle cell sarcomas. Molecular genetic studies for *SRF-RELA* may also be helpful.

Prognosis and prediction

Most myopericytomas do not recur even if marginally or incompletely excised. Local recurrences probably represent persistent rather than truly recurrent growth. Extremely rare malignant myopericytomas have shown aggressive growth and distant spread, with poor clinical outcome {2046}. The overall prognosis for solitary myofibromas is excellent, and these tumours do not recur locally or metastasize. Infants with multicentric or generalized myofibromatosis involving viscera and brain have a worse outcome {604}.

Angioleiomyoma

Matsuyama A

Definition

Angioleiomyoma is a benign tumour that typically arises in the dermis or subcutis and is composed of well-differentiated perivascular smooth muscle cells arranged around numerous vascular channels. A morphological continuum exists between angioleiomyoma and myopericytoma.

ICD-O coding

8894/0 Angioleiomyoma

ICD-11 coding

2E86.1 & XH7CL0 Leiomyoma of other or unspecified sites & Angiomyoma

Related terminology

Acceptable: angiomyoma; vascular leiomyoma.

Subtype(s)

None

Localization

The tumours occur most commonly in the subcutis or dermis of the extremities, followed by the head and neck (including the sinonasal or oral cavities) and the trunk {1265,2017,51,27}. The most common solid form usually arises in the lower extremities, with less common venous forms more often involving the head and neck region {1265}. Rare cavernous forms most often occur in the upper extremities {1265}.

Clinical features

The lesion presents as a firm, well-circumscribed, and slow-growing nodule. Approximately half of angioleiomyomas are painful {1265,2017}.

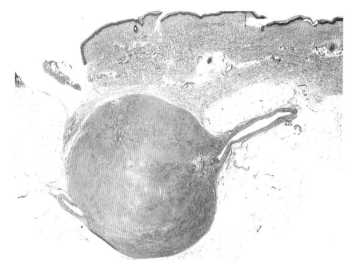

Fig. 1.207 Angioleiomyoma. This lesion has an attached vein and shows sharp circumscription.

Epidemiology

Angioleiomyoma affects a wide age range, peaking in the fourth through sixth decades of life {1265,2017}. The overall M:F ratio is about 0.7:1. The solid type is significantly more common in women, whereas the venous and cavernous types show a slight male predominance {1265}.

Etiology

No established etiology exists, although minor trauma and venous stasis have been proposed as potential causal factors {2573}.

Pathogenesis

Angioleiomyoma is believed to arise from vascular smooth

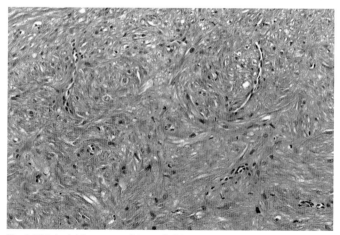

Fig. 1.206 Angioleiomyoma, solid type. Solid-type angioleiomyoma is composed of a proliferation of smooth muscle cells with slit-like vascular channels.

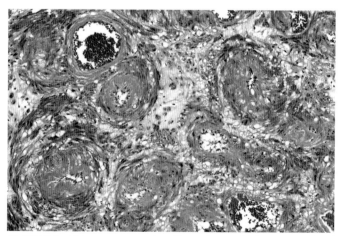

Fig. 1.208 Angioleiomyoma, venous type. Venous-type angioleiomyoma consists of thick muscle-coated blood vessels with intervascular smooth muscle bundles.

muscle {1265}. Cytogenetic abnormalities, including monosomy of chromosome 13 and loss of 6p, 21q, and 13q, have been reported {3271,2297,2308}. *NOTCH2* gene rearrangement, frequently identified in glomus tumours, has been detected in a single case of angioleiomyoma {2206}.

Macroscopic appearance
The tumours are typically solitary, sharply circumscribed, and relatively small (< 3 cm in diameter). An attached blood vessel wall may be identified.

Histopathology
Angioleiomyomas are subclassified into the three histological subtypes (solid, venous, and cavernous) on the basis of their vascular morphologies. Angioleiomyomas are composed of bundles of bland, well-differentiated smooth muscle cells and intervening variably sized blood vessels. Mitotic figures are absent. Solid-type angioleiomyoma has closely compacted bundles of smooth muscle cells with intervening thin-walled, slit-like vascular channels. Venous-type angioleiomyoma is characterized by thick muscle-coated blood vessels with smooth muscle cells of the vascular walls swirling and blending with intervascular smooth muscle bundles. Cavernous-type tumour is composed of dilated vascular channels with a proliferation of smooth muscle bundles in the intervascular spaces. Tumours showing mixed morphologies may be seen. Some tumours contain myopericytoma-like elements, with a concentric perivascular proliferation of less eosinophilic spindled or ovoid myoid cells {2017}. Other minor histological variations include adipocytic metaplasia (often erroneously described as cutaneous/subcutaneous angiomyolipoma), prominent hyalinization and calcification {1265}, and degenerative atypia {1993}.

Immunohistochemically, the tumour cells are diffusely positive for SMAs and calponin, and usually strongly positive for h-caldesmon {2017}. Desmin expression is variable and may be focal or absent in a minority of tumours {2017}. HMB45 and/or melan-A are negative even in tumours with adipocytic metaplasia {1265,2017,27}.

Cytology
Not clinically relevant

Diagnostic molecular pathology
Not clinically relevant

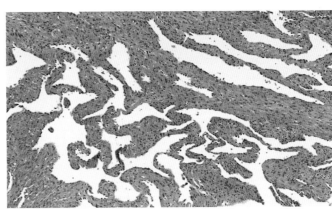

Fig.1.209 Angioleiomyoma, cavernous type. This lesion is composed of cavernously dilated vascular channels with attenuated walls of smooth muscle cells.

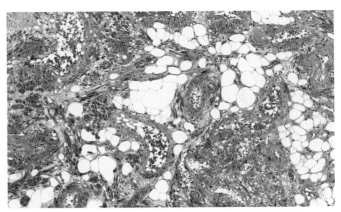

Fig.1.210 Angioleiomyoma with adipocytic metaplasia.

Essential and desirable diagnostic criteria
Essential: well-circumscribed tumour composed of cytologically bland smooth muscle cells showing concentric growth around vascular channels of varying calibre.

Staging
Not clinically relevant

Prognosis and prediction
Angioleiomyoma is a benign tumour that very seldom recurs after surgical excision.

Leiomyoma

Billings SD
Panagopoulos I

Definition
Leiomyoma is a benign smooth muscle tumour that occurs in the deep somatic soft tissue or the retroperitoneum-abdominal cavity.

ICD-O coding
8890/0 Leiomyoma NOS

ICD-11 coding
2E86.1 Leiomyoma of other or unspecified sites

Related terminology
None

Subtype(s)
None

Localization
Leiomyomas of somatic soft tissue mostly occur in extremities and arise in deep subcutis or skeletal muscle {321,1627}. Although the retroperitoneum is the most common location in the other group, they may also occur in abdominal wall, omentum, mesentery, and peritoneal surface {321,2407}. In the inguinal region, leiomyomas may arise from the round ligament {2463}.

Clinical features
Although usually solitary, retroperitoneal tumours may be multiple {321}. Somatic tumours often have calcification and may be detected radiographically {1627,321,2145,2674}. No recurrence has been reported for somatic leiomyomas {1627,321}. Recurrence was reported in < 10% of leiomyomas of retroperitoneum-abdominal cavity {321,2407}.

Epidemiology
Leiomyomas of somatic soft tissue occur primarily in middle-aged adults, with no sex difference {1627,321}. Leiomyomas of retroperitoneum-abdominal cavity are much more common in women, often of perimenopausal age {321,2407}.

Etiology
The causation of somatic leiomyomas is unknown. The fact that > 40% of retroperitoneal leiomyomas were reported in patients who had concurrent uterine leiomyomas or had undergone previous hysterectomy for uterine leiomyomas may support a theory of multifocal origin {579,1402,321,2407}.

Pathogenesis
Retroperitoneal / abdominal cavity leiomyomas carry some of the same genetic changes as uterine leiomyomas {2417,2415, 2419}. Genetic analysis of 8 leiomyomas of the retroperitoneum-abdominal cavity showed 3 tumours with 12q rearrangements, 3 with 8q rearrangements, 1 with deletion of 7q, and 1 with aberrations of chromosome bands 3q21-q23 and 11q21-q22. The target genes of the 12q and 8q aberrations were *HMGA2* and *PLAG1*, respectively {2419}. In other studies, mutations in exon 2 of *MED12* were reported in retroperitoneal leiomyomas {2586,2794}. *KAT6B-KANSL1* and *EWSR1-PBX3* fusion genes were found in retroperitoneal leiomyomas with t(10;17)(q22;q21) and t(9;22)(q33;q12) chromosomal translocations, respectively {2417,2415}.

Macroscopic appearance
Somatic leiomyomas are circumscribed masses that are tan-grey to white in colour and often have a rubbery texture and a whorled cut surface. Degenerative mucoid-cystic change is occasionally present {1627,321}. The size ranges from < 1 to 15 cm {321}. Leiomyomas of retroperitoneum-abdominal cavity are reddish-tan, greyish-tan, or white circumscribed masses, often having a trabecular surface resembling that commonly seen in uterine leiomyomas {321,2407}. They range in size from 2.5 to 37 cm {321,2407}.

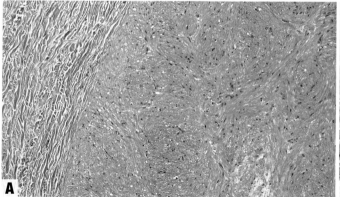 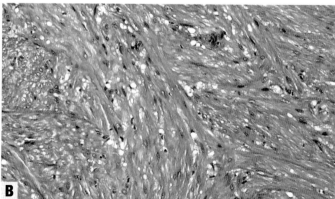

Fig. 1.211 Leiomyoma. **A** Low-power view shows clear distinction from surrounding tissue and broad interlacing fascicles of smooth muscle cells. **B** Higher magnification of leiomyoma of somatic soft tissue, showing fascicles of smooth muscle cells.

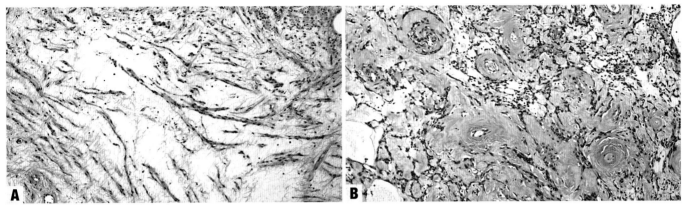

Fig. 1.212 Leiomyoma. **A** Retroperitoneal leiomyoma with myxoid change. **B** Retroperitoneal leiomyoma with hyalinization.

Histopathology

Leiomyomas of deep soft tissue are composed of cells that closely resemble normal smooth muscle cells with eosinophilic cytoplasm and uniform blunt-ended, cigar-shaped nuclei. They are arranged in orderly intersecting fascicles. They are highly differentiated, have little or no nuclear atypia, and have at most an extremely low level of mitotic activity. Limb lesions and intra-abdominal lesions in males show almost no mitoses. In peritoneal/retroperitoneal lesions in females (showing positivity for hormonal receptors), there may be a few mitoses visible. Necrosis is not found in deep leiomyoma. Most lesions are paucicellular, and degenerative or regressive changes, such as fibrosis, hyalinization, calcification, and myxoid change, are common in large tumours. Leiomyomas of retroperitoneum-abdominal cavity display a spectrum of patterns similar to those of uterine leiomyomas. They show macrotrabecular and microtrabecular organization, hyalinization, and focal myxoid or cystic change. Focal epithelioid change, clear cell change, metaplastic bone, and fatty differentiation are also occasionally seen {2059}. Focal degenerative nuclear atypia should always prompt a careful search for mitoses and additional sampling, because some leiomyosarcomas may have only focal atypia and very low mitotic activity.

Tumour cells are positive for SMA, desmin, and h-caldesmon, at least focally, but they are negative for S100. Leiomyomas of retroperitoneum-abdominal cavity are almost always positive for ER, PR, and WT1 {321,2407,2463}. Leiomyomas of somatic soft tissue do not express ER or PR {1627,2407}.

Cytology

Large mass-forming leiomyomas may be sampled by EUS-guided FNA. Fragments of spindle cells with bland cytology are noted in adequate samples. Confirmatory immunohistochemical staining can be performed on cell block material {2939}.

Diagnostic molecular pathology

Not clinically relevant

Essential and desirable diagnostic criteria

Essential: intersecting fascicles of benign smooth muscle.
Desirable (in selected cases): expression of SMA and desmin.

Staging

Not clinically relevant

Prognosis and prediction

These tumours are benign, and patients are cured by complete excision. There is no metastatic risk, but local recurrences have been reported in some patients with retroperitoneal tumours {321,2407}. None of the patients with recurrence have demonstrated disease progression or metastasis in follow-up.

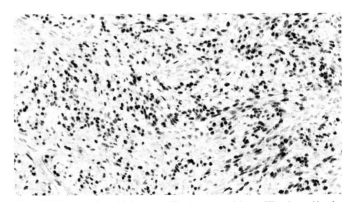

Fig. 1.213 Retroperitoneal leiomyoma with hydropic change. Retroperitoneal leiomyoma composed of thin fascicles of bland smooth muscle separated by an oedematous stroma. Hydropic change is often seen in retroperitoneal leiomyomas.

Fig. 1.214 Retroperitoneal leiomyoma. The tumour nuclei are diffusely positive for ER, typical of retroperitoneal leiomyomas.

EBV-associated smooth muscle tumour

Watanabe R
Schafernak KT
Soares FA

Definition

EBV-associated smooth muscle tumour is a smooth muscle tumour associated with EBV infection, usually in the setting of immunosuppression.

ICD-O coding

8897/1 Smooth muscle tumour of uncertain malignant potential

ICD-11 coding

2F7Y & XH00B4 Neoplasms of uncertain behaviour of other specified site & Smooth muscle tumour NOS

Related terminology

Not recommended: AIDS-associated EBV-positive smooth muscle tumour; EBV-associated posttransplant smooth muscle tumour; smooth muscle tumour in immunocompromised patient.

Subtype(s)

None

Localization

EBV-associated smooth muscle tumours can occur anywhere in the body, including sites unusual for sporadic leiomyomas and leiomyosarcomas. HIV-associated smooth muscle tumours have a particular predilection for the intra-axial or extra-axial CNS (41% of cases), whereas posttransplant smooth muscle tumours most commonly involve the liver (56%; the donor liver in liver transplant recipients and the native liver in recipients of other solid organs), followed by the lungs (31%) and gastrointestinal tract (15%); they have also been reported in kidney, lung, and heart allografts. Tumours are multicentric in 71%, 54%, and 29% of primary immunodeficiency, posttransplant, and HIV-positive patients, respectively.

Clinical features

Presenting features may be nonspecific (pain) or related to the site of involvement: neurological symptoms with intra-axial or extra-axial CNS tumours; bleeding, abdominal pain, obstruction, and perforation when involving the gastrointestinal tract; and cyanosis, fever, and lung infections with endobronchial lesions.

Epidemiology

Occurring over a wide age range (1–66 years) and with a slight female predominance, most cases occur in one of three main settings: immunodeficiency due to HIV/AIDS, immunodeficiency after transplantation of a solid organ (63% kidney, 15% heart, 12% liver) or haematopoietic stem cells, and (least commonly) congenital or primary immunodeficiency. Most primary immunodeficiency patients (88%) with EBV-associated smooth muscle tumours have been children {1936}; reported

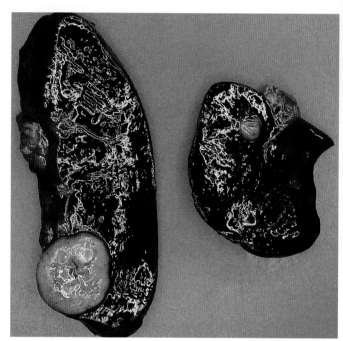

Fig. 1.215 EBV-associated smooth muscle tumour. Gross autopsy photograph of multiple splenic tumours in a child who underwent haematopoietic stem cell transplantation for a primary immune disorder 10 months earlier; a monomorphic B-cell posttransplant lymphoproliferative disorder was found concurrently in the liver.

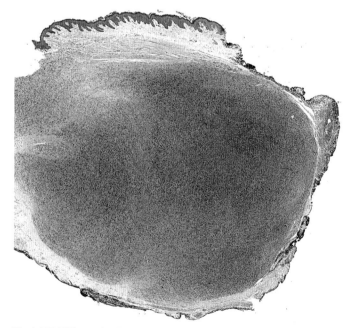

Fig. 1.216 EBV-associated smooth muscle tumour. Whole-mount section of EBV-associated smooth muscle tumour developing in penile skin.

adult primary immunodeficiency patients had GATA2 deficiency {632}. In contrast, 68% of posttransplant and 72% of HIV/AIDS patients are adults. Tumours are found several months to years after the onset of the patient's immunodeficiency syndrome or transplantation. The epidemiology is similar to that of the immunodeficiency-associated lymphoproliferative disorders, which are frequently EBV-positive, although they tend to occur as a later consequence than the EBV-positive lymphoproliferative disorders observed in a subset of smooth muscle tumour patients (particularly in children in the posttransplant and primary immunodeficiency settings). Rarely, these tumours are associated with iatrogenic immunosuppression for autoimmune disease {2183}. If these tumours are encountered outside of any of these settings, a thorough immunological work-up and close follow-up for opportunistic infections are warranted.

Etiology

The etiology involves EBV infection in the setting of T-lymphocyte immunosuppression.

Pathogenesis

During latent infection, as many as 10 of the nearly 100 genes in the EBV genome are expressed, another mechanism to evade T-cell immune surveillance. The latency pattern remains controversial and is perhaps unique to this entity, although many authors describe a type III–like pattern with positivity for EBV-encoded small RNA (EBER), EBNA2, and LMP1 despite somewhat inconsistent EBNA2 results and absence of LMP1 from most posttransplant and some HIV-associated cases. MYC overexpression and AKT/mTOR pathway activation appear to be main mediators of EBV-induced smooth muscle tumour proliferation {2384,3035}. Tumour multicentricity is related to multiple infection events, with viral episomal analysis showing independent viral clones rather than dissemination or metastasis of a single clone, which is far less common {811}. Furthermore, short tandem repeat (STR) analysis has revealed that posttransplant smooth muscle tumours can be derived from either recipient or donor {1548}.

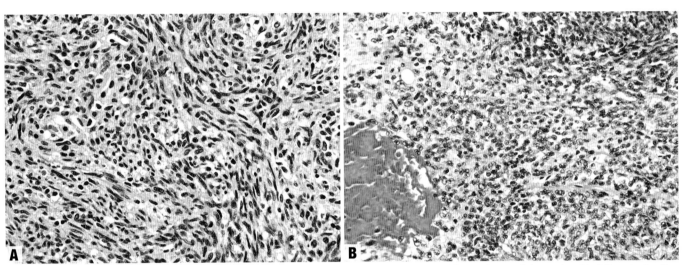

Fig. 1.217 EBV-associated smooth muscle tumour. **A** Intersecting fascicles of spindled cells with ample eosinophilic cytoplasm and elongated nuclei. **B** Round cells with a more primitive appearance accompany the spindled cells in about one half of cases.

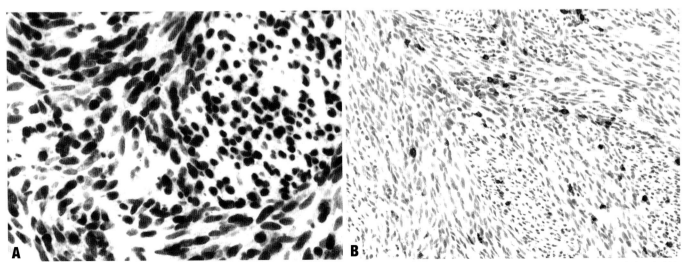

Fig. 1.218 EBV-associated smooth muscle tumour. **A** The nuclei are positive with in situ hybridization for EBV-encoded small RNA (EBER). **B** T cells are commonly found within the tumour, although they are usually sparse.

Macroscopic appearance

Tumours range from subcentimetre to > 20 cm {1444,1548}, with white to grey cut surfaces, a firm to rubbery consistency, and well-circumscribed to infiltrative borders.

Histopathology

The tumour is composed of intersecting fascicles of spindled cells with ample eosinophilic cytoplasm and elongated nuclei; in about half of cases, a second population of round, more primitive-appearing smooth muscle cells is seen. A subset of these tumours exhibit a haemangiopericytoma-like pattern. Cytological atypia is usually mild to moderate but can be marked in HIV-positive patients, whose tumours also show higher mitotic activity and/or necrosis. An intratumoural T-lymphocytic infiltrate is common and usually sparse but can be more pronounced {811}. Neoplastic cells are diffusely positive for SMA and h-caldesmon. Desmin is sometimes positive but expression is usually focal. EBER is consistently positive {1444}.**Cytology**
Not clinically relevant

Diagnostic molecular pathology

Diagnostic molecular pathology involves demonstration of EBV, usually by in situ hybridization for EBER.

Essential and desirable diagnostic criteria

Essential: clinical history of immunosuppression; neoplasm with smooth muscle differentiation; positivity for EBER transcripts by in situ hybridization.

Staging

Not clinically relevant

Prognosis and prediction

Prognosis is mainly dependent on the condition of the individual patient's immune system. Most of these tumours do not metastasize. Intracranial posttransplant smooth muscle tumours (but not HIV/AIDS-associated or primary immunodeficiency–associated smooth muscle tumours) have an adverse prognosis. Some posttransplant cases respond to reduced immunosuppression, which partially restores immune function, and complete resolution of EBV-associated smooth muscle tumours has been reported in a patient with GATA2 deficiency after haematopoietic stem cell transplantation {2454}.

Inflammatory leiomyosarcoma

Fletcher CDM
Mertens F

Definition

Inflammatory leiomyosarcoma (LMS) is a malignant neoplasm showing smooth muscle differentiation, a prominent inflammatory infiltrate, and near-haploidization.

ICD-O coding

8890/3 Leiomyosarcoma NOS

ICD-11 coding

2B58 & XH7ED4 Leiomyosarcoma, primary site & Leiomyosarcoma NOS

Related terminology

None

Subtype(s)

None

Localization

Most inflammatory LMSs arise in deep soft tissue, most commonly in the lower limb, followed by the trunk and retroperitoneum. Isolated cases have arisen at visceral locations {536, 2321}.

Clinical features

Most cases present as an enlarging deep soft tissue mass of variable duration and with no specific features. Isolated cases have been associated with inflammatory-type symptoms {536}.

Epidemiology

Inflammatory LMS is very rare. The majority of cases occur in adults (with a median age of 35–40 years and an age range of 12–64 years in published cases) {2093,536,2321,150}. There is a relative male predominance.

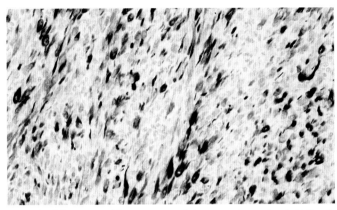

Fig. 1.220 Inflammatory leiomyosarcoma. Between numerous lymphohistiocytic cells, the spindled tumour cells are highlighted by immunopositivity for desmin.

Etiology

Unknown

Pathogenesis

The pathogenesis is not fully understood, but these tumours have a distinctive near-haploid genotype, with or without subsequent whole-genome doubling, and they are associated with striking myogenic gene expression. The near-haploidization is thought to be pathogenetically important {150}. When analysed by chromosome banding or genomic arrays, 10 of 11 inflammatory LMSs displayed near-haploidization, with or without subsequent whole-genome doubling(s) {721,536,2321,150}. Although most chromosomes thus showed loss of heterozygosity, there was always retained heterozygosity for chromosomes 5 and 22, and often for chromosomes 18, 20, and 21. Apart from mutation of the *NF1* gene in a subset of the cases, no additional somatic variants that could serve as driver mutations have been detected {150}. Gene expression profiling has shown prominent

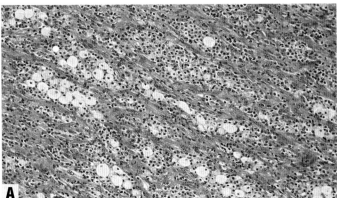 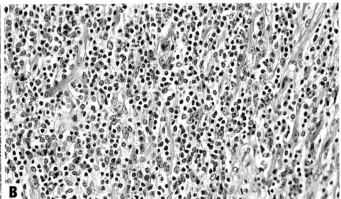

Fig. 1.219 Inflammatory leiomyosarcoma. **A** In this tumour there is a mixed lymphohistiocytic infiltrate with prominent xanthomatous cells. **B** Tumour cells are largely obscured by the prominent lymphoid infiltrate.

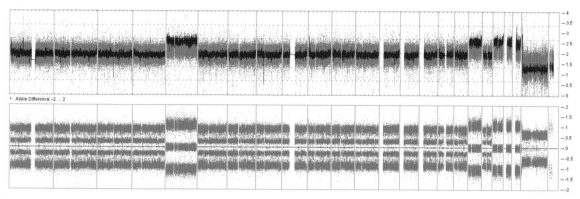

Fig. 1.221 Inflammatory leiomyosarcoma. Genomic array findings in an inflammatory leiomyosarcoma showing relative copy-number gain of chromosomes 5, 18, and 20–22 (top, red) and loss of heterozygosity for all other chromosomes (bottom, grey).

differential expression of genes involved in muscle development and function {150}.

Macroscopic appearance
Most tumours appear well circumscribed, with a maximum diameter of 3–12 cm. Cut surfaces are tan-yellow or red and soft/fleshy.

Histopathology
These tumours consist of eosinophilic spindle cells with blunt-ended elongated nuclei, arranged in fascicles or sometimes in a storiform fashion. The degree of nuclear atypia and pleomorphism varies, as does mitotic count, depending on histological grade. However, most cases appear to be low-grade. The striking and characteristic feature is the presence of a prominent, usually diffuse, inflammatory infiltrate, which often obscures the neoplastic cell population. The inflammatory component is usually dominated by small lymphocytes, sometimes admixed with plasma cells. Histiocytes are also often prominent and may have a xanthomatous appearance. In a minority of cases, the inflammatory infiltrate may consist mainly of neutrophils or eosinophils. Calcospherites (psammomatous calcifications) are a striking feature in some cases. Virtually all cases show immunopositivity for some combination of SMA, desmin, and caldesmon.

Cytology
Not clinically relevant

Diagnostic molecular pathology
Not clinically relevant

Essential and desirable diagnostic criteria
Essential: fascicular proliferation of variably atypical eosinophilic spindle cells, which show mitotic activity; dense inflammatory infiltrate, most often lymphoid or histiocytic/xanthomatous, but the composition is variable; immunopositivity for smooth muscle antigens.

Staging
The American Joint Committee on Cancer (AJCC) or Union for International Cancer Control (UICC) TNM system is appropriate.

Prognosis and prediction
Published follow-up data in inflammatory LMS are limited due to its rarity. Among 20 cases with follow-up, only 4 have been reported to metastasize, but duration of follow-up is < 5 years in most cases. Of the cases in which a near-haploid genotype has been well documented, the prognosis seems generally to be very good {150}.

Leiomyosarcoma

Dry SM
Fröhling S

Definition

Leiomyosarcoma (LMS) is a malignant neoplasm composed of cells showing smooth muscle differentiation.

ICD-O coding

8890/3 Leiomyosarcoma NOS

ICD-11 coding

2B58.0 & XH7ED4 Leiomyosarcoma of retroperitoneum or peritoneum & Leiomyosarcoma NOS

2B58.Y & XH7ED4 Leiomyosarcoma, other specified primary site & Leiomyosarcoma NOS

2B58.Z & XH7ED4 Leiomyosarcoma, unspecified primary site & Leiomyosarcoma NOS

Related terminology

None

Subtype(s)

None

Localization

Soft tissue LMSs most commonly arise in the extremities (particularly the lower extremities), retroperitoneum, abdomen/pelvis, and trunk {1164,3290}. A distinctive subgroup originates in large blood vessels, most commonly the inferior vena cava, its major tributaries, and the large veins of the lower extremity. Tumours occur at intramuscular and subcutaneous localizations in approximately equal proportions, and many originate from a small to medium-sized vein {1829,972}.

Clinical features

Soft tissue LMS generally presents as a mass lesion that is often associated with nonspecific symptoms caused by the displacement of structures rather than invasion. The symptoms produced by inferior vena cava LMS depend on location. In the upper portion, it obstructs the hepatic veins and can evince Budd–Chiari syndrome with hepatomegaly, jaundice, and ascites. Tumours of the middle portion may block the renal veins. Involvement of the lower portion may cause leg oedema. Imaging studies of LMS (MRI and contrast-enhanced CT) are nonspecific but helpful in delineating the relationship to adjacent structures, particularly in the retroperitoneum.

Epidemiology

The incidence of soft tissue LMS increases with age and peaks in the seventh decade of life, although this neoplasm may develop in young adults and children {795}. LMS accounts for about 11% of all newly diagnosed soft tissue sarcomas {865}. It is the predominant sarcoma arising from larger blood vessels {3182,1829,1617,275,1754}. Gastrointestinal LMSs are very rare, with < 80 cases reported in the English-language literature

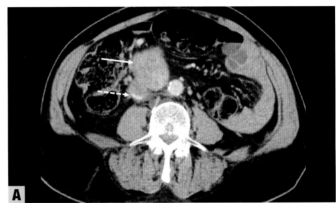

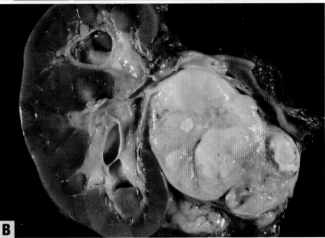

Fig. 1.222 Leiomyosarcoma. **A** Axial contrast-enhanced CT shows a right-sided retroperitoneal mass (solid arrow), which is clearly arising from the inferior vena cava. The lumen of the inferior vena cava is partially occluded (slit-like residual lumen indicated by dashed arrow). **B** Leiomyosarcoma arising from the inferior vena cava.

since 2000 {2133,2134,2124,2136,3336,1366}. LMS accounts for 10–15% of limb sarcomas, with preference for the thigh {2001}. Women constitute the clear majority of patients with retroperitoneal and inferior vena cava LMSs, but not among patients with tumours at other sites.

Etiology

Predisposing factors recognized for LMS include Li–Fraumeni syndrome, hereditary retinoblastoma, and radiation exposure {3187,2354,426,1133}.

Pathogenesis

Cytogenetic, molecular cytogenetic, and next-generation sequencing studies show that LMSs display extensive genomic instability, including chromothripsis and whole-genome duplication in subsets of cases {594}. Recurrent DNA copy-number alterations include losses involving tumour suppressors *PTEN* (10q23.31), *RB1* (13q14.2), and *TP53* (17p13.1), as well as

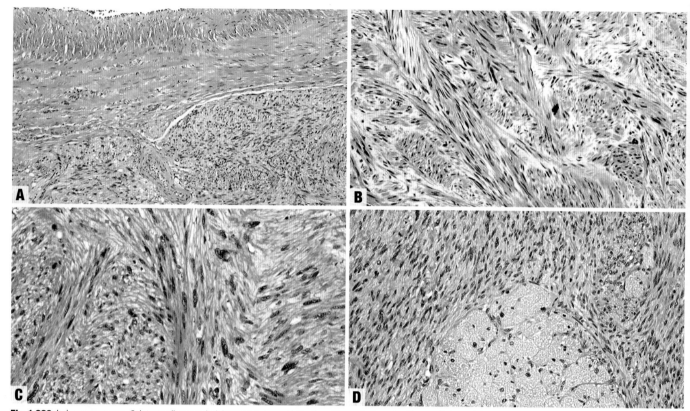

Fig. 1.223 Leiomyosarcoma. **A** Intermediate-grade leiomyosarcoma, arising from the wall of a vein. Many soft tissue leiomyosarcomas arise from vascular smooth muscle, and such tumours may be deceptively well circumscribed. **B** Low-grade leiomyosarcoma, composed of well-differentiated smooth muscle, with nuclear hyperchromatism and identifiable mitotic activity. **C** Intermediate-grade leiomyosarcoma. The tumour cells show classic features of smooth muscle differentiation, with variably pleomorphic, elongated nuclei; perinuclear vacuoles; and distinctly eosinophilic cytoplasm. **D** Low-grade leiomyosarcoma with granular cell change. Leiomyosarcomas with this unusual morphological feature may be confused with granular cell tumours.

amplification of *MYOCD* at 17p12, which encodes a smooth muscle–specific transcriptional coactivator {899,1962,3238, 1657,3348,1150,472,594}.

Whole-exome/genome and RNA sequencing studies have demonstrated that LMSs are characterized by a modest burden of somatic mutations and substantial mutational heterogeneity {472,594}. *TP53* is mutated in as many as 50% of sporadic LMSs; approximately 90% of samples present with biallelic *TP53* inactivation through mutations, deletions, chromosomal rearrangements, or protein-damaging microalterations {2525, 2492,1493,37,3346,472,594}. Similarly, the function of RB1 is disrupted in nearly all cases of soft tissue LMS by diverse mechanisms that either target RB1 itself or result in altered expression of *CDKN2A, CCND1, CCND2*, or *CDK4* {775,1595, 2963,472,594}. Potentially deleterious *ATRX* alterations have been observed in 16–49% of cases and probably contribute to the high prevalence of alternative lengthening of telomeres in LMS {3346,1812,472,594}. *ALK* rearrangements have been identified in a small subset of LMSs (9 of 377 cases; 2.4%) arising in males and females (soft tissue and uterine), imparting potential for clinically actionable opportunities {744}.

Gene expression studies suggest that there are multiple subgroups of LMS, including a muscle-enriched subtype and less-differentiated groupings, with indications of differing frequencies of specific genomic changes and varying prognoses {2291,244,575,1150,1257,1256,1818,594,1490}. Interestingly, some tumours classified as undifferentiated pleomorphic sarcoma cluster closely with a subset of LMSs {794,2291,1817, 2804,1751,244,1150,2150}.

Macroscopic appearance

LMS of soft tissue typically forms a fleshy, grey to white to tan mass. A whorled appearance may be evident. Larger examples often display haemorrhage, necrosis, or cystic change. The tumour border frequently appears well circumscribed, although grossly infiltrative tumours are also seen.

Histopathology

Typical LMS shows spindle-shaped cells with plump, blunt-ended nuclei and moderate to abundant, pale to brightly eosinophilic fibrillary cytoplasm. The cells are set in long intersecting fascicles parallel and perpendicular to the plane of section, although this pattern may be ill defined or subtle; some tumours show areas with storiform or palisaded patterns {3290}. Moderate nuclear pleomorphism is usually noted, although pleomorphism may be focal, mild, or occasionally absent. Mitotic figures, including atypical ones, are typically easy to find. LMS usually shows diffuse hypercellularity, although focal fibrosis, myxoid change, and hyalinized hypocellular areas can be seen. Tumour cell necrosis is often present in larger tumours {3290}. The majority of LMSs are high-grade {1164,921}. Unusual features in soft tissue LMS include myxoid stroma, multinucleated osteoclast-like giant cells, and granular cytoplasmic change {3290,2682}. Epithelioid morphology is exceedingly rare.

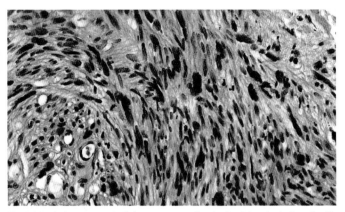

Fig. 1.224 Leiomyosarcoma. Leiomyosarcoma showing fascicles of spindle cells with hyperchromatic nuclei with scattered moderate pleomorphism and abundant eosinophilic cytoplasm.

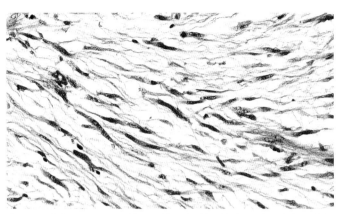

Fig. 1.226 Leiomyosarcoma with myxoid matrix. Myxoid change in soft tissue leiomyosarcomas is unusual but may be seen.

Osseous or chondro-osseous areas are rarely reported in pleomorphic/dedifferentiated LMS {554}. Lymph node metastases are very rare {860,921}.

By immunohistochemistry, at least one myogenic marker (i.e. SMA, desmin, or h-caldesmon) is positive in 100% of cases, and > 70% of cases are positive for more than one of these markers. None of these is absolutely specific for smooth muscle, and positivity for two myogenic markers is more supportive. Other markers, such as keratin, EMA, and CD34, may also be positive, often focally. In general, the diagnosis of LMS should not be made on the basis of immunohistochemical stains alone in the absence of appropriate morphological features.

As many as 8% of soft tissue LMSs exhibit a nonspecific, poorly differentiated, pleomorphic appearance in addition to typical areas. These tumours are called pleomorphic LMS or dedifferentiated LMS {2280,2347,1016,554}. For this diagnosis to be established, morphological features characteristic of classic LMS must be present, or the patient must have a prior history of LMS. The area of typical LMS may be exceedingly focal, constituting far less than 5% of the tumour. The typical and pleomorphic components may form discrete areas or may comingle. Pleomorphic LMSs most often show polygonal cells, but spindled, epithelioid, and rhabdoid cells may also be seen, and multiple cell types may be present. Pleomorphic areas usually have higher mitotic counts. By immunohistochemistry, about

50–75% of pleomorphic LMSs are positive for at least one myogenic marker, although staining is often weaker and more focal than in the typical leiomyosarcomatous areas {2280,2347}. The term "dedifferentiated" has been used for pleomorphic LMSs that lack immunohistochemical staining for myogenic markers in the pleomorphic areas {2280,2347,554}. Dedifferentiation is often seen in the primary tumour, but some cases present in recurrent or metastatic disease.

Cytology
Not clinically relevant

Diagnostic molecular pathology
Not clinically relevant

Essential and desirable diagnostic criteria
Essential: fascicles of eosinophilic spindled cells with blunt-ended nuclei showing variable pleomorphism; immunolabelling for SMA, desmin, and/or caldesmon.

Staging
LMS should be staged using the sarcoma staging information from the eighth edition (2017) of the Union for International Cancer Control (UICC) TNM classification {423}.

Prognosis and prediction
LMSs are clinically aggressive neoplasms with frequent local recurrences and distant metastases. The most important prognostic factors are histological grade and tumour location and size {642,2518}. Retroperitoneal LMSs are very often fatal; they are typically large (> 10 cm), often difficult or impossible to excise with clear margins, and prone to both local recurrence and metastasis {1933,2585,3290,1164}. LMSs of large vessels also tend to have a poor prognosis, although local control rates are higher. Non-retroperitoneal LMSs are generally smaller than those in the retroperitoneum, are more amenable to local control, and have a better prognosis. In some studies, intramuscular rather than subcutaneous location {1316} and larger tumour size {972,2163,1164} were related to increased metastasis and poorer survival. Metastases most commonly occur in lung, liver, and soft tissue, and more rarely in bone {3290,1164}. LMS is the most common sarcoma to produce skin metastases {3239}.

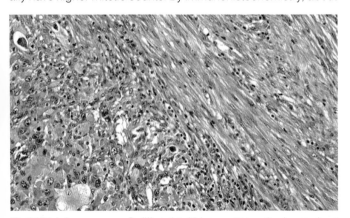

Fig. 1.225 Leiomyosarcoma. Dedifferentiated leiomyosarcoma, showing an abrupt transition from conventional grade 2 leiomyosarcoma to an essentially undifferentiated-appearing pleomorphic sarcoma. These undifferentiated areas lacked expression of muscle markers.

Rhabdomyoma

Parham DM

Definition
Rhabdomyoma is a benign soft tissue neoplasm showing skeletal muscle differentiation.

ICD-O coding
8900/0 Rhabdomyoma NOS

ICD-11 coding
2E86.2 & XH8WG9 Rhabdomyoma & Rhabdomyoma NOS
2E86.2 & XH4729 Rhabdomyoma & Fetal rhabdomyoma
2E86.2 & XH4BG5 Rhabdomyoma & Adult rhabdomyoma
2E86.2 & XH5AF2 Rhabdomyoma & Genital rhabdomyoma

Related terminology
Not recommended: extracardiac rhabdomyoma; rhabdomyomatous hamartoma.

Subtype(s)
Fetal rhabdomyoma; adult rhabdomyoma; genital rhabdomyoma

Localization
Most adult and fetal rhabdomyomas arise in the head and neck (e.g. in the parapharyngeal space, salivary glands, larynx, mouth, and soft tissue) {80,1583}. Rarely, they arise from other locations, such as bladder {1188} and extremities {3006}. Fetal rhabdomyomas have a postauricular predilection. By definition, genital rhabdomyomas arise from the genitalia, predominantly the vagina {2779}, but paratesticular tumours are also described {3402}.

Clinical features
Rhabdomyomas usually present as slow-growing, painless masses, but some grow rapidly. Other symptoms include

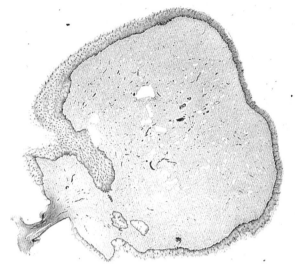

Fig. 1.228 Vaginal rhabdomyoma. Whole mount shows a polypoid configuration and fibrous stroma.

hoarseness, obstructive sleep apnoea, hearing loss, and dysphagia. Rare tumours are mistaken for parathyroid adenomas {1807,2144}. Adult rhabdomyomas arise as unifocal or multifocal lesions {805}, whereas fetal rhabdomyomas are usually solitary. Genital rhabdomyomas may present with menorrhagia, as vaginal polyps, or as scrotal masses.

Epidemiology
Rhabdomyomas are distinctly rare lesions; relatively few series exist. Adult rhabdomyomas are the most common {805} and occur in patients with a median age of 60 years (range: 33–80 years),

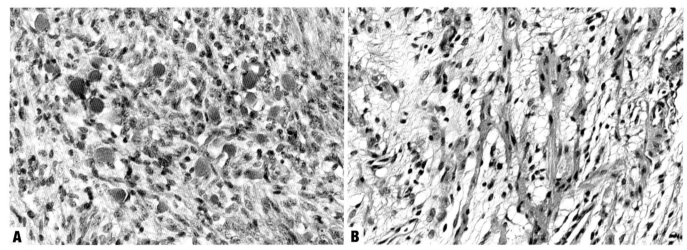

Fig. 1.227 Fetal rhabdomyoma. **A** Intermediate juvenile rhabdomyoma with increased cellularity and a mixture of mature rhabdomyoblasts and cells with smooth muscle features, lacking a myxoid component. **B** Fetal rhabdomyoma containing alternating bands of myotubes and loose myxoid stroma.

with an M:F ratio of 3:1. The mean age for fetal rhabdomyomas is 2.1 years, and the M:F ratio is about 1.7:1. Genital rhabdomyomas have been described in women with a mean age of 50 years and in males aged 8 months to 67 years {2766}.

Etiology
Fetal rhabdomyoma occurs in association with basal cell naevus syndrome, caused by loss-of-function mutations in the tumour suppressor gene *PTCH1* {1357}. Several cases have been reported with Birt–Hogg–Dubé syndrome {209}, caused by *FLCN* mutation.

Pathogenesis
PTCH1 encodes an inhibitory receptor in the sonic hedgehog signalling pathway. Inactivation of the second *PTCH1* allele in syndromic fetal rhabdomyoma may fully inactivate PTCH1 function and thereby activate hedgehog signalling. Non-syndromic fetal rhabdomyomas reveal evidence of hedgehog pathway activation by an unknown mechanism {1357}. Although adult rhabdomyomas are not associated with basal cell naevus syndrome, a few tumours show evidence of activation of the sonic hedgehog pathway {3093}. Cytogenetic analysis of one case revealed a t(15;17)(q24;p13) {1149}. SNP microarray has failed to reveal copy-number aberrations, including *PTCH1* deletion or loss of heterozygosity, in genital rhabdomyoma {2779}.

Macroscopic appearance
Adult rhabdomyomas form well-circumscribed, soft, nodular or lobular, deep-tan to reddish-brown masses. Tumour sizes range from 1.5 to 7.5 cm (median: 3 cm). Fetal rhabdomyomas may form sessile or pedunculated polyps on mucosal surfaces. Tumour sizes range from 1.0 to 12.5 cm (median: 3.0 cm). Genital rhabdomyomas in females form small, firm, lobulated, polypoid, non-ulcerated, epithelium-covered masses measuring 1–3 cm. Paratesticular rhabdomyomas may partially encase the testis and spermatic cord and have a pale, glistening surface.

Histopathology
Rhabdomyomas form unencapsulated, lobular masses. Adult rhabdomyomas consist of large polygonal cells with abundant granular eosinophilic cytoplasm, small round vesicular nuclei, and well-defined cellular borders. The cytoplasm may be vacuolated (spider cells) or may contain rod-like inclusions or cross-striations. Mitoses are rare.

Classic fetal rhabdomyomas contain irregular bundles of immature skeletal muscle fibres within a myxoid background. Cells have features of fetal myotubes, i.e. spindly contours, central oblong nuclei, and eosinophilic cytoplasm. An intermediate (juvenile) subset of cases show greater cellularity, less myxoid stroma, cells with a smooth muscle phenotype, and differentiated rhabdomyoblasts {1583}. The fetal cellular subtype contains a more uniform population of differentiating myoblasts. The myxoid subtype shows a predominance of stroma. Mitoses can be relatively frequent (as many as 5 per 50 mm²), but tumours lack substantial nuclear atypia, infiltrative margins, atypical mitoses, and necrosis {1583}.

Genital rhabdomyomas in females are relatively small lesions (< 2 cm) that contain loose fibrous connective tissue with differentiated spindled, polygonal, or elongated rhabdomyoblasts.

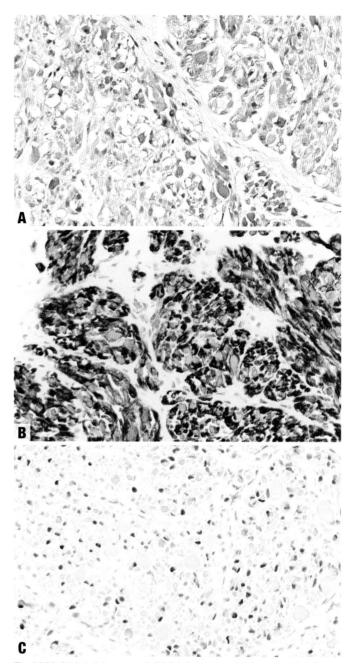

Fig. 1.229 Adult rhabdomyoma. **A** Adult rhabdomyoma showing mature rhabdomyoblasts with abundant eosinophilic cytoplasm. Scattered spider cells with cytoplasmic clearing are present. **B** Adult rhabdomyoma with strong, diffuse desmin expression. **C** Adult rhabdomyomas typically show variable degrees of myogenin expression.

Many contain eosinophilic cytoplasm with cross-striations. The cells generally appear bland and lack mitoses, but some degree of cytological atypia may be present {2779}. Vaginal lesions are polypoid in configuration but contain no cambium layer. Male genital tumours have features of adult or fetal rhabdomyomas.

Immunohistochemical stains used for ancillary diagnosis of rhabdomyoma include desmin, MSA, MYOD1, and myogenin. Desmin expression is generally strong and diffuse, whereas myogenin expression may be focal {2033}.

Cytology
Not clinically relevant

Diagnostic molecular pathology
Not clinically relevant

Essential and desirable diagnostic criteria
Essential: a well-circumscribed mass with no invasion of adjacent tissues; in the case of vaginal rhabdomyomas, small size (< 2 cm) and lack of cambium layer; mature rhabdomyoblasts lacking substantial atypia, mitotic activity, or necrosis; mitotic activity may be more prominent in fetal rhabdomyoma.

Staging
Not clinically relevant

Prognosis and prediction
Recurrences may occur in inadequately excised lesions, particularly with adult rhabdomyomas. Multifocal adult rhabdomyomas are seen in 3–10% of patients.

Embryonal rhabdomyosarcoma

Rudzinski ER

Definition

Embryonal rhabdomyosarcoma (ERMS) is a malignant soft tissue tumour with morphological and immunophenotypic features of embryonic skeletal muscle.

ICD-O coding

8910/3 Embryonal rhabdomyosarcoma NOS

ICD-11 coding

2B55.Z & XH83G1 Rhabdomyosarcoma & Embryonal rhabdomyosarcoma NOS

Related terminology

Not recommended: sarcoma botryoides; mixed embryonal and alveolar rhabdomyosarcoma.

Subtype(s)

Embryonal rhabdomyosarcoma, pleomorphic

Localization

Approximately one half of ERMSs occur within the head and neck region (including the orbit), and one half within the genitourinary system {3222,1324}. Less frequently, ERMS arises in the biliary tract, retroperitoneum, or abdomen. In contrast to alveolar rhabdomyosarcoma (ARMS), ERMS rarely involves the soft tissues of the extremities.

Clinical features

ERMS presents with a variety of clinical symptoms, generally related to mass effects, or it may be indolent. Head and neck lesions can cause proptosis, diplopia, or sinusitis; genitourinary lesions may produce a scrotal mass or urinary retention; biliary tumours may cause jaundice.

Epidemiology

Rhabdomyosarcoma is the most common soft tissue sarcoma in children and adolescents, with 4.5 cases per 1 million people aged 0–20 years {2885}. ERMS is the most common subtype, with one third of cases occurring in children aged < 5 years. About 4% of ERMSs affect infants. ERMSs also constitute 20% of all adult rhabdomyosarcomas. ERMS is slightly more common in males than females (M:F ratio: 1.5:1). About 80% of rhabdomyosarcomas in North America occur in white people, compared with 15% in African-Americans {2353}.

Etiology

ERMS is associated with several syndromes involving alterations of the RAS signalling pathway, for example, Costello syndrome (*HRAS* gene mutations), neurofibromatosis type 1 (*NF1* gene mutations), and Noonan syndrome (mutations in several genes). A few cases are reported in association with Beckwith–Wiedemann syndrome (dysregulation of imprinting in the

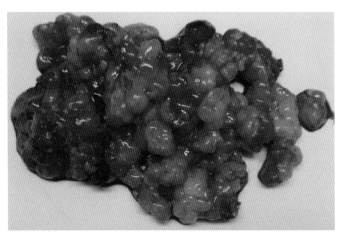

Fig. 1.230 Botryoid embryonal rhabdomyosarcoma. Gross photograph of a botryoid embryonal rhabdomyosarcoma showing multiple polypoid clusters of tumour.

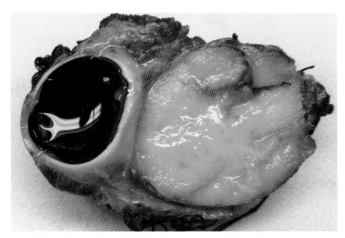

Fig. 1.231 Orbital embryonal rhabdomyosarcoma. An orbital embryonal rhabdomyosarcoma with a fleshy, pale-tan cut surface that resulted in proptosis of the overlying globe.

11p15.5 region). Uterine ERMSs occur in *DICER1* syndrome, and rhabdomyosarcoma of unclassified histology occurs in Li–Fraumeni syndrome (*TP53* mutations) {2885}.

Pathogenesis

Sporadic cases of ERMS are aneuploid with whole-chromosome gains including polysomy 8, followed by extra copies of chromosomes 2, 11, 12, 13, and/or 20. Whole-chromosome losses include monosomy 10 and 15. In most ERMSs, a genomic event such as chromosome loss, deletion, or uniparental disomy results in loss of one of the two alleles at many chromosome 11 loci. This loss of heterozygosity involves chromosomal region 11p15.5, which contains imprinted genes that encode a growth factor (*IGF2*) and growth suppressors (*H19* and *CDKN1C*)

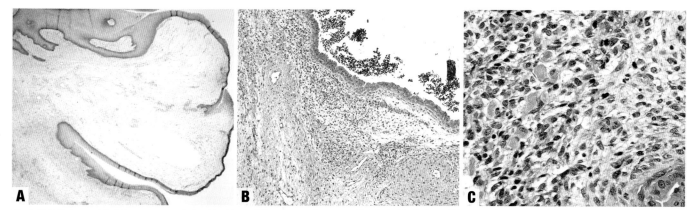

Fig. 1.232 Embryonal rhabdomyosarcoma, botryoid subtype. **A** Low-power microscopy. Histologically, the botryoid pattern of embryonal rhabdomyosarcoma shows a variably cellular tumour with a myxoid background and condensation of nuclei beneath an epithelial surface. **B** This tumour presented as a polypoid submucosal mass in the bladder of a boy. **C** Primitive round to slightly spindled cells with several differentiating rhabdomyoblasts.

{2835}. Genomic amplification in the form of double minutes or as ascertained by comparative genomic hybridization is frequent in ERMS with anaplasia {414,2558}.

Genomic studies of ERMS have identified somatic driver mutations involving the RAS pathway (*NRAS*, *KRAS*, *HRAS*, *NF1*, *FGFR4*), involving effectors of PI3K (*PTEN*, *PIK3CA*), or in genes that control the cell cycle (*FBXW7*, *CTNNB1*) {2834,2885}. Mutation of a RAS isoform occurs in one third of ERMSs, and mutation of a RAS pathway member has been found in < 50% of ERMSs. Within this group, *HRAS* mutations are enriched in the infant population (70% of infants aged < 1 year had *HRAS*

or *KRAS* mutations), and *NRAS* mutations are enriched in adolescents. *NF1* mutations occur in 10% of cases. Epigenetic modifications may also play a role, and *BCOR* point mutations or focal homozygous deletions are described in 15% of ERMSs. Mutations in *TP53* occur in approximately 10% of ERMSs and may be associated with anaplasia {1356}. About 30% of ERMSs harbour more than one driver mutation, whereas one quarter have no driver mutation identified. Expression studies have identified markers that distinguish *FOXO1* fusion–negative rhabdomyosarcoma (HMGA2 and EGFR [HER1] overexpression)

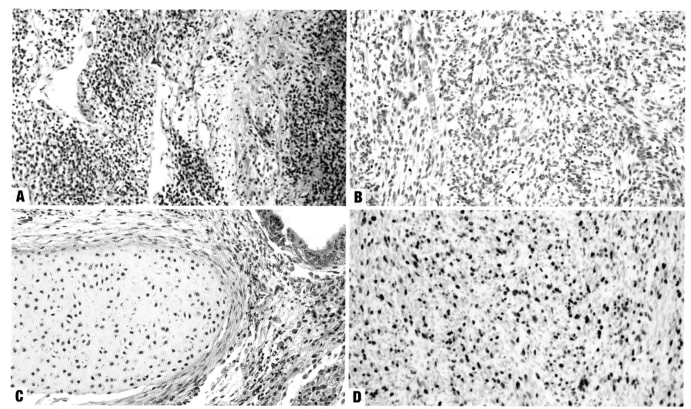

Fig. 1.233 Embryonal rhabdomyosarcoma. **A** The typical histological pattern of embryonal rhabdomyosarcomas recapitulates skeletal muscle development, with alternating areas of loose and dense cellularity. **B** Embryonal rhabdomyosarcoma in this example is composed of short, irregular fascicles of ovoid to spindled cells with focal myotube formation. **C** Cartilaginous differentiation – a rare but well-recognized phenomenon. **D** Myogenin staining confirms skeletal muscle differentiation.

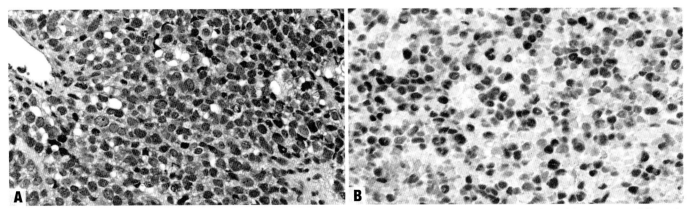

Fig. 1.234 Dense embryonal rhabdomyosarcoma. **A** This pattern with sheets of round cells may show similarity to the solid pattern of alveolar rhabdomyosarcoma. **B** Myogenin expression confirms the diagnosis of rhabdomyosarcoma, although nuclear staining in 50–90% of tumour cells may be seen in either embryonal or alveolar rhabdomyosarcoma.

from *FOXO1* fusion–positive rhabdomyosarcoma (AP-2β and P-cadherin overexpression) {1210,2687}.

Macroscopic appearance

ERMS forms poorly circumscribed, fleshy, pale-tan masses that impinge upon neighbouring structures. Botryoid tumours have a characteristic polypoid appearance with clusters of small, sessile or pedunculated nodules that abut an epithelial surface.

Histopathology

Analogous to embryonic skeletal muscle, ERMS contains primitive mesenchymal cells in various stages of myogenesis. Stellate cells with sparse, amphophilic cytoplasm represent the most primitive end of this spectrum. Differentiating rhabdomyoblasts acquire more cytoplasmic eosinophilia and elongation, manifested by tadpole or spider cells. Terminal differentiation with cross-striations or myotube formation may be evident. Differentiation often becomes more evident after therapy {170}. Typical ERMSs are composed of variably differentiated rhabdomyoblasts within a loose, myxoid mesenchyme, with alternating areas of dense and loose cellularity. The relative amount of myxoid matrix and spindled cells is highly variable. Occasional poorly differentiated ERMSs consist largely of primitive round cells, simulating ARMS (so-called dense pattern) {2689}.

Botryoid ERMS contains linear aggregates of tumour cells (the cambium layer) that tightly abut an epithelial surface, along with hypocellular polypoid nodules that may appear deceptively benign. ERMS may also have prominent spindle cell morphology, particularly in paratesticular tumours, although small foci of more-typical ERMS are usually present as well {2267}. Very rare tumours display mixed embryonal and alveolar morphologies; however, these cases typically lack the *FOXO1* gene rearrangements {2689}. Heterologous cartilaginous differentiation is occasionally present.

Anaplastic ERMS is defined by the presence of markedly enlarged, atypical cells with hyperchromatic nuclei, often with bizarre, multipolar mitotic figures {2558}. Anaplastic features may be focal or diffuse.

By immunohistochemistry, ERMSs are essentially always positive for desmin, although the extent of immunoreactivity is variable. The skeletal muscle–specific nuclear regulatory proteins myogenin (MYF4) and MYOD1 are also positive in essentially all cases, although the number of positive nuclei may be highly

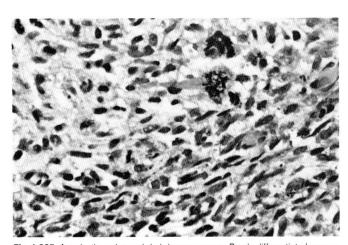

Fig. 1.235 Anaplastic embryonal rhabdomyosarcoma. Poorly differentiated appearance with a large, atypical mitotic figure.

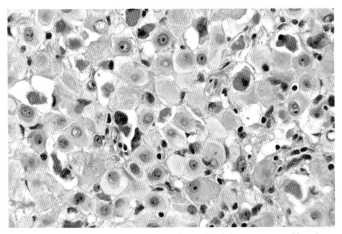

Fig. 1.236 Posttherapy differentiation in embryonal rhabdomyosarcoma. After chemotherapy, embryonal rhabdomyosarcoma may show extensive differentiation.

variable {2198}. MSA and SMA are frequently positive. Aberrant expression of keratins, S100, and NFP may be seen {638}.

Cytology

Cytological preparations demonstrate primitive round, spindled and stellate cells with scattered rhabdomyoblasts.

Diagnostic molecular pathology

Lack of *FOXO1* gene fusion distinguishes ERMS from ARMS {737}.

Essential and desirable diagnostic criteria

Essential: primitive round and spindle cell morphology with scattered differentiated rhabdomyoblasts; positivity for desmin and heterogeneous nuclear staining for myogenin and/or MYOD1.

Desirable (in selected cases): lack of *FOXO1* gene rearrangements to distinguish poorly differentiated ERMS from solid ARMS.

Staging

Rhabdomyosarcoma may be staged based on site of origin using the American Joint Committee on Cancer (AJCC) / Union for International Cancer Control (UICC) system for soft tissue sarcomas, with the exception of head and neck tumours, which are excluded from this system {101}. In children, a modified TNM staging system is used (the Intergroup Rhabdomyosarcoma Study Group [IRSG] grouping system). This system is heavily reliant on site of origin, with risk stratification based on favourable site (e.g. bile ducts, orbit, head and neck, or genitourinary [excluding bladder, prostate, and parameningeal]) or unfavourable (other) site. The IRSG grouping system is used for surgicopathological evaluation, including assessment of margins and residual disease {2105}.

Prognosis and prediction

Age and tumour stage are the most important risk factors in ERMS. Patients aged 1–9 years have better outcomes than infants or adolescents {1363}. Similarly, children have a better outcome than adults.

Alveolar rhabdomyosarcoma

Kohashi K
Bode-Lesniewska B

Definition

Alveolar rhabdomyosarcoma (ARMS) is a malignant neoplasm composed of a monomorphic population of primitive round cells showing skeletal muscle differentiation. The presence of either a *PAX3-FOXO1* or a *PAX7-FOXO1* fusion gene is detected in the majority of cases.

ICD-O coding

8920/3 Alveolar rhabdomyosarcoma

ICD-11 coding

2B55.Z & XH7099 Rhabdomyosarcoma & Alveolar rhabdomyosarcoma

Related terminology

Not recommended: mixed embryonal and alveolar rhabdomyosarcoma; fusion-negative alveolar rhabdomyosarcoma.

Subtype(s)

None

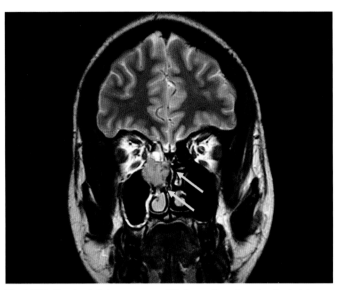

Fig. 1.237 Alveolar rhabdomyosarcoma. CT of a maxillary sinus alveolar rhabdomyosarcoma (arrows).

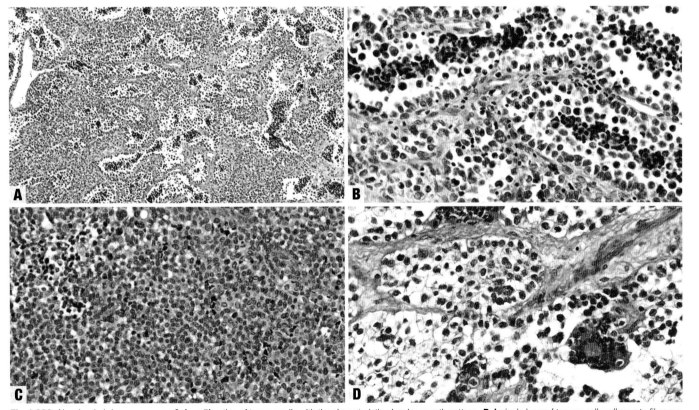

Fig. 1.238 Alveolar rhabdomyosarcoma. **A** A proliferation of tumour cells with the characteristic alveolar growth pattern. **B** A single layer of tumour cells adheres to fibrovascular septa. **C** Solid subtype shows a proliferation of small round tumour cells arranged in a sheet-like pattern without fibrovascular septa. **D** Multinucleated giant cells with multiple and peripherally placed nuclei.

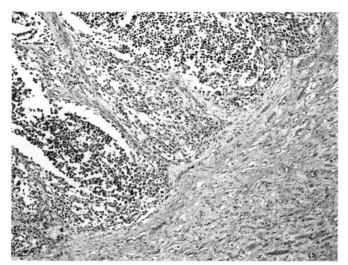

Fig. 1.239 Rhabdomyosarcoma with embryonal and alveolar components. Foci of small round tumour cells and differentiating rhabdomyoblasts. Most of these tumours lack the presence of a *FOXO1*-related fusion and probably represent embryonal rhabdomyosarcoma.

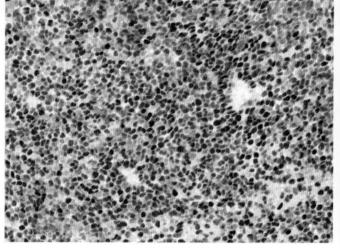

Fig. 1.240 Alveolar rhabdomyosarcoma. Diffuse and strong immunoexpression of myogenin.

Localization

ARMS most commonly arises in the deep soft tissue of the extremities {1303}. Other sites include the head and neck, paraspinal region, and perineal region {1329,2576,3358,171}.

Clinical features

ARMS is a highly aggressive and rapidly growing malignant soft tissue tumour, presenting at diagnosis with distant or locoregional metastases via lymphatic or haematogenous spread in 25–30% of patients {2339,1953,2686}. Symptoms are typically related to tumour location and size. Head and neck tumours with meningeal extension often cause cranial nerve deficits {3120}, paraspinal tumours may result in spinal nerve compression {1882,3067}, and perirectal or pelvic tumours may lead to constipation or symptoms of bowel obstruction {1084}. Primary disseminated tumours resembling leukaemia may rarely occur {1612,1467}.

Epidemiology

ARMS is the second most common type of rhabdomyosarcoma, constituting about 25% of these tumours. ARMS occurs in a slightly older population than embryonal rhabdomyosarcoma (ERMS), with a peak incidence among individuals aged 10–25 years and roughly equal incidence in male and female patients {2686,3152,1953,361}. A subset of cases have also been observed in adults aged > 40 years {3358,870}.

Etiology

Unknown

Pathogenesis

A t(2;13)(q36;q14) translocation is found in the majority of ARMSs, and a t(1;13)(p36;q14) is seen in a smaller subset. These translocations juxtapose *PAX3* (at 2q36.1) or *PAX7* (at 1p36.13) with the *FOXO1* gene at 13q14.11, to generate chimeric genes that encode PAX3-FOXO1 and PAX7-FOXO1 fusion proteins {222,746,1106}. PAX3 and PAX7 represent transcription factors that play essential roles in myogenesis {442}. The

PAX-FOXO1 fusion proteins function as oncoproteins affecting growth, survival, differentiation, and other pathways through activation of numerous downstream target genes such as *MET, ALK, FGFR4, MYCN, IGF1R,* and *MYOD1* {270,252,476,1239, 2885}. Less common fusion gene variants include the fusion of *PAX3* to *FOXO4, NCOA1,* or *INO80D* and the fusion of *FOXO1* to *FGFR1* {223,2986,1878,2834}.

Amplification of genomic regions 2p24 (containing the *MYCN* oncogene) and 12q13-q14 (including *CDK4*) occur most often in *PAX3-FOXO1* ARMSs, and amplification of regions 1p36 (which encompasses the *PAX7* locus) and 13q31 (which includes *MIR17HG*) are associated specifically with *PAX7-FOXO1* tumours {1266,106,221,2591,1192,2885}. Analyses of individual genes in sporadic ARMS have implicated several important oncogenetic pathways. Inactivating mutations of *TP53* and *CDKN2A/CDKN2B* and activating mutations of *FGFR4* are present in a small subset {1475,3026,3058}. *ALK* gene copy-number gain and cytoplasmic overexpression of ALK protein

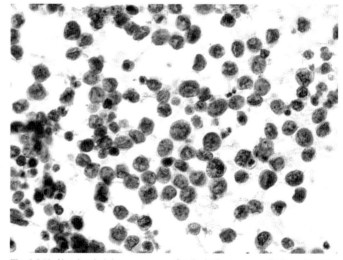

Fig. 1.241 Alveolar rhabdomyosarcoma. Cytologically, tumour cells form dyscohesive clusters, with comparatively monomorphous round nuclei and scant cytoplasm.

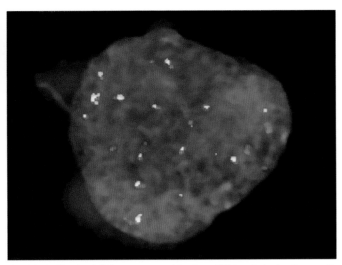

Fig. 1.242 Alveolar rhabdomyosarcoma. Interphase FISH analysis showing amplification of the *PAX7-FOXO1* fusion gene (juxtaposed red and green signals) by 1;13 translocation breakpoint-flanking probes.

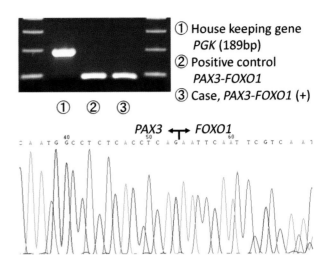

① House keeping gene *PGK* (189bp)
② Positive control *PAX3-FOXO1*
③ Case, *PAX3-FOXO1* (+)

Fig. 1.243 Alveolar rhabdomyosarcoma. Detection of *PAX3-FOXO1* fusion gene by RT-PCR and direct sequencing.

occur in the vast majority of ARMSs; however, targeting this kinase in vivo does not yield therapeutic efficacy {3158,3289}. The presence of recurrent somatic mutations (fusion-positive ARMSs have few to none) and distinct gene expression and DNA methylation profiles characterize fusion-positive and fusion-negative rhabdomyosarcomas (fusion-negative ARMS profiles are similar to those of ERMS) {223,738,1732,3298,2989, 1944,2809,3364,2273,2988}.

Macroscopic appearance
ARMS is soft, fleshy, and grey, with variable amounts of fibrous tissue and occasional necrotic areas and haemorrhage. Deep-seated tumours involving the musculature commonly infiltrate surrounding tissues.

Histopathology
ARMS is highly cellular and composed of primitive round cells with scant cytoplasm and hyperchromatic nuclei. Tumour cells are arranged in nests separated by fibrovascular septa, which frequently exhibit loss of cellular cohesion in the centre, conferring a pattern of irregular alveolar spaces and a varying degree of cystic change {2686,2438}. The solid subtype of ARMS is composed of sheets of neoplastic cells that have cytomorphological features of ARMS but lack septa or discohesion. Mitotic activity is often brisk. Occasionally, recognizable rhabdomyoblastic differentiation can be discerned. Multinucleated tumour giant cells are a common feature of ARMS. Rare cases may show clear cell morphology, with pale-staining and glycogen-containing cytoplasm. Tumours with mixed embryonal and alveolar features were previously considered to be a subtype of ARMS, but most such cases lack PAX-*FOXO1* fusions, thus appearing to be clinically and biologically more akin to ERMS. However, fusion genes have been detected in rare cases of so-called mixed ERMS/ARMS, which therefore represent examples of ARMS {2689,171}.

Rhabdomyoblastic differentiation of ARMS is shown immunohistochemically with positive reactions to desmin, myogenin, and MYOD1. The nuclear expression of myogenin is strong and diffuse, unlike in ERMS and other rhabdomyosarcoma subtypes

in which the staining pattern is focal {818,1418,2604}. MYOD1 expression may be focal. Occasional expression of keratin or neuroendocrine markers (CD56, synaptophysin, and chromogranin) may also be observed.

Cytology
Fine-needle biopsies are highly cellular and consist of uniform round cells with scant cytoplasm and variable rhabdomyoblastic differentiation. Wreath-like multinucleated giant cells are a common feature {1654,1066,2333,3216}.

Diagnostic molecular pathology
Approximately 85% of histologically diagnosed ARMSs contain characteristic fusion genes. In fusion-positive ARMSs, *PAX3-FOXO1* and *PAX7-FOXO1* account for about 70–90% and 10–30% of the fusions, respectively {2686,861}. Rare cases show alternative novel gene fusions (see *Pathogenesis*, above), which can be detected by various molecular strategies. The

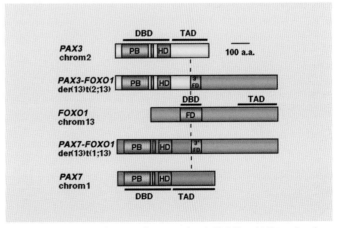

Fig. 1.244 Wildtype and fusion products associated with 2;13 and 1;13 translocations. The paired box (PB), octapeptide, homeobox domain (HD), and forkhead domain (FD) are shown as grey boxes. Transcriptional domains (DNA-binding domain [DBD] and transcriptional activation domain [TAD]) are indicated as solid horizontal bars. The translocation fusion point is shown as a vertical dashed line.

absence of one of these gene fusions suggests a diagnosis of ERMS with a primitive phenotype (formerly known as fusion-negative ARMS or mixed ERMS–ARMS).

Essential and desirable diagnostic criteria

Essential: uniform primitive round cell morphology with features of arrested myogenesis; an alveolar growth pattern is common but not required; strong, homogeneous nuclear immunoexpression for myogenin; heterogeneous staining for desmin and/or MYOD1; detection of *PAX3/7-FOXO1* fusion genes by molecular analysis.

Staging

See *Embryonal rhabdomyosarcoma* (p. 201).

Prognosis and prediction

Risk stratification predictive of outcome has been addressed with surgicopathological staging and fusion-based classification (the Intergroup Rhabdomyosarcoma Study Group [IRSG] grouping system) {1325,2885,2273}. The prognosis for patients with fusion-positive ARMS is worse than for those with fusion-negative rhabdomyosarcoma and ERMS, and the prognosis for patients with *PAX3-FOXO1* ARMS is inferior to that for patients with *PAX7-FOXO1* ARMS {2884,3298,2159,861,2813}. Amplification of *MYCN*, *CDK4*, and *MIR17HG* has also been correlated with poor outcomes {414,221,2591}.

Pleomorphic rhabdomyosarcoma

Montgomery EA
Dry SM

Definition

Pleomorphic rhabdomyosarcoma is a high-grade pleomorphic sarcoma, usually of adults, composed of bizarre brightly eosinophilic polygonal, round, and spindle cells that display skeletal muscle differentiation.

ICD-O coding

8901/3 Pleomorphic rhabdomyosarcoma NOS

ICD-11 coding

2B55.Z & XH5SX9 Rhabdomyosarcoma, primary site & Pleomorphic rhabdomyosarcoma NOS

Related terminology

None

Subtype(s)

None

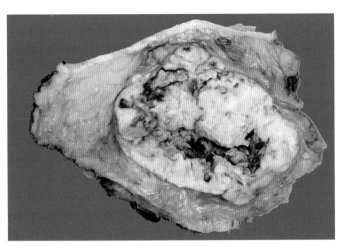

Fig. 1.245 Pleomorphic rhabdomyosarcoma. In this gross image, a firm and centrally necrotic tumour is present in the subcutaneous adipose tissue, although such lesions are frequently deep.

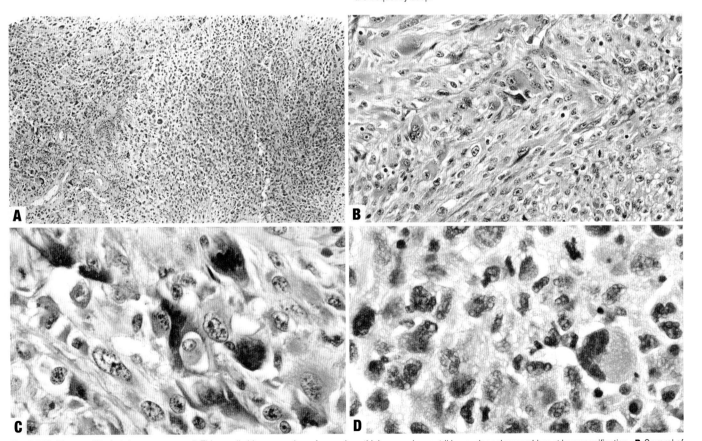

Fig. 1.246 Pleomorphic rhabdomyosarcoma. **A** This needle biopsy specimen from a deep thigh mass shows striking nuclear pleomorphism at low magnification. **B** Several of the cells in this image feature macronucleoli. **C** Note the nuclear pleomorphism. A malignant cell in the centre of the image appears to have cannibalized another cell. There is an atypical mitosis at the upper right. **D** There is striking variability in the sizes and shapes of the nuclei, and many feature macronucleoli.

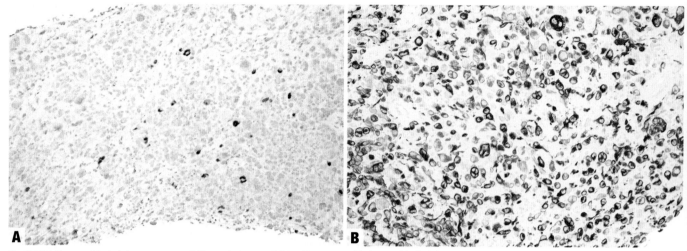

Fig. 1.247 Pleomorphic rhabdomyosarcoma. **A** Myogenin immunostaining. Not every cell is immunolabelled, but the pattern depicted here is sufficient to confirm the diagnosis. **B** These tumours are generally diffusely reactive with desmin antibodies.

Localization

These tumours arise in the deep soft tissue, with occasional exceptions {2329}, most often in the lower extremity but also in the chest/abdominal wall, upper extremity, abdomen/retroperitoneum, and head and neck {2329,1097,1104}.

Clinical features

Patients present with rapidly growing, usually deep, variably painful soft tissue swelling {1097}.

Epidemiology

These are tumours of adults and are most common in the sixth to seventh decades of life (mean age: ~72 years), occurring more frequently in men than in women, with an M:F ratio of 1.8:1 {2329}.

Etiology

Unknown

Pathogenesis

Pleomorphic rhabdomyosarcomas have complex karyotypes with numerical and unbalanced structural changes but no recurrent structural alterations {1843}. Genome-wide surveys have identified recurrent losses of DNA (e.g. 10q23), gains (e.g. 1p22-p23), and amplifications {1191}. This copy-number pattern differs from that found in either alveolar or embryonal rhabdomyosarcoma. The genetic profiles of pleomorphic rhabdomyosarcomas are indistinguishable from those of undifferentiated pleomorphic sarcomas {501}.

Macroscopic appearance

Pleomorphic rhabdomyosarcomas are usually large, well-marginated tumours {2329}, with a pseudocapsule and a whitish or fleshy cut surface, often with necrosis.

Histopathology

The tumours are composed of sheets of large, atypical, and frequently multinucleated polygonal, spindled, or rhabdoid cells with eosinophilic cytoplasm. Tumours typically display strong desmin expression and often limited expression of MYOD1 and myogenin.

Cytology

Not clinically relevant

Diagnostic molecular pathology

Not clinically relevant

Essential and desirable diagnostic criteria

Essential: pleomorphic cells with copious brightly eosinophilic cytoplasm; immunolabelling for desmin and myogenin.

Staging

See *Embryonal rhabdomyosarcoma* (p. 201).

Prognosis and prediction

These are highly aggressive sarcomas. The median survival was 7.3 months in the largest study to date, and about 80% of patients died of disease {2329}. Patients with superficial tumours (~20%) had a favourable outcome. Metastases to lungs are common {2329,1097,1104}.

Spindle cell / sclerosing rhabdomyosarcoma

Agaram NP
Szuhai K

Definition
Spindle cell / sclerosing rhabdomyosarcoma is a type of rhabdomyosarcoma that has fascicular spindle cell and/or sclerosing morphology.

ICD-O coding
8912/3 Spindle cell rhabdomyosarcoma

ICD-11 coding
2B55.Z & XH7NM2 Rhabdomyosarcoma, primary site & Spindle cell rhabdomyosarcoma

Related terminology
None

Subtype(s)
Congenital spindle cell rhabdomyosarcoma with *VGLL2/NCOA2/CITED2* rearrangements; *MYOD1*-mutant spindle cell / sclerosing rhabdomyosarcoma; intraosseous spindle cell rhabdomyosarcoma (with *TFCP2/NCOA2* rearrangements)

Localization
The head and neck region is the most common site of involvement, followed by the extremities. In the paediatric population, spindle cell / sclerosing rhabdomyosarcoma arises most often in the paratesticular region, followed by the head and neck and other regions. Rarely, other locations including viscera (uterus, prostate), retroperitoneum, or bone are affected {2251,518,1241, 1629,2032,38,1056,3253,175,1767,735,2172,2085,3401}.

Clinical features
Spindle cell / sclerosing rhabdomyosarcoma presents as a rapidly growing, painless soft tissue mass with symptoms related to local compression at the tumour site.

Epidemiology
Spindle cell / sclerosing rhabdomyosarcoma accounts for 3–10% of rhabdomyosarcomas. It affects infants, children, and adults. Although it affects both sexes overall, there is a decreased M:F ratio for the *MYOD1*-mutant genetic subtype {32,2251,518}.

Etiology
Unknown

Pathogenesis
The genetic abnormalities identified in spindle cell / sclerosing rhabdomyosarcoma can be categorized into three groups. The first group, congenital/infantile spindle cell rhabdomyosarcoma, shows gene fusions involving the *VGLL2*, *SRF*, *TEAD1*, *NCOA2*, and *CITED2* genes. The gene fusions include *SRF-NCOA2*, *TEAD1-NCOA2*, *VGLL2/NCOA2*, and *VGLL2-CITED2* {2207,

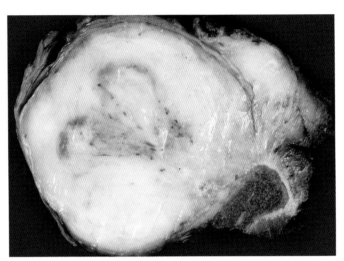

Fig. 1.248 Spindle cell rhabdomyosarcoma. Gross image showing a well-circumscribed tumour with tan-yellow cut surface with central necrosis, involving soft tissue and abutting the bone.

61}. The second group, which comprises most spindle cell / sclerosing rhabdomyosarcomas in adolescents and young adults, as well as a subset of tumours in older adults, shows the presence of *MYOD1* p.Leu122Arg gene mutation. The mutation, which occurs in the DNA-binding domain of MYOD1, leads to blocking of the wildtype MYOD1 function and imparts a MYC-binding capability {3012,1677,30,61,32,3147}. The third group of spindle cell / sclerosing rhabdomyosarcoma shows no recurrent identifiable genetic alterations. The recently described intraosseous spindle cell rhabdomyosarcoma shows two gene fusions, one involving either the *EWSR1* or the *FUS* gene being fused to the *TFCP2* gene. The other is the *MEIS1-NCOA2* gene fusion {3253,735,38}.

Macroscopic appearance
Spindle cell / sclerosing rhabdomyosarcomas present as variably circumscribed tumours, with sizes ranging from 1.5 to 35 cm. They show a white to tan cut surface with a whorled appearance. Necrosis and cystic degeneration may be present.

Histopathology
Spindle cell / sclerosing rhabdomyosarcoma shows variable morphology. Spindle cell rhabdomyosarcoma is characterized by cellular fascicles of spindle cells with an intersecting or herringbone growth pattern, resembling leiomyosarcoma or fibrosarcoma. The spindled neoplastic cells have pale eosinophilic cytoplasm and blunted, ovoid or fusiform, centrally located nuclei with small inconspicuous nucleoli. Mitotic figures, nuclear atypia, and hyperchromatic nuclei are often present. Primitive undifferentiated areas with round cells and hyperchromatic nuclei may also be present focally. Tadpole or strap cells, rhabdomyoblasts with elongated eosinophilic tails

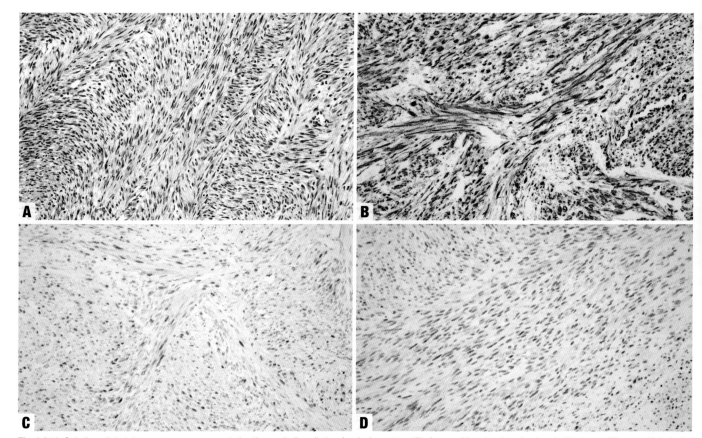

Fig. 1.249 Spindle cell rhabdomyosarcoma composed of uniform spindle cells in a fascicular pattern (**A**). Immunohistochemistry for desmin (**B**) shows diffuse positivity in the tumour cells. Myogenin staining (**C**) shows focal positivity, and MYOD1 staining (**D**) shows diffuse positivity.

with cross-striations, can be observed in some cases. Sclerosing rhabdomyosarcomas show prominent hyalinization/sclerosis, with tumour cells arranged in cords, nests, microalveoli, or trabeculae in a pseudovascular growth pattern. Prominent intervening sclerosis is noted. Sclerosing areas may mimic osteosarcoma due to the extensive matrix formation {32,2251, 518,1830,2085}. The recently described intraosseous spindle cell rhabdomyosarcomas show, apart from the typical spindle cell morphology, areas of distinctly epithelioid cells arranged in sheets and fascicles {3253,735,38}.

Immunohistochemically, spindle cell / sclerosing rhabdomyosarcoma is characterized by diffuse expression of desmin in all cases, with only focal expression of myogenin (MYF4) in most cases. MYOD1 staining can be focal or diffuse in the spindle cell tumours, but it is usually present in a diffuse pattern in the sclerosing cases. Staining for SMA and MSA is usually not present. A subset of the recently described intraosseous spindle cell rhabdomyosarcoma can also show positivity for cytokeratin and ALK.

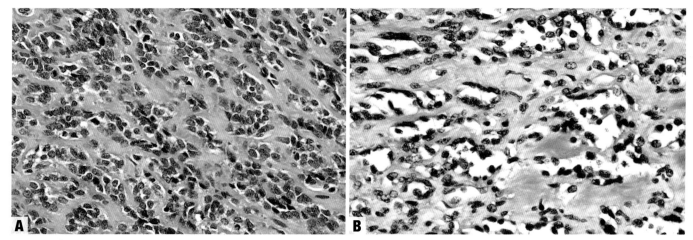

Fig. 1.250 Sclerosing rhabdomyosarcoma. **A** Clusters of tumour cells in a sclerotic collagenous background. **B** Pseudovascular pattern of arrangement of the tumour cells.

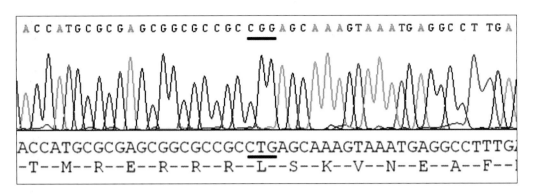

ACC ATG CGC GAG CGG CGC CGC **CGG** AGC AAA GTA AAT GAG GCC CT TGA

ACCATGCGCGAGCGGCGCCGCCTGAGCAAAGTAAATGAGGCCTTTG
-T--M--R--E--R--R--R--L--S--K--V--N--E--A--F--

Fig. 1.251 Spindle cell rhabdomyosarcoma. *MYOD1* p.Leu122Arg homozygous mutation represented on direct sequencing.

Cytology
Not clinically relevant

Diagnostic molecular pathology
VGLL2, *CITED2*, *NCOA2*, *MEIS1*, *EWSR1*, and *TFCP2* gene rearrangements can be detected by FISH studies, using break-apart probes or fusion probes. Alternatively, the gene fusion can be detected by targeted RNA sequencing using next-generation sequencing platforms. *MYOD1* mutations can be identified by PCR and Sanger sequencing of the hotspots or by targeted DNA sequencing on next-generation sequencing platforms.

Essential and desirable diagnostic criteria
Essential: cellular spindle cell fascicles or tumour cells in a variably sclerotic collagenous background; positivity for desmin, myogenin (focal), and MYOD1.
Desirable in selected cases: MYOD1 mutations and/or various gene rearrangements (see above).

Staging
See *Embryonal rhabdomyosarcoma* (p. 201).

Prognosis and prediction
Congenital / infantile spindle cell / sclerosing rhabdomyosarcomas with gene fusions show a favourable clinical course {61}. *MYOD1*-mutant spindle cell / sclerosing rhabdomyosarcomas follow an aggressive course despite multimodality therapy and have a poor prognosis in children and adults, with 3-year and 4-year survival rates of 36% and 18%, respectively {30,61,2608,32}.

Ectomesenchymoma

Huang SC
Antonescu CR

Definition
Ectomesenchymoma is an exceedingly rare multiphenotypic sarcoma consisting of both mesenchymal and neuroectodermal lines of differentiation. This biphasic neoplasm is composed of areas resembling rhabdomyosarcoma intermixed with variable neuronal/neuroblastic components.

ICD-O coding
8921/3 Ectomesenchymoma

ICD-11 coding
2F7C & XH0S12 Neoplasms of uncertain behaviour of connective or other soft tissue & Ectomesenchymoma

Related terminology
Not recommended: gangliorhabdomyosarcoma.

Subtype(s)
None

Localization
The common sites include pelvis/perineum, urogenital organs, and intra-abdominal or retroperitoneal soft tissue; less commonly, the head and neck, extremities, and mediastinum are affected {1596,372,731,1430}.

Clinical features
Tumours present as a superficial or deep soft tissue mass.

Epidemiology
Ectomesenchymomas are exceedingly rare, with approximately 50 cases reported to date if only composite rhabdomyosarcomas and neuroblastic tumours are included {1596, 372,731,1430}. Most patients are infants or children in the first two decades of life (range: birth to 15 years), frequently aged < 5 years, and there is a slight male preponderance (M:F ratio: 1.38:1) {1596,372,731,1430}.

Etiology
Unknown

Pathogenesis
Cytogenetic and array comparative genomic hybridization findings of ectomesenchymoma show overlap with those of embryonal rhabdomyosarcoma, with common trisomies of chromosomes 2, 8, and 11 {1424}. Frequent *HRAS* mutations at codon 13 or 61 and upregulated myogenesis-related genes, such as *MYOG*, *CHRND*, and *MRLN*, have been demonstrated, further underscoring the shared alterations seen in embryonal rhabdomyosarcoma {1430}.

Macroscopic appearance
The masses are multilobulated and thinly encapsulated, with a tan cut surface and variable necrosis and haemorrhage {372}. The tumours can vary widely in size (range: 3–18 cm), with most being > 5 cm in diameter {372}.

Histopathology
The prototypical morphology is that of an embryonal rhabdomyosarcoma with intermixed neuroectodermal elements. The latter cover the entire spectrum of neuroblastic phenotype, ranging from scattered ganglion cells to mature ganglioneuroma, intermediate ganglioneuroblastoma, and primitive neuroblastoma. The appearances of embryonal rhabdomyosarcoma vary, spanning botryoid, classic fascicular spindle cell with alternating myxoid-cellular areas, and the so-called dense pattern of primitive round cells {372,1424,1430}. Immunophenotypically, ectomesenchymoma is a multiphenotypic tumour, with the rhabdomyosarcomatous component expressing MSA, desmin, MYOD1, and myogenin, whereas the neuroblastic component is highlighted

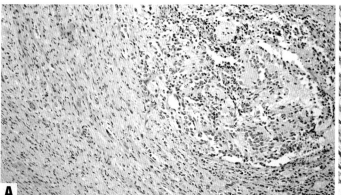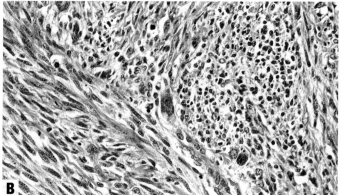

Fig. 1.252 Ectomesenchymoma. **A** Intimate and composite growth of embryonal rhabdomyosarcoma and ganglioneuroblastoma is seen in this ectomesenchymoma. The former is evident by myogenin immunoreactivity (shown in Fig. 1.253). **B** This example shows rhabdomyosarcoma of spindle cell morphology with scattered neurons.

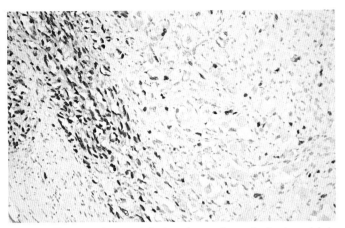

Fig. 1.253 Ectomesenchymoma. Intimate and composite growth of embryonal rhabdomyosarcoma and ganglioneuroblastoma is seen in this ectomesenchymoma (shown in Fig. 1.252A). The former is evident by myogenin immunoreactivity (shown here).

by NSE, synaptophysin, and chromogranin A, and the Schwannian or satellite cells by S100 {372,1430}. Pure rhabdomyosarcoma cases with aberrant expression of neuroendocrine markers should not be considered ectomesenchymomas {372,204}.

Cytology
Not clinically relevant

Diagnostic molecular pathology
Not clinically relevant

Essential and desirable diagnostic criteria
Essential: composite morphology with areas mostly resembling embryonal rhabdomyosarcoma, intermixed with unequivocal neuroblastic elements (neurons, ganglioneuroma, ganglioneuroblastoma, or neuroblastoma); immunoprofile highlighting the two components, with positivity for desmin/myogenin and synaptophysin, respectively.

Staging
Ectomesenchymoma is staged according to the American Joint Committee on Cancer (AJCC) staging system for rhabdomyosarcoma or the Union for International Cancer Control (UICC) TNM system.

Prognosis and prediction
Patients treated with multimodality strategies including rhabdomyosarcoma-based protocols have a comparable outcome to patients with embryonal rhabdomyosarcoma {372,731}. Favourable prognostic factors include age ≤ 3 years, size < 10 cm, and superficial location. Localized stage and the presence of a primitive neuroblastic element do not appear to have a substantial impact on outcome {372}.

Gastrointestinal stromal tumour

Dei Tos AP
Hornick JL
Miettinen M
Wanless IR
Wardelmann E

Definition

Gastrointestinal stromal tumour (GIST) is a mesenchymal neoplasm with variable behaviour, characterized by differentiation towards the interstitial cells of Cajal.

ICD-O coding

8936/3 Gastrointestinal stromal tumour

ICD-11 coding

2B5B & XH9HQ1 Gastrointestinal stromal tumour, primary site & Gastrointestinal stromal sarcoma

Related terminology

Not recommended: leiomyoblastoma; gastrointestinal autonomic nerve sheath tumour (GANT); gastrointestinal pacemaker cell tumour (GIPACT).

Subtype(s)

Succinate dehydrogenase–deficient gastrointestinal stromal tumour

Localization

GIST can occur anywhere in the gastrointestinal tract; however, approximately 54% of all GISTs arise in the stomach, 30% in the small bowel (including the duodenum), 5% in the colon and rectum, and about 1% in the oesophagus {2669}. Rarely, GISTs arise in the appendix. About 10% of cases are primarily disseminated, and the site of origin cannot be established with certainty. Extragastrointestinal GISTs occur predominantly in the mesentery, omentum, and retroperitoneum; they most probably represent a metastasis from an unrecognized primary or a detached mass from the gastrointestinal tract.

Clinical features

The most common presentations include vague abdominal symptoms, as well as symptoms related to mucosal ulceration, acute and chronic bleeding, an abdominal mass, and tumour perforation. Smaller GISTs are detected incidentally during endoscopy, surgery, or CT. Advanced GISTs spread into the peritoneal cavity and retroperitoneal space and often metastasize to the liver. Bone, skin, and soft tissue metastases are infrequently observed, whereas lung metastases are exceedingly rare. Systemic spread can occur years after detection of the primary tumour. Gastric GISTs exhibit a higher local recurrence rate than do small bowel GISTs, but the latter have a higher rate of abdominal dissemination and metastasis.

Epidemiology

Population-based studies in Scandinavia indicate an incidence of 1.1–1.5 cases per 100 000 person-years {2299}. However, incidental subcentimetre GISTs (called microGISTs) seem to be remarkably common. A frequency of 10% was reported in a study of oesophagogastric junction carcinoma resection specimens {8}, and even higher frequencies in autopsy and entirely embedded gastrectomy series (22.5% and 35%, respectively) {28,1598}. Approximately 25% of GISTs (excluding microGISTs) are clinically malignant. SEER Program data (interpolated from data on leiomyosarcomas) indicate that GISTs account for 2.2% of all malignant gastric tumours {3065}.

Sporadic GISTs can occur at any age, with a peak incidence in the sixth decade of life (median age: 60–65 years) and a slight male predominance {2135}. A small fraction of GISTs affect children and adolescents; such tumours are usually succinate dehydrogenase (SDH)-deficient (and *KIT/PDGFRA*-wildtype). SDH-deficient GISTs arise in the stomach, are more common in females, and affect younger patients {2126,1513}.

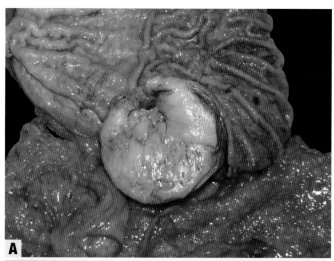
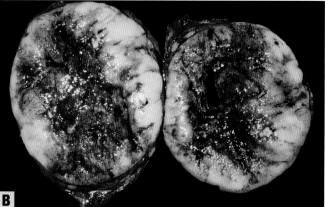

Fig. 1.254 Gastrointestinal stromal tumour (GIST). **A** Gross image of localized gastric GIST. Ulceration of the gastric mucosa is present. **B** Gross image of metastatic GIST to the liver. The cut surface features areas of haemorrhage and necrosis.

Etiology

Most GISTs are sporadic; 5–10% occur in association with a variety of syndromes. Most syndromic GISTs are SDH-deficient, including those associated with the non-hereditary Carney triad (GIST, pulmonary chondroma, paraganglioma) {483} and the autosomal dominant Carney–Stratakis syndrome (GIST and paraganglioma in the context of SDH germline mutations) {2455,2962}.

Rarely, GISTs are associated with neurofibromatosis type 1 (NF1); such cases are often multifocal, and most are located in the small bowel {2122,1121}. The extremely rare familial GISTs are caused by germline mutations of *KIT* or (far more rarely) *PDGFRA* {249,1840,1972}. Patients with these tumours tend to develop multiple GISTs, throughout the gastrointestinal tract, that can behave aggressively.

Pathogenesis

Most GISTs harbour gain-of-function mutations of the *KIT* or *PDGFRA* oncogene and progress by the stepwise inactivation of tumour suppressor genes. See *Diagnostic molecular pathology*, below, for full details, which are of clinical significance.

Macroscopic appearance

Localized GIST presents as a well-circumscribed mass of highly variable size (ranging from incidental, submillimetre lesions to > 20 cm). In larger lesions, the cut surface may show foci of haemorrhage, cystic change, and/or necrosis. Gastric GISTs often feature an intraluminal component and may produce umbilicated mucosal ulcers. In the small bowel, GISTs more frequently present as external masses. Some GISTs feature a narrow pedicle linked to the serosal surface, the interruption of which may contribute to the generation of extragastrointestinal GISTs {2135,2130,2119}.

Advanced disease most often presents as a main lesion associated with multiple smaller nodules that may extend from the diaphragm to the pelvis. Invasion of surrounding organs such as the spleen and pancreas can be observed in aggressive tumours. SDH-deficient GISTs are often associated with a distinctive multinodular pattern of growth.

Histopathology

Microscopically, GISTs exhibit a broad morphological spectrum. Anatomical location (gastric vs small bowel) seems to influence

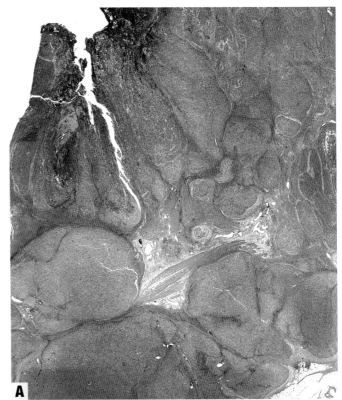

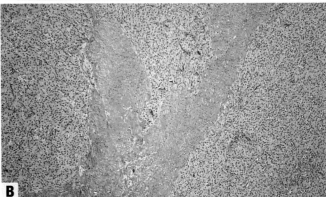

Fig. 1.256 Succinate dehydrogenase–deficient gastrointestinal stromal tumour. **A** The tumour shows a multinodular growth pattern through the wall of the stomach. **B** Muscularis propria separates tumour nodules.

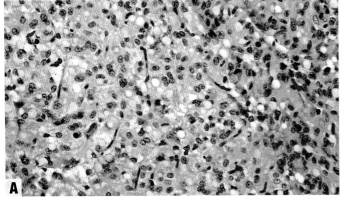

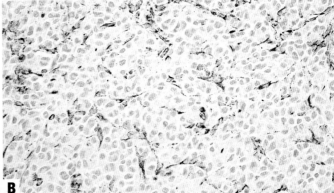

Fig. 1.255 Succinate dehydrogenase–deficient gastrointestinal stromal tumour. **A** The tumour shows epithelioid morphology. Note the uniform nuclei and cytoplasmic vacuoles. **B** The tumour cells show loss of staining for SDHB. Endothelial cells serve as an internal positive control.

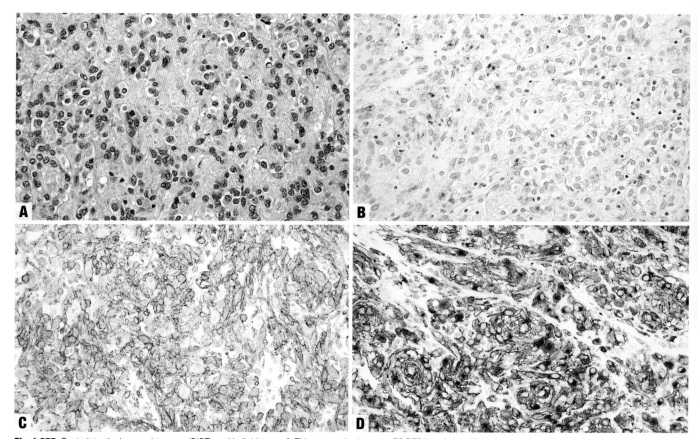

Fig. 1.257 Gastrointestinal stromal tumour (GIST), epithelioid type. **A** This tumour harbours a *PDGFRA* mutation. Note the round nuclei and abundant eosinophilic cytoplasm. **B** *PDGFRA*-mutant GISTs often show limited expression of KIT by immunohistochemistry (or are entirely KIT-negative). **C** Immunohistochemistry for ANO1/DOG1 is helpful to confirm the diagnosis of *PDGFRA*-mutant GIST. **D** *PDGFRA*-mutant GISTs typically show strong and diffuse expression of PDGFRA.

the histological appearance. Most gastric GISTs are spindle cell tumours, with epithelioid morphology seen in approximately 20–25% of cases. Some cases feature a combination of spindle cell and epithelioid histology. Nuclear pleomorphism is uncommon. Distinctive histological patterns among spindle cell GISTs exist. One example is the sclerosing type, seen especially in small tumours that often contain calcifications. The palisaded-vacuolated subtype is one of the most common, whereas some examples show a diffuse hypercellular pattern. Very rarely, sarcomatoid features with substantial nuclear atypia and high mitotic activity can be observed. Epithelioid GISTs may show sclerosing, discohesive, hypercellular (sometimes with a pseudopapillary pattern), or sarcomatous morphology with substantial atypia but low mitotic activity. Myxoid stroma is rarely observed {2135}.

Small intestinal and colonic GISTs are usually spindle cell tumours with diffuse sheets or vague storiform arrangements of tumour cells. Tumours with low biological potential often contain extracellular collagen globules (skeinoid fibres). Intestinal GISTs may feature anuclear areas (somewhat mimicking Verocay bodies or neuropil) composed of cell processes. Nuclear palisading, perivascular hyalinization, and regressive vascular changes (e.g. dilated and thrombosed vessels, haemosiderin deposition, and fibrosis) similar to those in schwannomas can be seen. Rectal GISTs most often feature spindle cell morphology {1177,397,2124,2135,2130}.

SDH-deficient GISTs characteristically show epithelioid morphology and are typically multinodular with plexiform mural involvement. Unlike in conventional GISTs, lymphovascular invasion and lymph node metastases are common {2141,853}.

Extremely rarely, morphological progression to high-grade (KIT-negative) sarcomatous morphology can be observed either de novo or after therapy with imatinib (dedifferentiated GIST). Dedifferentiation can also be associated with heterologous epithelial, myogenic, or angiosarcomatous differentiation {1856,135}.

Immunophenotypically, most GISTs show strong and diffuse expression of KIT (CD117), which appears as cytoplasmic, membrane-associated, or sometimes perinuclear dot-like staining. However, a small minority (< 5%), especially GISTs with *PDGFRA* mutations, may lack KIT expression or show very limited staining {2050}. The chloride-channel protein ANO1/DOG1 is an equally sensitive and specific marker and may rescue diagnostically as many as 50% of KIT-negative GISTs {3275, 934,2139,2330}. KIT and DOG1 are also expressed in the interstitial cells of Cajal, whose precursors are believed to be the histogenetic origin of GISTs. Most spindle cell GISTs (especially gastric tumours) are positive for CD34, whereas epithelioid examples are less consistently positive. Some GISTs express h-caldesmon; a minority express SMA; and rare examples show positivity for desmin, keratins (CK18), or S100 {2130}. SDH-deficient GISTs exhibit loss of SDHB protein expression irrespective of which SDH gene is mutated {1152,2141,1100}. SDHA loss is

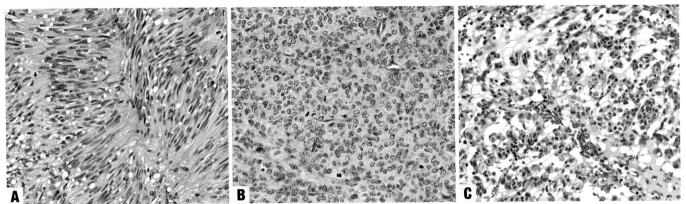

Fig. 1.258 Gastrointestinal stromal tumour (GIST). **A** GISTs are often composed of cytologically bland spindle cells that may feature distinctive perinuclear vacuolization. **B** Rarely, GIST may feature a high-grade morphology that is associated with high mitotic count. **C** The presence of myxoid change of the stroma is seen in this example of epithelioid GIST.

specific for *SDHA*-mutant tumours {3213}. Loss of expression of neurofibromin (NF1; using an antibody specific to the C-terminus) may help in identifying NF1-associated GISTs {2667}.

Cytology

Not clinically relevant

Diagnostic molecular pathology

About 85% of GISTs harbour gain-of-function mutations of the *KIT* or *PDGFRA* oncogene located on chromosome 4 (4q12), encoding for type III receptor tyrosine kinases {1374,1637, 1342,1535}. With exceedingly rare exceptions, they are mutually exclusive and result in the constitutive activation of either KIT or PDGFRA. Normally, KIT and PDGFRA are activated by the binding of their respective ligands (i.e. stem cell factor and PDGFA). Downstream oncogenic signalling involves the RAS/MAPK and PI3K/AKT/mTOR pathways {659,1534,2755}.

About 75% of GISTs harbour activating mutations of *KIT*, most often in exon 11 (66% overall) or exon 9 (6%); mutations in exons 13 and 17 are rare (~1% each) {1374,2683,902,1535}. Even more uncommon are mutations in exon 8 {1443A,1493A}.

KIT exon 11 mutations include deletions (45%), substitution mutations (30%), and insertion/deletion (indel) mutations (15%) including duplications. Nearly all *KIT* exon 9 mutations are duplications (p.Ala502_Tyr503); 80% of GISTs with such mutations arise in the small intestine. *KIT* exon 13 and 17 mutations are most often p.Lys642Glu and p.Asn822Lys, respectively {1641,1763}.

About 10% of GISTs harbour *PDGFRA* activating mutations (most often in the stomach), usually in exon 18 (8% overall); mutations in exons 12 and 14 are rare {1342,660}. The most common *PDGFRA* mutations are p.Asp842Val (55%) and p.Val561Asp (10%). Patients with *PDGFRA*-mutant tumours have a lower risk of metastasis than patients with *KIT*-mutant tumours {1535}. Given these differences in metastatic risk, nearly 85% of advanced GISTs harbour *KIT* mutations and only 2% harbour *PDGFRA* mutations {902}.

Many GISTs that are wildtype for *KIT* and *PDGFRA* harbour alterations in SDH subunit genes (5–10% overall) {1513,351}; 60% harbour inactivating mutations (nearly always germline); and 40% harbour *SDHC* promoter methylation (epimutation) {2141,1623}, leading to SDH dysfunction (SDH-deficient GIST). Patients with SDH-deficient GISTs are younger than those with tyrosine kinase receptor gene–mutant tumours; nearly all paediatric GISTs are SDH-deficient {351}. Tumours from patients with Carney triad usually show *SDHC* epimutation {1623}. *SDHA* is the most commonly mutated subunit gene (~35% of SDH-deficient GISTs) {3213}, followed by *SDHB*, *SDHC*, and *SDHD*. Rare

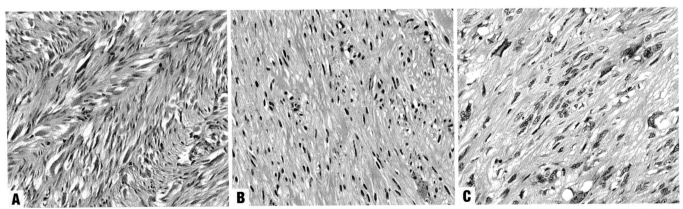

Fig. 1.259 Gastrointestinal stromal tumour (GIST). **A** Small bowel GISTs most often feature a spindle cell morphology that may be associated with the presence of skeinoid fibres. **B** GISTs sometimes appear microscopically hypocellular with neoplastic cells embedded in abundant fibrous stroma. **C** The presence of nuclear pleomorphism represents a rare morphological feature of GIST.

Table 1.03 Relationship of mitotic count and tumour size to prognosis of gastrointestinal stromal tumour (GIST), based on large follow-up studies conducted by the US Armed Forces Institute of Pathology (AFIP)

Category	Size (cm)	Mitotic count (mitoses/5 mm²)	% progression[a]	
			Stomach	Small bowel[b]
1	≤ 2	≤ 5	0	0
2	> 2 to ≤ 5	≤ 5	1.9	4.3
3a	> 5 to ≤ 10	≤ 5	3.6	24
3b	> 10	≤ 5	12	52
4	≤ 2	> 5	0	50
5	> 2 to ≤ 5	> 5	16	73
6a	> 5 to ≤ 10	> 5	55	85
6b	> 10	> 5	86	90

[a]The given numbers for GISTs of each size indicate the percentages of progressive disease (metastasis or death due to disease) observed in the patient cohorts during a long-term follow-up. [b]Prognostic assessment of GISTs of all non-gastric sites follows the criteria for small bowel GISTs.
Data based on Miettinen and Lasota, 2006 {2125}.

GISTs are associated with mutations of *NF1* (which are usually germline alterations in patients with NF1 or rarely somatic mutations), *BRAF*, or *KRAS* {2153,262,1121}. Like *KIT* and *PDGFRA* mutations, these alterations also result in RAS/RAF/MEK pathway activation.

Most GISTs (with the exception of SDH-deficient tumours) progress through a stepwise acquisition of chromosomal alterations, each of which probably inactivates tumour suppressor genes: loss of 14q (as many as 70%), followed by loss of 22q (~50%), 1p (~50%), and 15q (~40%) {2755}. *MAX* is the 14q GIST tumour suppressor gene, inactivated early (in microscopic and low-risk tumours) {2757}. Inactivating mutations in *CDKN2A*, *TP53*, and *RB1* are found in GISTs of higher-risk categories {2773}. *DMD* inactivation is a late event in GIST progression, identified in nearly all metastatic GISTs {3247}. Very rare GISTs harbour *NTRK3* or *FGFR1* gene fusions {406,2838}.

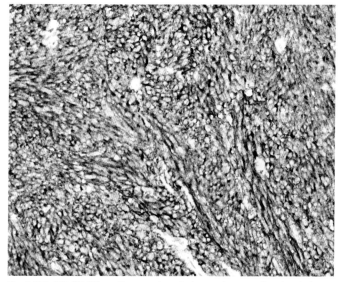

Fig. 1.260 KIT (CD117)-positive gastrointestinal stromal tumour. Cytoplasmic immunopositivity is associated with perinuclear dot-like accentuation.

Essential and desirable diagnostic criteria

Essential: an intramural, submucosal, or subserosal mass; spindle cell, epithelioid, or mixed morphology; KIT and/or DOG1 immunopositivity; SDHB loss in SDH-deficient GISTs.
Desirable: KIT or PDGFRA gene mutations in approximately 85% of tumours.

Staging
Risk stratification is preferred to anatomical staging.

Prognosis and prediction
The best-documented prognostic parameters for GIST are mitotic activity, tumour size, and anatomical site (see Table 1.03). Mitotic counting is for an area of 5 mm², which in most modern microscopes corresponds to 20–25 fields with the 40× objective and standard eyepiece diameter {2125}. This prognostic assessment applies best to *KIT/PDGFRA*-mutant GISTs. In general, intestinal GISTs and SDH-deficient GISTs are more unpredictable {3395,1998}. Tumours with low mitotic counts can metastasize, whereas tumours with higher mitotic counts may remain indolent for extended periods. Many patients with SDH-deficient GISTs with liver metastases can survive for years or decades without specific treatment, in contrast to patients with *KIT/PDGFRA*-mutant GISTs, which are rapidly progressive when metastatic. Tumour rupture is an additional adverse factor in GIST {1394}. The grading principles for soft tissue sarcomas do not apply to GIST. In order to refine risk assessment for consideration of adjuvant therapy, it has been suggested to include size and mitotic counts as continuous variables to be incorporated along with anatomical site into prognostic tools such as nomograms {2669} or prognostic contour maps {1536}.

Mutation status represents a prognostic as well as predictive factor {1765}. In general, *KIT*-mutant tumours tend to behave more aggressively than *PDGFRA*-mutant or triple-negative (*KIT/PDGFRA/BRAF*-wildtype) tumours. The best outcome seems to be associated with *PDGFRA* exon 12, *BRAF*, and *KIT* exon 12 mutations. An intermediate risk seems to be associated with *KIT/PDGFRA/BRAF*-wildtype status and with *KIT* exon 17, *PDGFRA* exon 18 (p.Asp842Val), and *PDGFRA* exon 14 mutations.

The worst outcome seems to be associated with *KIT* exon 9 and 11 and *PDGFRA* exon 18 (non-p.Asp842Val) mutations {2668}.

Mutation status also predicts response to imatinib, with *KIT* exon 11–mutant tumours exhibiting the highest rate of response and *PDGFRA* exon 18 (p.Asp842Val) mutants showing primary resistance {1537}. Molecular status also influences imatinib dose selection, with *KIT* exon 9 mutants benefiting from a higher dose (800 mg instead of 400 mg) {770}.

Subsequent mutations are associated with acquired resistance to imatinib. Secondary *KIT* gene mutations are most often found in the ATP-binding pocket of the kinase domain (exons 13 and 14) or in the kinase activation loop (exons 17 and 18) {127,1199}. Both *KIT/PDGFRA/BRAF/*SDH-wildtype and NF1-associated GISTs are also characterized by a lack of sensitivity to imatinib {503}.

Soft tissue chondroma

Rosenberg AE

Definition
Soft tissue chondroma is a benign neoplasm composed of chondrocytes that produce hyaline or myxoid cartilage that arises in the extraosseous and extrasynovial soft tissues.

ICD-O coding
9220/0 Chondroma NOS

ICD-11 coding
2E89.1 & XH0NS4 Benign tumours of uncertain differentiation, soft tissue & Chondroma NOS

Related terminology
Acceptable: chondroma of soft parts; extraskeletal chondroma.

Subtype(s)
Chondroblastoma-like soft tissue chondroma

Localization
Approximately 80% of cases occur in the region of the fingers {580,2334}. The remainder of cases arise most commonly in the hands, followed by the toes and feet, with origin in the trunk and the head and neck region {957} being uncommon. Rare examples have been described in the skin {235}, lip {1816}, dura {2977}, and tongue {827}.

Clinical features
The tumour is solitary and presents as a painless, firm, slowly enlarging mass {580}. Radiographically, it is well demarcated, is separated from bone, and has spiculated or ring-like calcifications. The cartilage is bright on T2-weighted MRI.

Epidemiology
Patients are usually middle-aged (average: 34.5 years), and males are affected more frequently than females (M:F ratio: 1.5:1) {601}.

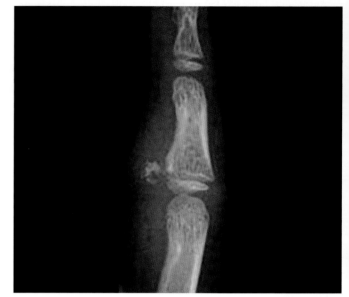

Fig. 1.261 Soft tissue chondroma. Small oval mineralized mass in soft tissues separate from the phalange.

Etiology
Unknown

Pathogenesis
Cytogenetic analyses of limited numbers of soft tissue chondromas reveal several different aberrations, including rearrangements of 12q13-q15 and trisomy 5, and in a set of tumours with rearrangements of 12q13-q15, a truncated or full-length HMGA2 transcript was found {410,2820,3033,710,2977}. In about 50% of the cases, *FN1* gene rearrangements were reported, with *FGFR1* and *FGFR2* as fusion partners {92}.

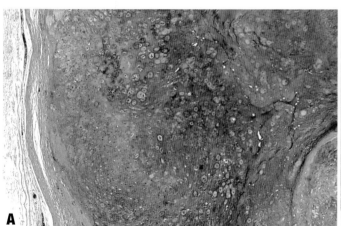
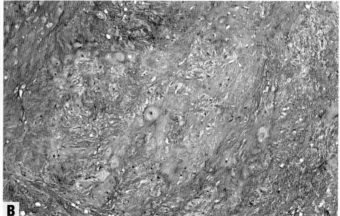

Fig. 1.262 Soft tissue chondroma. **A** Mass is well circumscribed by fibrous pseudocapsule. **B** Chondrocytes in lacunae and surrounded by abundant well-formed hyaline matrix.

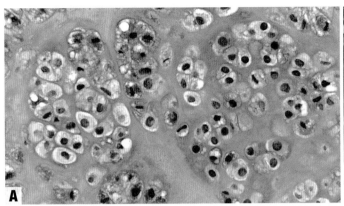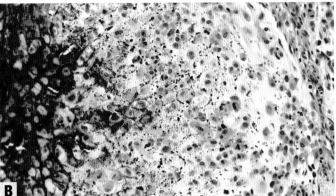

Fig. 1.263 Soft tissue chondroma. **A** Cellular tumour with chondrocytes that have mildly enlarged nuclei. **B** Chondroblastoma-like soft tissue chondroma is cellular, the chondrocytes are large, and the matrix contains calcification around individual cells.

Macroscopic appearance

Soft tissue chondroma is a well-circumscribed, nodular, solid mass that is greyish-bluish-white and sometimes focally myxoid. Most tumours are solid and 1–2 cm in size.

Histopathology

The tumour is composed of lobules of well-formed hyaline and/or myxoid cartilage that are delineated by fibrous septa {601}. The cartilage is often hypercellular and the chondrocytes are arranged in clusters and reside within lacunar spaces or float in a flocculent myxoid matrix. The nuclei are usually small, round, and dark, but they may be large with fine or coarse chromatin and small nucleoli and exhibit mild to moderate pleomorphism. Coarse calcifications and endochondral ossification may be present. The chondrocytes in the mineralized areas undergo necrosis, and heavily calcified tumours may have an infiltrate of histiocytes that may obscure the nature of the lesion. The chondroblastoma-like subtype is hypercellular and contains chondrocytes with nuclei that are often grooved or cleaved and have moderate amounts of eosinophilic cytoplasm; the matrix contains calcifications that surround individual chondrocytes, thereby mimicking chondroblastoma {514}. Regardless of the morphology, mitotic activity is limited and abnormal mitotic figures are not observed.

Differential diagnosis

The tumour is distinguished from synovial chondromatosis because it lacks an association with synovium. It is separated from juxtacortical chondroma because it lacks attachment to bone. Soft tissue chondrosarcoma exhibits greater cellularity, cytological atypia, and mitotic atypia.

Cytology

Not clinically relevant

Diagnostic molecular pathology

Not clinically relevant

Essential and desirable diagnostic criteria

Essential: a soft tissue mass composed of nodules of well-delineated cartilage; matrix is hyaline or myxoid and may calcify; chondrocytes show limited atypia and little mitotic activity.

Staging

Not clinically relevant

Prognosis and prediction

Treatment is marginal excision, and the recurrence rate is 15–20% {601}.

Extraskeletal osteosarcoma

Yamashita K
Hameed M

Definition
Extraskeletal osteosarcoma is a malignant tumour characterized by the production of osteoid or bone matrix by neoplastic cells, and it arises without connection to the skeletal system.

ICD-O coding
9180/3 Osteosarcoma, extraskeletal

ICD-11 coding
2B5F.2 & XH2CD6 Sarcoma, not elsewhere classified of other specified sites & Osteosarcoma, extraskeletal

Related terminology
Acceptable: extraosseous osteosarcoma; soft tissue osteosarcoma.

Subtype(s)
None

Localization
The majority of the tumours present as deep-seated soft tissue masses, but occasionally they originate in the dermis or subcutis. The lower extremity is commonly involved, with thigh as the most common location (27–52%); other frequent sites include the buttock, shoulder, trunk, and retroperitoneum {602, 217,1808,1851}.

Clinical features
Most patients present with a progressively enlarging mass that may be associated with pain. Some patients present with lung metastases. Plain radiographs, CT, and MRI usually reveal a large deep-seated soft tissue mass with variable mineralization. By definition these tumours do not arise from bone, but they may subsequently involve osseous structures.

Epidemiology
Extraskeletal osteosarcoma accounts for < 1% of all soft tissue sarcomas and approximately 4% of all osteosarcomas {2911, 2024,583,3318,2582}. It typically arises during midlife and late adulthood, with most patients being in the fifth to seventh decades of life at diagnosis; occurrence in children is uncommon. Males may be affected more frequently than females (M:F ratio: 0.8–1.9:1) {602,1808,1891,3064}.

Etiology
Most cases develop de novo, but approximately 5–10% of cases are associated with previous exposure to radiation {602, 1808,583}.

Pathogenesis
Conventional karyotyping has shown clonal chromosomal and highly complex aberrations {2095,1964,2168}. Recurrent

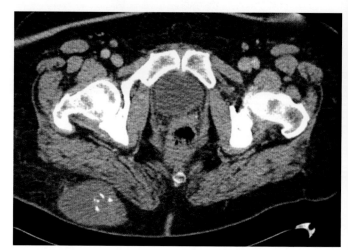

Fig. 1.264 Extraskeletal osteosarcoma. Axial contrast-enhanced CT of the pelvis shows a subcutaneous soft tissue mass superficial to the right gluteal musculature. Dense mineralization is seen centrally.

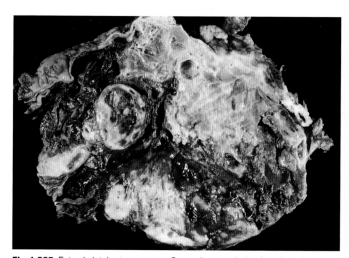

Fig. 1.265 Extraskeletal osteosarcoma. Gross photograph showing a large heterogeneous tan-white fleshy tumour with haemorrhagic and cystic spaces.

copy-number losses in tumour suppressor genes (*CDKN2A, TP53, RB1, PTEN, NF1, LSAMP*); gains and amplifications in oncogenes (*RUNX2, CDC5L, COPS3, EGFR, MDM2, CDK4, PMP22*); mutations involving tumour suppressor genes (*TP53, PTEN, RB1, NF1, SMARCA4*), chromatin-remodelling genes (*ATRX, DAXX, BRCA1, DAXX2, CHEK2, ARID5B*), histone methylation and demethylation genes (*BCOR, DNMT3A, MKK3 [MAP2K3]*), and WNT/β-catenin and sonic hedgehog pathway genes (*AMER1, AXIN2, GSK3B, GLI1, NOTCH3*); and in some cases *TERT* promoter mutation and *PIK3CA* mutations have been reported. The genomic signature of this tumour shows features overlapping those of conventional skeletal osteosarcoma {1554}.

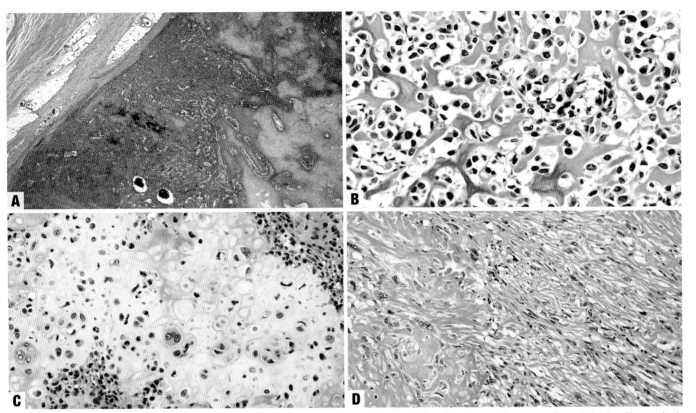

Fig. 1.266 Extraskeletal osteosarcoma. **A** The bone is more prominent in the centre of the tumour. **B** Osteoblastic type with tumour cells producing lace-like neoplastic bone. **C** Chondroblastic type. Condensation and spindling of the tumour cells are shown at the periphery of the cartilaginous area. **D** Fibroblastic type composed of intersecting fascicles of tumour cells with focus of neoplastic bone.

Macroscopic appearance

These tumours range in size from 1 to 50 cm (mean: 8–10 cm) and vary considerably in gross appearance; many tumours are circumscribed, tan-white, haemorrhagic, and focally necrotic gritty masses {602,217}. Extensive haemorrhagic cystic change is present in a minority of cases.

Histopathology

Extraskeletal osteosarcoma shows an extremely broad spectrum of morphology, and all the major histological patterns of osteosarcoma in bone can be seen. The osteoblastic type is the most common {602,217,1808,1851,1554}. In general, the tumours are composed of spindle or polygonal cells that are variously pleomorphic, cytologically atypical, and mitotically active and frequently demonstrate atypical mitotic figures. Tumour necrosis is also a common feature.

Identification of the neoplastic bone intimately associated with tumour cells, which may be deposited in lace-like, trabecular, or sheet-like patterns, is necessary for diagnosis. SATB2 immunoreactivity could be useful to detect osteoblastic differentiation when immature osteoid is difficult to distinguish from collagenous stroma {654,3342}. The amount and distribution of the neoplastic bone vary from tumour to tumour and even between different portions of the same tumour. The bone is sometimes more prominent in the centre of the tumour, with the more densely cellular areas located in the periphery, a pattern that is the reverse of myositis ossificans.

The rare well-differentiated subtype contains abundant bone deposited in well-formed trabeculae, surrounded by a minimally atypical spindle cell component similar to parosteal osteosarcoma; high-grade transformation or dedifferentiation has been reported in several cases {3361,9}.

Cytology

Cytologically, a hypercellular smear consists of mostly individually dispersed and small clusters of atypical cells. Most cases could be recognized as malignant, and fragments of osteoid-like matrix material might be observed in association with the individual cells and cell clusters {2278,2238}.

Diagnostic molecular pathology

Not clinically relevant

Essential and desirable diagnostic criteria

Essential: no connection to the skeletal system; identification of neoplastic bone/osteoid in association with malignant cells in otherwise unclassified soft tissue sarcoma.

Staging

Union for International Cancer Control (UICC) and American Joint Committee on Cancer (AJCC) TNM staging can be applied.

Prognosis and prediction

The prognosis is usually poor, and recent large series reported the 5-year overall survival rate to be 37–52% {1891,2872,3064}. Distant metastasis, old age (> 60 years), large tumour size (> 10 cm), and positive margin status were associated with poor prognosis in more than one study {2872,3064,1891,1554}.

Schwannoma

Perry A
Jo VY

Definition
Schwannoma is a nerve sheath tumour composed entirely or nearly entirely of differentiated neoplastic Schwann cells.

ICD-O coding
9560/0 Schwannoma NOS

ICD-11 coding
2F38 & XH98Z3 Benign neoplasm of other or unspecified sites & Schwannoma (neurilemmoma)

Related terminology
Acceptable: neurilemmoma.

Subtype(s)
Ancient schwannoma; cellular schwannoma; plexiform schwannoma; epithelioid schwannoma; microcystic/reticular schwannoma

Localization
Common sites of origin are peripheral nerves in the skin and subcutaneous tissues of the head and neck or along the flexor surfaces of the extremities. Spinal intradural extramedullary examples are also common and form so-called dumbbell tumours when growing through neural foramina, with multiple paraspinal schwannomas being commonplace in neurofibromatosis type 2 (NF2). Cranial nerve involvement is not uncommon, with cerebellopontine angle tumours emanating from the vestibular division of the eighth cranial nerve encountered most often and bilateral involvement being a definitional criterion for NF2 {937}. Spinal intramedullary and CNS sites are rare {502}, as are those involving viscera (such as the gastrointestinal tract) and bone {3205}.

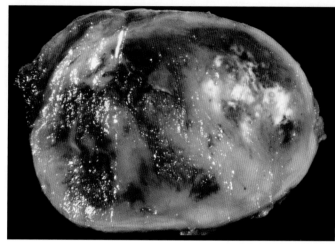

Fig. 1.267 Schwannoma. Cut surface showing an encapsulated tan-grey tumour with foci of haemorrhage, yellowish-white foci of xanthic change, and cystic degeneration.

Clinical features
Schwannomas are slow-growing tumours. They often present as asymptomatic masses or incidental findings on imaging studies, and they may be painful, particularly in the setting of schwannomatosis. Spinal schwannomas may elicit sensory symptoms such as radicular pain and motor signs if growing intraspinally. Vestibular schwannomas often present with hearing loss and vertigo.

Epidemiology
More than 90% of these lesions are solitary and sporadic and may affect all ages but have a peak incidence in the fourth to sixth decades of life. There is no known predisposition with regard to race or sex.

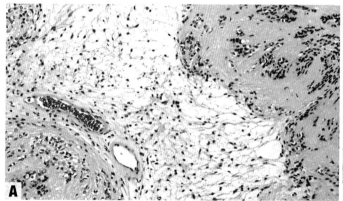
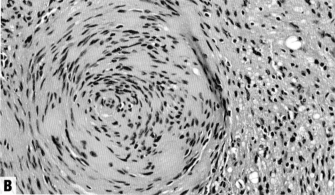

Fig. 1.268 Schwannoma. **A** Alternating compact Antoni A (periphery) and loose Antoni B (centre) areas. Nuclear palisades, known as Verocay bodies, are noted in the Antoni A area on the right. **B** The formation of Schwannian whorls can raise the differential with meningioma.

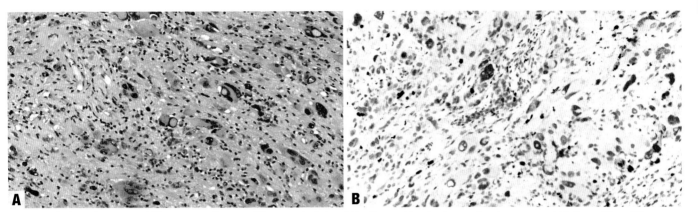

Fig. 1.269 Ancient schwannoma. **A** The presence of scattered bizarre or atypical nuclei is often considered a degenerative phenomenon, which does not impact the prognosis. **B** Despite the nuclear atypia, the Ki-67 proliferation index is low, with the majority of bizarre nuclei being negative.

Etiology

The etiology of most sporadic schwannomas is not known, although there is an established increased incidence associated with prior irradiation {2654,2540}. There is an association with neurofibromatosis in some cases (see *Pathogenesis*, below).

Pathogenesis

A causal relationship exists between schwannoma tumorigenesis and loss of expression of merlin (NF2, schwannomin), the growth inhibitory protein product of the *NF2* tumour suppressor gene located at 22q12.2 {2943}. *NF2*-inactivating mutations have been detected in approximately 50–75% of sporadic cases {1503,1766,2360,1323}. Underlying genetic events are predominantly frameshift and nonsense mutations, with loss of the remaining wildtype allele on chromosome 22. Other common mutations involve the *LATS1*, *LATS2*, *ARID1A*, *ARID1B*, and *DDR1* genes, whereas a recurrent in-frame *SH3PXD2A-HTRA1* fusion is found in roughly 10% of cases {2360,42}.

Multiple schwannomas are a feature of NF2 and schwannomatosis, both of which can also occur in mosaic or segmental forms {337,1607}. NF2-associated schwannomas commonly

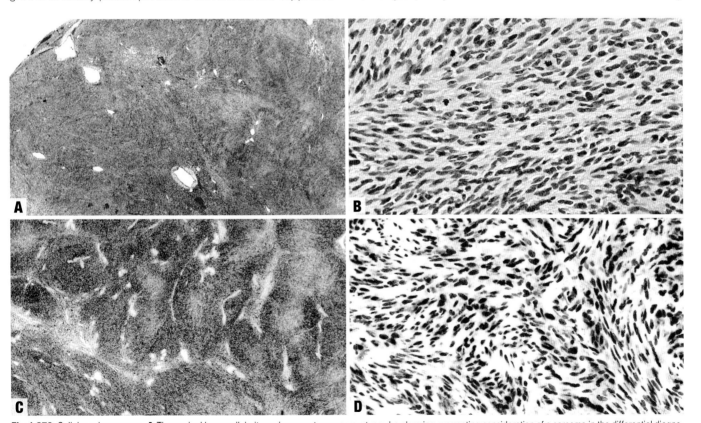

Fig. 1.270 Cellular schwannoma. **A** The marked hypercellularity and compact arrangement may be alarming, warranting consideration of a sarcoma in the differential diagnosis. **B** Mitotic figures are common, but the mitotic count is < 5 mitoses/mm² in most examples. **C** Diffuse S100 positivity is typical and helps distinguish this schwannoma subtype from malignant peripheral nerve sheath tumour. **D** Retained H3K27me3 expression differs from the complete loss of staining in tumour nuclei of most malignant peripheral nerve sheath tumours.

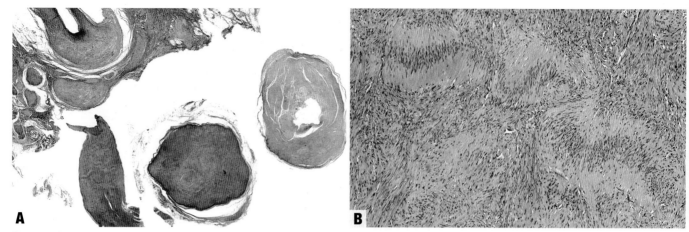

Fig. 1.271 Plexiform schwannoma. **A** The presence of tumour within multiple nerve fascicles defines this subtype and often raises the differential of plexiform neurofibroma at low magnification. **B** At higher magnification, typical features of schwannoma are seen, including Verocay bodies.

present before the age of 30 years, whereas tumours usually manifest in adulthood in schwannomatosis. Bilateral vestibular schwannoma is a hallmark of NF2, often showing multifocal nerve involvement and a nodular microscopic growth pattern. In addition, patients with the more severe Wishart form of NF2 typically have meningiomas, which are often multiple and associated with increased morbidity and mortality. Gliomas, most frequently cervical spinal ependymoma, develop less commonly {937}. NF2 is inherited in an autosomal dominant manner, with 50% of cases representing new or sporadic mutations.

Schwannomatosis is characterized by the presence of multiple schwannomas, mostly (but not invariably) in the absence

of vestibular nerve involvement and meningiomas. Cranial and cutaneous nerves are infrequently affected. Germline mutations of either the *SMARCB1* or *LZTR1* tumour suppressor gene are found in 86% of familial and 40% of sporadic schwannomatosis patients {1607}. Nevertheless, the tumorigenesis appears to be more complex given that these tumours arise from a 3-hit or 4-hit mechanism that involves two genes. One common pattern is a germline *SMARCB1* or *LZTR1* mutation followed by a somatic *NF2* mutation on the same chromosome 22 and a deletion of the entire other chromosome 22, leading to biallelic inactivation of both tumour suppressor genes simultaneously (i.e. 3 hits). Not surprisingly, therefore, the somatic *NF2* mutation often differs

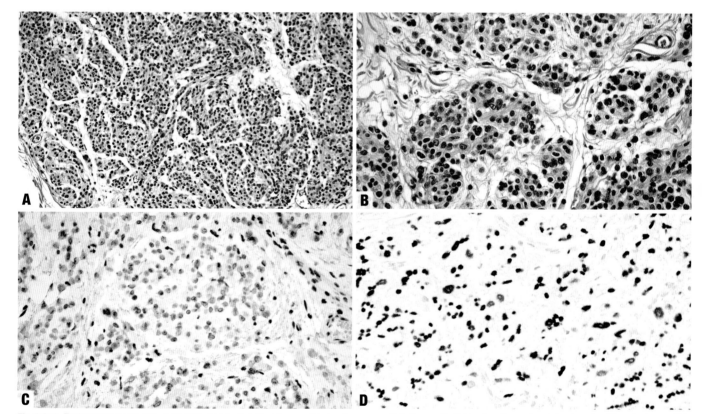

Fig. 1.272 Epithelioid schwannoma. **A** Multilobular growth pattern is appreciated on low power. **B** Uniform epithelioid cells with round nuclei and amphophilic cytoplasm, within a myxoid or fibrous stroma. **C** SMARCB1 (INI1) loss occurs in 40% of cases, as in this case. **D** Extensive SOX10 immunoreactivity, similar to other schwannomas.

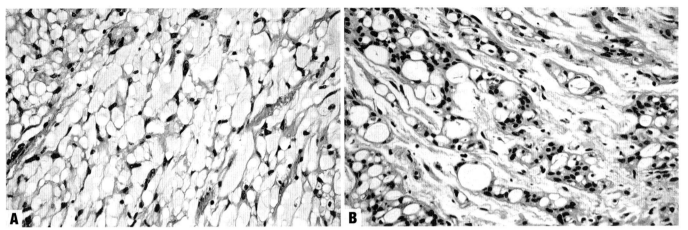

Fig. 1.273 Microcystic/reticular schwannoma. **A** Reticular growth pattern with formation of microcysts within an abundant myxoid stroma. **B** Microcysts may appear pseudoglandular.

among schwannomas from any one patient, as well as between the schwannomas of different family members.

Macroscopic appearance
These tumours are mainly solitary and globoid, have a smooth surface, and measure < 10 cm in greatest dimension, except for giant schwannomas, which are mostly encountered in the lumbosacral region. Fewer than half have an evident attached nerve, which is most often small. The uninvolved nerve fascicles are often found draped over the tumour capsule. Except for those arising in CNS parenchyma, skin, viscera, and bone, the tumours are usually encapsulated. Sectioned tumours reveal firm, light-tan, glistening tissue, interrupted by white/yellow areas and/or patches of haemorrhage.

Histopathology
Conventional schwannoma is usually an encapsulated spindle cell tumour that is composed nearly entirely of well-differentiated Schwann cells. Schwannomas have a broad morphological range. The large majority are biphasic tumours with compact areas (Antoni A tissue) showing occasional nuclear palisading (Verocay bodies), alternating with loosely arranged foci (Antoni B tissue). Cells of Antoni A tissue possess modest eosinophilic cytoplasm, no discernible cell borders, and normochromatic elongated tapered nuclei. Cytoplasmic nuclear inclusions, nuclear pleomorphism, and mitotic figures may be seen. Palisading (Verocay bodies) takes the form of parallel rows of Schwann cell nuclei separated by their aligned cell processes. Antoni B tissue commonly contains a cobweb-like network of tumour processes with collections of lipid-laden histiocytes and thick-walled, hyalinized blood vessels. Lymphoid aggregates are often present in a subcapsular distribution, or at the periphery in unencapsulated tumours.

A minority of schwannomas deviate from the description above. Tumours of the eighth cranial nerve show predominantly Antoni A tissue, and intestinal schwannomas typically lack Antoni B tissue. The most extreme deviation is seen in the morphological subtypes (see below).

Diffuse staining for S100 in cell nuclei and cytoplasm, which is more prominent in Antoni A than in Antoni B areas, is found in all tumours and subtypes. Similarly, SOX10 immunoreactivity is usually extensive {2315,1584}. Expression of GFAP is less frequent and more variable. Retroperitoneal and mediastinal lesions are commonly positive for keratin AE1/AE3 due to cross-reactivity with GFAP. In contrast to the lattice-like staining pattern in neurofibromas, CD34 is commonly positive only in subcapsular areas, although a small subset of cases show more-extensive positivity. Staining for NFP is helpful in identifying entrapped intratumoural axons, found in many sporadic schwannomas, albeit most often at their periphery {2252}. EMA highlights perineurial cells in the capsule, if present.

Ancient schwannoma
This subtype differs from the conventional schwannoma only by its presence of scattered atypical to bizarre-appearing nuclei, a feature that is often considered degenerative. Such cases may show extensive hyalinization or central ischaemic changes.

Cellular schwannoma
This subtype is composed exclusively or predominantly of Antoni A tissue and is devoid of Verocay bodies. The tumours most commonly involve large nerves and nerve plexuses at paravertebral sites, mediastinum, retroperitoneum, and pelvis {3308,3281,2476}. Cranial nerves can rarely be affected {928}. In addition to the cells being closely packed, they are not uncommonly hyperchromatic and mitotically active. Small areas of microscopic necrosis may be seen. These features may raise concern for malignant peripheral nerve sheath tumour (MPNST); however, the presence of conventional features of schwannoma aid in this distinction, including encapsulation, subcapsular lymphocytes, hyalinized blood vessels, and Schwannian whorls. Cellular schwannoma shows Ki-67 labelling hotspots (rather than diffuse increases), with an index still < 20%, and p16 and H3K27me3 expression are both retained {2476}. Tumour erosion of nearby bone may occur.

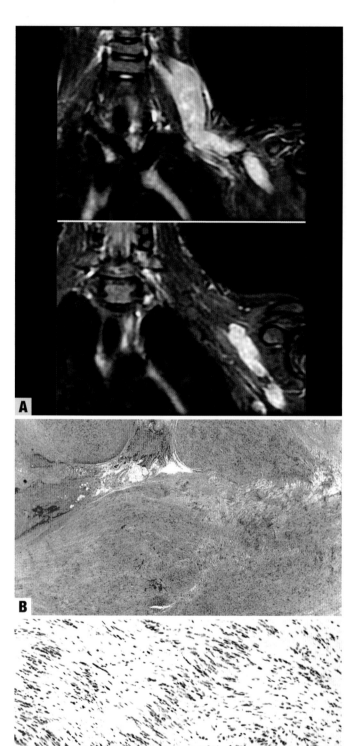

Fig. 1.274 Syndrome-associated schwannoma. **A** On MRI, a longitudinally extensive and/or multicentric/discontinuous-appearing nerve sheath tumour such as this should raise suspicion of a tumour predisposition syndrome such as schwannomatosis or neurofibromatosis type 2. **B** The histology from the same case similarly showed a multicentric or multinodular appearance. **C** The mosaic pattern of SMARCB1 (INI1) immunostaining in this same case further suggests that this schwannoma is arising as part of a syndrome, such as schwannomatosis or neurofibromatosis type 2.

Plexiform schwannoma

These conventional or cellular subtypes often arise in skin or subcutaneous tissue, growing as thinly encapsulated plexiform or multinodular tumours {272,1022}. More infrequently these tumours can occur in the deep soft tissues {34}. The tumours come to clinical attention earlier in life, often in childhood and even at birth {3309}, with some predilection for the trunk and head and neck region. Most are sporadic, but they have also been occasionally reported in patients with NF2 or schwannomatosis. Biphasic plexiform schwannomas are more readily identified pathologically than plexiform cellular examples. The latter are composed of solid nodules separated by thin fibrous bands, or of more-infiltrative nodules with entrapped axons. The tumours generally differ from the conventional schwannoma in their absence of a well-formed capsule and thick-walled vessels.

Epithelioid schwannoma

Most epithelioid schwannomas are sporadic, although some may be multiple and/or arise in the setting of schwannomatosis {1308,1533}. Tumours show multilobulated growth of epithelioid cells, arranged singly or in nests within a myxoid and/or hyalinized stroma. Tumour cells show eosinophilic cytoplasm and uniform, round nuclei with small or inconspicuous nucleoli, occasionally with pseudoinclusions. Conventional areas of spindled morphology, Antoni A or Antoni B tissue, and vessels with hyalinized walls may be present. Loss of SMARCB1 expression is observed in approximately 40% of cases, and such cases are associated with *SMARCB1* inactivation {1533,2751}. Some examples show increased cytological atypia, and rare examples show malignant transformation to epithelioid MPNST.

Microcystic/reticular schwannoma

This is the rarest subtype of schwannoma, and tumours seem to preferentially arise in visceral sites, most commonly in the gastrointestinal tract {1854}. Most lesions are encapsulated except in visceral sites. Microscopically, tumours are characterized by a microcyst-rich network of interconnected bland spindle cells with eosinophilic cytoplasm, associated with a myxoid, fibrillary, and/or hyalinized collagenous stroma. Antoni A tissue is frequent, and tumours show strong and diffuse expression of S100. However, conventional features of hyalinized blood vessels, foamy histiocytes, and Verocay bodies are generally absent.

Other patterns

Although most syndrome-associated schwannomas are not histologically distinguishable from their sporadic counterparts, several clinicopathological clues may indicate a setting of NF2 or schwannomatosis: young patient age, multiple tumours, extensive longitudinal involvement of a nerve, discontinuous or multinodular growth pattern, and a mosaic SMARCB1 immunostaining pattern defined by an admixture of positive and negative nuclei {2465,464}. Some schwannomas feature predominantly small blue round cells with or without structures resembling Homer Wright rosettes or giant rosettes surrounding collagen fibres resembling those of low-grade fibromyxoid sarcoma; these cases are often referred to as neuroblastoma-like, although they lack increased proliferative activity and show a typical schwannoma immunoprofile {1688}. Another rare pitfall is a schwannoma with neuromelanin-like pigment accumulation that is positive on Fontana–Masson staining. Nevertheless, the histology is otherwise typical of schwannoma and the tumour cells are negative for more-specific melanocytic markers, such as HMB45 {1086}; therefore, these should not be equated with the more aggressive and Carney complex / PRKAR1A–associated malignant melanotic nerve sheath tumour (previously termed melanotic schwannoma).

Cytology

Aspirate smears of schwannoma typically yield cohesive syncytial fragments of spindle cells {549}. Within the fragments, variably wavy and bent tumour cell nuclei with tapered edges and fibrillary cytoplasm are seen. Nuclear pleomorphism or degenerative atypia and intranuclear inclusions may be seen. Schwannomas may be difficult to distinguish from other spindle cell neoplasms on cytological preparation alone, and their diagnosis requires correlation with core biopsy and/or immunohistochemical staining {46}.

Diagnostic molecular pathology

Despite frequent *NF2* alterations in schwannomas, this is not specific, and a pathognomonic molecular signature has not been found.

Essential and desirable diagnostic criteria

In most examples, a diagnosis of schwannoma is readily made on histopathology alone, which is further supported by extensive S100 and SOX10 expression.

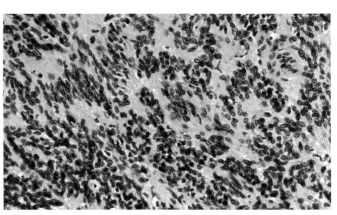

Fig. 1.275 Schwannoma with neuroblastoma-like features. The small cell cytology and vague structures resembling Homer Wright rosettes are reminiscent of neuroblastoma.

Staging

Not clinically relevant

Prognosis and prediction

Schwannomas are benign and do not usually recur if treated by gross total resection. Cellular and plexiform examples are least amenable to total removal and sometimes can only be debulked. Malignant transformation of conventional schwannoma is exceptionally rare. In the small number of cases reported to date, it has most often taken the form of epithelioid MPNST {3310, 2045,494}. Less common examples feature foci of conventional MPNST, primitive neuroectodermal cells, rhabdomyosarcoma, and/or angiosarcoma {3310,3096,2045,1719,494,41}.

Neurofibroma

Perry A
Reuss DE
Rodriguez F

Definition

Neurofibroma is a benign peripheral nerve sheath tumour consisting of differentiated Schwann cells, perineurial/perineurial-like cells, fibroblasts, mast cells, and residual interspersed myelinated and unmyelinated axons embedded in a myxoid and collagenous extracellular matrix.

ICD-O coding

9540/0 Neurofibroma NOS

ICD-11 coding

2F38 & XH87J5 Benign neoplasm of other or unspecified sites & Neurofibroma NOS

2F24 & XH87J5 Benign cutaneous neoplasms of neural or nerve sheath origin & Neurofibroma NOS

Related terminology

None

Subtype(s)

Ancient neurofibroma; cellular neurofibroma; atypical neurofibroma; plexiform neurofibroma

Localization

The most common site of involvement is the skin, where the tumours are associated with small nerves. Less often involved are more-deeply situated medium-sized nerves, a nerve plexus, or a major nerve trunk. Tumours may also arise from spinal nerve roots, with multiple paraspinal tumours being particularly common in neurofibromatosis type 1 (NF1). Cranial nerve examples are exceptional.

Clinical features

Cutaneous neurofibromas are usually asymptomatic (rarely painful) and most commonly present as a mass. They are mobile soft lesions without a particular anatomical distribution. Deep tumours often present with motor or sensory symptoms in the distribution of the affected nerve. Least commonly, the tumour

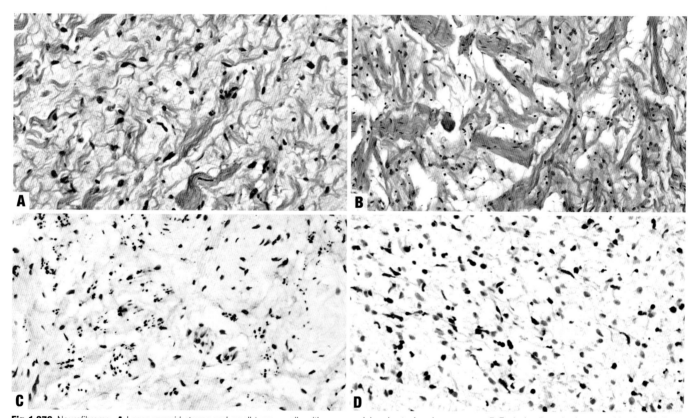

Fig. 1.276 Neurofibroma. **A** Loose myxoid stroma and small tumour cells with wavy nuclei and cytoplasmic processes. **B** Foci of collagenization resemble shredded carrots. **C** NFP immunostaining highlights entrapped axons. **D** A SOX10 immunostain highlights numerous neoplastic Schwann cells, whereas the non-neoplastic components in the tumour (e.g. fibroblasts, perineurial cells, mast cells) are negative.

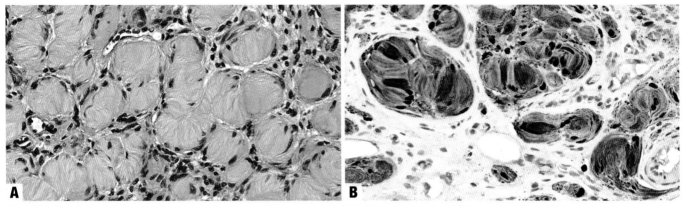

Fig. 1.277 Neurofibroma. **A** Pseudomeissnerian bodies. **B** An S100 immunostain highlights the parallel stacks of Schwann cell cytoplasm within pseudomeissnerian bodies.

presents as a plaque-like cutaneous and subcutaneous mass, mainly in the head and neck region, or as massive soft tissue enlargement of a body region such as the shoulder or pelvic girdle. The presence of multiple neurofibromas or a plexiform neurofibroma should raise suspicion of underlying NF1. Associated findings of NF1 include pigmented cutaneous macules (café-au-lait spots in fair-skinned individuals but brown spots in those of African descent), axillary or inguinal freckling, Lisch nodules, optic pathway gliomas, and bone dysplasia.

Epidemiology

Neurofibromas are the most common peripheral nerve sheath tumours, with the majority occurring sporadically as solitary lesions. Less often, they occur as multiple or numerous tumours in individuals with NF1. The diffuse cutaneous and plexiform tumours are presumably of congenital origin and, in NF1, the localized cutaneous and localized intraneural neurofibromas begin to appear in the second half of the first decade of life. All demographic groups are affected and there is no sex predilection.

Etiology

Unknown

Pathogenesis

Conventional neurofibromas (including subtypes)

Only a subpopulation of Schwann cells is considered neoplastic within neurofibromas {2494}, and biallelic genetic inactivation of the tumour suppressor gene *NF1* in this Schwann cell population is generally the only recurrent somatic event detectable {904,2482}. Therefore, complete loss of function of the *NF1* gene product, neurofibromin (NF1), is considered prerequisite for tumour development. Neurofibromin (NF1) is a negative regulator of RAS oncogenes acting as RAS-GAP {2862}. The best-characterized effector pathways in the context of NF1 tumorigenesis are the RAS/RAF/MEK/ERK and PI3K/AKT/mTOR pathways, both of which play important roles in cell growth, survival, (de)differentiation, and migration {1892}. However, inactivation of *NF1* alone is insufficient for neurofibroma development in several mouse models unless a specific microenvironment is also present. There is increasing evidence that inflammatory signals mediated by various components of the microenvironment, such as mast cells, macrophages, lymphocytes, and dendritic cells, as well as Schwann cell interactions with axons, are important for tumour development {2532,1029,1850,1849}. *NF1* haploinsufficiency of the microenvironment and nerve injury may promote tumorigenesis {1849,2619}. Dermal and plexiform neurofibromas exhibit distinct DNA methylation profiles, suggesting different cells of origin {2647}. Consistent with

Fig. 1.278 Diffuse cutaneous neurofibroma. This example is characterized by a plaque-like pattern of growth expanding the dermis and the superficial subcutis. Note the lack of a discrete mass.

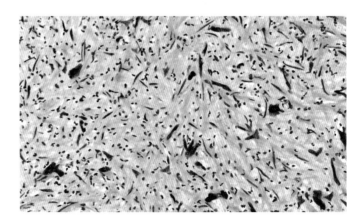

Fig. 1.279 Neurofibroma with atypia (ancient neurofibroma). Other than the scattered cytologically atypical cells, no worrisome features are present in this neurofibroma to warrant consideration of atypical neurofibromatous neoplasm of uncertain biological potential or malignant peripheral nerve sheath tumour.

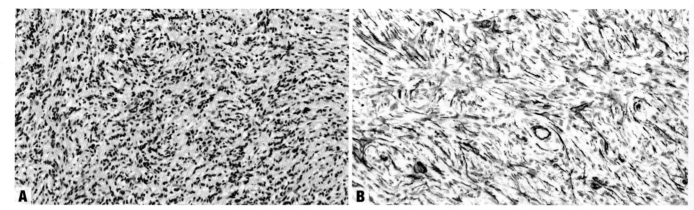

Fig. 1.280 Cellular neurofibroma. **A** Other than hypercellularity, this neurofibroma shows no worrisome features to warrant consideration of atypical neurofibromatous neoplasm of uncertain biological potential or malignant peripheral nerve sheath tumour. **B** A CD34 stain reveals the normal lattice-like architecture encountered in neurofibromas.

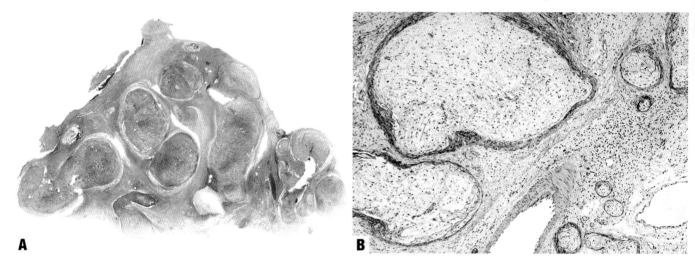

Fig. 1.281 Plexiform neurofibroma. **A** Multiple nerve fascicles are involved by this tumour, imparting a multinodular or bag-of-worms appearance at low magnification. **B** EMA immunostaining highlights the perineurium surrounding multiple individual nerve fascicles involved by the tumour.

this assumption, dermal skin–derived precursors and Schwann cell precursors in embryonic nerve roots were identified as cells of origin for dermal and plexiform neurofibromas, respectively, in transgenic mouse models {565,1791}.

Atypical neurofibroma / atypical neurofibromatous neoplasm of uncertain biological potential

Histological features of atypical neurofibroma (AN) / atypical neurofibromatous neoplasm of uncertain biological potential (ANNUBP) described mainly in the setting of NF1 are strongly associated with deletions of the *CDKN2A/CDKN2B* locus encoding cell-cycle regulators p16 (p16INK4a) and p14ARF (both encoded by *CDKN2A*) and p15 (p15INK4b; encoded by *CDKN2B*) {248,2647,2142,489,2481}. One study reported the association of heterozygous *CDKN2A/CDKN2B* deletion with cytological atypia alone, and of homozygous *CDKN2A/CDKN2B* deletion with AN/ANNUBP histology in different parts of the same tumour {489}. Another study reported additional heterozygous loss of *SMARCA2* in a portion of AN/ANNUBP, either as part of a larger deletion together with *CDKN2A/CDKN2B* or in the form of a separate, smaller deletion event {2481}.

Macroscopic appearance

Five macroscopic forms are distinguished: localized cutaneous, diffuse cutaneous, localized intraneural, plexiform intraneural, and massive diffuse soft tissue tumour. Localized cutaneous neurofibromas are nodular or polypoid lesions, as large as 2 cm in size. Diffuse cutaneous neurofibromas can have a variety of gross appearances, including flat, sessile, globular, and pedunculated {2388}. Intraneural neurofibromas present as solitary fusiform masses or as ropy to worm-like growths when plexiform. Massive soft tissue neurofibromas range in shape from a relatively uniform regional soft tissue enlargement to pendulous bag-like or cape-like masses. The skin overlying massive tumours commonly shows hyperpigmentation. Cut surfaces of neurofibromas are most often uniformly tan or greyish-tan, glistening, mucoid, semitranslucent, and firm. On neuroimaging, ANNUBP or malignant peripheral nerve sheath tumour (MPNST) arising from a plexiform neurofibroma is suspected when there is a distinct growing nodule and/or increased PET activity {1365}.

Histopathology

Neurofibromas are relatively common benign nerve sheath tumours that are characterized by bland spindle cells with thin, wavy nuclei representing the neoplastic Schwann cell, immersed in a variably loose myxoid stroma. The tumour cells are typically smaller than those of schwannoma. Stromal collagen is characteristic, often likened in classic pathology descriptions to shredded carrots. A variety of other cell components are also identifiable in neurofibroma, including perineurial and perineurial-like cells, fibroblasts, and mast cells. Even when localized at the gross level, they lack a capsule and tend to infiltrate underlying soft tissues and parent nerves, in contrast to the more circumscribed schwannoma. Nerve fibres are easily identifiable in intraneural subtypes, which are characterized by expansion of single (localized) or multiple (plexiform) nerve fascicles, but they may be rare in cutaneous and soft tissue locations. Entrapped ganglion cells may be conspicuous in neurofibromas that infiltrate dorsal root ganglia, and these should not be mistaken for ganglioneuroma. The individual fascicles are recognized by the limiting perineurium that is composed of EMA-positive cells.

Neurofibroma with atypia (ancient neurofibroma) is characterized by scattered atypical or bizarre nuclei and smudgy chromatin in the absence of other worrisome features. This is not considered a premalignant lesion, and it therefore should not be confused with AN/ANNUBP as described below.

Cellular neurofibroma is defined by hypercellularity in the absence of other worrisome features. Increased cell crowding in the absence of mitotic activity or atypia may also be found

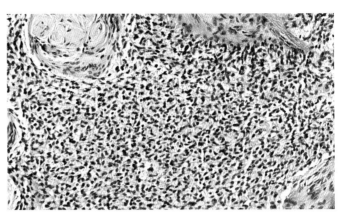

Fig. 1.283 Massive soft tissue neurofibroma. A typical finding is a cellular component composed of cells with high N:C ratios but rare to absent mitotic activity. Pseudomeissnerian corpuscles are also common (present in upper-left corner).

in individual tumours. These cellular neurofibromas may even show a fascicular growth pattern, but they lack the uniform cytological atypia, chromatin morphology, and mitotic activity seen in MPNST.

Plexiform neurofibroma is a multinodular subtype with involvement of multiple nerve fascicles, each surrounded by perineurium. It most often involves a large nerve or plexus, imparting a bag-of-worms or ropy gross appearance. It is highly associated

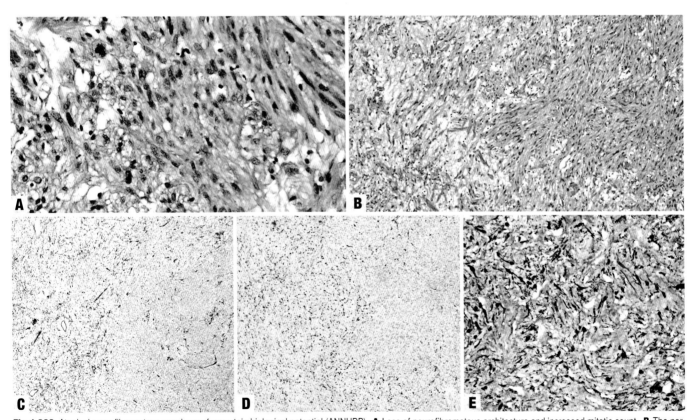

Fig. 1.282 Atypical neurofibromatous neoplasm of uncertain biological potential (ANNUBP). **A** Loss of neurofibromatous architecture and increased mitotic count. **B** The normally loose and myxoid neurofibroma architecture is seen on the left, but it is replaced by a more compact fascicular pattern in the focus of ANNUBP on the right. Compare with the CD34 and p16 immunohistochemistry figures on the same case (Panels C and D, respectively). **C** A CD34 immunostain reveals the normal lattice-like pattern of positivity in the conventional neurofibroma component (left), with loss of this architectural pattern in the focus of ANNUBP (right). **D** Loss of p16 expression is seen in the focus of ANNUBP on the right. At higher magnification within the neoplasm, there is retained expression in vascular cells but no expression in tumour cells. **E** In contrast to frankly malignant transformation (i.e. malignant peripheral nerve sheath tumour), foci of ANNUBP typically retain their extensive S100 positivity.

with NF1 and an increased risk of transformation to MPNST {2594}.

Pseudomeissnerian bodies or corpuscles are a typical feature of diffuse and plexiform neurofibromas. They represent delicate round layered structures and are strongly labelled by S100 immunohistochemistry. In the rare massive soft tissue subtype limited to individuals with neurofibromatosis, extensive infiltration of soft tissue and even skeletal muscle may be present. Pseudomeissnerian corpuscles are frequent in this subtype, as are cellular areas containing cells with high N:C ratios. Although they may be alarming at first glance, proliferative activity is very low. Other histological features that may be identifiable in individual neurofibromas include Schwann cell nodules, onion bulbs (S100-positive in contrast to EMA expression in perineurioma), melanin pigment, metaplastic bone, epithelioid change, and overt glandular differentiation.

The neoplastic cell in neurofibroma is the Schwann cell, and therefore markers of Schwann cell differentiation are positive, including S100, SOX10, and collagen IV, albeit with a variable fraction of Schwann cells that is often less extensive than in schwannomas. Non-neoplastic cell components are also present in neurofibroma, including a limited number of EMA-positive and GLUT1-positive perineurial cells, as well as CD34-positive stromal cells; the latter often form a lattice-like network that is typical of neurofibroma but usually absent in schwannoma, ANNUBP, and MPNST. Similarly, p16 is typically expressed in a subset of tumour cells of neurofibroma, whereas expression is lost in foci of ANNUBP and MPNST. NFP highlights entrapped axons. Staining for p53 is usually negative, and the Ki-67 proliferation index is low.

ANNUBP or AN is characterized by at least two of the following worrisome features: cytological atypia, hypercellularity, loss of neurofibroma architecture (on H&E and/or CD34 immunostaining), and a mitotic count as described in Table 1.04 (p. 256). This is considered a premalignant or early malignant stage that falls short of the diagnostic criteria for MPNST but is associated with increased risk of progression to MPNST {1365}. The concept of ANNUBP, discussed in detail in the MPNST section, has been mainly developed and used in NF1 patients and not applied in sporadic lesions.

Cytology

Intraoperative smears and FNA specimens are often paucicellular due to the increased collagen matrix in neurofibromas. Nevertheless, the presence of a mucin-rich background and small spindled cells with thin wavy nuclei can provide diagnostic clues.

Diagnostic molecular pathology

Molecular analyses do not have an established role in the diagnosis of neurofibroma. However, chromosomal copy-number profiling may be helpful for the evaluation of AN/ANNUBP (*CDKN2A/CDKN2B* deletion) and its differentiation from MPNST (complex highly rearranged genome). Of note, conventional dermal and plexiform neurofibromas, AN/ANNUBP, and MPNST all exhibit distinct DNA methylation profiles {2647}.

Essential and desirable diagnostic criteria

Essential: infiltrative, low-cellularity spindle cell neoplasm associated with a variably myxoid to collagenous stroma.

Desirable: immunoprofile includes S100 positivity in the Schwannian cell population, whereas CD34 highlights the stromal component; the presence of nuclear atypia raises the possibility of an AN/ANNUBP in the setting of NF1, which typically shows loss of p16 expression.

Staging

Staging is not applicable, although one study showed that AN/ANNUBP is associated with low recurrence rates even when surgical margins are positive, suggesting that an overly aggressive surgical approach may not be necessary {281}.

Prognosis and prediction

Localized cutaneous neurofibromas are consistently benign. Plexiform neurofibroma, ANNUBP, and solitary intraneural neurofibroma arising in sizeable nerves are precursor lesions of MPNST. The lifetime risk for MPNST in NF1 patients is estimated at 9–13% {938}. Diffuse cutaneous neurofibromas rarely undergo malignant transformation {2752}. Massive soft tissue neurofibromas, invariably benign, may nevertheless overlie an intraneural or plexiform neurofibroma-derived MPNST.

Perineurioma

Hornick JL
Carter JM
Creytens D

Definition
Perineuriomas of soft tissue are nearly always benign peripheral nerve sheath tumours composed entirely of perineurial cells. Intraneural and mucosal perineuriomas also exist.

ICD-O coding
9571/0 Perineurioma NOS

ICD-11 coding
2F38 & XH0XF7 Benign neoplasm of other or unspecified sites
   & Perineurioma NOS
2C41 Malignant perineurioma

Related terminology
Acceptable: benign fibroblastic polyp.

Subtype(s)
Perineurioma, malignant; reticular perineurioma; sclerosing perineurioma

Localization
Soft tissue perineuriomas most commonly arise on the lower limbs, followed by the upper limbs and trunk {1414}. The head and neck region, visceral organs, and central body cavity sites are rarely affected. Sclerosing perineuriomas are commonly found on the fingers and palms {999} and rarely at other sites {933}.

Clinical features
Perineuriomas of soft tissue usually present as painless masses. Subcutaneous tissue is involved more often than deep soft tissue. About 10% of cases are limited to the dermis {1414,2642}.

Epidemiology
Perineuriomas of soft tissue are rare. About 300 cases have been reported {3107,2082,1147,2578,1414}. These tumours are slightly more common in females than males and occur over a wide age range, with a peak in middle-aged adults {1414}. Children are rarely affected. Sclerosing perineuriomas are more common in males and usually affect young adults {999,3335}.

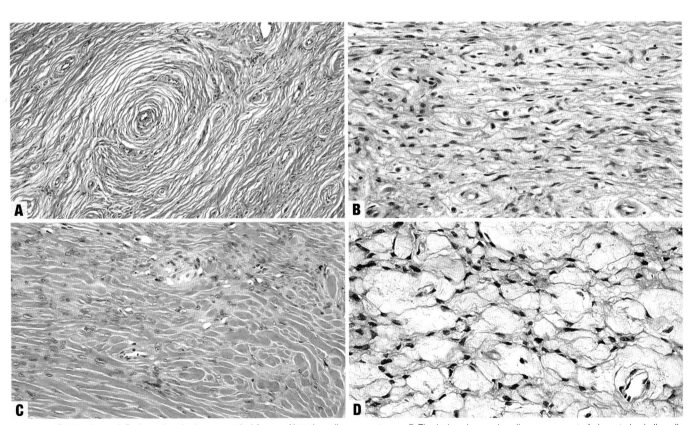

Fig. 1.284 Perineurioma. **A** Perivascular whorls are a typical feature. Note the collagenous stroma. **B** The lesion shows a lamellar arrangement of elongated spindle cells with tapering nuclei in a somewhat myxoid stroma. **C** Sclerosing perineurioma composed of cords of epithelioid cells in a dense collagenous stroma. **D** Reticular perineurioma composed of anastomosing elongated spindle cells with a lacy architecture.

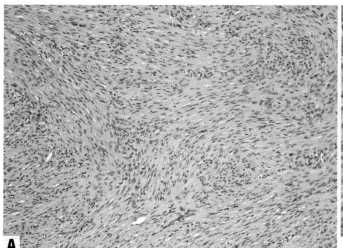
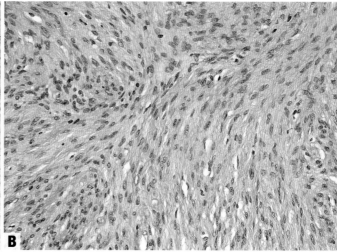

Fig. 1.285 Perineurioma of soft tissue. **A** The tumour shows a storiform growth pattern. **B** The tumour cells contain uniform ovoid to elongated nuclei. Note the fibrillary stroma.

Etiology

Soft tissue perineuriomas are nearly always sporadic. Very rare cases have been reported in patients with neurofibromatosis type 1 or neurofibromatosis type 2 {2520,184,2756}.

Pathogenesis

Soft tissue perineuriomas share pathogenetic mechanisms with other nerve sheath tumours. Deletion of 22q12 and mutations in *NF2* (encoding the tumour suppressor merlin [NF2]) are the most frequently reported genetic alterations {1147,499,1764}, similar to in schwannomas and meningiomas. Deletion of 17q11 (including *NF1*) is also a recurrent event in soft tissue perineurioma. Other reported chromosomal alterations include a three-way chromosome 2, 9, and 4 translocation involving *ABL1*; various chromosomal losses; and a rearrangement involving 10q24 in a soft tissue perineurioma of the foot. Alterations in 10q24 are recurrent events in sclerosing perineuriomas {429}. Malignant perineurial tumours have been less well characterized: loss of chromosome 13q and small deletions of chromosomes 3, 6, and 9 have been reported in 2 cases of low-grade malignant perineurial tumour {2746,499}.

Macroscopic appearance

Soft tissue perineuriomas are well circumscribed but unencapsulated. The cut surface is usually firm or rubbery and yellow, tan, or white. A small subset of tumours show a gelatinous appearance. Size ranges from < 1 to 20 cm, although most tumours are between 1.5 and 8 cm. The mean size of superficial tumours is 3 cm, compared with 7 cm for deep-seated tumours {1414}.

Histopathology

Soft tissue perineuriomas typically show a predominantly storiform or whorled growth pattern. Other distinctive architectural features include long fascicles with tumour cells arranged in a lamellar fashion and perivascular growth. The tumour cells are usually slender spindle cells with wavy or tapering nuclei, indistinct nucleoli, and characteristic delicate bipolar cytoplasmic processes. Some perineuriomas contain shorter, ovoid tumour cells. The stroma is usually collagenous; about 20% of cases contain at least focally myxoid matrix, which is occasionally abundant {1414}. Mitotic activity is typically scarce or absent. Occasional soft tissue perineuriomas show degenerative

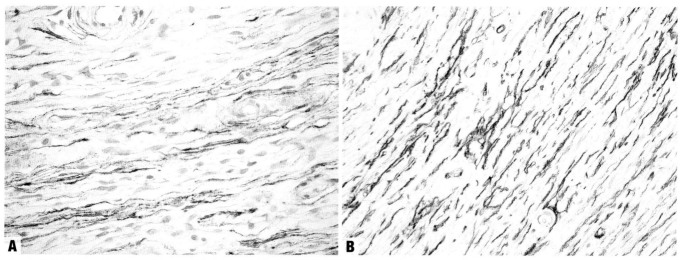

Fig. 1.286 Soft tissue perineurioma. **A** Immunohistochemical staining for EMA highlights the delicate bipolar cytoplasmic processes of the tumour cells. **B** Expression of CD34 is often more diffuse than that of EMA.

nuclear atypia, including pleomorphic and multinucleated cells, some with nuclear pseudoinclusions {1414}. Plexiform architecture has rarely been reported {3390,2086}. Sclerosing perineuriomas are composed of cords of small epithelioid to spindle cells in a dense collagenous stroma {999}. Reticular perineuriomas are composed of interconnected, elongated spindle cells with a lacy or reticular architecture {1202}. Rare perineuriomas contain cells with intracytoplasmic vacuoles, mimicking lipoblasts {3092}. The very rare malignant perineuriomas (perineurial malignant peripheral nerve sheath tumours) show cytoarchitectural features similar to benign soft tissue perineuriomas, in addition to hypercellularity, nuclear atypia and hyperchromasia, and a high mitotic count {1373}.

By immunohistochemistry, perineuriomas consistently express EMA, which ranges from weak and focal to strong and diffuse {1414}. Claudin-1 and GLUT1 are also often positive {1045,3335}. CD34 is expressed in about 60% of soft tissue perineuriomas {1414}. Staining for S100, SOX10, and GFAP is negative. In addition to EMA, sclerosing perineuriomas may show limited staining for keratin {999}.

Cytology
There is little experience with cytological diagnosis of these lesions, but FNA specimens are said to be paucicellular, with smears containing fragments of myxoid stroma {1809}.

Diagnostic molecular pathology
Not clinically relevant

Essential and desirable diagnostic criteria
Essential: storiform, whorled, and lamellar architecture; elongated, slender spindle cells with bipolar cytoplasmic processes; expression of EMA; variable claudin-1, GLUT1, and CD34.

Staging
Not clinically relevant

Prognosis and prediction
Conventional perineuriomas of soft tissue (and sclerosing and reticular subtypes), including those with degenerative nuclear atypia, are benign and only rarely recur locally {999,1202,1414}. Malignant perineuriomas may sometimes metastasize, but they appear to behave in a less aggressive fashion than conventional malignant peripheral nerve sheath tumours {1373}.

Granular cell tumour

Rubin BP
Lazar AJ
Reis-Filho JS

Definition

Granular cell tumour is a tumour showing neuroectodermal differentiation and composed of epithelioid to polygonal cells with copious eosinophilic, distinctively granular cytoplasm.

ICD-O coding

9580/0 Granular cell tumour NOS

ICD-11 coding

2E89.1 & XH09A9 Benign tumours of uncertain differentiation, soft tissue & Granular cell tumour NOS

2B5F.2 & XH90D3 Sarcoma, not elsewhere classified of other specified sites & Granular cell tumour, malignant

Related terminology

Not recommended: granular cell schwannoma; granular cell nerve sheath tumour; granular cell myoblastoma; Abrikossoff tumour.

Subtype(s)

Granular cell tumour, malignant

Localization

Most cases affect deep dermis and subcutaneous tissue, particularly of the head and neck, trunk, and proximal extremities {19,2502}. The single most common site is the tongue, representing 25% of cases, followed by breast (5–15%) {783,19}. Visceral involvement of the gastrointestinal tract (oesophagus, large bowel, perianal area) and respiratory tract (larynx) is also common {2870,3154}. Although most granular cell tumours are solitary, as many as 10% are multifocal, and these can be regional or involve multiple organ sites {318,1727}. Most bona fide malignant granular cell tumours occur in the deep soft tissue, with a predilection for the trunk and extremities, the thigh being the single most common site. Head and neck and oral locations are less common for malignant tumours {966}.

Clinical features

Although usually asymptomatic, granular cell tumour can be pruritic to painful in the skin and tongue. Cutaneous lesions are firm, flesh-coloured to reddish-brown, and 0.5–3.0 cm in size. Tumour growth is usually indolent.

Epidemiology

Granular cell tumours usually occur in adults in the fourth to sixth decades of life, but they can be encountered at any age. They are more prevalent in males than females (M:F ratio: 2–3:1), as well as in African-Americans {318,1727}, in whom multiple lesions are also more common. Malignant granular cell tumour is very rare and occurs with a female predominance and an age range of 3–70 years (mean: 40 years) {966}.

Etiology

Multiple granular cell tumours have been reported in association with various syndromes, such as neurofibromatosis type 1, Noonan syndrome, and LEOPARD syndrome (multiple lentigines, electrocardiographic conduction abnormalities, ocular hypertelorism, pulmonic stenosis, abnormal genitalia, retardation of growth, and sensorineural deafness), mostly characterized by aberrant signalling within the RAS/MAPK pathway through inactivating mutations {1890,2780,2572,2856}.

Pathogenesis

Loss-of-function mutations affecting the V-ATPase accessory genes, *ATP6AP1* (61%) and *ATP6AP2* (11%), are found in 72% of granular cell tumours collectively {2436,2810}. These genes

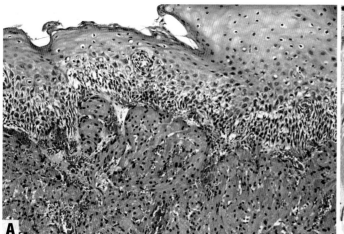
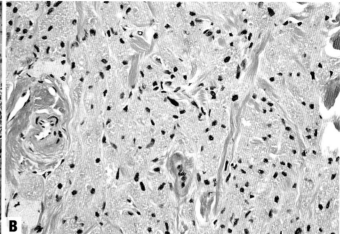

Fig. 1.287 Granular cell tumour. **A** The squamous epithelium overlying the tumour shows basal cell hyperplasia. **B** The tumour is composed of polygonal cells with hyperchromatic nuclei and abundant granular eosinophilic cytoplasm. Note the occasional cells with degenerative nuclear atypia.

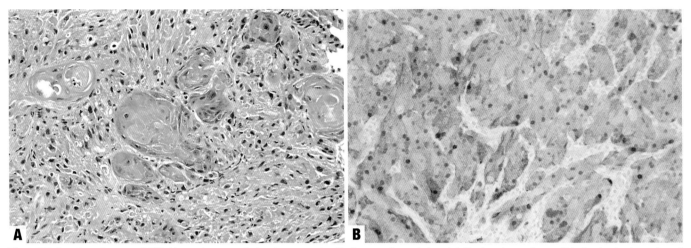

Fig. 1.288 Granular cell tumour. **A** This biopsy of a tongue lesion shows pseudoepitheliomatous hyperplasia, mimicking invasive carcinoma. Note the sheets of granular cell tumour cells with extensive granular cytoplasm surrounding the nests of hyperplastic squamous epithelium. **B** As seen here, S100 immunohistochemistry is diffusely and strongly positive in granular cell tumour.

play pivotal roles in endosomal pH regulation {2436}; loss-of-function mutations affecting these genes are found irrespective of anatomical site or whether the lesions are benign or malignant, and they have not been detected in other neoplasms. Therefore, loss-of-function *ATP6AP1* or *ATP6AP2* mutations appear to be pathognomonic for the diagnosis of granular cell tumour. Granular cell tumours lacking mutations in these genes have been reported to harbour mutations affecting other V-ATPase-related genes {2810}. Inactivation of either *ATP6AP1* or *ATP6AP2* in Schwann cells leads to the accumulation of intracytoplasmic granules that are characteristic of granular cell tumour. Analysis of the granules revealed that they display ultrastructural and immunophenotypic features of early and recycling endosomes {2436}. The mechanism by which loss-of-function mutations in endosomal regulatory proteins drive oncogenesis is currently unknown.

Macroscopic appearance

Granular cell tumours are uninodular, firm masses involving the skin/subcutis or submucosa, often with an overlying epithelial hyperplasia. On sectioning, the tumour has a yellowish, finely granular texture. Malignant granular cell tumours range in size from 1 to 18.2 cm, usually being > 5 cm {966,1456}. Grossly, tumours are pale grey and firm, often deeper (subcutaneous/intramuscular) than their benign counterparts.

Histopathology

Granular cell tumour has ill-defined borders and is composed of sheets, nests, and trabeculae of large, monotonous epithelioid to polygonal cells with intensely eosinophilic, granular cytoplasm. Cell borders may be indistinct, producing a syncytial appearance. Nuclei are usually centrally situated and range from uniformly small and mildly hyperchromatic to larger and vesicular with distinct nucleoli. Mitoses are variable in number but usually not prominent.

The finely granular appearance of the cytoplasm is due to massive accumulation of lysosomes including larger intracytoplasmic granules highlighted by clear haloes {922}. Perineural infiltration is common. For cutaneous granular cell tumour and granular cell tumour arising in sites such as the tongue and

oesophagus with overlying squamous epithelium, pseudoepitheliomatous hyperplasia is sometimes seen and when extensive can raise the consideration of squamous cell carcinoma.

Malignant granular cell tumours are rare and their features vary from overtly sarcomatous to morphologically bland on rare occasions. Histological features associated with malignancy include increased cellularity, prominent spindling, high N:C ratio, vesicular nuclei with prominent nucleoli, marked pleomorphism, increased mitotic activity (> 2 mitoses per 2 mm²), and geographical necrosis {966,1456,3229}. Although most malignant granular cell tumours show necrosis and/or high mitotic activity, these parameters alone may not identify all tumours that metastasize {689}.

Granular cell tumours are generally reactive for S100, SOX10, nestin, inhibin, and calretinin {2437,531}. Tumours are also positive for CD68, CD63 (NKI/C3), and NSE, probably nonspecific due to the cytoplasmic lysosomal content {1004}. MITF and TFE3 (in the absence of gene rearrangements) show diffuse nuclear reactivity in most cases, but HMB45 is uniformly negative and only very rarely is there focal reactivity for melan-A {1169,531}.

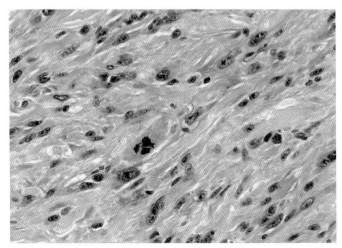

Fig. 1.289 Malignant granular cell tumour. This malignant granular cell tumour shows cytological pleomorphism and extensive mitotic activity, including atypical mitotic figures.

Cytology

In FNA samples, the characteristic granular cytoplasm and bland nuclei are useful features {1151,890}, but carcinomas (particularly apocrine) and histiocytic processes must be considered.

Diagnostic molecular pathology

Not clinically relevant

Essential and desirable diagnostic criteria

Essential: nests and sheets of epithelioid to polygonal cells; abundant, intensely eosinophilic, granular cytoplasm; positive for S100 and SOX10 by immunohistochemistry.

Staging

Malignant granular cell tumour of somatic soft tissue can be staged according to the American Joint Committee on Cancer (AJCC) eighth-edition TNM staging system for soft tissue sarcoma of the trunk and extremities, although given the rarity of this entity, there is not current evidence demonstrating prognostic power for this approach.

Prognosis and prediction

Although granular cell tumour is benign in the vast majority of cases, local recurrence can sometimes be seen after incomplete excision. Malignant granular cell tumour has a 50% rate of metastasis {966}. Local recurrence, metastasis, larger tumour size, and older patient age are adverse prognostic factors for malignant granular cell tumour {966}.

Dermal nerve sheath myxoma

Dry SM

Definition
Dermal nerve sheath myxoma is a benign peripheral nerve sheath tumour composed of small epithelioid, ring-like, and spindled Schwann cells embedded within an abundant myxoid matrix. It typically arises in the skin or subcutis and often has a multinodular growth pattern.

ICD-O coding
9562/0 Nerve sheath myxoma

ICD-11 coding
2F24 & XH3L35 Benign cutaneous neoplasms of neural or nerve sheath origin & Neurothekeoma
2F24 & XH6Q84 Benign cutaneous neoplasms of neural or nerve sheath origin & Myxoma NOS

Related terminology
Previous terminology included "classic or myxoid variant of neurothekeoma" {1107}. However, pathological data {1756,993, 995,1407} and molecular data {2837} have demonstrated the Schwann cell derivation of dermal nerve sheath myxoma, which is clinically and biologically distinct from neurothekeoma.

Subtype(s)
None

Localization
Tumours predominantly occur in the distal extremities, particularly involving the fingers/toes and lower extremities {995,1756}. The fingers are the most common site, accounting for approximately 36% of cases. Rare locations include the spinal canal {3343}.

Clinical features
Dermal nerve sheath myxomas typically present as small, superficial, slow-growing masses. The lesions are often asymptomatic, but some tumours may be painful {995}.

Epidemiology
Dermal nerve sheath myxomas are rare. The two largest modern series, using immunohistochemistry to confirm the diagnosis,

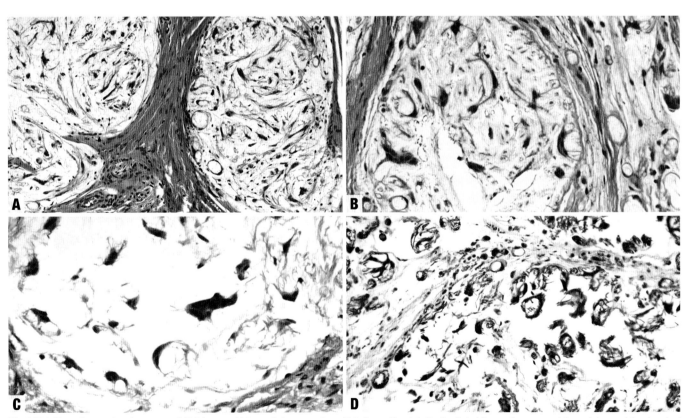

Fig. 1.290 Dermal nerve sheath myxoma. **A,B,C** Low- and intermediate-power views. Note the multinodularity, the rind of fibrous tissue around the nodules, and the abundant myxoid matrix. The neoplastic Schwann cells are arranged in cords and syncytial-like aggregates. Some have a ring-like appearance and resemble fat cells. **D** The neoplastic Schwann cells express S100.

describe 68 tumours arising in patients with a wide age range (8–72 years), with a peak in young adults in their mid-30s and a slight male predominance {995,1756}.

Etiology
Unknown

Pathogenesis
No genetic abnormality has been described to date; however, a microarray-based expression profile analysis has shown that nerve sheath myxomas have a similar gene signature to dermal schwannomas. In contrast, cellular neurothekeomas have a genetic signature that more closely resembles that of cellular fibrous histiocytomas {2837}.

Macroscopic appearance
The tumours generally range from 0.4 to 4.5 cm in greatest dimension, with most lesions being < 2.5 cm in size. Because the lesions are located in the dermis or subcutis, the resection specimens often include overlying epidermis. The tumours have a rubbery to firm consistency, and on cut section they show well-demarcated, glistening, white to translucent mucoid nodules within skin and subcutis {995}.

Histopathology
Tumours typically involve the dermis, subcutis, or both, although rare tumours may extend to underlying skeletal muscle. They often have a multinodular growth pattern and an abundant myxoid matrix, usually bordered by dense fibrous connective tissue. The lesional cells are composed of small epithelioid, ring-like, stellate, and spindled neoplastic Schwann cells. The epithelioid Schwann cells are arranged in cords, nests, and syncytial-like aggregates. Some of the Schwann cells with ring-like morphology may superficially resemble lipoblasts. Infrequent Schwann cells may be multivacuolated and have spider-like cytoplasmic processes. Rare examples may show focal nuclear palisading or Verocay body–like structures. There is generally only mild nuclear atypia, although scattered moderate pleomorphism, akin to that seen in so-called ancient schwannomas, may be present. Mitoses are typically very few to absent. A small number of delicate intralesional fibroblast-like cells may be evident. Scattered small-calibre vessels are present {995}.

The neoplastic Schwann cells are diffusely immunoreactive for S100, and most cases show moderate to diffuse reactivity for GFAP and CD57 {118,345,995,1756}. Strong immunoreactivity for collagen IV is typically present around the tumour cells. Rare cells have been reported positive for AE1/AE3 keratin cocktail, and scattered EMA-positive epineurial cells can be found in the fibrous capsule. Occasional delicate CD34-positive fibroblasts may be present. Infrequent cases may have rare detectable NFP-positive axons {995}.

Cytology
Not clinically relevant

Diagnostic molecular pathology
Currently, there are no molecular tests used in the diagnosis of dermal nerve sheath myxoma.

Essential and desirable diagnostic criteria
Essential: typical clinical presentation includes young adults with small superficial lesions in the distal extremities (commonly fingers/toes); myxoid neoplasm with multilobulated growth, composed of bland spindle and epithelioid Schwann cells; immunopositivity for S100.

Staging
Not clinically relevant

Prognosis and prediction
Dermal nerve sheath myxomas are benign tumours. Incomplete removal is associated with a high rate of local recurrence. In the largest modern study, 47% of patients treated by local excision experienced local recurrence. Although most had only one recurrence in the follow-up period, nearly one third of patients experienced more than one and as many as five local recurrences, and 25% of patients who had experienced local recurrences had active disease at last follow-up. Local recurrences were most common in tumours arising in the fingers {995}.

Solitary circumscribed neuroma

Scolyer RA
Ferguson PM

Definition
Solitary circumscribed neuroma (SCN) is a benign, often cutaneous nodular proliferation of nerve fibres with Schwann cells predominating over axons, showing a strong predilection for the face.

ICD-O coding
9570/0 Solitary circumscribed neuroma

ICD-11 coding
2F24 & XH90Y8 Benign cutaneous neoplasms of neural or nerve sheath origin & Solitary circumscribed neuroma

Related terminology
Acceptable: palisaded encapsulated neuroma; palisaded and encapsulated neuroma.

Subtype(s)
Plexiform solitary circumscribed neuroma {164}

Localization
The skin of the face hosts approximately 90% of SCNs, particularly the nose, forehead, and lips. Many lesions occur in proximity to mucocutaneous junctions or even affect oral mucosa; the latter represents the most common non-cutaneous site {1689}.

Clinical features
SCN usually presents as a slow-growing, firm, painless, circumscribed dermal-based nodule. SCN is mostly solitary, but rare examples of multiple SCNs have been reported with no evidence of any associated systemic disease {1876}.

Epidemiology
SCN is most common in the fifth to seventh decades of life, but it can occur in patients of any age. There is no sex predilection.

Etiology
Unknown

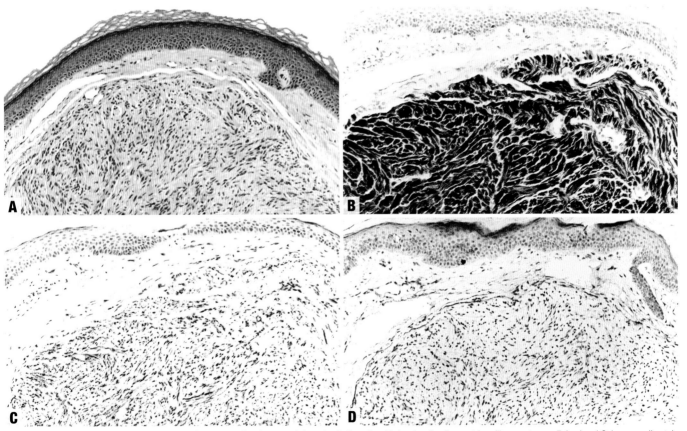

Fig. 1.291 Solitary circumscribed neuroma. **A** Higher magnification reveals banal spindle cells with focal palisading, set in a fibrous stroma. **B** Lesional Schwann cells stain diffusely positively with S100. **C** NFP is expressed by variable numbers of small intratumoural axons. **D** EMA staining highlights perineurial cells in the capsule.

Pathogenesis

SCN is a benign tumour of nerve fibres with slow growth over many years and is unrelated to trauma {1017}.

Macroscopic appearance

SCN usually presents as a flesh-coloured papule < 1 cm in diameter. It is a circumscribed dermal-based nodule with a firm, pale-grey cut surface.

Histopathology

SCN is a circumscribed dermal-based tumour composed of bland spindle-shaped cells with wavy nuclei in a background of hyalinized collagen. The cells often form well-developed fascicles, and some palisading of nuclei within the tumour is characteristically present. A thin perineurial-derived fibrous capsule may surround the lesion, but it is often incomplete at the superficial aspect. Artefactual clefting is a frequent finding, and extension into the subcutis may be present on occasion {2589}. No cytological atypia is present and mitoses are inconspicuous. Occasional cases showed degenerative nuclear changes or focal epithelioid cytology. The overlying epidermis is usually normal or attenuated. The spindle cells are strongly and diffusely positive for S100. NFP staining typically identifies the presence of small nerve fibres within the tumour {163}. Perineurial cells in the capsule stain for EMA, claudin-1, and GLUT1 {1689}. Occasionally, SCNs may have a multinodular or plexiform growth pattern {1542}.

Cytology

FNA of SCN shows a nonspecific paucicellular pattern of bland spindle cells.

Diagnostic molecular pathology

No diagnostic molecular findings have been described.

Essential and desirable diagnostic criteria

Essential: circumscribed cutaneous lesion of Schwann cell–rich fascicles of nerve fibres with or without partial encapsulation; focal palisading and artefactual clefting; S100 positivity with focal NFP staining; the peripheral capsule is highlighted by perineurial markers (EMA, GLUT1).

Staging

Not clinically relevant

Prognosis and prediction

SCN is a benign tumour with no capacity for metastasis.

Ectopic meningioma and meningothelial hamartoma

Perry A

Definition

Ectopic meningioma is a meningothelial neoplasm occurring entirely outside intracranial and intraspinal cavities. Meningothelial hamartoma represents a developmental rest, composed of non-neoplastic arachnoid cells. In both, a CNS connection must be excluded.

ICD-O coding

9530/0 Meningioma NOS

ICD-11 coding

2A01.0Z Meningeal tumours, unspecified

Related terminology

Acceptable: extradural, extracranial/extraspinal, extraneuraxial, heterotopic, cutaneous, calvarial, or intraosseous meningioma; meningothelial choristoma; rudimentary meningocoele; sequestrated meningocoele; meningothelial rest; meningothelial heterotopia.

Subtype(s)

None

Localization

More than 90% of ectopic meningiomas present in the head and neck region. Orbital examples have no dural connection. Other locations include the skull, sinonasal tract, oropharynx, lung, mediastinum, middle ear, scalp, parotid gland, and neck. Meningothelial hamartomas most commonly present as solitary scalp masses, usually in the occiput. Rests have also been described in the lung (meningothelial-like nodules) and lymph nodes, among other sites {2621,2378}.

Clinical features

The presenting signs and symptoms of ectopic meningiomas vary greatly, with the most common pattern being that of a painless, slow-growing mass. Meningothelial hamartoma is typically detected as an incidental scalp mass or dimple, sometimes with alopecia and/or tenderness.

Epidemiology

Ectopic meningiomas are rare. In one review, they accounted for 1.6% of all resected meningiomas and presented at all ages, with bimodal peaks in the second decade of life and in the fifth to seventh decades {1744}. There was a slight female predominance. Meningothelial hamartomas are typically found in neonates or infants, with no known sex or racial predisposition {694}.

Etiology

Four histogenetic hypotheses have been postulated for ectopic meningiomas: meningothelial cells carried along nerve sheaths

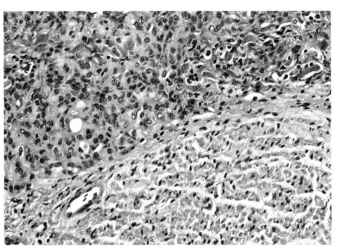

Fig. 1.292 Ectopic (meningothelial) meningioma. This epidural tumour surrounded and tracked along a paraspinal nerve root. Invasion of adjacent skeletal muscle was seen in other sections.

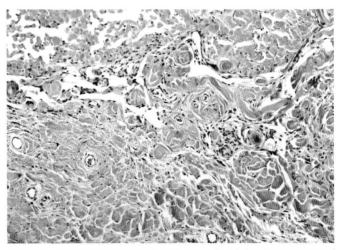

Fig. 1.293 Meningothelial hamartoma of the scalp. Occipital scalp mass resected from a neonate. The lesion involves the dermis and subcutaneous soft tissue. Note the slit-like spaces mimicking subarachnoid spaces, in association with occasional more easily recognizable meningothelial clusters and psammoma bodies.

exiting the skull or vertebral column, ectopic arachnoid cells, meningothelial cells displaced during trauma, and pluripotent mesenchymal cells capable of undergoing meningothelial differentiation or metaplasia. Meningothelial hamartomas in the scalp are considered pathogenetically related to meningocoeles and meningoencephalocoeles, but without an intracranial connection. In other locations, they are often incidental, possibly representing ectopic rests or metaplastic meningothelial-like cells (e.g. pulmonary nodules).

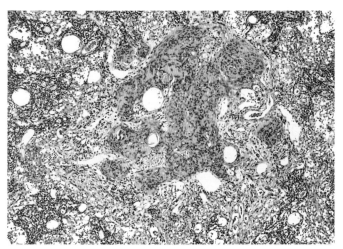

Fig. 2.194 Meningothelial rest. This ectopic rest was an incidental microscopic finding within a lymph node.

Pathogenesis
Molecular studies are lacking, but one intranodal rest in a Cowden syndrome patient indirectly implicated the *PTEN* gene {2378}.

Macroscopic appearance
Ectopic meningiomas are similar to their CNS counterparts, except for greater invasive qualities. Colour and consistency vary with cellularity, collagen deposition, and tumour grade, but a rubbery tan-white mass is most common. Calvarial meningiomas are typically hyperostotic {1465}. Hamartomas are solitary nodules; plaques; or spongy tan-grey, red, or flesh-coloured lesions in cutaneous and/or subcutaneous scalp.

Histopathology
The same range of histological appearances and grades encountered intracranially may be seen in ectopic meningiomas, with benign meningothelial tumours being most common. In the scalp, hamartomas usually show slit-like spaces resembling lymphatics. However, they are lined by meningothelial (rather than endothelial) cells. Well-formed meningothelial clusters and psammoma bodies can also be encountered. Highly sensitive and specific immunohistochemical markers are generally lacking, with coexpression of vimentin, EMA, and progesterone used most consistently {3066}. The newer marker, SSTR2A {2075}, can be expressed in pulmonary meningothelial-like nodules {2621}. Because meningiomas may express p63, this marker does not reliably distinguish epithelial neoplasms {1064}. Ultrastructurally, they contain overlapping cytoplasmic processes resembling interlocking pieces of a jigsaw puzzle, as well as desmosomes and other intercellular junctions.

Cytology
The cytological features of ectopic meningothelial lesions resemble those of their CNS counterparts.

Diagnostic molecular pathology
Not clinically relevant

Essential and desirable diagnostic criteria
Essential: meningothelial rest or neoplasm located entirely outside of and with no connection to the CNS.

Staging
Not clinically relevant

Prognosis and prediction
As with other meningiomas, tumour grade and extent of resection play important prognostic roles. Intraosseous skull base cases have higher recurrence rates than those of the convexity. Distant metastases have been reported in about 6% of cases, mostly in anaplastic (malignant) examples {1744}. Hamartomas are usually cured by surgery alone, with only rare recurrences.

Benign triton tumour / neuromuscular choristoma

Perry A

Definition
Benign triton tumour / neuromuscular choristoma (NMC) is an expansile intraneural mass characterized by the intimate interposition of mature skeletal muscle and nerve fibres within the endoneurium.

ICD-O coding
None

ICD-11 coding
None

Related terminology
Acceptable: benign triton tumour; neuromuscular hamartoma; nerve rhabdomyoma; rhabdomyoma/choristoma; ectomesenchymal hamartoma.

Subtype(s)
None

Localization
Classic cases involve large nerves or plexuses, most commonly the sciatic nerve and the brachial plexus, although cranial nerve and intraorbital examples have also been reported {643}.

Clinical features
Patients present most often with progressive pain or features of peripheral neuropathy/plexopathy. There may be atrophy of the involved limb, as well as superimposed desmoid fibromatosis (NMC-fibromatosis) in as many as 80% of cases, with the latter seen mostly after biopsy {493}. On MRI, NMC features T1- and

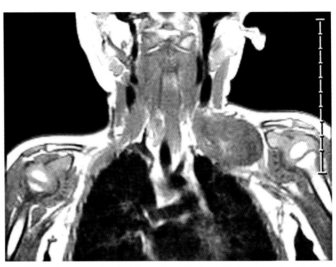

Fig. 1.296 Neuromuscular choristoma. Coronal T1-weighted MRI showing a fusiform mass of the left brachial plexus with signal density resembling that of adjacent skeletal muscle.

T2-weighted signals similar to those of adjacent skeletal muscle, with no interfascicular fat (unlike fibrolipomatous hamartoma) and minimal contrast enhancement. In contrast, when a fibromatosis component develops, it is contrast-enhancing with hypointense T1/T2 signals compared with muscle. Of interest, a review of MRI features in one study suggested that as many as 5% of sporadic limb-associated desmoids show evidence of an occult NMC precursor, suggesting that the NMC-fibromatosis combination may be currently underdiagnosed {2958}.

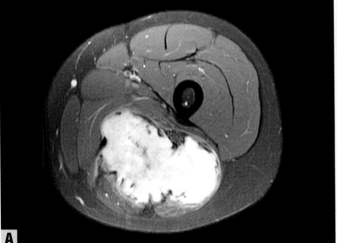 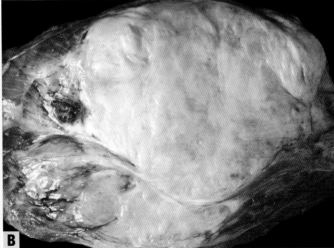

Fig. 1.295 Neuromuscular choristoma-fibromatosis. **A** Postcontrast MRI of the thigh showing an enhancing and invasive mass diagnosed as a desmoid-type fibromatosis on histopathology. This was seen in association with a neuromuscular choristoma of the sciatic nerve. **B** Gross pathology from the resection specimen of the patient shown in Panel A. On cut surface, the desmoid showed a firm, irregular, glistening greyish-white mass that invades into adjacent skeletal muscle.

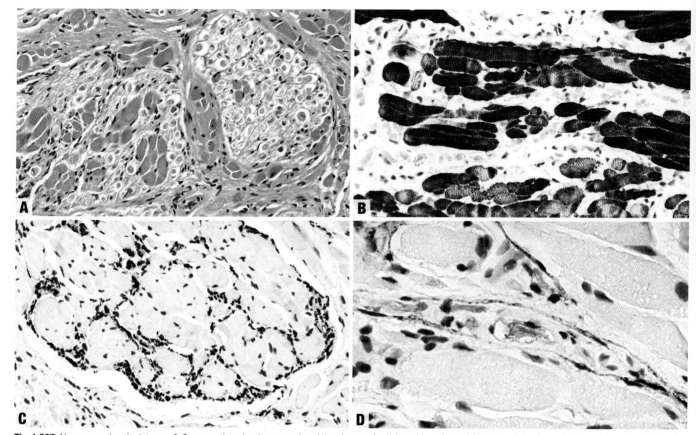

Fig. 1.297 Neuromuscular choristoma. **A** Cross-section showing several peripheral nerve fascicles with endoneurial mature skeletal muscle fibres intertwined with native neural elements. **B** Longitudinal section showing several peripheral nerve fascicles with endoneurial mature skeletal muscle fibres highlighted by desmin positivity, intertwined with native neural elements. **C** Cross-section highlighting axons with NFP immunostaining. **D** Tangential section with small involved peripheral nerve fascicles surrounded by perineurial cells, the latter highlighted with an EMA immunostain.

Epidemiology

NMC is an extremely rare disorder, with as many as 40–50 cases reported, depending on diagnostic stringency {493,643,2442}. It presents mostly in infancy or childhood, although adult onset has also been seen. The sexes are roughly equally represented.

Etiology

Published etiological hypotheses have included hamartomatous overgrowth of muscle spindles, a developmental lesion with intraneural entrapment of skeletal muscle during embryogenesis, myogenic metaplasia of nerve sheath elements, and a benign intraneural neoplasm (rhabdomyoma).

Pathogenesis

Although studies have been limited to date, most cases of NMC and NMC-fibromatosis show *CTNNB1* exon 3 (p.Thr41Ala and p.Ser45Phe) mutations, similar to those of sporadic desmoids; this possibly reflects somatic mosaicism in the patient {493}.

Macroscopic appearance

Fusiform nerve enlargement with multifascicular involvement is typical. On cut surface, a subset of nerve fascicles appear beefy red like skeletal muscle. Intraoperative stimulation of the involved nerve causes contraction of not only the innervated muscle but also the abnormal nerve. When present, foci of desmoid fibromatosis are grossly identical to their sporadic counterparts.

Histopathology

Haphazardly arranged bundles of mature skeletal muscle with cross-striations are intercalated between intraneural elements; smooth muscle elements have also been encountered rarely {3157}. Some cranial nerve examples have reported adipose tissue as well, although this probably represents a different entity. In terms of immunostains, the myogenic component expresses markers of mature skeletal muscle, including desmin. Residual nerve includes NFP-positive axons surrounded by S100-positive Schwann cells. The intraneural location of myocytes is elucidated by EMA, which highlights perineurium surrounding individual fascicles. Nuclear β-catenin may be seen in a subset of both the neural and myogenic cells within the NMC, as well as in adjacent fibromatosis components when present.

Cytology

The cytology has not been studied to date.

Diagnostic molecular pathology

The presence of *CTNNB1* exon 3 (p.Thr41Ala and p.Ser45Phe) mutations supports the diagnosis of NMC with or without associated desmoid fibromatosis {493}.

Essential and desirable diagnostic criteria

Essential: skeletal muscle intercalated between intraneural elements; immunohistochemical validation of both endoneurial myogenic and neural elements; intact perineurium surrounding individual fascicles; the presence of nuclear β-catenin expression in either NMC alone or NMC-fibromatosis.

Staging
Not clinically relevant

Prognosis and prediction
Because these lesions typically involve large functional nerves, accurate intraoperative diagnosis is critical to prevent an overly aggressive approach. Although benign triton tumour / NMC is considered benign, there is frequent development of desmoid fibromatosis (mostly postsurgical), identical to that seen in these lesions' sporadic counterparts {493}. It is hypothesized that trauma/surgery stimulates *CTNNB1*-mutated fibroblasts/myofibroblasts to form a desmoid-type fibromatosis, akin to that forming after abdominal surgery in Gardner syndrome patients. Unfortunately, NMC-fibromatosis often necessitates radical resection or limb amputation {1337}. For this reason, a no-touch approach has been advocated for patients with classic clinical and radiological features. Rare examples of NMC regression have also been reported. Additional follow-up is needed to establish the long-term prognosis.

Hybrid nerve sheath tumour

Stemmer-Rachamimov AO
Hornick JL

Definition
Hybrid nerve sheath tumours are benign peripheral nerve sheath tumours with combined features of more than one conventional type (neurofibroma, schwannoma, perineurioma).

ICD-O coding
9563/0 Hybrid nerve sheath tumour

ICD-11 coding
2F24 & XH01G0 Benign cutaneous neoplasms of neural or nerve sheath origin & Hybrid nerve sheath tumour

Related terminology
Acceptable: benign nerve sheath tumour NOS.

Subtype(s)
Perineurioma/schwannoma; schwannoma/neurofibroma; perineurioma/neurofibroma

Localization
Tumours show a wide anatomical distribution in somatic soft tissue, most commonly occurring in the dermis or subcutaneous tissue {1405,976}. Rare cases arise in cranial nerves. The most commonly reported site for hybrid schwannoma / reticular perineurioma is on the fingers {2112}.

Clinical features
The clinical presentation is similar to that of other benign peripheral nerve sheath tumours (neurofibromas and schwannomas); hybrid nerve sheath tumours present most often as painless masses in subcutaneous tissue or dermis. When large peripheral nerves or spinal nerves are involved, the tumours may be associated with pain or neurological deficit.

Epidemiology
Hybrid nerve sheath tumours are rare. The most common examples are tumours showing hybrid features of schwannoma and perineurioma, followed by hybrid neurofibroma/schwannoma. These tumours occur over a wide age range, with a peak in young adults and an equal sex distribution {1405}. Hybrid neurofibroma/perineurioma is rare.

Etiology
Hybrid schwannoma/perineurioma occurs sporadically {1405}, whereas hybrid neurofibroma/schwannoma is strongly associated with neurofibromatosis type 1, neurofibromatosis type 2, and schwannomatosis {1302}. A high prevalence of hybrid schwannoma/neurofibroma morphology was found in tumours from schwannomatosis patients (71%), often leading to misdiagnosis as neurofibroma {1302,1927}. Hybrid neurofibroma/perineurioma has been described in association with neurofibromatosis type 1 {1469,1558}.

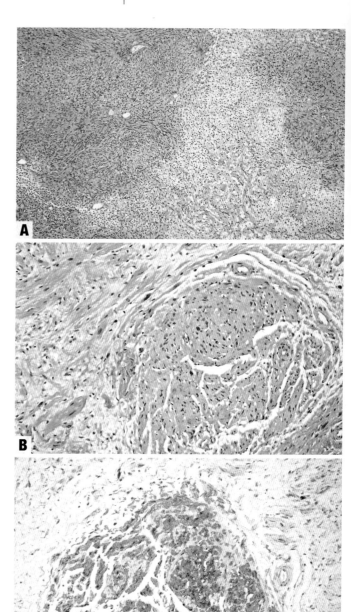

Fig. 1.298 Hybrid schwannoma/neurofibroma. **A** Hybrid schwannoma/neurofibroma with areas of solid Schwann cell proliferation and loose areas of neurofibroma appearance. **B** Solid nodule of Schwann cell proliferation surrounded by loose hypocellular tumour. **C** S100 stain showing diffuse staining in the solid Schwann cell nodule and mixed population of cells (S100-positive and S100-negative) in surrounding loose areas.

Pathogenesis
Unknown

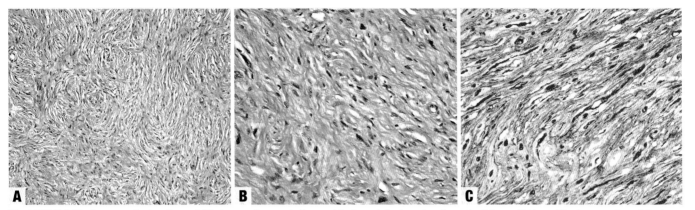

Fig. 1.299 Hybrid schwannoma/perineurioma. **A** The tumour shows a storiform architecture, similar to perineurioma of soft tissue. **B** Many of the tumour cells contain plump, tapering nuclei and eosinophilic cytoplasm, typical of Schwann cells. The perineurial cell component is often inconspicuous. **C** Double immunolabelling for S100 (red) and EMA (brown) highlights alternating Schwann cells and perineurial cells, respectively.

Macroscopic appearance
The gross appearance is similar to that of other benign peripheral nerve sheath tumours. Grossly, the tumours are well circumscribed, with a firm cut surface.

Histopathology
Hybrid schwannoma/perineurioma shows a storiform or fascicular growth and is usually composed of an intimate admixture of alternating Schwann cells with plump nuclei and eosinophilic cytoplasm and perineurial cells with slender nuclei and delicate elongated cytoplasmic processes. The Schwann cell component is often prominent. The tumours may show degenerative nuclear atypia (ancient change). Mitoses are rare. Rare cases show a biphasic appearance and a lobulated growth pattern, either with separate schwannomatous and perineurial nodules or with schwannomatous nodules surrounded by a perineurial component with a reticular growth pattern and myxoid stroma. The two components can be highlighted by immunohistochemistry: S100-positive Schwann cells and EMA-positive perineurial cells. Perineurial cells may also be immunoreactive for claudin-1 and GLUT1 {1405}.

Hybrid neurofibroma/schwannoma is composed of schwannomatous nodules within an otherwise typical neurofibroma or Schwann cell bundles dispersed in a myxoid background. The tumours may have a plexiform architecture. The Schwann cell nodular proliferations may exhibit Verocay body formation or fascicular growth, and the neurofibroma component may demonstrate myxoid change, collagen bundles, and mixed cellular composition. Tumours may contain entrapped NFP-positive axons. Immunostaining highlights the mixed population of cells in the neurofibromatous component, including fibroblasts (CD34), Schwann cells (S100 and SOX10), and perineurial cells (EMA, claudin-1, and GLUT1), and the monomorphic Schwann cell populations in the Schwann cell solid nodules (highlighted by diffuse expression of S100 and SOX10) {976,1302}.

Hybrid neurofibroma/perineurioma contains a plexiform neurofibroma with areas of perineurial differentiation. These areas are often only recognizable with the aid of immunohistochemistry. The perineuriomatous areas are immunopositive for EMA, GLUT1, and claudin-1, and the neurofibroma areas show a mixed population of cells including fibroblasts (CD34), Schwann cells (S100 and SOX10), and perineurial cells (EMA, claudin-1, and GLUT1) {1558,22}.

Cytology
Not clinically relevant

Diagnostic molecular pathology
Not clinically relevant

Essential and desirable diagnostic criteria
Essential: intermingled features of two types of benign nerve sheath tumours; appropriate immunohistochemical staining for each component.

Staging
Not clinically relevant

Prognosis and prediction
The tumours are benign and rarely recur locally {1405}.

Malignant peripheral nerve sheath tumour

Nielsen GP
Chi P

Definition

Malignant peripheral nerve sheath tumour (MPNST) is a malignant spindle cell tumour often arising from a peripheral nerve, from a pre-existing benign nerve sheath tumour, or in a patient with neurofibromatosis type 1 (NF1). In the absence of these settings, particularly in sporadic de novo or radiotherapy-associated tumours, the diagnosis can be more challenging and is based on the histological and immunohistochemical features suggesting Schwannian differentiation.

ICD-O coding

9540/3 Malignant peripheral nerve sheath tumour NOS

ICD-11 coding

2B5E & XH2XP8 Malignant nerve sheath tumour of peripheral nerves or autonomic nervous system, primary site & Malignant peripheral nerve sheath tumour

2B5E & XH4V81 Malignant nerve sheath tumour of peripheral nerves or autonomic nervous system, primary site & Malignant peripheral nerve sheath tumour, epithelioid

2B5E & XH2VV8 Malignant nerve sheath tumour of peripheral nerves or autonomic nervous system, primary site & Malignant peripheral nerve sheath tumour with rhabdomyoblastic differentiation

Related terminology

Not recommended: malignant schwannoma; neurofibrosarcoma; neurogenic sarcoma.

Subtype(s)

Malignant peripheral nerve sheath tumour, epithelioid

Localization

The most common locations are the trunk and extremities, followed by the head and neck area {1783,863}. When arising in a peripheral nerve, MPNST most frequently affects the sciatic nerve.

Clinical features

MPNSTs are typically seen in patients aged 20–50 years; rarely do they arise in children, usually in the setting of NF1. Patients with NF1 are usually younger at the time of diagnosis than patients with sporadic tumours. The presenting symptoms are an enlarging painful or painless mass that may be palpable or identified on imaging studies. When the tumour involves a nerve, the patient may present with neuropathic symptoms such as motor weakness, paraesthesia, or radicular pain. There are no specific imaging characteristics that distinguish MPNST from other sarcomas, except possible origin from a large nerve or from neurofibromas in patients with NF1. The FDG PET imaging technique is sensitive but not specific in detecting MPNSTs in patients with NF1 {403}.

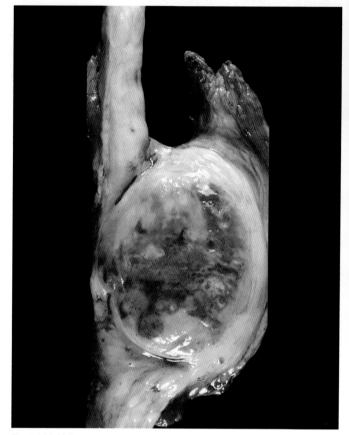

Fig. 1.300 Malignant peripheral nerve sheath tumour arising in plexiform neurofibroma. Malignant peripheral nerve sheath tumour arising in a nerve involved by a plexiform neurofibroma (proximal and distal to tumour) in a patient with neurofibromatosis type 1. The tumour has variegated tan, red, and yellow areas.

Epidemiology

MPNST is a rare tumour accounting for approximately 3–5% of soft tissue sarcomas.

Etiology

MPNST may be associated with irradiation or NF1.

Pathogenesis

Conventional MPNSTs have complex karyotypes. Despite different clinical presentations (e.g. NF1-associated, sporadic de novo, or radiotherapy-associated), recent genomic studies of MPNSTs demonstrated highly frequent and concurrent inactivating mutations in three pathways: *NF1*, *CDKN2A/CDKN2B*, and PRC2 core components (*EED* or *SUZ12*), resulting in complete loss of function {1815,761,3396,2481}. In NF1-associated peripheral nerve sheath tumours, as benign precursor plexiform neurofibroma progresses into atypical neurofibroma / atypical neurofibromatous neoplasm of uncertain biological potential

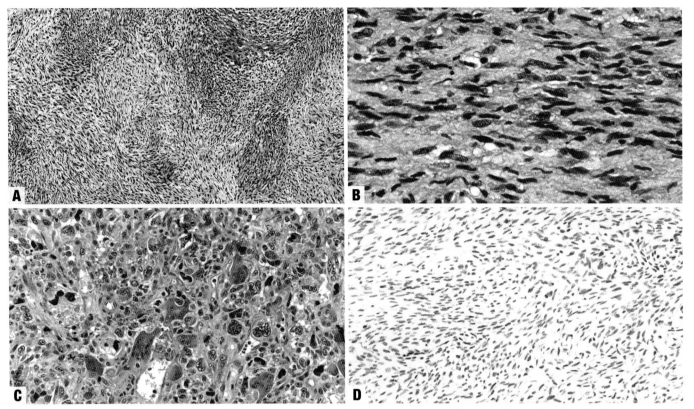

Fig. 1.301 Malignant peripheral nerve sheath tumour. **A** The tumour is composed of alternating cellular and less cellular areas (marble-like pattern). **B** High-power view demonstrating the spindle-shaped and wavy nuclei characteristic of malignant peripheral nerve sheath tumour. **C** High-grade malignant peripheral nerve sheath tumour arising in a patient with neurofibromatosis type 1. The sarcoma shows marked pleomorphism, mimicking an undifferentiated pleomorphic sarcoma. **D** Malignant peripheral nerve sheath tumour demonstrating loss of H3K27me3.

and/or transforms to high-grade MPNST, it is accompanied by progressive genomic alterations that inactivate the neurofibromin (NF1), p16/p15 (CDKN2A/CDKN2B), and PRC2 pathways and increased genomic copy-number variations, respectively {248,1815,2481}. About 80% of all high-grade MPNSTs exhibit complete loss of PRC2 activity through loss of the PRC2 core component (*EED* or *SUZ12*) and complete loss of H3K27me3 expression {2545,1815,2754}. The loss of H3K27me3 expression has become a useful diagnostic tool in high-grade MPNST. Given the critical role of PRC2 in development and cell-lineage specification, PRC2 loss may underlie the molecular mechanisms of the histological phenotype of heterologous differentiation in MPNSTs.

Epithelioid MPNSTs are distinct from conventional MPNSTs molecularly. *SMARCB1* gene inactivation resulting in SMARCB1 loss by immunohistochemistry is observed in approximately 75% of cases {2751}. They rarely have genetic alterations in the neurofibromin (NF1), p16/p15 (CDKN2A/CDKN2B), and PRC2 pathways {1815,1533}.

Macroscopic appearance

When the tumour arises in a nerve, there is a fusiform enlargement of the nerve. In patients with NF1, a tumour can be seen usually in association with a plexiform neurofibroma. MPNSTs are usually > 5 cm at the time of diagnosis and have a tan-white, fleshy cut surface, often with areas of haemorrhage and necrosis.

Histopathology

Tumours are typically composed of fascicles of spindle-shaped cells, often with a haemangiopericytoma-like vascular pattern, and alternating hypercellular and hypocellular areas (tapestry appearance). There are often areas of geographical necrosis and conspicuous mitotic figures. The cells are spindle or serpentine in shape, with hyperchromatic nuclei and pale wavy cytoplasm. MPNST may occasionally show extensive pleomorphism, simulating an undifferentiated pleomorphic sarcoma. Perivascular accentuation of tumour cells may be seen; in those areas, the cells frequently become plumper. Heterologous

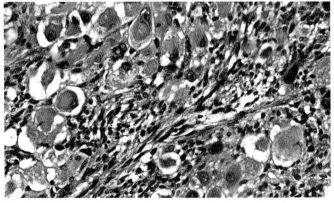

Fig. 1.302 Malignant triton tumour. Malignant peripheral nerve sheath tumour with extensive rhabdomyoblastic differentiation (malignant triton tumour).

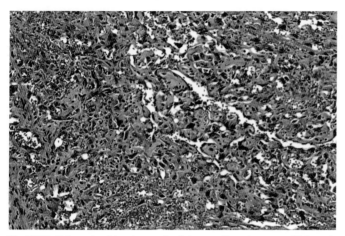

Fig. 1.303 Malignant peripheral nerve sheath tumour with angiosarcoma. High-grade angiosarcomatous component in a malignant peripheral nerve sheath tumour arising in a patient with neurofibromatosis type 1.

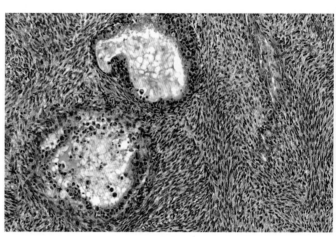

Fig. 1.304 Malignant peripheral nerve sheath tumour with glands. Malignant peripheral nerve sheath tumour with glandular differentiation.

differentiation, such as skeletal muscle, bone, cartilage, and blood vessels, is seen in about 15% of tumours. A malignant triton tumour is an MPNST with skeletal muscle differentiation. Glandular differentiation, with or without mucin production, is rarely seen (glandular MPNST); almost all of these tumours arise in patients with NF1. When involving a large nerve, the neoplastic cells may track along the nerve bundles. In NF1-related MPNST arising in a pre-existent neurofibroma, the distinction between a low-grade MPNST and an atypical neurofibroma / atypical neurofibromatous neoplasm of uncertain biological potential is often problematic, especially on small biopsies. Recently, diagnostic criteria to distinguish these tumours from other types of NF1-associated nerve sheath tumours have been established (see Table 1.04) {2142}.

Epithelioid MPNST is a rare subtype of MPNST (< 5% of the tumours) that is composed of plump, epithelioid cells with abundant eosinophilic cytoplasm, sometimes embedded in an abundant extracellular myxoid or hyalinized matrix and typically demonstrating a lobulated growth pattern {1762}. Although rare, this subtype of MPNST is the most common type to arise

ex-schwannoma {2751}. Epithelioid MPNST is not associated with NF1.

Immunohistochemically, MPNST may be positive for S100 (< 50% of tumours), SOX10 (< 70%), and GFAP (20–30%) {1569}. Importantly, staining for S100 and SOX10 is patchy or focal. Diffuse staining for S100 or SOX10 is not usually compatible with the diagnosis of conventional MPNST. Complete loss of staining for H3K27me3 may be helpful in the diagnosis of MPNST, with high-grade tumours (and radiation-induced MPNST) showing more-frequent loss than low-grade tumours {2475,2545,2754,2397}. The heterologous components (e.g. skeletal muscle differentiation or angiosarcomatous areas) stain for appropriate markers. The glands in glandular MPNST show positive staining for keratin and CEA and may be positive for neuroendocrine markers. Unlike conventional MPNSTs, epithelioid MPNSTs show strong and diffuse staining for S100 and SOX10, in the absence of melanoma markers. They retain expression of H3K27me3 and most show loss of SMARCB1 expression {2751}. Epithelioid MPNST may also be positive for keratin.

Table 1.04 Proposed nomenclature for the spectrum of neurofibromatosis type 1–associated nerve sheath tumours

Diagnosis	Proposed definition
Neurofibroma	Benign Schwann cell neoplasm with thin (often wavy) nuclei, wispy cell processes, and a myxoid to collagenous (shredded carrots) matrix; immunohistochemistry includes extensive but not diffuse S100 and SOX10 positivity and a lattice-like CD34+ fibroblastic network
Plexiform neurofibroma	Neurofibroma diffusely enlarging and replacing a nerve, often involving multiple nerve fascicles, delineated by EMA+ perineurial cells
Neurofibroma with atypia (ancient neurofibroma)	Neurofibroma with atypia alone, most commonly manifesting as scattered bizarre nuclei
Cellular neurofibroma	Neurofibroma with hypercellularity but retained neurofibroma architecture and no mitoses
ANNUBP	Schwann cell neoplasm with ≥ 2 of the following 4 features: cytological atypia, loss of neurofibroma architecture, hypercellularity, and < 1.5 mitoses/mm^2 (< 3 mitotic figures per 10 HPFs[a])
MPNST, low-grade	Features of ANNUBP, but with a mitotic count of 1.5–4.5 mitoses/mm^2 (3–9 mitotic figures per 10 HPFs[a]) and no necrosis
MPNST, high-grade	MPNST with ≥ 5 mitoses/mm^2 (≥ 10 mitotic figures per 10 HPFs[a]) or 1.5–4.5 mitoses/mm^2 (3–9 mitotic figures per 10 HPFs[a]) combined with necrosis

ANNUBP, atypical neurofibromatous neoplasm of uncertain biological potential; HPF, high-power field; MPNST, malignant peripheral nerve sheath tumour.
[a]1 mm^2 = approximately 5 HPFs of field diameter 0.51 mm.

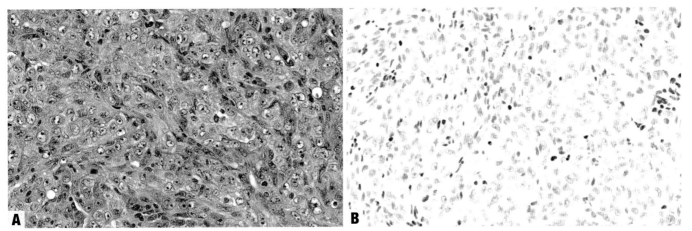

Fig. 1.305 Epithelioid malignant peripheral nerve sheath tumour. **A** The neoplastic cells are epithelioid, with eosinophilic cytoplasm and nuclei with prominent nucleoli. **B** Epithelioid malignant peripheral nerve sheath tumour showing loss of SMARCB1 (INI1) staining. Normal cells in the background show nuclear staining.

Cytology
Not clinically relevant

Diagnostic molecular pathology
Not clinically relevant

Essential and desirable diagnostic criteria
Essential: sarcoma arising from a nerve or pre-existing nerve sheath tumour or in a patient with NF1; tumours with a spindle fascicular growth, geographical necrosis, and often a limited degree of nuclear pleomorphism; in the sporadic setting, diagnosis is most often based on the identification of Schwann cell differentiation (S100/SOX10 focal positivity) and/or loss of H3K27me3 expression in a soft tissue mass; heterologous elements in a sarcoma should suggest MPNST; epithelioid MPNSTs occur outside the NF1 setting and often show diffuse S100 and SOX10 positivity and loss of SMARCB1 expression.

Staging
Not clinically relevant

Prognosis and prediction
MPNST is an aggressive tumour with a poor prognosis. Truncal location, tumour size > 5 cm, local recurrence, and high-grade morphology are all adverse prognostic factors; patients with NF1-associated MPNST appear to have a worse prognosis than patients with sporadic tumours {1783}. Malignant triton tumours are particularly aggressive.

Malignant melanotic nerve sheath tumour

Folpe AL
Hameed M

Definition

Malignant melanotic nerve sheath tumour (MMNST) is a rare peripheral nerve sheath tumour composed uniformly of Schwann cells showing melanocytic differentiation, usually arising in association with spinal or autonomic nerves. It is variably associated with Carney complex and frequently shows aggressive clinical behaviour. *PRKAR1A* mutations and loss of PRKAR1A protein expression are seen in the overwhelming majority of cases.

ICD-O coding

9540/3 Melanotic malignant peripheral nerve sheath tumour

ICD-11 coding

2B5E & XH2XP8 Malignant nerve sheath tumour of peripheral nerves or autonomic nervous system, primary site & Malignant peripheral nerve sheath tumour

Related terminology

Acceptable: melanotic schwannoma; psammomatous melanotic schwannoma; malignant melanotic Schwannian tumour.

Subtype(s)

None

Localization

MMNST most often arises from the spinal or autonomic nerves near the midline. However, cases have been reported in the gastrointestinal tract {564,571}, as well as in bone, soft tissues, heart, bronchus, liver, and skin.

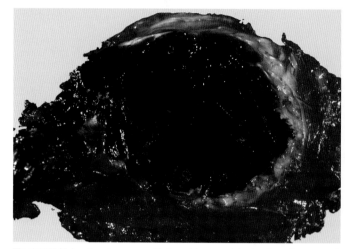

Fig. 1.306 Melanotic schwannoma. Malignant tumour arising in a thoracic nerve root. The sectioned tumour had the appearance and texture of dried tar, and it was circumscribed except for a portion (left) that invaded nearby soft tissues and vertebral bone.

Clinical features

Presenting symptoms include pain, sensory abnormalities, and mass effect. Bone erosion may be seen in spinal nerve root tumours. Parenchymal symptoms, such as respiratory and liver failure, may be seen in patients with metastatic disease.

Epidemiology

MMNST is rare and occurs chiefly in adults. The tumour typically develops at an earlier age (average: 22.5 years) in patients with Carney complex than in those without this complex (average: 33.2 years) {484,3091}. Multiple tumours are seen in about

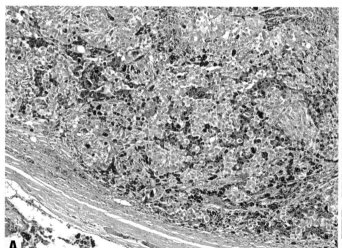
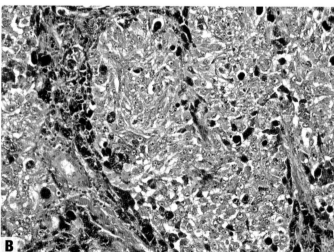

Fig. 1.307 Malignant melanotic nerve sheath tumour. **A** Malignant melanotic nerve sheath tumour presenting as an encapsulated posterior mediastinal mass in a 31-year-old woman. **B** Higher-power view showing heavily pigmented, vaguely syncytial epithelioid cells with visible nucleoli.

20% of patients; in such patients, there is a higher probability that other manifestations of Carney complex will also be present {484,3091}.

Etiology

In some series, > 50% of patients with MMNSTs have evidence of the Carney complex, an autosomal dominant, sometimes familial multiple neoplasia syndrome {484}. However, other series have noted an association with Carney complex in ≤ 5% of affected patients {3145,3091,3393,3233}.

Pathogenesis

Two genetic loci have been identified in Carney complex: *PRKAR1A* (*CNC1*) and *CNC2*, mapping to 17q22-q24 and 2p16, respectively. *PRKAR1A* inactivation is seen in roughly 50% of Carney complex kindreds {2020,1643}. *PRKAR1A* encodes a tumour suppressor; *PRKAR1A* mutations and loss of PRKAR1A protein expression are seen in the overwhelming majority of studied MMNSTs, almost all of which have occurred in patients lacking other stigmata of Carney complex {3091,3233}. SNP arrays typically show hypodiploidy, with monosomies of chromosomes 1, 2, and 17. Inactivation of both alleles of *PRKAR1A* through mutations and/or loss of heterozygosity of 17q has been reported {3233}. Gene expression analyses show MMNST to clearly segregate from conventional schwannomas and melanomas {3091}.

Macroscopic appearance

Most MMNSTs are solitary, although multiple and multicentric tumours may be seen in patients with Carney complex. Grossly, the tumours appear circumscribed or partially encapsulated, and they are frequently heavily pigmented, with the appearance of dried tar.

Histopathology

The neoplastic cells grow in short fascicles or sheets, vary in shape from polygonal to spindled, and often have a syncytial appearance. Vague palisading or formation of whorled structures may be present. Cellular detail is often difficult to discern,

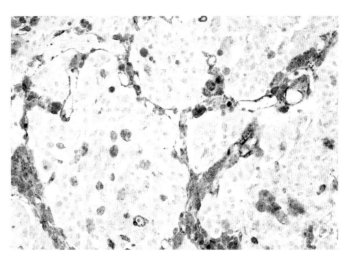

Fig. 1.309 Malignant melanotic nerve sheath tumour. Although this patient was not known to have Carney complex, there was complete loss of PRKAR1A expression.

owing to the heavy pigment deposits. The melanin pigment may be coarsely clumped or finely granular and varies from area to area. It stains positively with the Fontana stain and negatively for iron and PAS. In less pigmented areas, the tumour cells have eosinophilic to amphophilic cytoplasm, round to ovoid nuclei (often with nuclear grooves and pseudoinclusions), and usually small nucleoli. Occasional tumours show marked nuclear hyperchromatism with prominent macronucleoli. Mitoses and necrosis can be present, but they are not clearly associated with outcome. Psammoma bodies are present in roughly 50% of cases, although extensive sampling may be required to identify them. There are no clinical differences between psammomatous and non-psammomatous MMNSTs, with both showing a variable association with Carney complex, loss of PRKAR1A expression, and similar clinical behaviour {3091,3233}. Immunohistochemically, MMNSTs strongly express S100; SOX10; and various melanocytic markers, including HMB45, melan-A, and tyrosinase. PRKAR1A expression is typically lost {3091, 3233}. Ultrastructurally, the cells resemble Schwann cells with elaborate cytoplasmic processes that interdigitate or spiral in

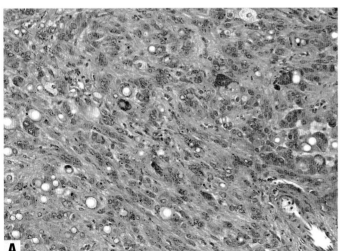
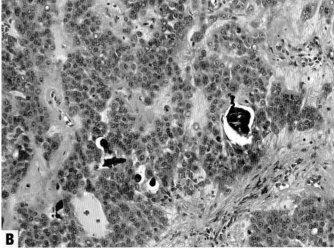

Fig. 1.308 Malignant melanotic nerve sheath tumour. **A** Malignant melanotic nerve sheath tumour presenting as a perigastric mass in a 45-year-old woman. Portions of this tumour showed pigmented spindle cell morphology. **B** Other areas in this tumour had a trabecular, epithelioid appearance, with scattered psammoma bodies.

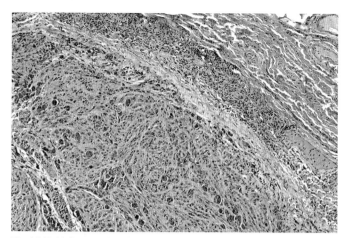

Fig. 1.310 Malignant melanotic nerve sheath tumour. Cervical lymph node metastasis in a 46-year-old man with malignant melanotic nerve sheath tumour. Neither the primary tumour nor the metastasis showed features that might have suggested an increased risk of metastasis.

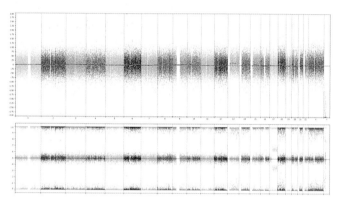

Fig. 1.311 Malignant melanotic nerve sheath tumour. SNP array (OncoScan) analysis demonstrating copy-neutral loss of heterozygosity of the long arm of chromosome 17; *PRKAR1A* is localized to 17q24.2.

the manner of mesaxons; premelanosomes and melanosomes are routinely present {3393,1429}.

Cytology
Not clinically relevant

Diagnostic molecular pathology
PRKAR1A expression is typically lost, corresponding to mutations of the gene {3091,3233}.

Essential and desirable diagnostic criteria
Essential: frequent origin from paraspinal or visceral autonomic nerves; fascicular to sheet-like proliferation of heavily pigmented, relatively uniform plump spindled cells; coexpression of S100/SOX10 and melanocytic markers (e.g. HMB45, melan-A).
Desirable: loss of PRKAR1A expression.

Staging
Not clinically relevant

Prognosis and prediction
The behaviour of MMNST is difficult to predict, and metastases can occur in the absence of morphologically malignant features. In the past, it was thought that most of these lesions had a benign, indolent course, with a < 15% metastatic risk {484}. However, more-recent reports have shown frequently aggressive behaviour, with a local recurrence rate and metastatic risk of 26–44% {3145,3091,3233,1620}. Additionally, only 53% of patients followed for > 5 years have been reported to be disease-free, suggesting that long-term follow-up is required to fully judge metastatic risk. In general, histopathological features are not predictive of outcome, although there are limited data suggesting more-aggressive behaviour in mitotically active tumours {3091}.

Intramuscular myxoma

Liegl-Atzwanger B
Hogendoorn PCW
Nielsen GP

Definition
Intramuscular myxoma is a benign hypocellular soft tissue tumour composed of bland spindle-shaped cells embedded in a usually abundant myxoid and hypovascular stroma.

ICD-O coding
8840/0 Myxoma NOS

ICD-11 coding
2E84.Z & XH6Q84 Benign fibrogenic or myofibrogenic tumour, site unknown & Myxoma NOS

Related terminology
Acceptable: cellular myxoma.

Subtype(s)
Cellular myxoma

Localization
The most common locations are the large muscles of the thigh, shoulder, buttock, and upper arm {914,1479,2286,3179}.

Clinical features
Intramuscular myxoma is a slow-growing painless mass {914, 1479,2286,3179}. On MRI, it is bright in T2-weighted images and shows low signal intensity compared with skeletal muscle in T1-weighted images {2788}. Intramuscular myxomas are mainly sporadic but may occur in combination with fibrous dysplasia, a condition called Mazabraud syndrome {1479}.

Epidemiology
Intramuscular myxoma usually affects middle-aged individuals (40–70 years) and is more common in females (M:F ratio: ~0.3:1)

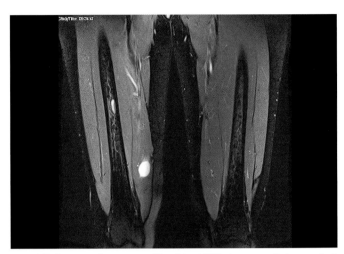

Fig. 1.313 Intramuscular myxoma. T2-weighted MRI shows a well-circumscribed, hyperintense tumour.

{914,1479,2286,3179}. Most lesions are sporadic but a minority are associated with fibrous dysplasia, which is most often polyostotic (Mazabraud syndrome) {1479,1947}. In Mazabraud syndrome, myxomas are often multiple.

Etiology
Unknown

Pathogenesis
Activating point mutation in *GNAS* (exons 8 and 9) is detected in > 90% of sporadic intramuscular and cellular myxomas {2996, 781}, as well as in cases of Mazabraud syndrome {2368}. Mutations in *GNAS* lead to downstream activation of FOS (c-FOS) {3294}.

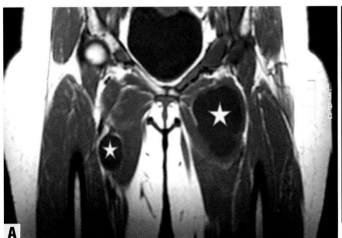

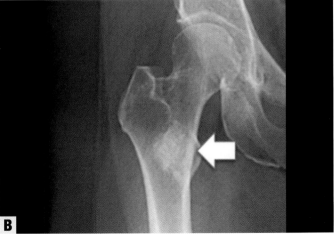

Fig. 1.312 Mazabraud syndrome. **A** Intramuscular myxomas are seen in the proximal muscles of the lower extremities (stars). **B** Fibrous dysplasia is present in the proximal femur (arrow).

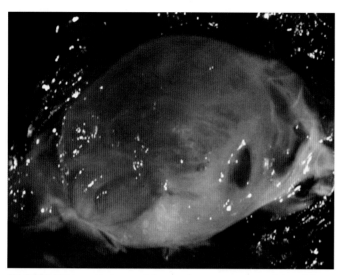

Fig. 1.314 Intramuscular myxoma. Intramuscular myxoma composed of a gelatinous mass with internal septa. The tumour is well circumscribed overall but shows some infiltration of the surrounding skeletal muscle (left of tumour).

Macroscopic appearance

On gross examination, the tumour size ranges from 5 to 10 cm {914,1479,2286,3179}; however, examples as large as 20 cm have been documented. The larger ones are usually cellular myxomas {1317}. Although these tumours appear well circumscribed, close examination can demonstrate ill-defined borders where the tumour merges with the surrounding skeletal muscle. The cut surface is gelatinous and lobulated and may have cystic, fluid-filled areas.

Histopathology

Classic intramuscular myxoma is a cytologically bland, hypocellular lesion composed of uniform spindle to stellate-shaped cells with uniform small oval nuclei and indistinct palely eosinophilic cytoplasm embedded in an abundant extracellular myxoid stroma. Only sparse capillary-sized blood vessels are seen. Cystic change and vacuolation may be seen in the stroma. Necrosis and mitotic figures are not seen. At the edge of the lesion, infiltration of the tumour between and around individual skeletal muscle cells is often observed.

A subset of tumours show hypercellular areas occupying 10–90% of the tumour. These tumours show an increased number of cells and a more prominent vascular pattern with capillary-sized, occasionally thick-walled vessels, sometimes focally in a more collagenous background {2286,3179,2996}. Mitoses are very rare and pleomorphism or necrosis is absent. There may sometimes be morphological overlap between cellular myxoma and low-grade myxofibrosarcoma (also on immunohistochemistry) {2996,3294}, although nuclear atypia and hyperchromasia usually exclude the former.

Immunohistochemically, the tumour cells are commonly positive for CD34 and rarely stain for SMA. Desmin and S100 are

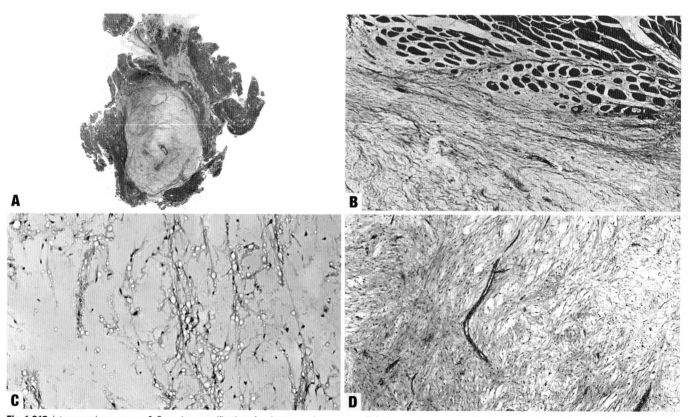

Fig. 1.315 Intramuscular myxoma. **A** Scanning magnification of an intramuscular myxoma. **B** Intramuscular myxoma with entrapment of skeletal muscle fibres in the periphery. **C** Intramuscular myxoma with extracellular matrix with frothy appearance, mimicking lipoblasts. **D** Cellular intramuscular myxoma is a more cellular and more collagenous neoplasm, with bland uniform spindle cells lacking nuclear pleomorphism.

negative. There are often multifocally scattered muciphages immunopositive for CD163.

Cytology
Not clinically relevant

Diagnostic molecular pathology
GNAS mutation analysis may be a useful tool to differentiate cellular myxoma from a low-grade myxofibrosarcoma in diagnostically challenging cases or on limited biopsy material.

Essential and desirable diagnostic criteria
Essential: intramuscular mass in middle-aged predominantly female adults; hypocellular myxoid tumour composed of bland spindle cells; inconspicuous vessels; focal non-destructive infiltration of adjacent skeletal muscle; nuclear atypia, mitoses, and necrosis are absent; the cellular subtype is more cellular with areas of more-collagenous stroma and increased vasculature.
Desirable: detection of *GNAS* mutations (in selected cases).

Staging
Not clinically relevant

Prognosis and prediction
Classic intramuscular myxoma is typically a non-recurrent tumour, whereas the cellular subtype has a small risk for local non-destructive recurrence {3179,1947}. Malignant transformation does not occur.

Juxta-articular myxoma

Liegl-Atzwanger B
Hogendoorn PCW
Nielsen GP

Definition
Juxta-articular myxoma is a rare, benign myxoid soft tissue tumour morphologically similar to intramuscular/cellular myxoma (but lacking *GNAS* mutation), typically arising in the vicinity of large joints.

ICD-O coding
8840/0 Myxoma NOS

ICD-11 coding
2E84.Z & XH6Q84 Benign fibrogenic or myofibrogenic tumour, site unknown & Myxoma NOS

Related terminology
Acceptable: periarticular myxoma.

Subtype(s)
None

Localization
Juxta-articular myxoma usually arises adjacent to large joints, with the knee joint being the most commonly affected site (> 85%). Other locations affected are the shoulder, elbow, hip, and ankle {2058}, and rare locations include the temporomandibular joint {3360}.

Clinical features
Patients usually present with a swelling or a mass that may be associated with tenderness or pain in the vicinity of large joints. Duration of symptoms ranges from weeks to years. Imaging studies are similar to those of intramuscular myxoma {1638}.

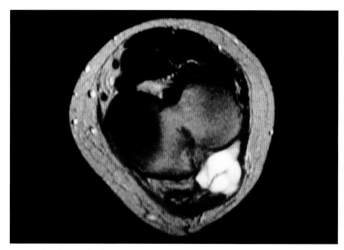

Fig. 1.316 Juxta-articular myxoma. MRI of a tumour located adjacent to the knee joint, showing a homogeneous bright signal, similar to intramuscular myxoma.

Epidemiology
These lesions occur over a wide age range, including rarely in children, but they typically affect patients in the fifth and sixth decades of life, with a male predominance {2058}.

Etiology
In most patients, the etiology is unknown. A minority of patients have a history of trauma or osteoarthritis, which may be coincidental.

Pathogenesis
Unknown

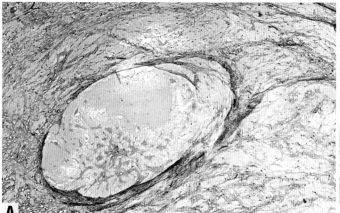
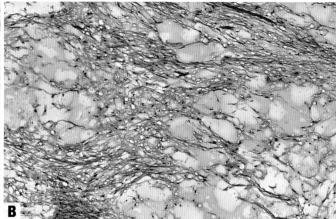

Fig. 1.317 Juxta-articular myxoma. **A** Cystic area filled with myxoid material surrounded by a more cellular proliferation. **B** Myxoid stroma with bland spindle cells resembling areas of cellular myxoma.

Macroscopic appearance

The tumour usually ranges in size between 2 and 6 cm, but tumours as large as 13 cm have been described {2058}. The cut surface is gelatinous and myxoid. Cystic degeneration is commonly seen.

Histopathology

The tumour is generally hypocellular and composed of bland spindle-shaped cells with uniform ovoid nuclei, inconspicuous nuclei, and palely eosinophilic cytoplasm embedded in a hypovascular myxoid stroma. Increased cellularity can be seen (similar to in cellular myxoma); however, mitoses are scarce. In the majority of cases, cyst-like spaces lined by a delicate fibrin layer or a thicker layer composed of collagen may be seen. The tumour is poorly circumscribed, demonstrating infiltration into the surrounding adipose or tendinous tissue. In a subset of cases, haemorrhage, chronic inflammation, and haemosiderin/fibrin deposition may be seen, probably due to trauma. These reactive changes may also be seen in recurrent tumours. Immunohistochemically, the lesional cells may express CD34 and/or SMA. S100 is negative. CD163-positive muciphages may be present.

Cytology

Not clinically relevant

Diagnostic molecular pathology

Unlike intramuscular myxomas, juxta-articular myxomas do not demonstrate *GNAS* mutations {2368}.

Essential and desirable diagnostic criteria

Essential: affects soft tissue around large joints, most commonly the knee (> 85%); hypocellular myxoid cytologically bland tumour; infiltrative growth pattern.
Desirable: lacks *GNAS* mutations (in selected cases).

Staging

Not clinically relevant

Prognosis and prediction

Local recurrence occurs in as many as one third of patients, sometimes more than once {2058}. Malignant transformation does not occur.

Deep (aggressive) angiomyxoma

Nucci MR
Bridge JA

Definition

Deep (aggressive) angiomyxoma is an infiltrative, benign, myxoid spindle cell neoplasm that occurs in the deep soft tissue of the pelviperineal region.

ICD-O coding

8841/0 Aggressive angiomyxoma

ICD-11 coding

2F7C & XH9HK9 Neoplasms of uncertain behaviour of connective or other soft tissue & Angiomyxoma

Related terminology

Acceptable: deep angiomyxoma; aggressive angiomyxoma.

Subtype(s)

None

Localization

Deep angiomyxoma typically occurs in the deep soft tissue of the pelvis and perineal region, including in the vulvovaginal and inguinoscrotal soft tissue in women {2937,250,994,1208} and men {3108,1463}, respectively.

Clinical features

Patients typically present with a slow-growing, deep-seated painless mass. Lesions may sometimes be associated with vague discomfort, pain, or mass effect on adjacent organs with associated symptoms. MRI may reveal an internal laminated appearance to the mass (the so-called swirl sign) {2998,2927}.

Epidemiology

Deep angiomyxoma occurs over a wide age range, with a peak in the fourth to fifth decades of life. It is much more common in women.

Etiology

Unknown

Pathogenesis

Karyotypic aberrations involving chromosome region 12q13-q15 predominate in aggressive angiomyxoma {2587}. Correspondingly, rearrangements of the HMGA2 (12q14.3) locus have been identified by FISH, with associated HMGA2 transcriptional upregulation and aberrant expression confirmed by RT-PCR and immunostaining in some studies {1602,2332, 2106,2051}. The target gene has been shown to be HMGA2 (previously designated HMGIC), which is a DNA architectural factor important in transcriptional regulation that is not typically expressed in non-neoplastic adult tissues. Aberrant expression of HMGA2 protein is also seen in other mesenchymal tumours, such as lipoma, pulmonary chondroid hamartoma, and uterine leiomyoma, with similar chromosomal aberrations {2332}. The molecular mechanism for aberrant expression appears multifactorial and tumour dependent; in some instances, deep (aggressive) angiomyxoma is due to fusion transcript production, whereas in others the gene is intact but shows deregulated expression via alterations affecting the 5′ regulatory region or the untranslated 3′ region. It is not clear how HMGA2 expression leads to tumour development, but presumably altered transcription of target genes is a potential mechanism.

Macroscopic appearance

Deep angiomyxomas are variably described as tan-yellow soft or gelatinous masses with ill-defined margins. The tumours can vary in size, but most are > 10 cm. Recurrent tumours may have a more fibrous appearance because they may be associated with scar tissue.

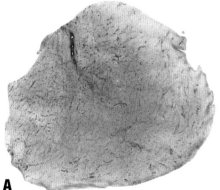 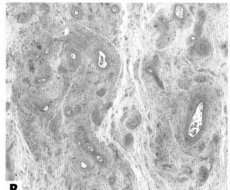 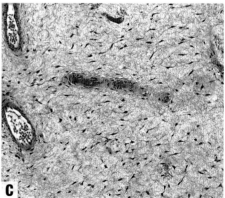

Fig. 1.318 Deep (aggressive) angiomyxoma. **A** This tumour is characteristically paucicellular and composed of bland spindle cells set within an abundant myxoid matrix interspersed with prominent vessels. **B** Medium-sized to large vessels can be seen, with thickened walls. Note the presence of particularly distinct myoid bundles wrapping about vessels of various calibres. **C** A higher-power view.

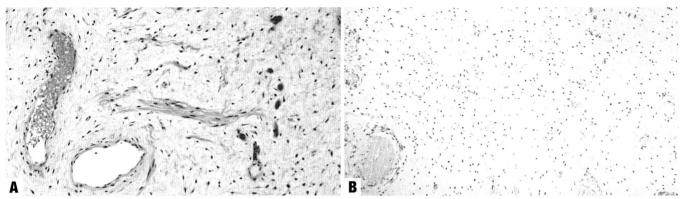

Fig. 1.319 Deep (aggressive) angiomyxoma. **A** The spindle-shaped cells have delicate cytoplasmic processes and ovoid bland nuclei. The myoid bundles are typically arranged in loose clusters or tight whorls around the vascular component. **B** When present, aberrant HMGA2 expression is a useful diagnostic marker for deep (aggressive) angiomyxoma. It is particularly helpful in defining the margin of the tumour, because non-neoplastic mesenchyme lacks expression.

Histopathology

Deep angiomyxoma is composed of spindled stromal cells and a prominent vascular component set within a copious myxoid matrix. On low-power examination, it is relatively hypocellular, and the vessels, which are characteristically medium-sized to large, are most often evenly dispersed throughout the tumour. Lesional spindle cells have delicate eosinophilic bipolar cell processes, and the nuclei are bland and ovoid or rounded. The vessel walls may be hyalinized and show perivascular concentric condensation of collagen fibres. In addition, collections of more eosinophilic smooth muscle cells (so-called myoid bundles) are commonly seen in stroma around the vessels. The tumour is infiltrative and the border may be difficult to delineate from surrounding non-neoplastic soft tissue.

The spindle cells are typically positive for desmin (more often diffusely than focally), and they may be positive for CD34 and SMA; SMA, when positive, is more commonly seen in the myoid bundles {1208,3168}. The spindle cells are also often positive for ER and PR (usually with moderate to strong positivity, > 50% nuclei) {316}. HMGA2 is a sensitive but not entirely specific marker for deep angiomyxoma {2030}. Positivity for CDK4 but not MDM2 has been described {3168}; of note, *CDK4* is in the same region as *HMGA2* on 12q.

Cytology
Not clinically relevant

Diagnostic molecular pathology
Not clinically relevant

Essential and desirable diagnostic criteria
Essential: poorly marginated lesion; relatively hypocellular with copious myxoid matrix; bland spindle-shaped stromal cells with eosinophilic processes; medium-sized to large vessels, often with hyalinized walls; collections of smooth muscle cells (myoid bundles) near vessels; desmin positivity.
Desirable: HMGA2 is often positive.

Staging
Not clinically relevant

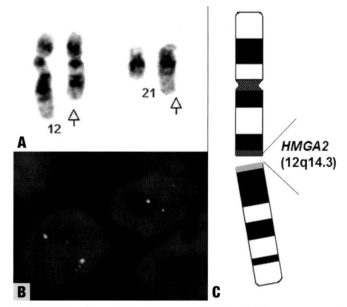

Fig. 1.320 Deep (aggressive) angiomyxoma. *HMGA2* (12q14.3) rearrangement. **A** Partial G-banded karyotype exhibiting a t(12;21)(q15;q21.1) in an aggressive angiomyxoma. **B,C** Dual-colour FISH with a probe set flanking *HMGA2* demonstrates the presence of a rearrangement of this locus in tumour interphase nuclei (split red and green signals).

Prognosis and prediction
Invasive local recurrence may occur, although this happens much less commonly than originally thought, which is reflected by the terminology change from "aggressive" to "deep" angiomyxoma, with the latter designation chosen to reflect lesional depth. Recurrence rates vary (ranging from 9% to 50%) {3168,1083,2990}; this wide range may reflect uncertainty regarding margin status, because the border of the tumour can be difficult to delineate. More than one recurrence is very uncommon. HMGA2 staining may be useful in determining margin status. Recurrent tumours that express hormone receptors have been successfully treated with surgery and adjuvant GnRH analogues {2791,44}.

Atypical fibroxanthoma

Mentzel TDW
Brenn T

Definition
Atypical fibroxanthoma (AFX) is a dermal-based mesenchymal neoplasm of uncertain differentiation, in a disease spectrum with pleomorphic dermal sarcoma in sun-damaged skin. Tumours that meet strict diagnostic criteria generally behave in a benign fashion.

ICD-O coding
8830/1 Atypical fibroxanthoma

ICD-11 coding
2F72.Y Other specified neoplasms of uncertain behaviour of skin (atypical fibroxanthoma)

Related terminology
None

Subtype(s)
None

Localization
AFX arises predominantly in sun-damaged skin of the head and neck region, whereas the extremities are rarely affected {1476, 2090,247,1916}.

Clinical features
AFX presents as a solitary, fast-growing, exophytic, dome-shaped nodule that is usually < 2 cm and often ulcerated. The neoplasms are red, flesh-coloured, or bluish-brown {1476,2090, 247,1916}.

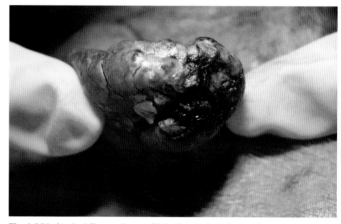

Fig. 1.321 Atypical fibroxanthoma. Clinically, atypical fibroxanthoma presents as a small, exophytic, often ulcerated dermal neoplasm.

Epidemiology
AFX represents a rare mesenchymal neoplasm that occurs most commonly in sun-damaged skin of elderly white patients; males are affected more often than females {1476,2090,247, 1916,2157}. Exceptionally rarely, AFXs have been reported in young patients with germline mutation of *TP53* or with xeroderma pigmentosum {541,1814}.

Etiology
Ultraviolet (UV) radiation plays a central role in the development of AFX, and UV radiation signature mutations in *TP53* have been found {776}. Rarely, AFX is seen in the field of prior radiation therapy and in patients with immunosuppression.

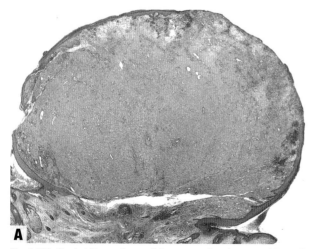

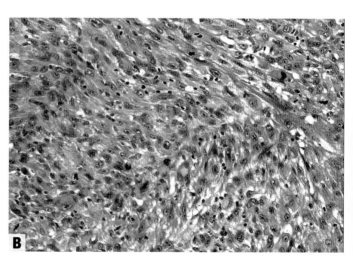

Fig. 1.322 Atypical fibroxanthoma. **A** Low-power view shows a nodular, well-circumscribed, dermal neoplasm with collarette formation of the hyperplastic epidermis. **B** Cellular neoplasm composed of atypical spindled, round, polygonal, and pleomorphic tumour cells; numerous mitoses are present.

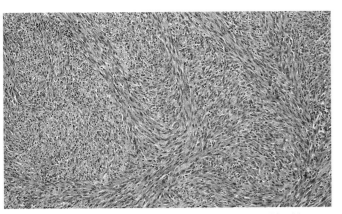

Fig. 1.323 Spindle cell atypical fibroxanthoma. Cellular bundles and fascicles composed of atypical spindled cells with numerous mitoses are noted.

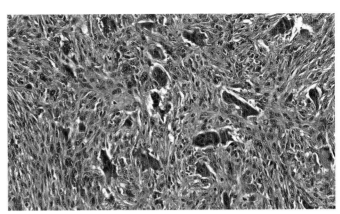

Fig. 1.325 Osteoclast-like giant cell–rich atypical fibroxanthoma. Numerous osteoclast-like giant cells with small, bland nuclei are admixed.

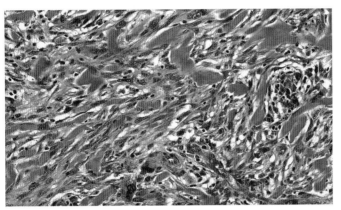

Fig. 1.324 Keloidal atypical fibroxanthoma. Thick bundles of hyalinized collagen masking nuclear atypia.

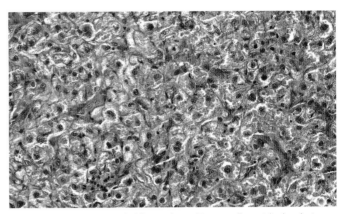

Fig. 1.326 Granular cell atypical fibroxanthoma. Tumour cells contain abundant granular cytoplasm and enlarged nuclei.

Pathogenesis

TP53 mutation due to UV irradiation is believed to be pathogenetically important. AFX shows abnormal accumulation of p53 and a characteristic *TP53* mutation pattern. Many AFXs show deletions but lack *HRAS*, *KRAS*, and *NRAS* gene mutations, in contrast to undifferentiated pleomorphic sarcoma {776,2711, 2143,2712}. Otherwise, activating mutations in the promoter region of the *TERT* gene, frequent *NOTCH1* and *FAT1* mutations, and a similar DNA methylation profile in AFX and pleomorphic dermal sarcoma suggest a close relationship {1218,1219,1669}.

Macroscopic appearance

AFXs are well-circumscribed nodular or polypoid tumours of the dermis. Ulceration of the epidermis is a common feature.

Histopathology

The histopathological criteria for the diagnosis of AFX must be used strictly, and the diagnosis of AFX should never be made on a biopsy only, or without the use of a panel of immunohistochemical antibodies. AFX represents an intradermal, usually symmetrical and well-circumscribed cellular neoplasm without involvement of the subcutis. Ulceration and collarette formation of the lateral hyperplastic epidermis are frequent. These cellular neoplasms are composed of sheets and fascicles of most often highly pleomorphic polygonal or histiocytoid cells, enlarged and atypical spindled and epithelioid cells, and variable numbers of atypical multinucleated tumour giant cells. Neoplastic cells contain enlarged atypical, vesicular, or hyperchromatic nuclei, and numerous mitoses (including atypical mitoses) are present. By definition, tumour necrosis, lymphovascular and/or perineural invasion, and subcutaneous invasion are absent. Scattered inflammatory cells, numerous vessels, and areas of haemorrhage may be present {247,1916,2090,2157}. A number of histological subtypes are described, as follows.

Spindle cell, non-pleomorphic AFX

Spindle cell AFX shows usual features of AFX but is composed of relatively monomorphic, eosinophilic, spindled tumour cells arranged in bundles and fascicles {463}.

Clear cell AFX

Clear cell AFX is rare and composed of pleomorphic tumour cells with foamy or clear cytoplasm and hyperchromatic nuclei; it must be distinguished from balloon cell melanoma, sebaceous or clear cell carcinoma, and signet-ring angiosarcoma {688,3049}.

Pigmented (haemosiderotic) AFX

Pigmented AFX may resemble melanoma and is characterized by abundant intratumoural haemorrhage with blood-filled, pseudovascular spaces. A variable number of osteoclast-like giant cells are present and abundant haemosiderin deposition is noted {819,3069}.

Myxoid AFX

Prominent myxoid stromal change is very rarely seen in AFXs. Such lesions must be distinguished from myxofibrosarcoma or myxoid leiomyosarcoma {2466}.

Osteoclast-like giant cell–rich AFX

AFX may contain numerous bland osteoclast-like giant cells and must be distinguished from giant cell tumour of soft tissue, as well as from leiomyosarcoma with osteoclast-like giant cells {3087}.

Keloidal AFX

AFX may rarely show thick bundles of hyalinized collagen, masking the nuclear atypia and worrisome morphology, mimicking keloid or keloidal dermatofibroma {1631}.

Granular cell AFX

Rarely, AFX is composed of atypical and pleomorphic tumour cells with abundant granular cytoplasm staining positively for CD68 and NKI/C3 {2685}. Granular cell tumour, non-neural granular cell tumour, and other neoplasms with prominent granular cell features must be distinguished.

Immunohistochemistry

No specific immunohistochemical marker for AFX is known, and a broad panel of antibodies must be used to exclude other neoplasms. Tumour cells in AFX usually stain positively for vimentin, CD10, and p53, and often for SMA, but these are nonspecific. AFX is consistently negative for keratins, S100, SOX10, CD34, ERG, and desmin. Cases of AFX occasionally may show at least focal nonspecific expression of melan-A, HMB45, MITF, EMA, p63, CD99, CD68, and CD31 {247,3034,1916,3068}.

Cytology

Not clinically relevant

Diagnostic molecular pathology

Not clinically relevant

Essential and desirable diagnostic criteria

Essential: usually pleomorphic (but variable) morphology; strict confinement to the dermis; immunonegativity for keratins, S100, and SOX10.

Staging

Not clinically relevant

Prognosis and prediction

When strict diagnostic criteria are applied, the vast majority of AFXs show benign behaviour after complete surgical excision. Local recurrence is rare and distant metastases exceptional {3244}. Cases with tumour necrosis, invasion into subcutis, and/or lymphovascular invasion have metastatic potential and should therefore be regarded as pleomorphic dermal sarcoma.

Angiomatoid fibrous histiocytoma

Rekhi B
Antonescu CR
Chen G

Definition

Angiomatoid fibrous histiocytoma (AFH) is a rare neoplasm of intermediate (rarely metastasizing) malignant potential, mostly occurring in subcutis and characterized by varying proportions of epithelioid, ovoid, or spindle cells arranged in a nodular and often syncytial growth pattern, with haemorrhagic pseudovascular spaces and frequently a peripheral fibrous pseudocapsule with a prominent lymphoplasmacytic cuff.

ICD-O coding

8836/1 Angiomatoid fibrous histiocytoma

ICD-11 coding

2F7C & XH9362 Neoplasms of uncertain behaviour of connective or other soft tissue & Angiomatoid fibrous histiocytoma

Related terminology

Acceptable: angiomatoid malignant fibrous histiocytoma.

Subtype(s)

None

Localization

Tumours occur as subcutaneous lesions, most frequently in the extremities, followed by the trunk and the head and neck. Nearly two thirds of cases occur in areas where lymph nodes are normally found (e.g. the antecubital fossa, popliteal fossa, axilla, inguinal area, and neck). These tumours are increasingly recognized in non-somatic sites, such as the ovary, vulva, lung, brain, bone, mediastinum, and retroperitoneum {555,872,1971}.

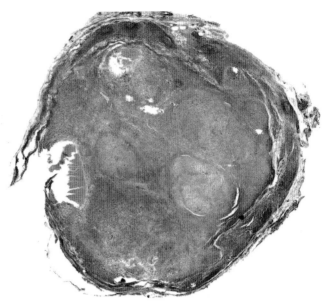

Fig. 1.328 Angiomatoid fibrous histiocytoma. A well-circumscribed tumour displaying multinodular fibrohistiocytic proliferation, pseudocystic spaces filled with blood, and a peripheral rim of lymphoid tissue, simulating a metastatic lymph node.

Clinical features

Patients typically present with a slow-growing, superficial, painless soft tissue mass, which may simulate a haematoma or a haemangioma {665,912}. Rarely, patients present with pyrexia, anaemia, malaise, and weight loss {665,912,1014}.

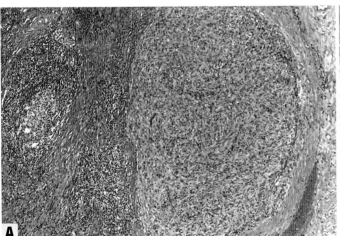
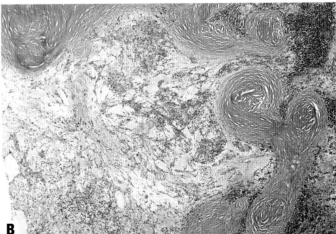

Fig. 1.327 Angiomatoid fibrous histiocytoma. **A** Tumour nodule surrounded by a characteristic lymphoplasmacytic cuff. **B** In this case from the retroperitoneum, tumour cells within a prominent myxoid stroma are surrounded by a lymphoplasmacytic cuff.

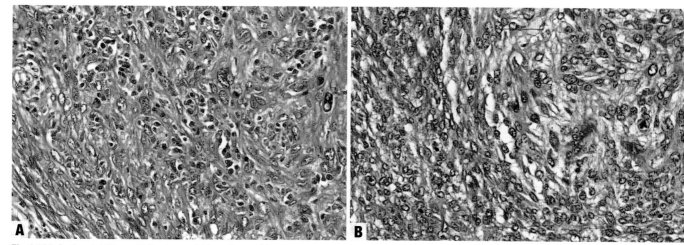

Fig. 1.329 Angiomatoid fibrous histiocytoma. **A** More-pleomorphic tumour cells containing a moderate amount of cytoplasm, vesicular nuclei, and focal intranuclear pseudoinclusions along with interspersed lymphocytes and plasma cells. **B** Mitoses are generally infrequent.

Epidemiology

AFH is a rare soft tissue neoplasm, accounting for 0.3% of all soft tissue tumours. There is no significant sex predilection. A wide age range is reported, from birth {165} to the ninth decade of life, with a peak incidence in the first two decades of life {665,129,2600}.

Etiology

Unknown

Pathogenesis

The most frequent genetic abnormality is the t(2;22)(q33;q12) translocation, resulting in an *EWSR1-CREB1* fusion, in > 90% of cases {129,2671,2600}. Less commonly, t(12;22)(q12;q12) translocation is detected, resulting in an *EWSR1-ATF1* fusion {1278}. Few cases harbouring a *FUS-ATF1* fusion have been reported {2565,3252}. *EWSR1-ATF1* is more frequently associated with AFH of extrasomatic soft tissues {555}. *EWSR1*–CREB family gene fusions have been recently reported in a subset of intracranial myxoid mesenchymal tumours that lack features typical of AFH, and thus it remains uncertain whether these represent a myxoid subtype of AFH or a novel entity {213,1580}.

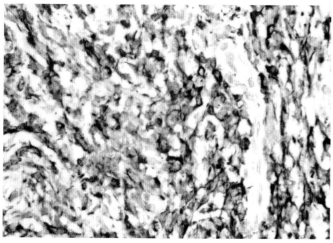

Fig. 1.330 Angiomatoid fibrous histiocytoma. Substantial desmin immunoreactivity in a case of angiomatoid fibrous histiocytoma.

Macroscopic appearance

These tumours appear as small, firm, nodular to cystic masses, with a wide size range (0.7–12 cm) and a median size of 2 cm {912,665}. The cut surface often shows multilocular haemorrhagic areas, simulating a haematoma, to a yellowish-tan or white fleshy appearance {912,665,3070}.

Histopathology

Tumours are circumscribed, lobulated, and characterized by four key morphological components, found in varying proportions: (1) solid nodules of epithelioid to spindle cells arranged in a syncytial pattern with moderate amounts of eosinophilic cytoplasm and mildly atypical vesicular nuclei; (2) pseudoangiomatous spaces containing blood and surrounded by tumour cells; (3) a thick fibrous pseudocapsule with haemosiderin deposition; and (4) a pericapsular rim of lymphoplasmacytic cells with germinal centres, simulating lymph node metastasis. Nearly one third of tumours lack cystic haemorrhagic spaces and show a completely solid appearance. Some cases lack any inflammatory component. Mitotic figures are generally few, although atypical mitotic figures may be present. A variable number of pleomorphic cells may be noted in some cases {3070,2600,1575}. A subtype of AFH is characterized by small blue round cells with hyperchromatic nuclei and scant eosinophilic cytoplasm, which can mimic an undifferentiated round cell sarcoma or epithelioid sarcoma {968,1314}. Myxoid forms have also been described, containing at least focal components of classic AFH {2753,555}.

Approximately 50% of cases are immunoreactive for desmin, which may be focal or diffuse. However, tumour cells are consistently negative for MYOD1 and myogenin. EMA, CD99, and CD68 are variably immunopositive in as many as 50% of cases {968}.

Cytology

The cytomorphological features of AFH are non-distinctive. Cellular smears show ovoid to spindled cells with moderate nuclear pleomorphism, arranged in loose clusters, containing moderate to abundant cytoplasm. Interspersed are blood products and a variable number of inflammatory cells {2557,1826}.

Diagnostic molecular pathology
The presence of *EWSR1-CREB1* or alternative gene fusions can be diagnostically helpful.

Essential and desirable diagnostic criteria
Essential: clinical presentation as a small subcutaneous painless nodule; nodules of epithelioid to ovoid cells arranged in syncytial-like sheets; pseudoangiomatoid spaces; peripheral rims of lymphoplasmacytic cells, including germinal centres; immunohistochemistry: variable desmin, CD99, and EMA immunoreactivity.
Desirable (in selected cases): molecular studies confirming *EWSR1* gene rearrangement.

Staging
Not clinically relevant

Prognosis and prediction
Most tumours follow an indolent course, with local recurrence in nearly 15% of cases and metastasis in < 2–5% of cases, predominantly to locoregional lymph nodes and rarely to lungs, liver, and brain {665,590,968}. Rare deaths have been reported from metastasis, although long-term survival after resection

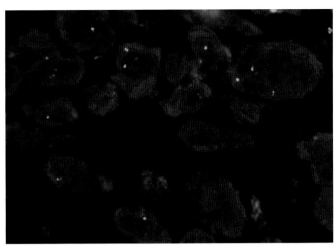

Fig. 1.331 Angiomatoid fibrous histiocytoma. *EWSR1* gene rearrangement detected, in the form of single red-green split signals, identified in the various tumour cells.

is reported in some metastatic cases {912,665}. There are no clinicopathological factors that correlate reliably with clinical outcome. However, cases with incomplete surgical clearance and those occurring in deeper locations and extrasomatic sites have been observed to show higher rates of recurrence and metastasis {665,555}.

Ossifying fibromyxoid tumour

Endo M
Mertens F
Miettinen M

Definition

Ossifying fibromyxoid tumour (OFMT) is a rare mesenchymal neoplasm of uncertain differentiation, with cords and trabeculae of ovoid cells embedded in a fibromyxoid matrix, often surrounded by a complete or incomplete peripheral shell of lamellar bone, having potential for local recurrence and metastasis (especially when showing malignant features).

ICD-O coding

8842/0 Ossifying fibromyxoid tumour NOS

ICD-11 coding

2F7C & XH1DA7 Neoplasms of uncertain behaviour of connective or other soft tissue & Ossifying fibromyxoid tumour

Related terminology

None

Subtype(s)

Ossifying fibromyxoid tumour, malignant

Localization

Lesions most frequently arise in the subcutis, but also not uncommonly within skeletal muscle of the extremities {1059,182}. Tumours may occur in all parts of the body; however, the relatively common sites are the thigh, head and neck, and trunk wall {918, 1059,2123}. More than 40% of cases arise in the lower extremity.

Clinical features

The tumour usually presents as a painless, slow-growing, elastic, hard mass. Radiologically, OFMT is usually a well-circumscribed, lobulated mass, occasionally surrounded by a partial peripheral calcification {905}. Intralesional mineralization may be present in some cases {918,1059,2123}.

Epidemiology

Tumours occur over a wide age range (5–88 years), with a median age of about 50 years {918,1205,1059,3387,182}. The M:F ratio is 1.5:1 {2123}. The malignant subtype shows the same epidemiological features as typical OFMT.

Etiology

Unknown

Pathogenesis

At least 85% of OFMTs, including typical, atypical, and malignant lesions, display a gene fusion, most commonly (in ~50% of cases) involving the *PHF1* gene; the most prevalent variants are *EP400-PHF1*, *MEAF6-PHF1*, *EPC1-PHF1*, and *PHF1-TFE3* {1127,1206,137,3005}. In addition, rare fusions involving *BCOR*, *BCORL1*, *CREBBP*, and/or *KDM2A* have been described, especially in malignant OFMT; the proteins encoded by these genes share with PHF1 direct or indirect involvement in processes affecting histone modification {1581}. Little is known about other genetic changes affecting the clinical behaviour of OFMT, but FISH studies have suggested that loss of chromosome 22 material might be more common in the malignant subgroup {1127}.

Macroscopic appearance

Grossly, lesions range from 0.5 to 21 cm in greatest diameter, with a median of about 4 cm {1059,1205,3387}. OFMTs are

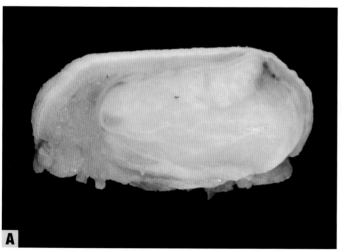
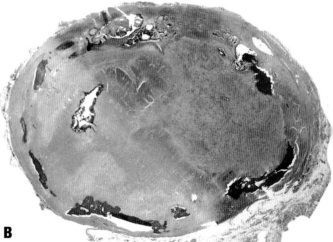

Fig. 1.332 Ossifying fibromyxoid tumour. **A** A well-demarcated tumour in the subcutis, whitish and translucent in gross appearance. **B** Low magnification reveals a partial rim of metaplastic bone.

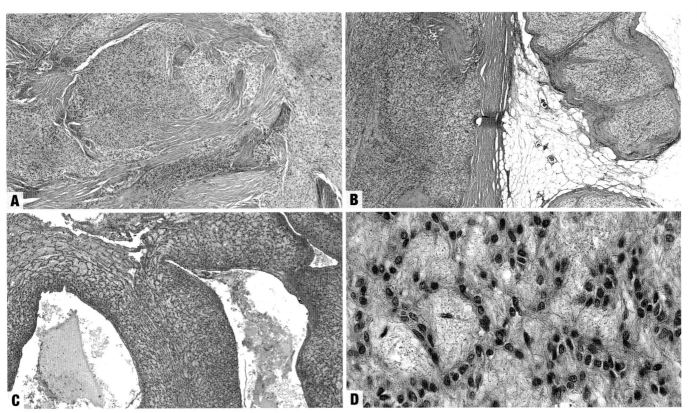

Fig. 1.333 Ossifying fibromyxoid tumour. **A** Multinodular pattern. **B** Satellite nodules in the surrounding fat. **C** Trabecular architecture with focal cystic change. **D** The characteristic architectural and cytological features of ossifying fibromyxoid tumour. Note the varying trabecular and solid patterns, delicate nucleoli, and mitotic figures.

usually well circumscribed and nodular or multinodular, and they are generally covered by a thick fibrous pseudocapsule with or without a shell of bone {918,2123,1059,3387}. The cut surface of the tumour is often glistening; white to tan in colour; and firm, hard, or rubbery in texture {1059,3387}.

Histopathology

Microscopically, OFMTs are generally well circumscribed, with a thick fibrous capsule or pseudocapsule {918,2123,1059}. Dense fibrous septa often extend into the tumour, producing a multinodular appearance. A complete or incomplete peripheral shell of metaplastic woven or lamellar bone is present in many cases {1059}. Bone may also be present in fibrous septa. Despite apparent circumscription at low power, tumour may invade through the capsule and form extracapsular nodules in adjacent tissue {2123}. The tumour is composed of lobules of uniform, round to spindle-shaped cells with bland round to ovoid nuclei and scant, pale eosinophilic cytoplasm {1059}. Tumour cells are usually arranged in cords, nests, or sheets, surrounded by variably fibrous or myxoid stroma. Cellularity

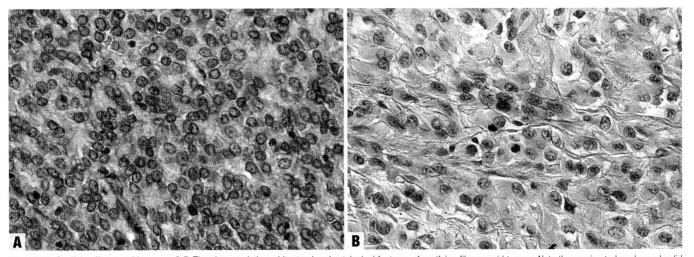

Fig. 1.334 Ossifying fibromyxoid tumour. **A,B** The characteristic architectural and cytological features of ossifying fibromyxoid tumour. Note the varying trabecular and solid patterns, delicate nucleoli, and mitotic figures.

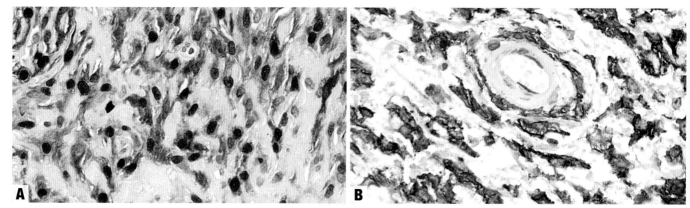

Fig. 1.335 Ossifying fibromyxoid tumour. **A** These tumours typically show both nuclear and cytoplasmic immunopositivity for S100. **B** CD10 immunoreactivity.

varies from low to moderate to high {2770}. Mitotic activity is usually low in typical OFMTs {2770}. About two thirds of OFMTs are positive for S100, although immunoreactivity is rarely diffuse {1206}. Desmin expression is observed in almost half of OFMTs. The lesions may also express MUC4, EMA, keratins, and SMA {1205}. SMARCB1 (INI1) expression is lost in a mosaic pattern in about three quarters of OFMTs {905,1206}. A malignant subtype has been proposed by some, as defined by cases with high nuclear grade or high cellularity and > 2 mitoses per 10 mm² (equating to ~50 high-power fields of 0.5 mm in diameter and 0.2 mm² in area) {1059,730}. In clinically malignant lesions, bone or osteoid deposition within tumour cell nodules may also be identified. OFMTs with histological findings deviating a little from typical OFMT, but not fulfilling these criteria for the malignant subtype, can be classified pragmatically as atypical OFMT.

Cytology
Not clinically relevant

Diagnostic molecular pathology
Demonstration of *PHF1* and/or *TFE3* gene rearrangement can be helpful.

Essential and desirable diagnostic criteria
Essential: lobulated growth pattern with frequent capsular ossification; usually very bland cytology with uniform round to ovoid nuclei; frequent (but not invariable) positivity for S100 and/or desmin.
Desirable: PHF1 gene rearrangement (in selected cases).

Staging
American Joint Committee on Cancer (AJCC) or Union for International Cancer Control (UICC) TNM staging can be applied to the malignant subtype.

Prognosis and prediction
Follow-up data indicate that even typical OFMT has the unpredictable potential for recurrence and metastasis. This is often delayed and may occur 10–20 years or more after the primary excision. The local recurrence rates for typical, atypical, and malignant OFMTs, respectively, are reported as 0–12%, 0–13%, and 0–60% {1059,182,730,1205}. The common metastatic sites are lung and soft tissue. The metastasis rates for typical, atypical, and malignant OFMTs, respectively, are reported as 0–4%, 0–6%, and 20–60% {1059,182,730,1205}.

Myoepithelioma, myoepithelial carcinoma, and mixed tumour

Jo VY
Antonescu CR
Hornick JL
Patel RM

Definition

Myoepithelioma, myoepithelial carcinoma, and mixed tumour are myoepithelial tumours of soft tissue – a group of uncommon neoplasms that share morphological, immunophenotypic, and genetic features with their counterparts in salivary gland and skin. Benign myoepithelial tumours of soft tissue include myoepithelioma and mixed tumour. Malignant myoepithelial tumours of soft tissue are designated myoepithelial carcinomas.

ICD-O coding

8982/0 Myoepithelioma NOS
8940/0 Mixed tumour NOS

ICD-11 coding

2F7C & XH3CQ8 Neoplasms of uncertain behaviour of connective or other soft tissue & Myoepithelioma

Related terminology

Not recommended: parachordoma.

Subtype(s)

Myoepithelial carcinoma; mixed tumour, malignant, NOS

Localization

Most myoepithelial tumours of soft tissue (75%) arise on the limbs and limb girdles (lower more frequently than upper); others arise on the trunk and less often the head and neck {1411, 1166,143}. Rarely, tumours arise in bone or visceral organs {143, 1790,1721}. Tumours may also arise primarily in the skin {1408, 1035,1531}.

Clinical features

Most patients present with a palpable mass, which is usually painless {1625,1411,1166}. Tumours arise in subcutaneous tissue somewhat more often than in deep soft tissue {2114,1411}.

Epidemiology

Myoepithelial tumours of soft tissue show equal distribution between the sexes and a wide age range, with peak incidence

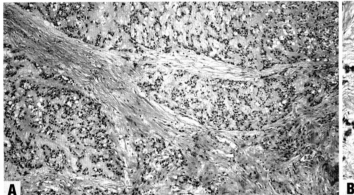
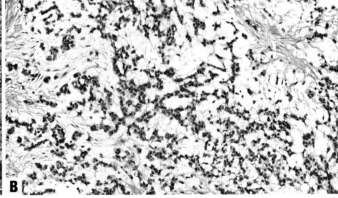

Fig. 1.336 Myoepithelial tumour of soft tissue. **A** Lobulated growth with reticular and trabecular patterns and myxoid stroma. **B** Epithelioid and spindle cells with eosinophilic cytoplasm arranged in trabeculae.

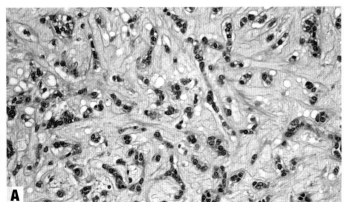
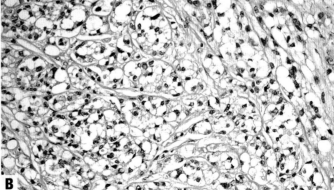

Fig. 1.337 Myoepithelioma. **A** Bland-appearing ovoid and epithelioid cells with uniform nuclei and eosinophilic cytoplasm. **B** Tumour cells may show clear cell change.

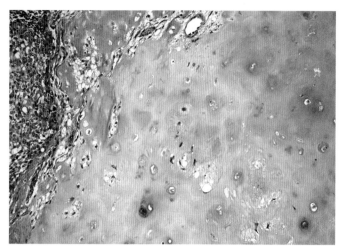

Fig. 1.338 Myoepithelioma. Cartilaginous and/or osseous differentiation is seen in about 10% of cases.

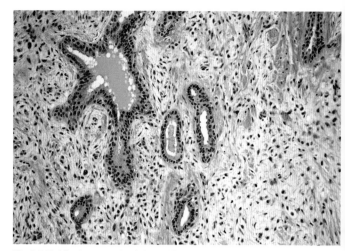

Fig. 1.340 Mixed tumour of soft tissue. Tumours show ductal differentiation and are indistinguishable from salivary pleomorphic adenoma.

in young to middle-aged adults (median age: 40 years) {1625, 2114,1411,1166}. About 20% of tumours, most of which are myoepithelial carcinomas, arise in the paediatric population {1166}.

Etiology
Unknown

Pathogenesis
EWSR1 gene rearrangements are common in myoepithelial tumours of soft tissue (as well as in those of skin and bone) {143}. The largest study to date reported *EWSR1* gene rearrangements in half of the soft tissue lesions tested, with the common fusion partners *POU5F1* and *PBX1* identified in 16% of cases each {143}. Rare fusion partners include *ZNF444*, *KLF17*, *ATF1*, and *PBX3*, and occasional cases show alternative *FUS* gene rearrangements with similar partner genes {143,1431,31,1034}. These studies have suggested some associations between genotype and phenotype. Most *EWSR1-POU5F1*–positive tumours present in deep soft tissues of the extremities in young patients and are composed of nests of epithelioid cells with clear cytoplasm; a subset of *EWSR1-PBX1*–positive tumours showed a deceptively bland and sclerotic appearance {143}. A

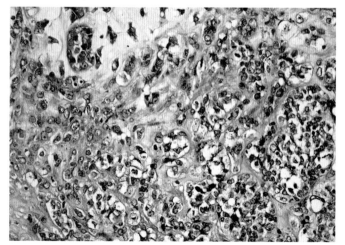

Fig. 1.339 Myoepithelial carcinoma. Nuclei show appreciable atypia and readily identifiable nucleoli.

subset of myoepithelial carcinomas have homozygous deletions of *SMARCB1* {1790}. Mixed tumours with ductal differentiation have *PLAG1* gene rearrangements (occasionally with *LIFR* as the fusion partner) {202,145}. The presence of rearrangements of *PLAG1* {1995} and *EWSR1* {2883}, respectively, in salivary gland pleomorphic adenoma and myoepithelial carcinoma emphasizes that soft tissue myoepithelial neoplasms are genetically related to their salivary gland counterparts.

Macroscopic appearance
Most benign myoepithelial tumours are grossly well circumscribed and nodular, whereas malignant tumours typically have infiltrative margins. The cut surface ranges from gelatinous and glistening to firm or fleshy. Tumour size range is broad (1–20 cm in greatest dimension), with a mean size of 4–6 cm {1166,1411, 2114}.

Histopathology
Myoepithelial tumours show a wide morphological spectrum of architectural and cytological heterogeneity, similar to their salivary gland and skin counterparts. Many show a predominantly reticular or trabecular growth pattern with prominent myxoid stroma; areas of more nested or solid growth and hyalinized stroma are commonly observed and occasionally predominate {1411,1166,143}. Tumour cells range from spindled to epithelioid with uniform nuclei and eosinophilic to clear cytoplasm. Studies have suggested some associations between genotype and phenotype (see *Pathogenesis*, above). Some tumours have large epithelioid cells showing prominent cytoplasmic vacuolation (and were classified as parachordoma in the past {700,1044}), whereas others may show predominantly spindled morphology, including the cutaneous syncytial subtype {1531}. Plasmacytoid cells with hyaline cytoplasmic inclusions may be prominent {991, 1625,1411}. Osseous or cartilaginous differentiation is observed in 10–15% of cases, whereas squamous or adipocytic metaplasia is more rare {1411}. Mixed tumours show a ductal component and account for approximately 10% of all myoepithelial lesions. Myoepithelial carcinomas are defined as having nuclear atypia with easily discerned nucleoli, often together with a high mitotic count and necrosis. Some such tumours (especially in children) may show undifferentiated round cell morphology {1411,1166}.

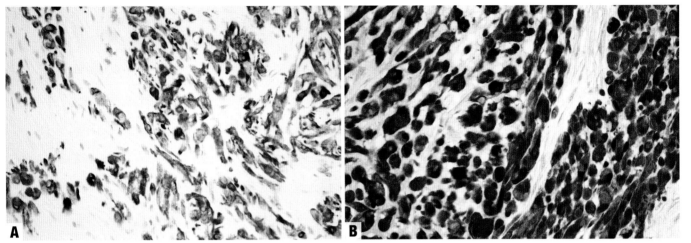

Fig. 1.341 Myoepithelioma. **A** Most cases show strong keratin immunoreactivity (CAM5.2 shown here). **B** S100 is positive in most cases.

Immunohistochemistry is necessary to confirm myoepithelial differentiation, although expression of myoepithelial markers is often variable. More than 90% of tumours express broad-spectrum keratins and S100 {1166,1411,2114}. Other frequently positive markers are EMA (~70%), GFAP (~50%), and SOX10 (~80%; lower in carcinomas) {1166,1411,2131}. p63 is positive in a subset of tumours {1411,1532}. Myogenic markers are more variable, with calponin being most frequent (90%), followed by SMA (60%) and desmin (0–20%) {1625,1411}. PLAG1 is positive in mixed tumours, correlating with *PLAG1* gene rearrangement {202}. Loss of expression of SMARCB1 (INI1) is observed in a subset of myoepithelial carcinomas {1166,1406,1790}.

Cytology

Aspirate smears of myoepithelial tumours of soft tissue, similar to those of their salivary gland counterparts, show variably spindle, epithelioid, and plasmacytoid cells embedded within fibrillary myxoid stromal fragments {3226,1928}. Rhabdoid morphology may be seen, and myoepithelial carcinoma shows appreciable cytological atypia {1928}.

Diagnostic molecular pathology

Rearrangements of *EWSR1*, *FUS*, or *PLAG1* (in mixed tumours) can be detected. *EWSR1* FISH alone may not be sufficient for distinguishing myoepithelial neoplasms from other tumours with *EWSR1* fusions.

Essential and desirable diagnostic criteria

Essential: trabecular, reticular, nested, and/or solid growth of variably spindled or epithelioid cells with a frequent myxoid or hyalinized stroma; mixed tumours in addition show ductal differentiation; myoepithelial carcinomas show increased cytological atypia and mitotic activity; positivity for EMA/keratin and S100, SOX10, or GFAP.

Desirable (in selected cases): EWSR1 rearrangements may be helpful.

Staging

Not clinically relevant

Prognosis and prediction

Most myoepithelial tumours of soft tissue show benign or indolent behaviour. The only reliable criterion for malignancy is the presence of moderate to severe nuclear atypia with discernible nucleoli {1411}. Histologically benign tumours have a 20% risk of recurrence, but they rarely metastasize, whereas myoepithelial carcinomas recur and metastasize in 40–50% of cases {1411, 1166}. Common sites of metastasis include lungs, lymph nodes, bone, and soft tissue {1411,1166}.

Pleomorphic hyalinizing angiectatic tumour of soft parts

Agaimy A
Dei Tos AP
Folpe AL

Definition

Pleomorphic hyalinizing angiectatic tumour (PHAT) of soft parts is a very rare, locally recurring, non-metastasizing neoplasm characterized by ectatic, fibrin-filled blood vessels surrounded by a cellular proliferation of pleomorphic, haemosiderin-laden cells with very few mitotic figures.

ICD-O coding

8802/1 Pleomorphic hyalinizing angiectatic tumour

ICD-11 coding

2F7C & XH2193 Neoplasms of uncertain behaviour of connective or other soft tissue & Pleomorphic hyalinizing angiectatic tumour

Related terminology

Acceptable: haemosiderotic fibrolipomatous tumour; early pleomorphic hyalinizing angiectatic tumour.

Subtype(s)

None

Localization

PHAT develops most often in subcutaneous tissue of the lower extremities, mainly in the region of the ankle/foot, and rarely as a deep-seated soft tissue mass in locations such as perineum, buttock, and arm {2895,1060}.

Clinical features

PHAT most often presents as a longstanding subcutaneous mass. Many cases clinically mimic a vascular tumour, such as haemangioma or Kaposi sarcoma.

Epidemiology

Affected patients have ranged from 10 to 79 years of age (median: 51 years). A slight female predilection is seen.

Etiology

Unknown

Pathogenesis

Many PHATs demonstrate peripheral zones of haemosiderotic fibrolipomatous tumour (HFLT), and foci resembling PHAT are frequently present in HFLT, findings suggesting that PHAT and HFLT represent different manifestations of a single entity {495, 1060}. This concept is also supported by genetic data, with TGFBR3 and/or OGA (MGEA5) rearrangements found in substantial subsets of both PHAT and HFLT {495,3407}. Tumours showing histological overlap between myxoinflammatory fibroblastic sarcoma and HFLT have been reported {353,3407,495, 1877,144}, suggesting a link between these two tumour types as well, but this remains incompletely understood and controversial.

Macroscopic appearance

Grossly, most PHATs appear lobulated, with a cut surface that varies from whitish-tan to maroon. Cystic or myxoid areas may be seen. Most tumours are 5–10 cm in size {2895,1060}.

Histopathology

At low-power magnification, PHAT is most notable for clusters of variably sized, thin-walled, ectatic blood vessels scattered throughout the lesion {2895,1060}. These ectatic vessels are surrounded by a thick rim of amorphous eosinophilic material, often with associated fibrosis. Organizing thrombi with papillary

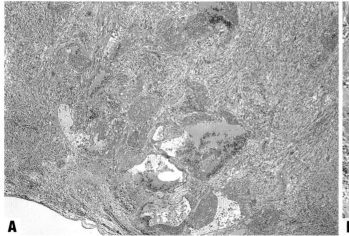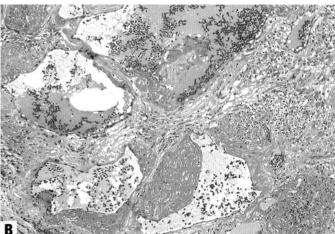

Fig. 1.342 Classic pleomorphic hyalinizing angiectatic tumour. **A** A dispersed mononuclear inflammatory component may be seen in the background stroma of pleomorphic hyalinizing angiectatic tumour. **B** Classic pleomorphic hyalinizing angiectatic tumour shows ectatic thin-walled vessels lined by fibrin-like hyaline material surrounded by paucicellular stroma containing spindled cells with variable nuclear pleomorphism.

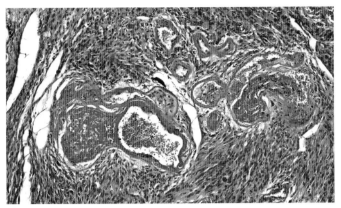

Fig. 1.343 Classic pleomorphic hyalinizing angiectatic tumour with *OGA* (*MGEA5*) gene fusion. Haemosiderotic changes are seen in the stromal cells.

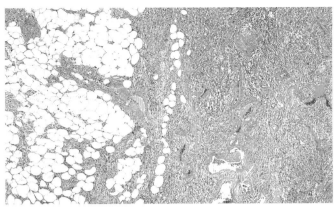

Fig. 1.345 Early pleomorphic hyalinizing angiectatic tumour. An example showing both haemosiderotic fibrolipomatous tumour–like features (left) and classic pleomorphic hyalinizing angiectatic tumour with increased cellularity and ectatic blood vessels (right).

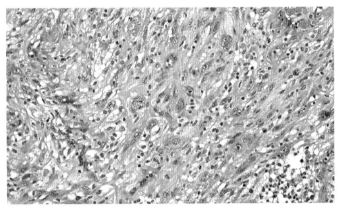

Fig. 1.344 Pleomorphic hyalinizing angiectatic tumour. Pleomorphic hyalinizing angiectatic tumour contains increased numbers of atypical stromal cells with lobulated large nuclei and prominent nucleoli.

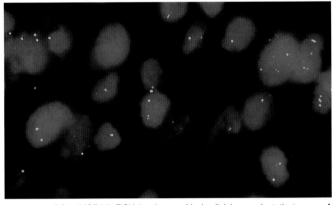

Fig. 1.346 *OGA* (*MGEA5*) FISH in pleomorphic hyalinizing angiectatic tumour. A subset of pleomorphic hyalinizing angiectatic tumours harbour *OGA* (*MGEA5*) gene fusions, as illustrated here by break-apart signals of the *OGA* (*MGEA5*) gene locus.

endothelial hyperplasia may be present. The tumour cells are arranged in sheets or fascicles and show epithelioid to spindled morphology, intracytoplasmic haemosiderin pigment, and strikingly pleomorphic nuclei with nuclear pseudoinclusions. Despite the pleomorphism, mitotic activity is very low. A mixed inflammatory infiltrate is frequently present, and psammomatous calcifications are sometimes seen. At the periphery, PHAT may show a variably myxoid proliferation of haemosiderin-laden, cytologically bland spindle cells with occasional nuclear pseudoinclusions, growing in an infiltrative fashion through adipose tissue – changes identical to those seen in HFLT (early PHAT) {1060}. Extremely rare PHATs showing mixed HFLT-like and classic morphology have shown morphological progression to mitotically active, pleomorphic myxoid sarcoma (myxofibrosarcoma-like) {495,2190,1601,1466}. By immunohistochemistry, PHAT expresses CD34.

Cytology
Not clinically relevant

Diagnostic molecular pathology
Some PHATs with a peripheral component of HFLT show rearrangements involving *TGFBR3* and/or *OGA* (*MGEA5*) {495,

1060}. One case of PHAT showing progression to myxoid sarcoma has been shown to be positive for *TGFBR3* and *OGA* (*MGEA5*) rearrangements {1060}. PHAT-like pleomorphic sarcomas are negative for these molecular genetic events.

Essential and desirable diagnostic criteria
Essential: clusters of ectatic vessels surrounded by pleomorphic, haemosiderin-laden cells with nuclear pseudoinclusions; very low to absent mitotic activity; peripheral component of HFLT often seen.
Desirable: *TGFBR3* and/or *OGA* (*MGEA5*) rearrangements (in selected cases).

Staging
Not clinically relevant

Prognosis and prediction
Roughly 50% of resected PHATs recur locally. Such local recurrences are usually curable with re-excision. The natural history of extremely rare PHATs showing morphological progression to myxoid sarcoma is not well defined.

Haemosiderotic fibrolipomatous tumour

Boland JM
Horvai AE
Mertens F

Definition

Haemosiderotic fibrolipomatous tumour (HFLT) is an unencapsulated, locally aggressive neoplasm composed of adipocytes, haemosiderin-laden spindle cells, and haemosiderin-laden macrophages.

ICD-O coding

8811/1 Haemosiderotic fibrolipomatous tumour

ICD-11 coding

2F7C & XH9526 Neoplasms of uncertain behaviour of connective or other soft tissue & Haemosiderotic fibrolipomatous tumour

Related terminology

Acceptable: haemosiderotic fibrohistiocytic lipomatous lesion.

Subtype(s)

None

Localization

The most dominant site by far is the foot, especially the dorsum and around the ankle, followed by the hand, calf, thigh, and cheek {437,1986}.

Clinical features

HFLT is a slow-growing, sometimes painful subcutaneous (or, less often, deeper) soft tissue mass {437,1986}. MRI shows an infiltrative fatty mass with haemosiderin deposition {2193, 2352}.

Epidemiology

HFLT has a female predominance, and it is most common in the fifth and sixth decades of life, but with a wide age range, including children {437,495}.

Etiology

Unknown

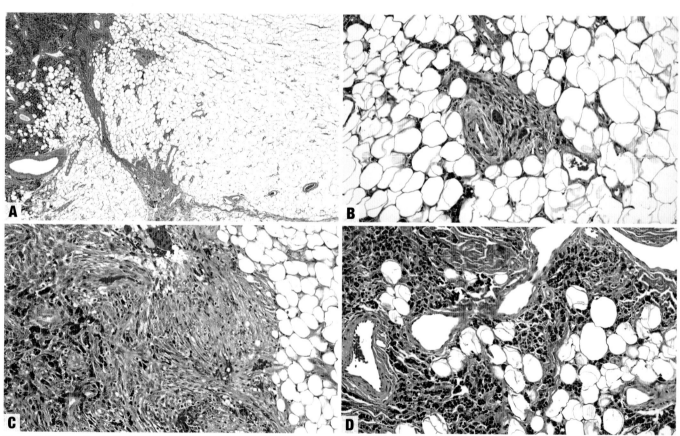

Fig. 1.347 Haemosiderotic fibrolipomatous tumour. **A** Low-magnification view of haemosiderotic fibrolipomatous tumour, containing mature adipose tissue and fibrous septa with spindled cells and macrophages containing conspicuous haemosiderin. **B** Perivascular collections of bland spindle cells and osteoclast-like giant cells. Note also haemosiderin in some spindle cells. **C** Collections of haemosiderin-laden macrophages are observed admixed with the bland spindle cells; mitotic activity is low and necrosis is absent. **D** The spindle cells can be present between individual adipocytes.

Pathogenesis

Cytogenetic analysis has shown near-diploid karyotypes with balanced or unbalanced t(1;10)(p22-p31;q24-q25), loss of material from 3p, and amplification of 3p11-p12 {3279,1279, 144}. The t(1;10) does not result in a fusion transcript but always targets *TGFBR3* in 1p22, demonstrates breakpoints in or near *OGA* (formerly *MGEA5*) in 10q24, and leads to transcriptional upregulation of neighbouring *FGF8* and *NPM3* {1279}. The t(1;10) has been found in as many as 85% of HFLTs {144}. The amplicon in 3p contains *VGLL3* and *CHMP2B*, which show increased expression {1279}. Similar karyotypes, rearrangement of *TGFBR3* and *OGA*, and amplification of *VGLL3* have also been observed in myxoinflammatory fibroblastic sarcoma {1279,144} and pleomorphic hyalinizing angiectatic tumour of soft parts {3261,3407}, suggesting a pathogenetic link between these entities {1877,495,3407}. *BRAF* fusions are present in some myxoinflammatory fibroblastic sarcomas, but they have not been detected in HFLT {1577}.

Macroscopic appearance

Tumour size averages 7.7 cm but can reach as large as 19 cm {437,1986}. HFLT is poorly circumscribed, dark yellowish-brown, and friable, with occasional haemorrhage.

Histopathology

HFLT consists of lobules of mature fat admixed in variable proportions with fascicles of fibroblastic spindle cells containing haemosiderin, haemosiderin-laden macrophages, and osteoclast-like giant cells {437,1986}. In areas, the spindle cells are distributed more loosely in smaller numbers and often extend between individual adipocytes and around vessels {1986,437}. Occasional larger cells with atypical nuclei are sometimes present. Mitotic activity is low and necrosis is absent. Nuclear pseudoinclusions and large, ectatic, partially thrombosed vessels with perivascular hyalinization are sometimes present, leading to morphological overlap with pleomorphic hyalinizing angiectatic tumour {437,1986}. Areas resembling HFLT may be observed at the edge of pleomorphic hyalinizing angiectatic tumour {1060}. Rare cases of HFLT may unpredictably recur as myxoid sarcoma with histological features of hybrid HFLT–myxoinflammatory fibroblastic sarcoma {3407,2903,144}. The spindled cells of HFLT are usually positive for CD34 and calponin {437,1986}.

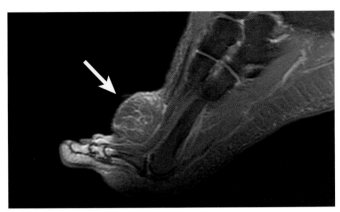

Fig. 1.348 Haemosiderotic fibrolipomatous tumour. Sagittal view of fat-saturated T1-weighted fast spin echo MRI sequences of the foot shows a heterogeneous, predominantly fatty subcutaneous soft tissue mass (arrow). The mass abuts but does not invade the dorsal neurovascular structures and extensor tendons.

Cytology

Aspirates typically show a variably cellular mixture of mature adipose tissue and bland, monotonous spindle cells, a subset of which contain haemosiderin, along with haemosiderin-laden macrophages {2190}.

Diagnostic molecular pathology

Demonstration of t(1;10)(p22;q24) or *OGA* and *TGFBR3* rearrangement may be helpful.

Essential and desirable diagnostic criteria

Essential: mature adipose tissue admixed with bland haemosiderin-laden spindle cells and macrophages.

Desirable: demonstration of t(1;10)(p22;q24), *OGA*, and/or *TGFBR3* rearrangement (in selected cases).

Staging

Not clinically relevant

Prognosis and prediction

The local recurrence rate is 30–50%, especially if the tumour is incompletely excised {1986,2193}. The recurrence rate can be reduced by complete surgical resection. Metastases have not been reported in pure HFLT, but rare tumours with transformation to sarcoma may result in distant metastasis {2903,2190}.

Phosphaturic mesenchymal tumour

Lee JC
Folpe AL

Definition
Phosphaturic mesenchymal tumours (PMTs) are morphologically distinctive neoplasms that cause tumour-induced osteomalacia (TIO) in most affected patients, usually through production of FGF23.

ICD-O coding
8990/0 Phosphaturic mesenchymal tumour NOS

ICD-11 coding
2F7C & XH9T96 Neoplasms of uncertain behaviour of connective or other soft tissue & Phosphaturic mesenchymal tumour, benign
2F7C & XH3B27 Neoplasms of uncertain behaviour of connective or other soft tissue & Phosphaturic mesenchymal tumour, malignant

Related terminology
Acceptable: phosphaturic mesenchymal tumour, mixed connective tissue type.

Subtype(s)
Phosphaturic mesenchymal tumour, malignant

Localization
PMTs may involve essentially any somatic soft tissue location {206,1049,3263,1806}. PMTs are extremely rare in the retroperitoneum, viscera, and mediastinum {3112,2806}. A substantial subset of cases occur in bone {206,1049,1806,25}.

Clinical features
Most PMTs present as small, inapparent lesions that may require very careful clinical examination and radionuclide scans (preferably 68Ga-DOTATATE PET-CT) for localization {2858,1116,619,897}. A long history of osteomalacia is usually present. PMTs are responsible for the overwhelming majority of previously reported cases of mesenchymal tumour–associated TIO, despite often being reported with other diagnoses {1049}. Severe hypophosphataemia and elevated serum levels of FGF23 can be demonstrated in patients with TIO. So-called non-phosphaturic PMTs in most instances represent small, superficial PMTs identified before the onset of TIO {206}.

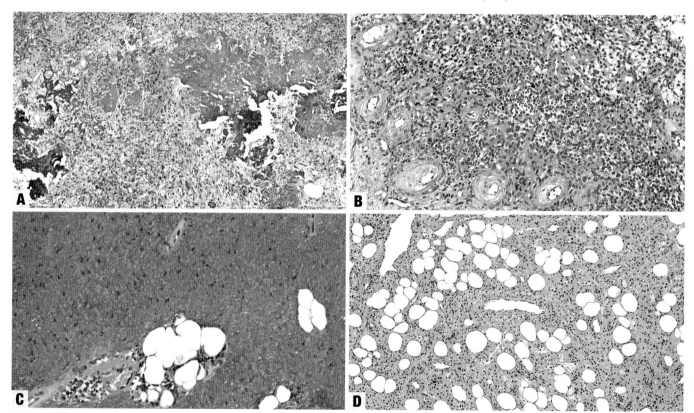

Fig. 1.349 Phosphaturic mesenchymal tumour is usually characterized by focal presence of grungy calcification (**A**) and composed of bland spindle cells with a rich vascular network (**B**). **C** Some cases are hypocellular and comprise mainly basophilic matrix. **D** Adipocytic component and/or staghorn vessels are common.

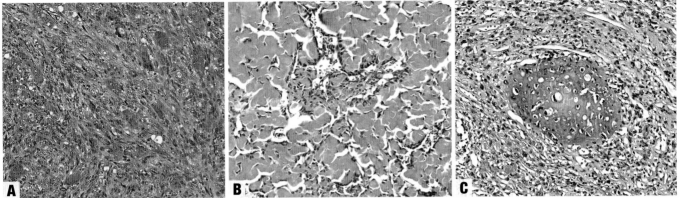

Fig. 1.350 Phosphaturic mesenchymal tumour. **A** Areas rich in osteoclastic giant cells may resemble giant cell tumour of bone or soft tissue. **B** Osteoblastoma-like phosphaturic mesenchymal tumour with prominent osteoid deposition. **C** Phosphaturic mesenchymal tumour with chondroid matrix and nuclear atypia, mimicking chondrosarcoma.

Epidemiology

PMTs are exceptionally rare, probably accounting for < 0.01% of all soft tissue tumours {206,1049,3263,1806,25}. They most commonly affect middle-aged adults of either sex (with approximately equal sex distribution), but they can also occur in paediatric or elderly patients {1049,25,492,3412}.

Etiology

The etiology of PMT is unknown. In a unique case, a germline chromosomal rearrangement causing α-Klotho upregulation may have predisposed the patient to later develop multiple PMTs {1806,438}.

Pathogenesis

Nearly half of all PMTs contain either *FN1-FGFR1* or, rarely, *FN1-FGF1* fusion {1806,1803}. FGFR1 expression is common in PMTs regardless of the fusion status {3023,1803}. These findings suggest that activated receptor tyrosine kinase FGFR1 signalling pathways could drive PMT tumorigenesis and upregulation of FGF23. Excess production of FGF23, a phosphaturic hormone that acts to inhibit renal proximal tubule phosphate reuptake, is responsible for TIO in most instances {2845,2846,388,1709, 1708}. However, low-level expression of FGF23 can also occasionally be identified in non-PMT tumours, including occasional cases of fibrous dysplasia {2634}, aneurysmal bone cyst, and chondromyxoid fibroma of bone {1204}. Rare cases of PMT with known TIO are FGF23-negative, presumably reflecting production of other phosphaturic hormones.

Macroscopic appearance

Most PMTs present as nonspecific soft tissue or bone masses, often with a component of fat. Some may be highly calcified.

Histopathology

PMTs are usually composed of bland, spindle to stellate cells, which produce an unusual hyalinized to smudgy-appearing matrix. A very well developed capillary network is typically present, with some cases also showing larger vessels arranged in a staghorn pericytoma-like pattern, or in a pattern resembling cavernous haemangioma. The matrix of PMT typically calcifies in an unusual grungy or flocculent fashion, sometimes forming flower-like slate-grey crystals, and in some instances it may

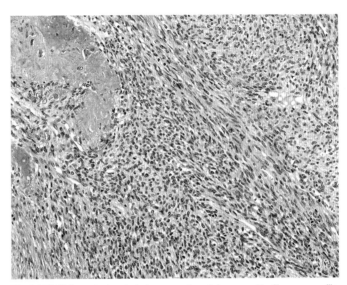

Fig. 1.351 Malignant phosphaturic mesenchymal tumour with fibrosarcoma-like pattern.

contain foci closely resembling primitive cartilage or osteoid {206,1049,3263,2830}. Osteoclasts, fibrohistiocytic spindled cells, mature adipose tissue, microcystic change, and a peripheral shell of woven bone may be present. Mitotic activity and necrosis are usually absent. In the jaws, PMTs with admixed epithelial (odontogenic) elements have been described. It is unclear whether these epithelial elements are neoplastic or entrapped/induced by the adjacent PMT {3314}.

Malignant PMT most often develops in lesions that have recurred locally, often more than once, and then show obvious features of malignancy including high nuclear grade, marked pleomorphism, high cellularity, necrosis, and elevated mitotic activity, resembling undifferentiated pleomorphic sarcoma or fibrosarcoma {1049,2355,3136}.

By immunohistochemistry, most PMTs express CD56, ERG, FGFR1, SATB2, and/or SSTR2A {1806,25,3327,3023}. Expression of FGF23 protein has been documented in some cases of PMT, although commercially available antibodies to FGF23 have questionable specificity and are not widely available {1049,206}.

Cytology

Isolated case reports have noted bland spindle cells with finely granular chromatin, indistinct nucleoli, and scant delicate cytoplasm; scattered osteoclasts associated with stromal matrix can also been found {2523,3296}.

Diagnostic molecular pathology

Detection of *FN1-FGFR1* or *FN1-FGF1* fusion is confirmatory but not required for routine diagnosis of PMT.

Essential and desirable diagnostic criteria

Essential: a usually bland spindle cell tumour with matrix deposition, grungy calcification, and/or a rich vascular network; clinical evidence of hypophosphataemia and/or osteomalacia, corrected by complete tumour excision.

Desirable: FGF23 overproduction in the serum or in the neoplastic tissue (in selected cases).

Staging

Not clinically relevant

Prognosis and prediction

The overwhelming majority of PMTs are histologically and clinically benign, with complete excision resulting in dramatic improvement of phosphate wasting and osteomalacia {1049, 1708,1141,755}. Malignant tumours may metastasize and cause death.

NTRK-rearranged spindle cell neoplasm (emerging)

Suurmeijer AJH
Antonescu CR

Definition
NTRK-rearranged spindle cell neoplasms (outside infantile fibrosarcomas) represent an emerging group of molecularly defined rare soft tissue tumours, spanning a wide spectrum of morphologies and histological grades and showing frequent coexpression of S100 and CD34 by immunohistochemistry. The tumours are most often characterized by a monomorphic spindle cell phenotype, variable stromal hyalinization, and infiltrative growth. This provisional category includes the recently described lipofibromatosis-like neural tumours and tumours that closely resemble peripheral nerve sheath tumours (PNSTs).

ICD-O coding
None

ICD-11 coding
None

Related terminology
Acceptable: lipofibromatosis-like neural tumour; NTRK-positive tumour resembling peripheral nerve sheath tumour.

Subtype(s)
None

Localization
Most tumours present as superficial or deep tumours in the extremities or trunk.

Clinical features
Most tumours present as a palpable, non-tender mass.

Epidemiology
Most tumours occur in the first two decades of life, with lipofibromatosis-like neural tumours presenting predominantly in children (median age: 13.5 years) {40}. More than half of the NTRK-rearranged tumours resembling PNSTs occur in the paediatric age group; the remaining cases have had a wide age range at diagnosis {3004}.

Etiology
Unknown

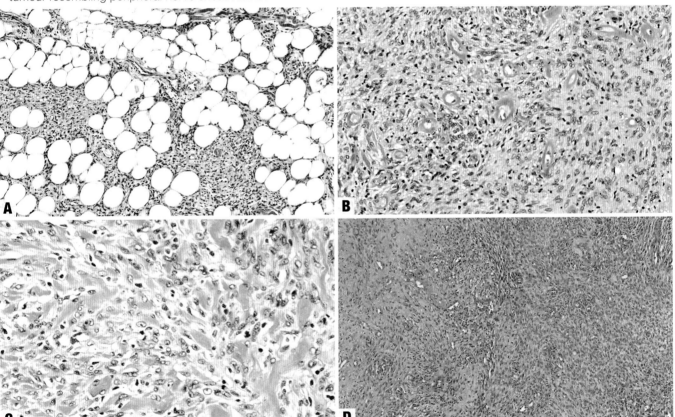

Fig. 1.352 NTRK-rearranged spindle cell neoplasm. **A** Spindle cell tumour infiltrating fat in a reticular fashion reminiscent of lipofibromatosis. **B** Monomorphic spindle cell tumour with patternless architecture and distinctive stromal and perivascular collagen deposition. **C,D** Areas with increased cellularity and thick stromal collagen bands.

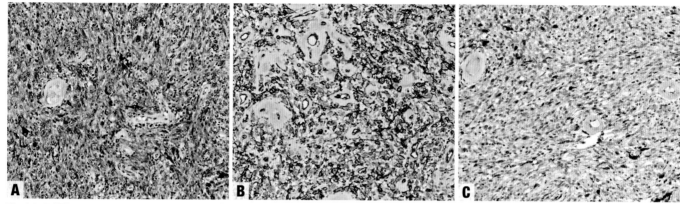

Fig. 1.353 NTRK-rearranged spindle cell neoplasm. **A** TRK-A/B/C expression by immunohistochemistry. **B** CD34 expression by immunohistochemistry. **C** S100 expression by immunohistochemistry.

Pathogenesis

Most tumours harbour *NTRK1* fusions with a variety of partners, resulting mostly from intrachromosomal interstitial deletions (*LMNA*) or inversions (*TPR*, *TPM3*) {40,3004,1275}. Rare cases involving *NTRK2* and *NTRK3* fusions have also been reported {3004,3344}. The NTRK fusions result in oncogenic pathway activation via chimeric proteins that contain the tropomyosin receptor kinase domains of TRK-A, TRK-B, and TRK-C {621}. Tumours with similar morphology resembling PNSTs have also been shown to harbour alternative *RAF1* and *BRAF* fusions {3004}. None of these tumours have been reported to be associated with neurofibromatosis type 1.

Macroscopic appearance

The macroscopic appearance of NTRK-rearranged spindle cell neoplasms has not yet been defined.

Histopathology

NTRK-rearranged spindle cell neoplasms appear to form a morphological spectrum. At one end of this spectrum is the so-called lipofibromatosis-like neural tumour, which is defined by haphazardly arranged monomorphic spindle cells, with tapering nuclei and indistinct cytoplasm. It shows a highly infiltrative pattern within subcutaneous fat, resembling lipofibromatosis {40}. Although some examples have areas of increased cellularity and mild cytological atypia, they are associated with a low mitotic count and lack necrosis.

Another subset of cases have a solid growth pattern, comprising a moderately to highly cellular proliferation of uniform spindle cells arranged in streaming or patternless patterns. A diagnostic hallmark of this subset is the prominent stromal bands and perivascular rings of keloid-like hyalinized collagen {3004}. A few cases showing infiltrative growth within the fat resembling lipofibromatosis-like neural tumour have also been reported, suggesting a potential pathogenetic link between these two phenotypes {3004}. Several tumours have a zoned appearance, where cellular areas merge with paucicellular zones with collagenous or myxoid stroma, resembling malignant PNST.

Tumours in this group encompass a wide histological spectrum, with most being of low grade, but some display a higher-grade phenotype, with markedly increased cellularity arranged in intersecting fascicles, with a high mitotic count. Necrosis may be present {743}. A less common presentation of *NTRK1*-rearranged sarcoma includes tumours with a myopericytoma-like architecture {1275}.

Immunohistochemically, most tumours show coexpression of S100 and CD34, in the absence of SOX10 reactivity {40,743}, whereas H3K27me3 expression is retained. The majority of tumours with NTRK fusions are reactive with an anti–pan-TRK monoclonal antibody {1442}; the staining can be either cytoplasmic or nuclear {1338,1442}. TRK-A immunohistochemistry is useful for the detection of *NTRK1*-rearranged tumours {2688}. Importantly, pan-TRK and TRK-A immunoreactivity is not completely specific, and additional molecular genetic testing is often required for a conclusive diagnosis. Tumours with similar morphology but alternative *RAF1* or *BRAF* fusions share a similar S100 and CD34 immunoprofile {743}.

Cytology

Not clinically relevant

Diagnostic molecular pathology

Molecular detection of NTRK fusions can be useful {743,3004}.

Essential and desirable diagnostic criteria

Essential: tumours span a wide spectrum of morphologies and histological grades; characterized by haphazardly arranged monomorphic spindle cells; infiltrative growth within fat resembling lipofibromatosis; distinctive stromal and perivascular keloid collagen; immunohistochemically tumours are positive for S100 and CD34 in many cases, whereas SOX10 is negative; tumours with *NTRK1* fusions will show NTRK1 immunoreactivity.

Desirable: detection of NTRK fusions is usually required for determination of therapy.

Staging

Staging is only applicable to the malignant subset. The American Joint Committee on Cancer (AJCC) or Union for International Cancer Control (UICC) TNM system may be used.

Prognosis and prediction

The prognosis of NTRK-rearranged adult tumours appears to be related to histological grade. Due to their infiltrative growth pattern, the benign lipofibromatosis-like neural tumours have a propensity for local recurrence if incompletely excised, but none were shown to metastasize {40}. Tumours with high-grade morphological features may show aggressive clinical behaviour, with metastatic spread to lungs and other organs. Importantly, the aberrantly expressed oncogenic receptor tyrosine kinases TRK-A, TRK-B, and TRK-C in NTRK-rearranged sarcomas have proven to be therapeutically targetable, which may potentially improve patient outcome.

Synovial sarcoma

Suurmeijer AJH
Ladanyi M
Nielsen TO

Definition

Synovial sarcoma (SS) is a monomorphic blue spindle cell sarcoma showing variable epithelial differentiation. SS is characterized by a specific *SS18-SSX1/2/4* fusion gene.

ICD-O coding

9040/3 Synovial sarcoma NOS

ICD-11 coding

2B5A.Y & XH9B22 Synovial sarcoma, other specified primary site & Synovial sarcoma NOS

Related terminology

Not recommended: synoviosarcoma.

Subtype(s)

Synovial sarcoma, spindle cell; synovial sarcoma, biphasic; synovial sarcoma, poorly differentiated

Localization

The majority (70%) of SSs arise in the deep soft tissue of the lower and upper extremities, often in juxta-articular locations. About 15% arise in the trunk and 7% in the head and neck region {2984}. Unusual sites of involvement include male and female external and internal reproductive organs, kidney, adrenal gland, retroperitoneum, stomach, small bowel, lung, heart, mediastinum, bone, CNS, and peripheral nerve {1010,251, 2762}.

Clinical features

SS usually presents as a swelling (sometimes longstanding), which may be painful. The initial growth of SS is often slow, and a small circumscribed tumour may give the wrong impression of a benign lesion by clinical examination and imaging {333}. SS may have radiologically detectable stippled or spiculated forms of calcification {3292}. SS with aggressive growth may erode or invade adjacent bone.

Epidemiology

SS may occur at any age and is equally distributed between the sexes {2984}. More than half of the patients are adolescents or young adults, and 77% of cases occur before the age of 50 years. The relative frequency of SS compared with other soft tissue sarcomas is age-dependent, ranging from 15% in patients aged 10–18 years to 1.6% in patients aged > 50 years {2984}.

Etiology

There are no known predisposing factors. Exceptionally, SS is associated with a history of previous radiotherapy {1353}. SS bears a unique chromosomal translocation that results in the formation of an oncogenic *SS18-SSX1/2/4* fusion gene. Otherwise, SSs have a very low mutation burden relative to other sarcomas {472}.

Pathogenesis

SS cells are dependent on SS18-SSX expression to maintain their transformed phenotype {557}. Conditional expression of SS18-SSX induces SSs in genetically engineered mouse models, supporting its function as an oncogene when expressed in permissive mesenchymal progenitor cells {1544,225}. Additionally, SS18-SSX1 has been shown to transform primary cell lines {2235}. Recent evidence suggests that the SS18-SSX fusion protein disrupts epigenetic control and blocks mesenchymal differentiation by complementary mechanisms including competitive binding with, and displacement of, native SS18 in the SWI/SNF chromatin-remodelling complex {1559}, inducing dependency on BRD9-containing alternative SWI/SNF complexes (ncBAF complexes) {2115,422} and colocalizing with factors such as the ATF2 transcription factor, TLE1 to repress ATF2 target genes {2290}, and the KDM2B lysine demethylase at unmethylated CpG islands to reactivate repressed genes {218,2022}.

Macroscopic appearance

Most SSs are 3–10 cm in diameter at diagnosis. Minute lesions < 1 cm occur especially in hands and feet {2110}. On cut surface, tumour colour and consistency are proportionate to cellularity, collagenization, and myxoid change or haemorrhage. Areas may be tan or grey, yellowish or pink, and soft or firm {946}. SS is frequently multinodular and can be multicystic. Calcification, metaplastic ossification, and necrosis may be present.

Histopathology

Histologically, SSs are classified as biphasic (in approximately one quarter to one third of cases) or monophasic (in the majority). Biphasic SS has epithelial and spindle cell components, in varying proportions. The epithelial cells are arranged in solid nests or cords, or in glands with a tubular or sometimes alveolar or papillary architecture. In glandular areas, epithelial cells are cuboidal or columnar and have ovoid vesicular nuclei, and they typically have more-abundant palely eosinophilic cytoplasm than in the dark-blue spindle cell component. Glandular lumina contain epithelial mucin. Focally, the glandular component can predominate, and it may be confused with adenocarcinoma; however, a scant spindle cell component is virtually always found. Rarely, epithelial cells show (keratinizing) squamous metaplasia or granular cell change.

The spindle cells in biphasic SS resemble the spindle cells found in monophasic SS. These delicate spindle cells are fairly uniform and relatively small, with sparse cytoplasm and ovoid, hyperchromatic nuclei with regular granular chromatin and inconspicuous nucleoli. The N:C ratio is so high that the nuclei can appear to overlap. Typically, in both monophasic and biphasic SSs, the spindle cells are arranged in dense cellular sheets or vague fascicles, with occasional tigroid nuclear palisading or a herringbone architectural pattern. The amount of collagen is variable and usually scant, but SS may contain strands of ropy or wiry collagen, bands of hyalinized collagen, or (especially after irradiation) foci of dense fibrosis. Myxoid change is usually only focally present and rarely predominates, with alternating hypocellular and more-cellular areas, as well as retiform cords or microcysts {1694}. Many SSs focally display a staghorn-shaped vascular pattern, reminiscent of solitary fibrous tumour / haemangiopericytoma. Mast cells are variably present. In as many as one third of SSs, areas with calcification and/or ossification are found, which are sometimes abundant. In areas with ossification, the osteoid has a lace-like pattern mimicking osteosarcoma, and bone tissue can mature to the point of being lamellar and trabecular {2146}. Metaplastic cartilage is rarely seen.

In otherwise typical biphasic or monophasic SS, poorly differentiated areas with increased cellularity, greater nuclear atypia, and high mitotic activity (> 6 mitoses/mm^2 or > 10 mitoses per 10 high-power fields of 0.17 mm^2) may be found {1244}. Poorly differentiated areas may be composed of fascicular spindle cells (reminiscent of malignant peripheral nerve sheath tumour), small round hyperchromatic tumour cells (reminiscent of Ewing sarcoma), or epithelioid cells {273}. Compared with typical biphasic or monophasic SS, poorly differentiated areas more often contain areas of necrosis, a branching vascular pattern, and thin fibrovascular septa separating groups of tumour cells {765}. Poorly differentiated lesions are disproportionately more common in elderly patients {533}.

Immunohistochemistry
By immunohistochemistry, EMA is expressed more often and more widely in SS than cytokeratins, especially in the monophasic and poorly differentiated subtypes {2480}. Epithelial cells in biphasic SSs consistently express EMA and cytokeratins and

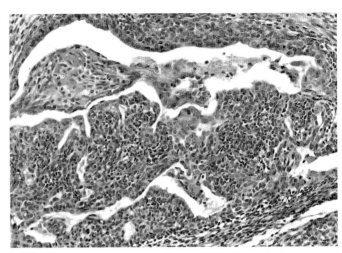

Fig. 1.355 Biphasic synovial sarcoma. Tumour with glandular epithelial component and spindle cell component.

may contain almost any cytokeratin subtype {2128}. Poorly differentiated areas of SS nearly always contain focal EMA, whereas cytokeratin expression is seen in only about 50% of these tumours {2128,2480}. Focal S100 expression may be detectable in as many as 40% of SSs {2480}. α-SMA is present in less than half of tumours, whereas focal desmin staining is exceptional and h-caldesmon is always negative {2480}. CD34 immunostaining is rare in monophasic SS {2480}. The large majority of SSs are positive for BCL2 and CD99 (which may show membranous staining like in Ewing sarcoma {2379}), but these markers are not specific. Moderate or strong nuclear

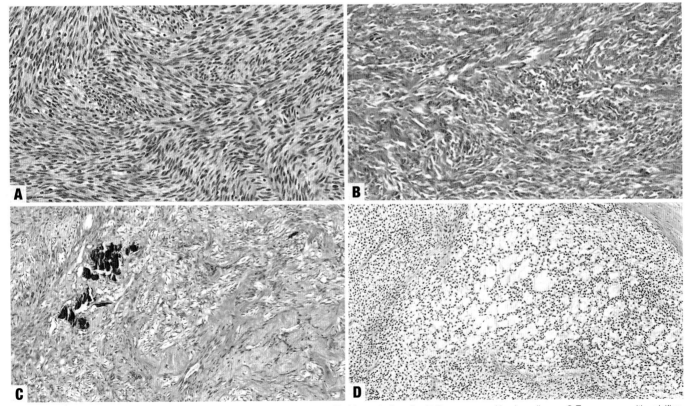

Fig. 1.354 Monophasic synovial sarcoma. **A** Tumour with fascicles of monomorphic blue spindle cells. **B** Tumour area with wiry collagen. **C** Tumour area with calcifications. **D** Tumour area with myxoid change.

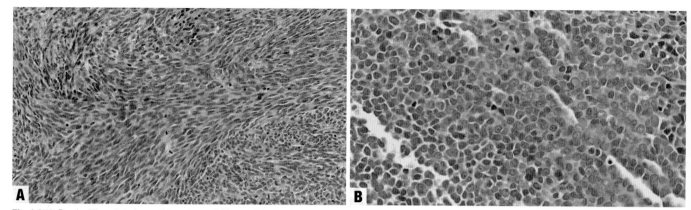

Fig. 1.356 Poorly differentiated synovial sarcoma. **A** Hypercellular fascicular tumour resembling malignant peripheral nerve sheath tumour. **B** Round cell tumour resembling Ewing sarcoma.

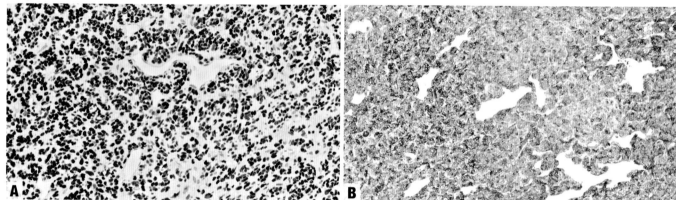

Fig. 1.357 Synovial sarcoma. **A** Immunohistochemistry: diffuse and strong TLE1 nuclear staining. **B** Immunohistochemistry: multifocal EMA expression.

staining for the transcriptional corepressor TLE1 is found in the large majority of biphasic, monophasic, and poorly differentiated SSs {1062}. However, TLE1 staining is not specific for SS, because it may also occur in histological mimics of SS, in particular malignant peripheral nerve sheath tumour and solitary fibrous tumour {2480,1062}.

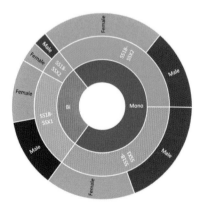

Fig. 1.358 Synovial sarcoma. Graphical representation of interrelationships of fusion type to tumour histology and patient sex in synovial sarcoma. Most synovial sarcomas are monophasic, and the *SS18-SSX1* fusion type is more common than *SS18-SSX2*. Men and women are affected in approximately even proportions, but men show a 3:2 ratio of *SS18-SSX1* to *SS18-SSX2*, whereas in women the ratio is close to 1:1. The vast majority of *SS18-SSX2* cases show monophasic histology, whereas most biphasic cases show *SS18-SSX1*. Biphasic synovial sarcomas harbouring the *SS18-SSX2* fusion are uncommon, and the diagnosis of such cases should therefore be well supported.

Cytology

For FNA material, preparation of a cell block is advocated, because a conclusive diagnosis of SS heavily relies on diagnostic molecular studies (e.g. FISH) {3176}.

Diagnostic molecular pathology

SS harbours a unique t(X;18)(p11;q11) translocation {1729}, by which *SS18* on chromosome 18 is fused to one of the SSX genes (*SSX1*, *SSX2*, or *SSX4*) on the X chromosome {842}. Although there is some variability, the most common fusion transcript links exon 10 of *SS18* with exon 6 of the partner SSX gene {94}. Approximately two thirds of SS cases carry an *SS18-SSX1* fusion, one third carry *SS18-SSX2*, and only rare cases carry *SS18-SSX4* {842,94} or *SS18L1-SSX1* – the latter arising from a t(X:20) {2959}. *SS18-SSX1* SSs show an approximately even sex ratio, whereas *SS18-SSX2* SSs are significantly more common in women {1544,1729}. Moreover, almost all *SS18-SSX2* cases show monophasic histology, whereas *SS18-SSX1* cases show an approximate 2:1 ratio of monophasic to biphasic histology {1544,132}. For optimal diagnostic accuracy, molecular confirmation (where available) of an *SS18-SSX1/2/4* fusion should ideally be performed {1489}.

Essential and desirable diagnostic criteria

Essential: monomorphic blue spindle cell sarcoma showing variable epithelial differentiation; diffuse and strong nuclear immunostaining for TLE1.

Desirable (in selected cases): demonstration of *SS18-SSX1/2/4* gene fusion.

Staging

The American Joint Committee on Cancer (AJCC) or Union for International Cancer Control (UICC) TNM system may be used.

Prognosis and prediction

SS has a variable prognosis. Metastatic disease commonly occurs in lungs and bone, but also in regional lymph nodes. Most distant tumour recurrences develop within a few years after initial diagnosis, but late recurrences do occur, even after 10 years {1700}. Major prognostic determinants are tumour stage at presentation, tumour size, and French Fédération Nationale des Centres de Lutte Contre le Cancer (FNCLCC) tumour grade {1244,3060,1700}. Tumours with > 20% poorly differentiated areas show more aggressive behaviour {3149, 1932,273}. The best outcomes are seen with tumours that are < 5 cm in diameter or that have < 6 mitoses/mm^2 (10 mitoses in 1.7 mm^2), with no necrosis {273,1244}. Minute SSs (< 1 cm) have an excellent prognosis {2110}. Children fare better than adults {2984}, and extremity-based SSs have a better prognosis than SSs involving the trunk or the head and neck area {2984,473}. A prognostic nomogram based on data available preoperatively in patients with SS has been developed {473}. Studies of the prognostic significance of *SS18-SSX1/2/4* fusion type have yielded inconsistent results, either positive for modest effects or negative {1703,473}; therefore, fusion type is not regarded as being prognostically useful. United States population-based SEER Program data indicate that the 5-year and 10-year disease-specific survival rates, respectively, are 83% and 75% in children and adolescents (age < 19 years) and 62% and 52% in adults {2984}.

Epithelioid sarcoma

Oda Y
Dal Cin P
Le Loarer F
Nielsen TO

Definition

Epithelioid sarcoma (ES) is a malignant mesenchymal neoplasm that exhibits partial or complete epithelioid cytomorphology and immunophenotype. Two clinicopathological subtypes are recognized: the classic (or distal) form, characterized by its proclivity for acral sites and pseudogranulomatous growth pattern, and the proximal-type (large cell) subtype, which arises mainly in proximal/truncal regions and consists of nests and sheets of large epithelioid cells.

ICD-O coding

8804/3 Epithelioid sarcoma

ICD-11 coding

2B5F.2 & XH4F96 Sarcoma, not elsewhere classified of other specified sites & Epithelioid sarcoma

Related terminology

None

Subtype(s)

Proximal or large cell epithelioid sarcoma; classic epithelioid sarcoma (also known as conventional or distal epithelioid sarcoma)

Localization

The classic subtype most commonly occurs in the distal upper extremity, predominantly arising in the fingers and hand {544, 3072}. Tumours of the foot and hand affect mainly volar surfaces. Proximal extremities and trunk are less frequent locations. The proximal-type subtype tends to arise in deep soft tissue, and it most often affects truncal (pelviperineal, genital, and inguinal) tissue, buttock, or hip {1249,1313}.

Clinical features

Superficially located examples of classic ES present as solitary or multiple, slow-growing, usually painless, firm nodules. Lesions often result in non-healing skin ulcers that can clinically mimic other ulcerative dermal processes. In comparison, classic and proximal-type tumours located in deep soft tissue are usually larger in size and more infiltrative {1249,1313}. This is one of the few sarcomas that regularly metastasize to lymph nodes.

Epidemiology

ES represents < 1% of all adult soft tissue sarcomas {1516} and between 4% and 8% of childhood non-rhabdomyosarcomatous soft tissue sarcomas {506}. The classic subtype is reported nearly twice as often as the proximal-type subtype {547,2603}. The M:F ratio is 2:1 for the classic subtype {3072} and 1.6:1 for the proximal-type subtype {1249,1313}. Both tumours affect patients over a wide age range. The classic subtype presents mainly in adolescents and young adults, whereas the proximal-type

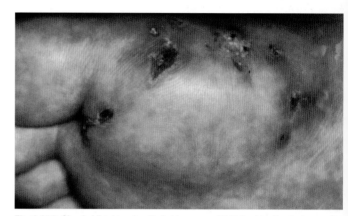

Fig. 1.359 Classic (distal-type) epithelioid sarcoma. Multiple ulcerating lesions on the sole of the foot.

subtype tends to affect a somewhat older population – young to middle-aged adults {3072}.

Etiology

The etiology is unknown. Three studies report (probably coincidental) antecedent trauma in 20% {544}, 27% {2535}, and 73% {701} of patients. There is no recurrent genetic predisposition.

Pathogenesis

Both classic and proximal-type ESs are associated with almost complete loss of SMARCB1 (INI1) nuclear protein expression, except for extremely rare SMARCB1-retained tumours. The *SMARCB1* gene (also called *BAF47, INI1*, or *SNF5*), located on 22q11.23, encodes a protein that is part of the SWI/SNF chromatin-remodelling complex present in normal cells. SWI/SNF has ATPase activity and functions to shift the position of nucleosomes, thereby modulating transcription of a large class of genes involved in stem cell biology and differentiation {2244}. By immunohistochemistry, recurrent loss of SMARCB1 (INI1) is seen in a limited variety of tumour types {3246,1672,23,109}, within which the mechanisms of protein loss can be distinct. In ES, *SMARCB1* biallelic deletions have been demonstrated by FISH analysis; less frequently, monoallelic deletions and heterogeneous FISH patterns have also been detected {2981, 1790,2739}. In some cases, decreased SMARCB1 (INI1) protein expression has been associated with negative regulation of *SMARCB1* transcripts by microRNAs {2434,1675,2739}. An extreme minority of ESs retain SMARCB1 (INI1) protein expression, instead exhibiting abnormal expression of other SWI/SNF chromatin-remodelling complex members, such as SMARCA4 (BRG1), SMARCC1 (BAF155), or SMARCC2 (BAF170); such cases have been correlated with rhabdoid morphology and with adverse prognosis, especially among proximal-type ESs {1676}. Unlike in many sarcomas that affect younger patients (especially malignant rhabdoid tumours {1538,595}), genomic

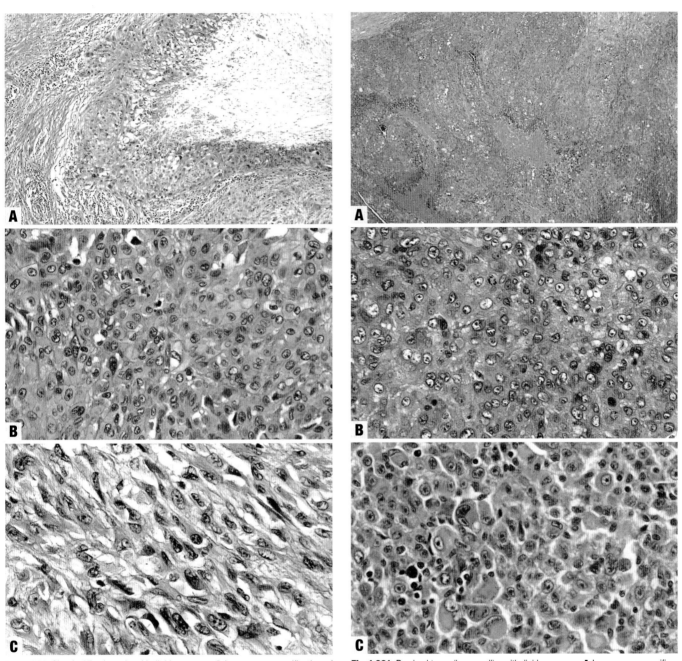

Fig. 1.360 Classic (distal-type) epithelioid sarcoma. **A** Low-power magnification of a nodular lesion centred in the dermis composed of tumour cells surrounding an area of necrosis (pseudogranulomatous growth pattern). **B** Epithelioid tumour cells with abundant eosinophilic cytoplasm. **C** Cells with a plump spindle-shaped morphology.

Fig. 1.361 Proximal-type (large cell) epithelioid sarcoma. **A** Low-power magnification shows a multinodular growth pattern of epithelioid cells with foci of tumour necrosis. **B** Pleomorphic epithelioid tumour cells with abundant, deeply eosinophilic cytoplasm and enlarged vesicular nuclei with prominent nucleoli. **C** Aggregates of rhabdoid cells with glassy intracytoplasmic hyaline inclusions and eccentrically located, vesicular nuclei.

analysis of ESs by next-generation sequencing has revealed complex copy-number aberrations (with 22q11.2 and 12p13 being the most frequent losses) and a high overall mutation burden {1512}, findings that support the differential diagnosis between ES and malignant rhabdoid tumour. *SMARCB1* is the most frequently mutated gene, with or without inactivation of its second allele. By RNA sequencing, the transcriptome shows a unique profile that does not cluster with any particular tissue type or with other SWI/SNF-aberrant model systems {1512, 1789}.

Macroscopic appearance

The classic subtype usually presents as one or more indurated, ill-defined, dermal or subcutaneous nodules measuring a few millimetres to 5 cm. Deep-seated tumours are multinodular masses that extend along nerves and fascial planes. The cut surface is glistening, with a greyish-white or greyish-tan colour punctuated by yellow and brown foci representing necrosis and haemorrhage, respectively. The proximal-type subtype presents as solitary or multiple whitish nodules ranging from 1 to 20 cm, with areas of haemorrhage and necrosis {1249,1313}.

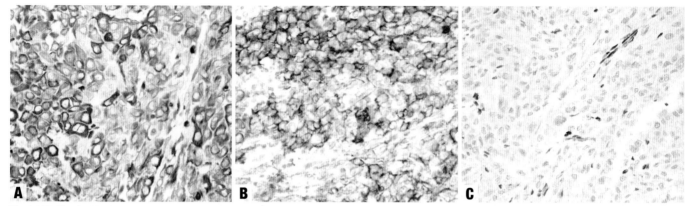

Fig. 1.362 Classic (distal-type) epithelioid sarcoma. **A** Diffuse expression of keratin (CAM5.2). **B** Strong membranous immunopositivity for CD34. **C** Complete loss of SMARCB1 (INI1) protein expression in the tumour cells (blood vessels being internal positive controls).

Histopathology

Classic ES consists of cellular nodules of epithelioid and spindled tumour cells with central degeneration and/or necrosis – a growth pattern that imparts a vaguely granulomatous appearance to the process {1340}. Fusion of necrotizing nodules results in a serpiginous mass with central geographical necrosis. Deep-situated lesions spread along the fascia as undulating bands of cells punctuated by foci of necrosis. Both types typically have infiltrative margins, and skip lesions are common in the classic type. Tumour nodules are composed of large ovoid or polygonal epithelioid cells and plump spindle-shaped cells with deeply eosinophilic cytoplasm and mildly atypical nuclei possessing vesicular chromatin and small nucleoli. The epithelioid cells, which are generally concentrated towards the centre of the nodule, gradually transition with the spindled element. Epithelioid cells may exhibit cytoplasmic vacuoles, mimicking a vascular tumour. Some cases have predominantly spindled morphology. Mitotic activity is usually low. Dystrophic calcification and metaplastic bone formation are detected in 20% of cases {544}, and aggregates of chronic inflammatory cells are usually present at the periphery of the tumour nodules.

The proximal type is characterized by a multinodular and sheet-like growth of large and sometimes pleomorphic epithelioid (carcinoma-like) cells with enlarged vesicular nuclei and prominent nucleoli {1249,1313}. Spotty foci of tumour necrosis are frequently encountered, but this feature does not generally result in a pseudogranulomatous pattern typical of classic ES. Cells with rhabdoid features occur in both forms, but they are more frequently observed in the proximal-type subtype, in which differentiation from extrarenal rhabdoid tumour becomes challenging when the rhabdoid cell is the predominant cell type {1249}. Occasional cases may have a prominent myxoid stroma {1033}. Additionally, rare cases of ES demonstrate hybrid histological features of both the classic and proximal types.

Both classic and proximal-type ESs show immunoreactivity for epithelial markers, including low- and high-molecular-weight cytokeratins and EMA {2118}. More specifically, most cases express CK8 and CK19 {2118} but are typically negative or only focally positive for CK5/6 {1759}. Unlike in carcinoma, CD34 is expressed in > 50% of cases. Loss of nuclear expression of SMARCB1 protein occurs in the vast majority of cases of both types {1406,1670,2716}. ERG expression is observed in 40–67%

of ESs, predominantly in classic-type cases, which can cause confusion with endothelial tumours {2137,2953,1674}.

Cytology
Not clinically relevant

Diagnostic molecular pathology
Not clinically relevant

Essential and desirable diagnostic criteria
Essential: tumour presenting as a soft tissue mass (so-called distal or proximal presentations); epithelioid to spindled cytomorphology with infiltrative growth; diffuse loss of SMARCB1 (INI1, BAF47) and staining for EMA and keratin.

Staging
The American Joint Committee on Cancer (AJCC) or Union for International Cancer Control (UICC) TNM system may be used.

Prognosis and prediction
Clinical series of ES patients have reported 5-year and 10-year overall survival rates of 45–70% and 45–66%, respectively {1833, 176,2533,2400}. Overall survival rates drop to 24% in patients with metastatic ES, whereas localized ES patients fare better, with an overall survival rate of 62–88% when patients are treated with R0 surgery {1313,1833,2533}. On multivariate analysis, deep location correlates with lower overall survival, accounting for the poorer survival associated with proximal-type ES, which is by definition deep-seated {1833,2533,2400}. Conversely, location in the hand correlates with good outcome in localized ES patients treated with R0 surgery {2533}. The rates of local recurrence, lymph node dissemination, and metastasis for localized ES are 14–25%, 34–52%, and 33%, respectively {1833,2533,2400}. A reported 22–30% of cases are metastatic at the time of diagnosis {1833,176,2533}. Multimodal management of localized ES is said to be associated with better local control rates when surgery is combined with isolated limb perfusion chemotherapy {1833} or neoadjuvant radiotherapy {2533}. Other adverse prognostic factors that have been reported include older age, high grade / high mitotic activity {1500,547,1120,1833}, nodal involvement {176, 2400,881}, tumour size > 5 cm {547,2603,1500}, and proximal-type histology with the presence of rhabdoid cells {1120,2603}.

Alveolar soft part sarcoma

Jambhekar NA
Ladanyi M

Definition

Alveolar soft part sarcoma (ASPS) is a rare tumour of uncertain histogenesis predominantly affecting the deep soft tissues of the extremities, featuring variably discohesive epithelioid cells arranged in nests, resulting in a distinct alveolar appearance. It is characterized by a specific translocation, der(17)t(X;17) (p11.2;q25), which results in *ASPSCR1-TFE3* gene fusion.

ICD-O coding

9581/3 Alveolar soft part sarcoma

ICD-11 coding

2B5F.2 & XH8V95 Sarcoma, not elsewhere classified of other specified sites & Alveolar soft part sarcoma

Related terminology

None

Subtype(s)

None

Localization

ASPS commonly involves deep soft tissues of the extremities (61%; predominantly the lower extremity [51%]), trunk (20%), internal organs (8%), and head and neck (9%) {3228}. Primaries in the head and neck region, particularly in the orbit and tongue, are seen in children {1061,970}. Uncommon locations include the female genital tract {2287}, bone {2450}, urinary bladder {102}, mediastinum {1030}, and spine {3399}.

Clinical features

ASPS presents as a slow-growing painless mass {581}. Proptosis or vaginal bleeding is seen with orbital or female genital tract tumours, respectively. At presentation the disease can be localized (38%), regional (11%), or metastatic (43%) {3228}. ASPS is isodense or hypodense on CT {3073}. MRI reveals flow voids, large vessels, moderate to intense postcontrast enhancement, and central necrosis {2029}. The vascular pattern is helpful for diagnosis {690}.

Epidemiology

ASPS accounts for < 1% of all soft tissue sarcomas. In a SEER Program data analysis, the patient age range was 1–78 years (median: 25 years); 72% of patients were aged < 30 years, and 58% were females {3228}. This female preponderance is well documented {591,1852,2356} but is less marked in patients aged > 30 years and in children {2529,2435,970}.

Etiology

The *ASPSCR1-TFE3* translocation appears to be the initiating genetic event in ASPS {1731}, but why the translocation occurs

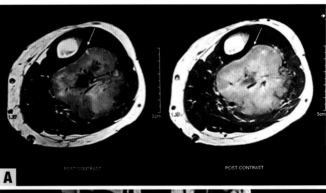
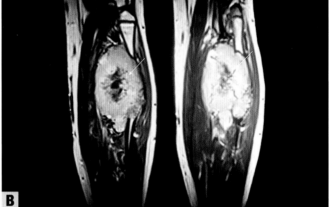

Fig. 1.363 Alveolar soft part sarcoma. Tumour involving fibula and calf muscles of a 13-year-old girl; postcontrast T1-weighted MRI images reveal a solid tumour with lobulated margins displaying inhomogeneous intense enhancement and a central non-enhancing component **A** Axial view. **B** Coronal view.

is unknown. There have been no cases reported in association with a history of irradiation or a germline cancer predisposition syndrome.

Pathogenesis

The ASPSCR1-TFE3 fusion protein localizes to the nucleus, where it functions as an aberrant transcription factor, causing c-Met overexpression and activation of c-Met signalling, rendering ASPS cells sensitive to c-Met inhibition in vitro {3109,1661} and in vivo {2212}. A recent clinical trial of the c-Met inhibitor crizotinib in ASPS reported disease stabilization in most patients, but tumour shrinkage was uncommon {2777}. Finally, a mouse model of ASPS driven by conditional expression of an *ASPSCR1-TFE3* transgene highlighted the exquisite dependence of ASPS on lactate for growth {1190}, which may be linked to its frequent occurrence in muscle and its high expression of the lactate transporter MCT1 and its associated protein, CD147 {1728}. Cytogenetically, ASPS is defined by a specific alteration, der(17)t(X;17)(p11;q25). Because the der(X) resulting

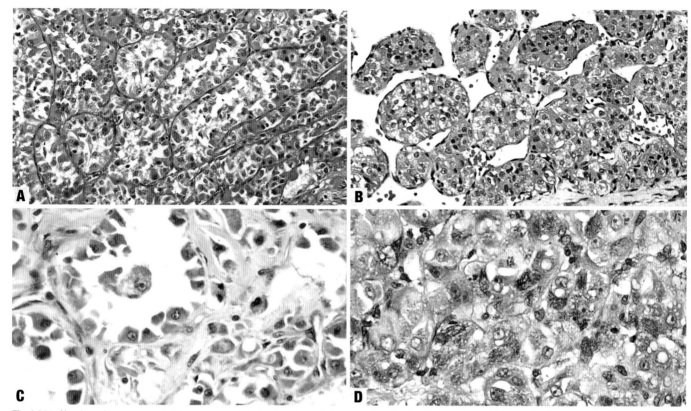

Fig. 1.364 Alveolar soft part sarcoma. **A** Typical organoid nests of eosinophilic tumour cells with abundant cytoplasm. **B** Compact cell nests outlined by sinusoidal vessels. **C** Alveolar-like structures, discohesive cells, and central or eccentric nuclei with prominent nucleoli. **D** PASD staining. A large centrally placed cell shows elongated rod-like intracytoplasmic crystals in a sheaf-like arrangement; numerous surrounding cells show intracytoplasmic PAS-positive, diastase-resistant granules.

from the t(X;17)(p11;q25) is rarely retained {3135}, the der(17) t(X;17) may be described in some cases as add(17)(q25), if the quality of the banding is not sufficient to allow for positive identification of the additional material as coming from the short arm of chromosome X. This translocation results in the fusion of the *TFE3* transcription factor gene (from Xp11) with *ASPSCR1* (also known as *ASPL*) at 17q25.3 {1731}. Depending on the *TFE3* intron involved in the genomic rearrangement, *ASPSCR1-TFE3* fusion transcripts can differ by the presence or absence of one additional exon of *TFE3*.

Macroscopic appearance

Tumours vary from 1.2 to 24 cm (median: 6.5 cm) {2529}. They are partially circumscribed and consist of multiple soft fleshy nodules and fibrotic bands. The centre of larger lesions often shows haemorrhage or necrosis.

Histopathology

ASPS is composed of large polygonal cells with well-defined cell borders, eosinophilic granular cytoplasm, a rounded

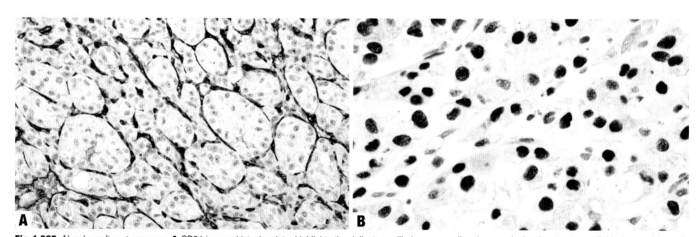

Fig. 1.365 Alveolar soft part sarcoma. **A** CD34 immunohistochemistry highlights the delicate capillaries surrounding the pseudoalveolar structures. **B** Nuclear staining with TFE3 is characteristic.

central/eccentric vesicular nucleus, and a prominent nucleolus. The cells are arranged in a uniform organoid or nest-like pattern, showing central discohesion resulting in the characteristic alveolar pattern. A rich sinusoidal capillary vasculature is seen throughout; this often encircles tumour nests and imparts a haemangiopericytomatous appearance focally. Vascular invasion is very common. Cytoplasmic clearing, rhabdoid cells, a pseudoglandular pattern, or cystic change with myxoid material may be seen {2605,1547}. Nuclear pleomorphism, hyperchromasia, giant cells, mitosis, necrosis {939,970}, calcification, lymphocytic infiltrate, and xanthomatous features are uncommon {1048,2605,3315}. Small cells, non-alveolar growth, and inconspicuous vessels are particularly seen in lingual tumours {970}. Many tumours show intracytoplasmic rod-like/rhomboid crystalline structures, focally or diffusely, in a sheaf-like or stacked configuration {970,1048,2605}. These crystals and the intracytoplasmic granules are PAS-positive/diastase-resistant and are immunoreactive for MCT1 and CD147 {1728,3111}. ASPS shows nuclear immunoreactivity for TFE3 {160,2427, 3297}. Immunopositivity for cathepsin K (100%) is also typical. Calretinin (46%) {1989,531} and focally desmin (50%) can be detected {1048}.

Cytology
In cytological preparations, smears reveal large cells, mainly distributed singly, with granularity or vacuoles {3214,2819}.

Diagnostic molecular pathology
Demonstration of *TFE3* rearrangement {1214} or *ASPSCR1-TFE3* fusion transcripts {1739,3405} may be diagnostically helpful. Although the presence of the *ASPSCR1-TFE3* fusion appears to be highly specific and sensitive for ASPS among sarcomas, the same gene fusion is also found in a small but unique subset of renal cell carcinomas, often affecting young patients {154}.

Essential and desirable diagnostic criteria
Essential: eosinophilic polygonal cells in an organoid/nested pattern; rich sinusoidal capillaries and intracytoplasmic crystals (in some cases); TFE3 nuclear expression by immunohistochemistry (strong and diffuse).
Desirable: demonstration of *TFE3* gene rearrangement or *ASPSCR1-TFE3* fusion (in selected cases).

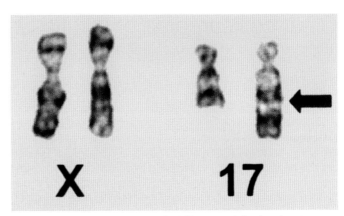

Fig. 1.366 Alveolar soft part sarcoma. Partial karyotype of alveolar soft part sarcoma showing the characteristic alteration, der(17)t(X;17)(p11.2;q25).

Staging
The Union for International Cancer Control (UICC) or American Joint Committee on Cancer (AJCC) TNM system can be used.

Prognosis and prediction
ASPS is not formally graded but is regarded as high-grade by definition. Local recurrence occurs in 11–50% of cases {3228}. Metastases involve the lungs, liver, bone, brain, and (rarely) lymph nodes, often ≥ 10 years after diagnosis {1031,2487,2529, 1852}. The overall survival rate is 82% at 2 years and 56% at 5 years {3228}. Negative prognostic factors include older age, tumour size > 10 cm, distant metastasis at diagnosis, and a primary site in the trunk {3228}. Tumours detected early, at a completely resectable stage, such as lingual ASPS, have a better prognosis {2435,970}.

Clear cell sarcoma of soft tissue

Fritchie KJ
van de Rijn M

Definition

Clear cell sarcoma (CCS) of soft tissue is a malignant mesenchymal neoplasm, typically involving deep soft tissue and most often characterized by *EWSR1-ATF1* fusion, harbouring a distinctive nested growth pattern and melanocytic differentiation.

ICD-O coding

9044/3 Clear cell sarcoma NOS

ICD-11 coding

2B5F.2 & XH77N6 Sarcoma, not elsewhere classified of other specified sites & Clear cell sarcoma

Related terminology

Not recommended: malignant melanoma of soft parts.

Subtype(s)

None

Localization

CCS occurs most commonly at deep-seated sites in the extremity, with almost 50% of cases arising in the distal lower extremity, ankle, or foot, where they can be associated with tendons or aponeuroses {605,772,880,1905}. CCS has also been reported in the head/neck, trunk, and viscera including the lung and gastrointestinal tract {11,1919,605,1905,1174}. Lesions arising in skin and oral mucosa are recognized. CCS-like tumour of the gastrointestinal tract (malignant gastrointestinal neuroectodermal tumour) most likely represents a distinct entity from CCS and is discussed in the *Digestive system tumours* volume {3282}.

Clinical features

Almost all patients present with a palpable mass of months' to years' duration. Pain and tenderness are reported in approximately one third to one half of cases {605,772,880,1905}.

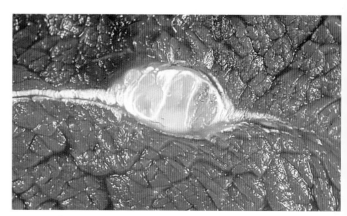

Fig. 1.367 Clear cell sarcoma. This well-circumscribed tumour arose in the plantaris tendon of an 18-year-old woman. Despite the small size of the tumour, she died from disseminated metastases 4 years later.

Epidemiology

CCS mainly affects young adults, with a peak incidence in the third and fourth decades of life {605,772,880,1905}. There is a slight female predominance {880,913,605,1905}.

Etiology

Unknown

Pathogenesis

The genetic hallmark of CCS is the reciprocal translocation t(12;22)(q13;q12), present in 70–90% of cases, which fuses *EWSR1* with *ATF1* {417,2945,2590,3099,2479,1746,2423, 1203,3350}. Exon 8 of *EWSR1* fuses with exon 4 of *ATF1* most frequently, and this has been designated as the type 1 fusion {3409,141,3241}. In the resultant EWSR1-ATF1 chimeric fusion protein, the N-terminus of EWSR1 and the basic leucine zipper (bZIP) domain of ATF1 are linked. Consequently, ATF1, a transcription factor normally regulated by cAMP, becomes

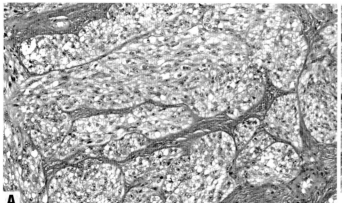
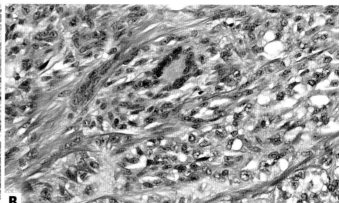

Fig. 1.368 Clear cell sarcoma. **A** Tumour cells have pale eosinophilic cytoplasm with prominent nucleoli. **B** Wreath-like multinucleated giant cells are a common finding.

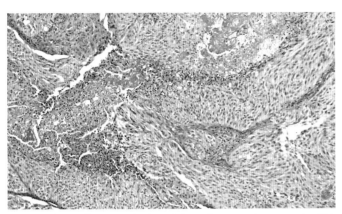

Fig. 1.369 Clear cell sarcoma. A subset of clear cell sarcomas have necrosis, which is an unfavourable prognostic factor.

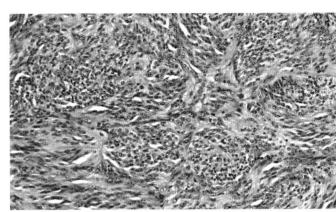

Fig. 1.371 Tumour with *CRTC1-TRIM11*. Newly recognized melanocytic neoplasms with *CRTC1-TRIM11* fusions exhibit morphological overlap with clear cell sarcoma.

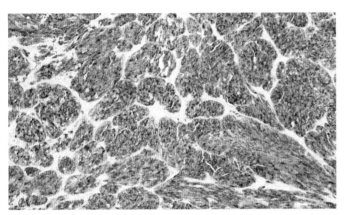

Fig. 1.370 Clear cell sarcoma. Tumour cells show strong and diffuse expression of S100.

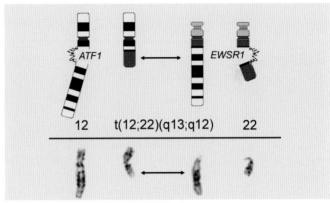

Fig. 1.372 Clear cell sarcoma of soft tissue. Schematic and partial G-banded karyotype of the 12;22 translocation in clear cell sarcoma.

a cAMP-independent transcriptional activator and constitutively activates the promoter for MITF, a target of the MSH pathway {741}. This activation is responsible for melanocytic differentiation and growth of CCS {741,434,1085}. ATF and CREB proteins are functionally similar, and a smaller subset of cases harbour a variant translocation, t(2;22)(q34;q12), resulting in an *EWSR1-CREB1* fusion {1378,3241}. An intradermal melanocytic neoplasm with a novel *CRTC1-TRIM11* fusion, substantial morphological overlap with CCS, and metastatic potential, provisionally termed cutaneous melanocytoma, was recently described {365,522}. Additional work is necessary to determine whether this tumour represents CCS with a novel fusion or a distinct entity. Although the majority of CCSs investigated have failed to show *BRAF* or *NRAS* mutations, *BRAF* p.Val600Glu mutations have been identified in a small subset of molecularly confirmed tumours {2424,1381, 3350,2262}.

Macroscopic appearance

Most CCSs measure 2–5 cm, but tumours > 15 cm have been reported {605,1905}. Gross examination reveals a circumscribed mass with a lobulated tan to greyish-white appearance, sometimes with a coarse or gritty texture {913}. A subset of CCSs may show melanin pigmentation, necrosis, or cystic change.

Histopathology

On low-power examination, CCS exhibits a characteristic nested or fascicular architecture with epithelioid to plump spindled cells partitioned by thin fibrous septa. Tumours typically show notably infiltrative growth through dense fibrous tissue. Despite its name, CCS typically has tumour cells with palely eosinophilic cytoplasm and vesicular nuclei with macronucleoli, with only rare examples showing true cytoplasmic clearing. Substantial nuclear pleomorphism is generally absent, although scattered wreath-like multinucleated giant cells are relatively common. Melanin pigment is present in more than half of cases but is difficult to appreciate on H&E staining. Rare cases may show junctional tumour nests at the dermoepidermal interface {1647,1098}. The mitotic count of CCS is frequently low (< 3 mitoses/mm², equating to < 5 mitoses per 10 high-power fields of 0.17 mm²), and necrosis is identified in roughly one third of cases {880,1905,913}. CCS shows consistent expression of S100, SOX10, melan-A, HMB45, and MITF {1378,1209,1381}.

Cytology

The cytological features of CCS are similar to those of melanoma, with aspiration specimens showing single or small clusters of round to polygonal cells with pale cytoplasm and prominent nucleoli {479,1498}. Pleomorphism is not prominent.

Diagnostic molecular pathology

Demonstration of *EWSR1* gene rearrangement or *EWSR1-ATF1* gene fusion may be helpful.

Essential and desirable diagnostic criteria

Essential: characteristic nested or fascicular low-power architecture; plump spindle or ovoid cells with palely eosinophilic cytoplasm and prominent nucleoli; multinucleated wreath-like giant cells are common; expression of melanocytic markers, including S100, SOX10, melan-A, and HMB45; 70–90% of cases harbour *EWSR1-ATF1* fusions, helping to differentiate these neoplasms from melanoma.

Staging

The American Joint Committee on Cancer (AJCC) or Union for International Cancer Control (UICC) TNM system may be used.

Prognosis and prediction

CCS is an aggressive malignancy with recurrence rates approaching 40% and pulmonary or lymph node metastasis in at least 30–50% of patients {880,772,1905,1378,1186,1381}. Metastasis often occurs more than a decade after initial diagnosis. Survival rates at 5, 10, and 20 years are approximately 60%, 35%, and 10%, respectively {1381,1378,1905,1186}. Tumour size > 5 cm, necrosis, and regional lymph node involvement are unfavourable prognostic factors {1905,772,1381,880,2740}. Fusion variant and transcript type have not been found to have prognostic significance {640}.

Extraskeletal myxoid chondrosarcoma

Horvai AE
Agaram NP
Lucas DR

Definition
Extraskeletal myxoid chondrosarcoma (EMC) is a malignant mesenchymal neoplasm of uncertain differentiation characterized by abundant myxoid matrix, multilobular architecture, and uniform cells arranged in cords, clusters, and reticular networks. These tumours are characterized by *NR4A3* gene rearrangement. Despite the name, there is no evidence of cartilaginous differentiation.

ICD-O coding
9231/3 Extraskeletal myxoid chondrosarcoma

ICD-11 coding
2B5F.2 & XH9344 Sarcoma, not elsewhere classified of other specified sites & Myxoid chondrosarcoma

Related terminology
Acceptable: NR4A3-rearranged myxoid sarcoma (provisional).

Subtype(s)
None

Localization
Most EMCs arise in the deep soft tissues of the proximal extremities and limb girdles, with the thigh being the most common site {917,2062}. Less common sites include the trunk, head and neck, paraspinal soft tissue, abdomen, pelvis, and foot. Rare tumours have also been reported in the finger {2367}, cranium {2745}, retroperitoneum {1087}, and pleura {1173}. Despite the current nomenclature, rare genetically confirmed cases of EMC have been described in bone {1626,1006}.

Clinical features
Patients most often present with an enlarging, deep-seated soft tissue mass, often accompanied by pain and tenderness. Some

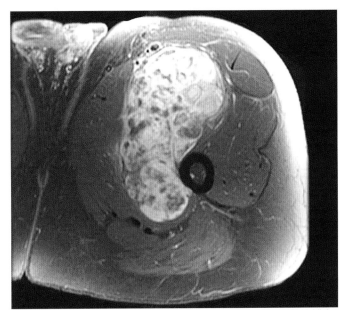

Fig. 1.373 Extraskeletal myxoid chondrosarcoma. T2-weighted axial MRI highlights the hyperintense signalling and pronounced lobular architecture in an extraskeletal myxoid chondrosarcoma of the thigh.

tumours may mimic a haematoma. Tumours around joints can restrict range of motion.

Epidemiology
EMC is rare, accounting for < 1% of soft tissue sarcomas. It usually occurs in adults, with a median age of 50 years {859, 2062}. Only rare cases in childhood or adolescence have been reported {1267}. The M:F ratio is 2:1.

Etiology
Unknown

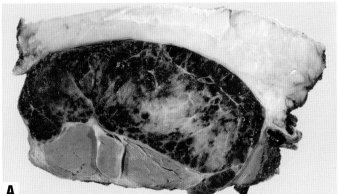
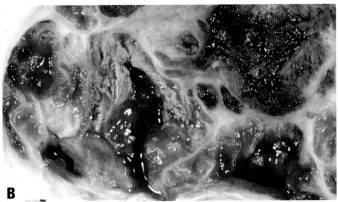

Fig. 1.374 Extraskeletal myxoid chondrosarcoma. **A** Grossly, these tumours are well demarcated, are contained by a pseudocapsule, and have a lobular architecture defined by fibrous septa. **B** Cystic cavities, haemorrhage, and necrosis are often found on the cut surface. Note the well-defined lobular architecture and thick fibrous septa.

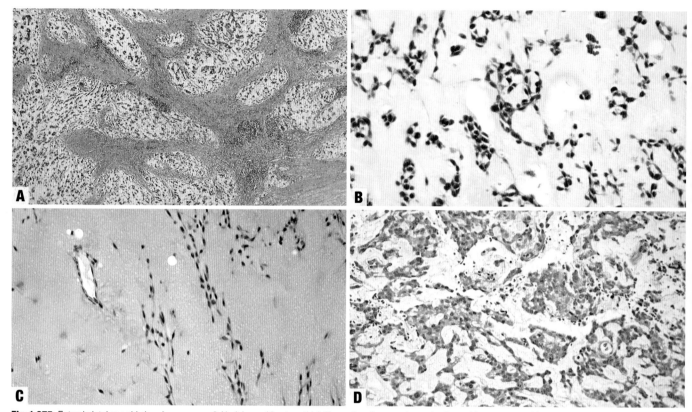

Fig. 1.375 Extraskeletal myxoid chondrosarcoma. **A** Nodular architecture; thick fibrous bands separate pools of myxoid stroma containing tumour cells. Chronic inflammation and focal haemorrhage may be seen. **B** The tumour is characterized by abundant myxoid matrix and interconnecting cords of uniform cells, often with long, delicate processes. **C** Spindle cell differentiation is common and when present can be either focal or diffuse. Note the interconnecting growth pattern. **D** The cells sometimes form cohesive clusters and ring-forms mimicking an epithelial neoplasm, most importantly a myoepithelial tumour.

Pathogenesis

Molecular characterization of the t(9;22) and subsequently also of the t(9;17) variant translocation has shown that they result in gene fusions in which the *NR4A3* gene is fused with either *EWSR1* at 22q12.2 or *TAF15* at 17q12 {183,1726,2422,2878}. The *NR4A3* fusions, which are present in > 90% of EMCs {1376, 2425,2879}, have not been found in any other sarcoma and may therefore be considered a hallmark of this disease. *NR4A3* (also known as *TEC*, *CHN*, and *NOR1*) encodes an orphan nuclear receptor belonging to the steroid/thyroid receptor gene family, whereas *EWSR1* and *TAF15* – also known as *TAF2N*, *RBP56*, and *TAF(II)68* – belong to the TET family of multifunctional proteins that bind both RNA and DNA. Two additional gene fusions, *TCF12-NR4A3* and *TFG-NR4A3*, have also been identified in isolated cases of EMC {1377,2881,39}.

The molecular consequences of the *NR4A3* gene fusions in EMC have only been partially elucidated. The EWSR1-NR4A3 and TAF15-NR4A3 fusion proteins are strong transcriptional activators {1633,1725}. There is evidence suggesting that coexpression of native NR4A3 and its coactivator SIX3 may be an alternative mechanism to gene fusion {1379}. The orphan receptor NR4A3 is a transcriptional target of p53 and interacts with the antiapoptotic BCL2 protein, presumably promoting apoptosis {978}.

Cytogenetically, EMC is characterized by a t(9;22)(q22;q12) translocation or less frequently a t(9;17)(q22;q11) or t(9;15)(q22;q21) translocation {183,2422,2798,2878,2879,2881,2944}. Although the t(9;22) has been found as the sole anomaly, most cases also show other chromosome changes, including trisomy for 1q25-qter, 7, 8, 12, and 19 {2425,2879}.

Macroscopic appearance

EMCs form large, well-demarcated tumours. Tumour size is variable and some very large tumours can reach 30 cm {2062}. On cut surface, EMC has a well-defined multinodular architecture comprising glistening, gelatinous areas separated by fibrous septa. Intratumoural haemorrhage, cystic cavities, and geographical areas of necrosis are common. Highly cellular tumours are fleshy.

Histopathology

EMC has a multinodular architecture defined by fibrous septa that divide the tumour into hypocellular lobules with abundant pale-blue myxoid or chondromyxoid matrix. Well-formed hyaline cartilage is virtually never seen. The stroma is strikingly hypovascular. The cells characteristically interconnect with one another to form cords, small clusters, and complex trabecular or cribriform arrays. The cells have a modest amount of deeply eosinophilic to vacuolated cytoplasm, as well as uniform round to oval nuclei, and delicate elongated cytoplasmic processes are common. The chromatin is evenly distributed, often with a small, inconspicuous nucleolus. Mitotic activity is usually low. Some tumours have prominent rhabdoid cytoplasmic inclusions. Rare cases are hypercellular with decreased myxoid matrix and have higher-grade, often epithelioid cytomorphology.

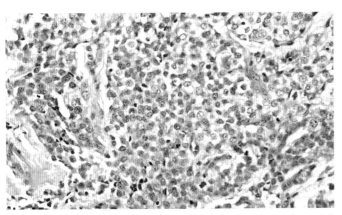

Fig. 1.376 Extraskeletal myxoid chondrosarcoma. The cellular subtype of extraskeletal myxoid chondrosarcoma is characterized by sheets and cords of cells with little intervening myxoid matrix. The cells frequently have an epithelioid morphology and large vesicular nuclei, prominent nucleoli, and brisk mitotic activity.

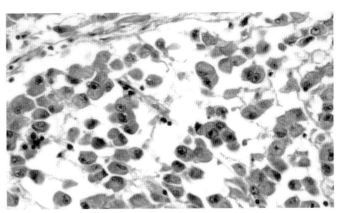

Fig. 1.377 Extraskeletal myxoid chondrosarcoma. Rhabdoid cells with eccentric eosinophilic cytoplasm and perinuclear hyaline globules are seen in some extraskeletal myxoid chondrosarcomas. These cells are frequently negative for SMARCB1 (INI1) by immunohistochemistry.

S100 is positive in as many as 20% of cases, and KIT (CD117, c-KIT) is positive in as many as 30%. Expression of synaptophysin and NSE has been demonstrated in some tumours {1305, 2367,2376}. Tumours with rhabdoid features are often negative for SMARCB1 (INI1). Notably, tumour cells only very rarely express keratins or GFAP, and muscle markers are negative.

Cytology
Not clinically relevant

Diagnostic molecular pathology
Identification of *NR4A3* gene rearrangement is diagnostically helpful.

Essential and desirable diagnostic criteria
Essential: generally bland cells with eosinophilic cytoplasm disposed in strands or cords in a predominantly myxoid stroma.
Desirable: NR4A3 rearrangement (in selected cases).

Staging
The American Joint Committee on Cancer (AJCC) or Union for International Cancer Control (UICC) TNM system may be used.

Prognosis and prediction
Although often associated with prolonged survival, EMC has high rates of distant recurrence and disease-associated death {859,2062,2721}. Metastases are usually pulmonary; however, extrapulmonary and disseminated metastases also occur

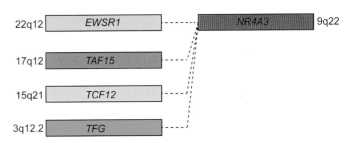

Fig. 1.378 Extraskeletal myxoid chondrosarcoma. Schematic of the four known *NR4A3* gene fusions and their respective chromosomal locations.

{2721}. Interestingly, prolonged survival even in the face of metastatic disease is not uncommon. Two large retrospective series {859,2062} report 5-year, 10-year, and 15-year overall survival rates of 82–90%, 65–70%, and 58–60%, respectively. Older age, large tumour size (especially > 10 cm), and proximal location are adverse prognostic factors {2062,2376}. Some studies suggest that tumours with increased cellularity and atypia are more aggressive {126,1902,2376}. Others suggest that the presence of rhabdoid cells represents an adverse histological finding {2376,2392}. EMCs with variant non-*EWSR1* gene fusions tend to show a higher incidence of rhabdoid phenotype, high-grade morphology, and aggressive outcome than the *EWSR1-NR4A3*–positive tumours {39}.

Desmoplastic small round cell tumour

Agaram NP
Antonescu CR
Ladanyi M

Definition
Desmoplastic small round cell tumour (DSRCT) is a malignant mesenchymal neoplasm composed of small round tumour cells associated with prominent stromal desmoplasia, polyphenotypic differentiation, and *EWSR1-WT1* gene fusion.

ICD-O coding
8806/3 Desmoplastic small round cell tumour

ICD-11 coding
2B5F.2 & XH5SN6 Sarcoma, not elsewhere classified of other specified sites & Desmoplastic small round cell tumour

Related terminology
Acceptable: intra-abdominal desmoplastic round cell tumour.

Subtype(s)
None

Localization
The vast majority of patients develop tumours in the abdominal cavity, frequently in the retroperitoneum, pelvis, omentum, and mesentery. Multiple serosal implants are common. Clinical presentation outside the abdominal cavity is rare and mainly restricted to the thoracic cavity and paratesticular region {692}. Very rare cases occur in the limbs, head and neck, kidney, and brain {3236}.

Clinical features
Clinical symptoms are usually related to the primary site of presentation, such as pain, abdominal distention, palpable mass, acute abdomen, ascites, and organ obstruction.

Epidemiology
DSRCT primarily affects children and young adults, who usually present with widespread abdominal/peritoneal involvement {1136}. There is a striking male predominance, with peak incidence in the third decade of life, although this tumour type occurs over a wide age range (first to fifth decades).

Etiology
Unknown

Pathogenesis
DSRCT is characterized by a recurrent chromosomal translocation t(11;22)(p13;q12) {2750,312,2645}, resulting in fusion of the *EWSR1* gene on 22q12.2 and the Wilms tumour gene, *WT1*, on 11p13 {1730,747,1137}. The most common chimeric transcript is composed of an in-frame fusion of the first seven exons of *EWSR1*, encoding the potential transcription-modulating domain, and exons 8–10 of *WT1*, encoding the last three zinc fingers of the DNA-binding domain. Rare variants including additional exons

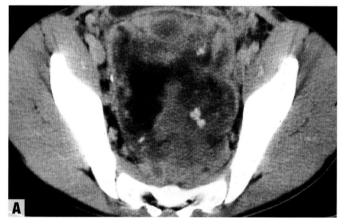
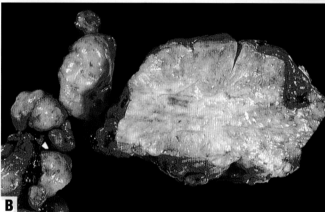

Fig. 1.379 Desmoplastic small round cell tumour. **A** CT image of a large pelvic desmoplastic small round cell tumour. **B** Desmoplastic small round cell tumour presenting as one dominant tumour mass and multiple smaller tumour nodules. The cross-section shows a solid whitish-tan cut surface, with foci of necrosis.

of *EWSR1* can also occur. Detection of the *EWSR1-WT1* gene fusion can be especially useful in cases with unusual clinical or histological features {1135}. Studies of the EWSR1-WT1 aberrant transcription factor have revealed deregulation of several target genes {1134} and activation of neural gene expression and partial neural differentiation via ASCL1 {1567}.

The serosal lining of body cavities, the most common site of DSRCT, has high transient fetal expression of the *WT1* gene. WT1 is expressed in tissues derived from the intermediate mesoderm, primarily those undergoing transition from mesenchyme to epithelium {2547,2571}. This pattern recapitulates the epithelial differentiation noted in DSRCT.

Macroscopic appearance
The typical gross appearance consists of multiple tumour nodules studding the peritoneal surface. Often there is a dominant tumour mass accompanied by satellite smaller nodules. The cut surface is firm and greyish-white, with foci of haemorrhage and necrosis.

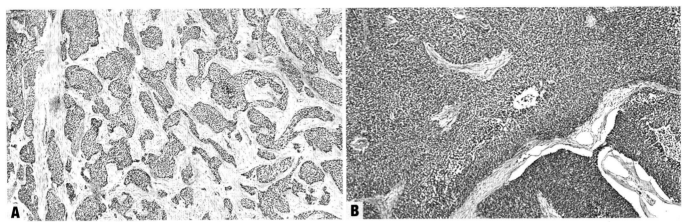

Fig. 1.380 Desmoplastic small round cell tumour. **A** Characteristic morphology with variably sized nests in a desmoplastic stroma. **B** Solid growth pattern with large confluent nests.

Histopathology

DSRCT is characterized by sharply outlined nests of small neoplastic round (more rarely epithelioid or even spindled) cells, usually surrounded by a prominent desmoplastic stroma. The nests can vary considerably in size, ranging from minute clusters to large irregular confluent sheets. Central necrosis is common and cystic degeneration can also be seen. Some tumours focally exhibit epithelial features, with glands or a rosette pattern. The tumour cells are typically uniform, with small hyperchromatic nuclei, scant cytoplasm, and indistinct cytoplasmic borders. In a subset of cases, tumour cells can show cytoplasmic eosinophilic rhabdoid inclusions. Some tumours have larger cells with greater pleomorphism. The chromatin is typically dispersed, with inconspicuous nucleoli. Mitoses are frequent and individual cell necrosis is common. The desmoplastic stroma is composed of fibroblasts or myofibroblasts embedded in a loose extracellular matrix or collagen. Prominent stromal vascularity is also present, ranging from complex capillary tufts to larger vessels with eccentric thickened walls.

Immunohistochemically, DSRCT shows a distinctive and complex pattern of multiphenotypic differentiation, expressing proteins associated with epithelial, muscular, and neural differentiation. Most cases are immunoreactive for cytokeratins, EMA, and desmin. A distinctive dot-like cytoplasmic localization is seen with desmin and occasionally with other intermediate filaments. Myogenin and MYOD1 are consistently negative. Nuclear expression of WT1 (using antibodies to the C-terminus but not the N-terminus) is usually seen {220,1367}.

Ultrastructurally, most tumour cells have a primitive/undifferentiated appearance, with minimal cytoplasm and scant organelles. A notable feature is the presence of paranuclear aggregates and whorls of intermediate filaments. Rare dense core granules can be also seen occasionally. Few cells are connected by cell junction complexes, including well-formed desmosomes.

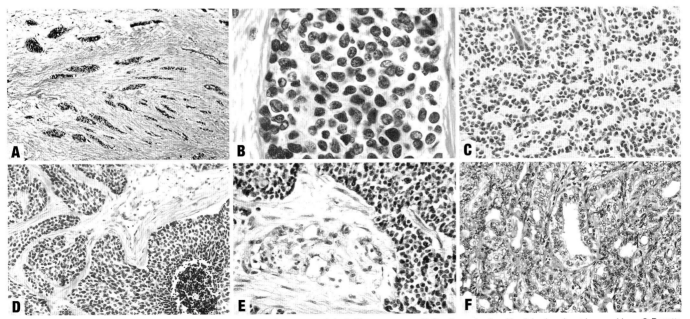

Fig. 1.381 Desmoplastic small round cell tumour. **A** Infiltrative growth pattern and single-file appearance. **B** Small round cells with minimal nuclear pleomorphism. **C** Rosette formation. **D** Focal necrosis. **E** Glomeruloid vascular proliferation. **F** Epithelial features with gland formation.

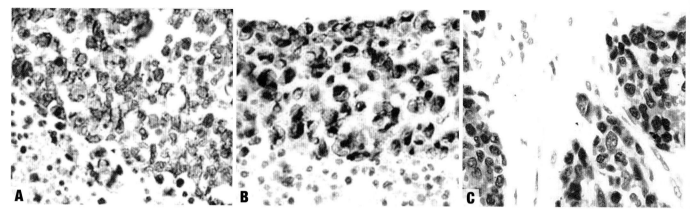

Fig. 1.382 Desmoplastic small round cell tumour. **A** Strong immunoreactivity for keratin. **B** Strong immunoreactivity for desmin. **C** Immunodetection of EWSR1-WT1 chimeric protein. Strong nuclear reactivity with the WT1 (C19) antibody directed to the C-terminus of WT1.

Cytology

Cytological specimens are cellular and show cells with a high N:C ratio, having granular chromatin, nuclear moulding, and variable nuclear membranes. Pseudorosettes are common {673}.

Diagnostic molecular pathology

The presence of *EWSR1* and *WT1* gene rearrangements or alternatively of the *EWSR1-WT1* chimeric transcript may represent a useful diagnostic tool.

Essential and desirable diagnostic criteria

Essential: nests of small round cells in a desmoplastic stroma; immunopositivity for cytokeratin, desmin (dot-like pattern), and WT1 (antibody to C-terminus).

Desirable (but often not required): molecular studies to demonstrate *EWSR1* gene rearrangement or *EWSR1-WT1* fusion transcript.

Staging

Not clinically relevant

Prognosis and prediction

The overall survival remains poor, despite multimodality therapy {2508,1738,2970}. The 5-year overall survival rate is about 10–15% at most.

Extrarenal rhabdoid tumour

Oda Y
Biegel JA
Pfister SM

Definition

Extrarenal rhabdoid tumour is a highly malignant soft tissue tumour, mainly affecting infants and children, that consists of characteristic rounded or polygonal neoplastic cells with glassy eosinophilic cytoplasm containing hyaline-like inclusion bodies, eccentric nuclei, and macronucleoli. Morphologically and genetically identical tumours also arise in the kidney and brain. The majority of tumours are characterized by biallelic alterations of the *SMARCB1* gene leading to loss of expression of SMARCB1 (INI1).

ICD-O coding

8963/3 Rhabdoid tumour NOS

ICD-11 coding

2B5F.2 & XH3RF3 Sarcoma, not elsewhere classified of other specified sites & Malignant rhabdoid tumour

Related terminology

Acceptable: rhabdoid tumour of soft tissue; malignant rhabdoid tumour.

Subtype(s)

None

Localization

This rare tumour seems to arise most often in deep, axial locations such as the neck, paraspinal region, perineal region, abdominal cavity or retroperitoneum, and pelvic cavity {1664, 3283,965,2348}. Lesions in the extremities (especially the thigh) and cutaneous lesions are also well documented. This tumour also often affects visceral organs such as the liver, thymus,

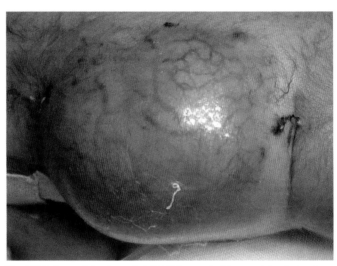

Fig. 1.383 Congenital extrarenal rhabdoid tumour. In this neonatal patient, a huge paravertebral and retroperitoneal tumour is evident. Multiple metastatic lesions were also identified at birth.

genitourinary tracts, and gastrointestinal system. The liver appears to be the single most common visceral location (73% of all cases {408,3103}).

Clinical features

Most cases present as a rapidly enlarging soft tissue mass – the associated clinical symptoms depend on the primary organ involvement. Occasional cases present with multiple cutaneous nodules {265}. Particularly in infants, some cases present with disseminated disease without an obvious primary tumour – such

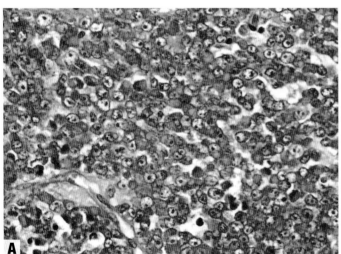
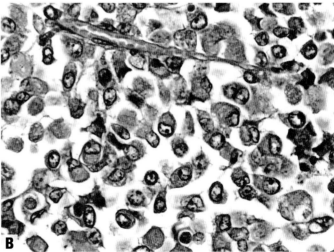

Fig. 1.384 Extrarenal rhabdoid tumour. **A** Characteristic rhabdoid cells with eosinophilic cytoplasm containing glassy inclusion-like bodies, eccentric vesicular nuclei, and prominent nucleoli. **B** Rhabdoid cells show a discohesive growth pattern.

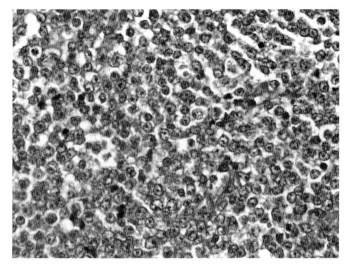

Fig. 1.385 Extrarenal rhabdoid tumour. Proliferation of undifferentiated small round cells, which is often observed in liver tumour.

cases are often associated with rhabdoid tumour predisposition {877}.

Epidemiology

Extrarenal rhabdoid tumour is exceedingly rare, and it is largely confined to infants and children. Among fetal and neonatal rhabdoid tumours, the extrarenal rhabdoid tumour is more common than those in the kidney or brain. Conversely, on average, patients with extrarenal, extracranial rhabdoid tumours tend to be older than patients with renal rhabdoid tumours {2983}.

Etiology

Familial cases are typically associated with germline mutations in *SMARCB1* (*INI1*, *hSNF5*, *BAF47*) in 22q11.23 {313,3199,877}. Germline mutations or deletions in *SMARCB1* (rhabdoid tumour predisposition syndrome 1) are present in approximately 13% of patients with extrarenal rhabdoid tumours {1398}. Patients with germline alterations in *SMARCB1* typically present in early childhood, but they are at increased risk for other soft tissue tumours, notably schwannomas, in later decades. A very small percentage of rhabdoid tumours are associated with *SMARCA4*

mutations, which may be present in the germline (rhabdoid tumour predisposition syndrome 2).

Pathogenesis

Extrarenal rhabdoid tumours arise as a consequence of homozygous inactivation of the *SMARCB1* gene in chromosome band 22q11.2. Approximately 98% of extrarenal rhabdoid tumours, malignant rhabdoid tumours of kidney, and atypical teratoid/rhabdoid tumours demonstrate genomic alterations of both copies of the gene, including coding-sequence mutations, partial- or whole-gene deletions, and copy-neutral loss-of-heterozygosity events that unmask a recessive allele on the remaining homologue {408}. There is some genotype–phenotype correlation, with rhabdoid tumours demonstrating truncating mutations or deletions throughout the coding sequence. Extrarenal rhabdoid tumours have a particularly high incidence of homozygous deletions of the *SMARCB1* gene. This is often a consequence of a chromosomal translocation between chromosome band 22q11.2 and a variety of different partner chromosomes. The translocation is unbalanced at the molecular level, resulting in deletion of *SMARCB1*. The second allele is usually lost as a result of an interstitial 22q11.2 deletion. Consistent with the function of *SMARCB1* as a classic tumour suppressor gene, initiating germline mutations or deletions in *SMARCB1* function as the first hit in patients who have a genetic predisposition to the development of rhabdoid tumours. Such patients are also at risk for malignant rhabdoid tumour of kidney and atypical teratoid/rhabdoid tumour. In rare rhabdoid tumours with retained SMARCB1 expression, mutation and/or loss of the *SMARCA4* gene in 19p13.2 has been reported {2775}. Inactivation of the SWI/SNF complex by targeting either *SMARCB1* or *SMARCA4* gives rise to both intracranial and extracranial rhabdoid tumours. The loss of this epigenetic remodeller leads to silencing of a variety of tumour suppressor and differentiation genes and pathways that are considered hallmarks in the pathogenesis of these tumours {927,2115,500}.

Macroscopic appearance

Most tumours are unencapsulated and measure > 5 cm in maximum diameter. The tumours are usually soft and grey to tan in colour on cut surface, and they are frequently accompanied by foci of coagulative and haemorrhagic necrosis.

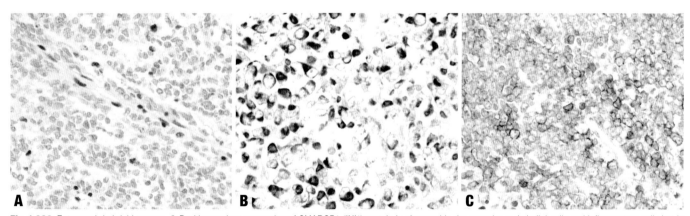

Fig. 1.386 Extrarenal rhabdoid tumour. **A** Positive nuclear expression of SMARCB1 (INI1) protein is observed in the vascular endothelial cells and inflammatory cells but is completely absent in the tumour cells. **B** Strong positive cytoplasmic immunoreactivity for keratin CAM5.2, which is confined to the inclusions. **C** Focal membranous positivity for EMA.

Histopathology

The tumour is characterized by rhabdoid cells with large vesicular rounded to bean-shaped nuclei, prominent nucleoli, and abundant cytoplasm, arranged in sheets or in a solid trabecular pattern. Many tumour cells have juxtanuclear eosinophilic, PAS-positive, diastase-resistant hyaline inclusions or globules. At the periphery, tumour cells infiltrate surrounding tissue. Nuclear pleomorphism is not evident, whereas mitotic figures are frequently observed. The tumour often shows loss of cellular cohesion. Some cases demonstrate predominant proliferation of undifferentiated small round cells, with only a small number of typical rhabdoid cells {1673,3204}. Immunohistochemically, most of these tumours show expression of epithelial markers such as keratins and EMA {965,2348}. The expression of neural or neuroectodermal markers such as CD99 and synaptophysin is also frequently observed in soft tissue tumours. Less commonly, the cells express MSA and focal S100 {965,1673}. SALL4 and glypican-3 (GPC3) immunoexpression is frequently observed {3369,1674,1671}. Characteristically, rhabdoid tumours show loss of SMARCB1 (INI1, BAF47) expression {1399A,1396A}.

Cytology

Not clinically relevant

Diagnostic molecular pathology

Not clinically relevant

Essential and desirable diagnostic criteria

Essential: primitive undifferentiated or rhabdoid cell morphology; loss of expression of SMARCB1 (INI1).

Staging

Not clinically relevant

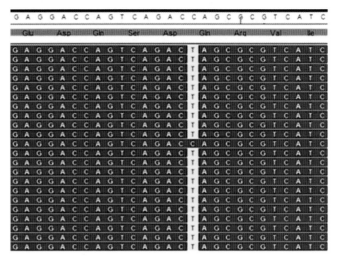

Fig. 1.387 Extrarenal rhabdoid tumour. Next-generation sequencing analysis demonstrating a *SMARCB1* nonsense mutation (NM_003073.4:c.778C>T, p.Gln260*) in a rhabdoid tumour with copy-neutral loss of heterozygosity of chromosome 22 (not shown). The mutant base is highlighted in yellow; sequencing reads are visualized with custom software (Genetrix).

Prognosis and prediction

Regardless of tumour location, patient outcome is dismal. Because of the entity's rarity, there are no large studies of survival analysis in uniformly treated patients with extrarenal tumours. The median age was 28 months, and the overall 5-year survival rate was < 15% {376,1934}. Patients with rhabdoid tumours of the liver have a worse survival than patients with other extracranial and extrarenal sites {3103,407}.

PEComa

Doyle LA
Argani P
Hornick JL

Definition
PEComas are mesenchymal neoplasms composed of perivascular epithelioid cells (PECs) – distinctive epithelioid cells that are often closely associated with blood vessel walls and that express both melanocytic and smooth muscle markers.

ICD-O coding
8714/0 Perivascular epithelioid tumour, benign

ICD-11 coding
2F7C & XH4CC6 Neoplasms of uncertain behaviour of connective or other soft tissue & Perivascular epithelioid tumour, benign
2B5F.2 & XH4CC6 Sarcoma, not elsewhere classified of other specified sites & Perivascular epithelioid tumour, malignant

Related terminology
Acceptable: angiomyolipoma; epithelioid angiomyolipoma; lymphangioleiomyomatosis
Not recommended: clear cell myomelanocytic tumour; sugar tumour of the lung.

Subtype(s)
Perivascular epithelioid tumour, malignant; angiomyolipoma; angiomyolipoma, epithelioid

Localization
PEComas show a wide anatomical distribution {1052,1057,269, 851,3175,2089,1857,3340}.

Clinical features
PEComas of soft tissue usually present as painless masses.

Epidemiology
PEComas are rare and are more frequent in females than males (M:F ratio: ~0.2:1), with a wide age range and a peak in young to middle-aged adults (mean age: 45 years) {1052,1057,851,1413}.

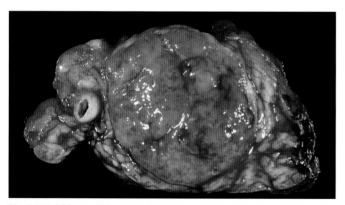

Fig. 1.388 PEComa. This pancreatic tumour is grossly well circumscribed, with a fleshy cut surface.

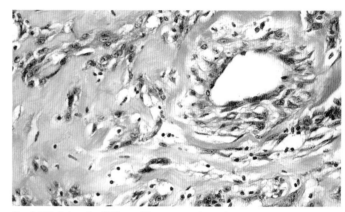

Fig. 1.389 Sclerosing PEComa. The tumour cells are focally situated within the wall of a dilated blood vessel.

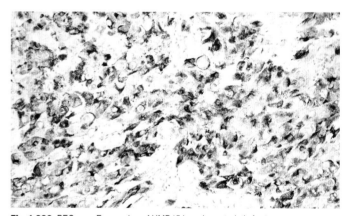

Fig. 1.390 PEComa. Expression of HMB45 is a characteristic feature.

Etiology
Most PEComas are sporadic; a small subset are associated with tuberous sclerosis {364,1057,1413}.

Pathogenesis
Loss of heterozygosity involving the *TSC2* locus has been found {2411}. Deletion of 16p, the location of the *TSC2* gene, indicates the oncogenetic relationship of PEComas and angiomyolipomas as *TSC2*-linked neoplasms. *TP53* mutations have been identified in 63% of *TSC2*-mutated PEComas {35}. A small subset of PEComas harbour *TFE3* gene fusions, which correlate with strong nuclear immunoreactivity for TFE3 {155}. The most common fusion partner with *TFE3* is *SFPQ* (*PSF*) {2580,3038,35}. *DVL2-TFE3* and *NONO-TFE3* gene fusions have also been identified in PEComa arising in soft tissue {162}. *TFE3*-rearranged PEComa lacks *TSC2* mutations / loss of heterozygosity and thus appears to be pathogenetically distinct {35,1956}.

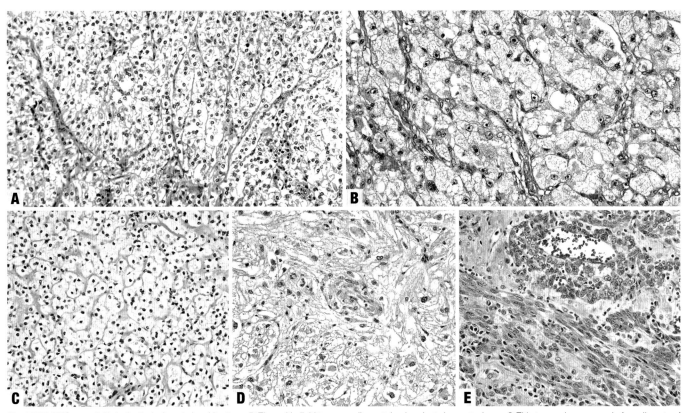

Fig. 1.391 PEComa. **A** Note the typical nested architecture. **B** The epithelioid tumour cells contain abundant clear cytoplasm. **C** This tumour is composed of small nests of clear cells with small round nuclei and sharply defined cell borders (sugar tumour). **D** A tumour with a sheet-like growth pattern. Note the granular to clear cytoplasm and uniform nuclear morphology. **E** Some tumours show spindle cell morphology.

Macroscopic appearance

PEComas are grossly well circumscribed, with a firm and fibrous or fleshy cut surface. Tumours show a wide size range (mean: 5–8 cm); cutaneous tumours are usually smaller than those arising at deep locations {1057,1857,1413,851,269}.

Histopathology

PEComas typically show a nested architecture and are composed of epithelioid cells with abundant granular eosinophilic or clear cytoplasm and round nuclei with small nucleoli. The nests or trabeculae are typically surrounded by thin-walled capillary vessels. A small subset of tumours have predominantly spindle cell morphology {1057,851}. PEComa usually shows

a distinctive perivascular pattern of growth, with tumour cells radially arranged around vessels, replacing the vessel wall and approaching the endothelium. The sclerosing subtype of PEComa is composed of cords and trabeculae of epithelioid cells in a densely collagenous stroma {1413}. Epithelioid angiomyolipoma is synonymous with PEComa {189,427}. Typical PEComa may contain occasional multinucleated cells and show limited pleomorphism (symplastic change), but mitotic figures are usually scarce or absent. Malignant PEComas are characterized by a variable combination of mitotic activity, necrosis, and pleomorphism {364,1057,851,269}.

PEComas characteristically express both melanocytic markers, such as HMB45 (the most sensitive immunomarker),

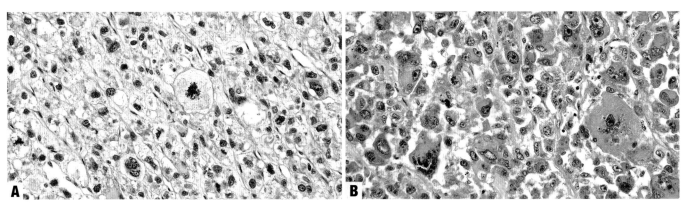

Fig. 1.392 PEComa. **A** Malignant PEComa composed of epithelioid tumour cells with clear cytoplasm, nuclear atypia, and mitotic activity. Note the trabecular architecture. **B** A malignant PEComa with marked nuclear atypia and pleomorphism. Note the abundant granular eosinophilic cytoplasm.

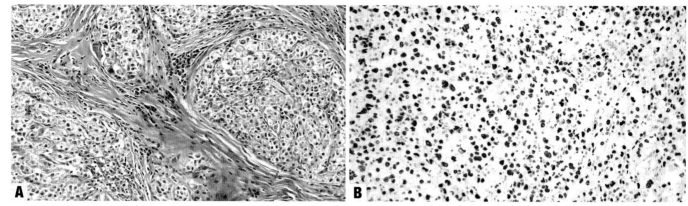

Fig. 1.393 PEComa with *TFE3* rearrangement. **A** PEComa with *TFE3* rearrangement showing nested and solid alveolar growth patterns and epithelioid tumour cells with moderate amounts of granular eosinophilic cytoplasm. **B** Nuclear TFE3 expression in PEComa corresponding to the presence of *TFE3* rearrangement.

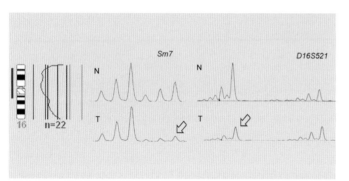

Fig. 1.394 PEComa. Loss of chromosome arm 16p demonstrated by comparative genomic hybridization and loss-of-heterozygosity analysis using microsatellite markers Sm7 and D16S521 (arrows), which flank the locus of the *TSC2* gene.

melan-A, and MITF, and muscle markers, such as SMA, desmin, and caldesmon {1054,1413,851,269,1949}. Expression of melanocytic markers is more common in epithelioid than spindled tumour cells. Desmin and h-caldesmon are often less extensively positive than SMA {1413}. Some tumours lack expression of muscle markers {1054}. Nuclear expression of S100 is generally not observed in PEComas. Approximately 15% of cases show strong nuclear staining for TFE3 {162,1057,851,155}. PEComas with *TFE3* rearrangement tend to occur in younger patients, have a prominent alveolar growth pattern and epithelioid morphology, and often lack expression of smooth muscle markers {162,1956,2580,35}. Occasional *TFE3*-rearranged epithelioid but non-epithelial neoplasms contain melanin pigment; these were initially described in the kidney as melanotic Xp11 translocation renal cancer, but they have also been described in soft tissue {156,162} and most closely fit into the category of *TFE3*-rearranged PEComa.

Cytology
Not clinically relevant

Diagnostic molecular pathology
For cases with strong TFE3 protein expression, identification of *TFE3* gene rearrangement or a corresponding fusion gene can help confirm the diagnosis.

Essential and desirable diagnostic criteria
Essential: epithelioid and/or spindle cells with granular eosinophilic to clear cytoplasm; nested, trabecular, or sheet-like architecture with frequent perivascular orientation; variable coexpression of melanocytic and smooth muscle markers.
Desirable: TFE3 expression if smooth muscle markers are negative.

Staging
Not clinically relevant

Prognosis and prediction
Clinically malignant tumours are typically large; show marked nuclear atypia and pleomorphism, conspicuous mitoses, necrosis, and infiltrative margins; and tend to pursue an aggressive clinical course {1057,269}. Tumour size > 5 cm has also been significantly associated with recurrence {341}. The most common metastatic sites are the liver, lymph nodes, lungs, and bone {1057,851,269}.

Intimal sarcoma

Bode-Lesniewska B
Debiec-Rychter M
Tavora F

Definition
Intimal sarcomas are malignant mesenchymal tumours arising in large blood vessels of the systemic and pulmonary circulation and also in the heart. The defining feature is predominantly intraluminal growth with obstruction of the lumen of the vessel of origin and seeding of emboli to peripheral organs.

ICD-O coding
9137/3 Intimal sarcoma

ICD-11 coding
2B5F.2 & XH36H7 Sarcoma, not elsewhere classified of other specified sites & Intimal sarcoma

Related terminology
None

Subtype(s)
None

Localization
Intimal sarcomas of the pulmonary circulation mainly involve the proximal vessels: the pulmonary trunk (80%), the right or left pulmonary arteries (50–70%), or both (40%) {450,2316}. Some tumours involve cardiac structures: the left heart, pulmonary valve, or right ventricular outflow {448,2266,1494,3156}. Direct infiltration or lung metastases are observed in 40% of cases, and extrathoracic spread occurs at presentation in 20% (brain, skin, lymph nodes) {450}. Aortic intimal sarcomas mostly arise in the abdominal aorta between the celiac artery and the iliac bifurcation, and 30% are located in the thoracic aorta {2931, 450,2738,2801}.

Clinical features
Clinical presentation is nonspecific and often related to tumour emboli {1628,2803,1088,3413}, with recurrent pulmonary embolic disease being the most common primary diagnosis. Proper diagnosis is often delayed or made after death. Imaging is nonspecific, but the neoplastic nature of the tissue occluding the lumen can be suspected on the basis of some diagnostic procedures (CT, MRI, PET) {1628,2803,2396,3299}.

Epidemiology
Intimal sarcomas are very rare tumours, with major pulmonary vessel sarcomas being twice as common as aortic tumours {349,450,808,2485,2801}. Intracardiac intimal sarcomas are rare, although this is the most common type of heart sarcoma {2266}. Pulmonary and heart intimal sarcomas are slightly more common in females (M:F ratio: ~0.7:1), whereas aortic tumours may be more common in males {2931}. The mean age at diagnosis is 48 years for pulmonary, 50 years for heart, and 62 years for aortic intimal sarcomas {1628,3156,2931,450}.

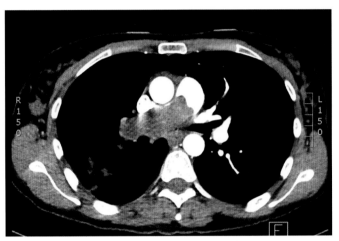

Fig. 1.395 Intimal sarcoma. CT of a patient with intimal sarcoma of the right pulmonary artery demonstrating a solid intraluminal mass, which showed metabolic activity on PET-CT (not pictured).

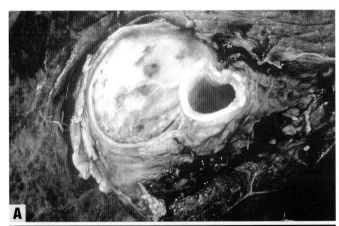

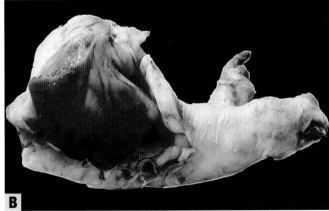

Fig. 1.396 Intimal sarcoma. **A** View of the hilum of the resected lung of a patient with obstruction of the lumen of the pulmonary artery by tumour tissue. **B** Endarterectomy specimen of another patient with intimal sarcoma of the pulmonary artery.

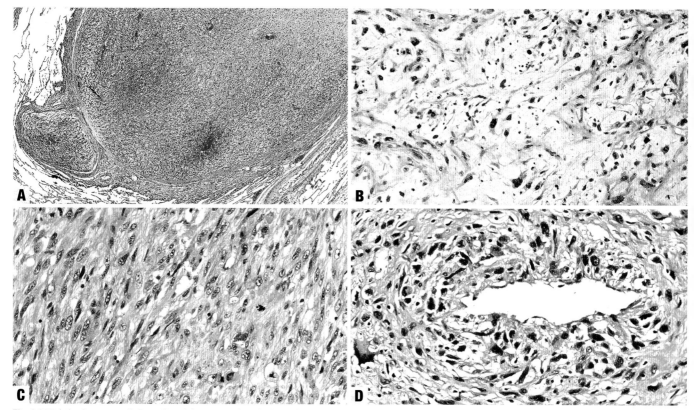

Fig. 1.397 Intimal sarcoma. **A** Spreading of the tumour along the intrapulmonary branches of the pulmonary artery. **B** Myxoid tumour with low cellular density. **C** Bundles of tumour cells resembling leiomyosarcoma. **D** An endothelium-lined vascular cleft surrounded by pleomorphic tumour cells.

Etiology

Unknown

Pathogenesis

By comparative genomic hybridization (CGH) and array comparative genomic hybridization (aCGH), gains/amplifications of 12q12-q15 (*CDK4, TSPAN31, MDM2, GLI1* [*GLI*]) and 4q12 were reported as the most consistent aberrations {349,3392,3399A}.

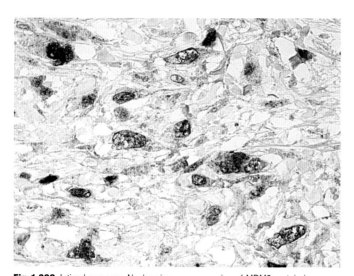

Fig. 1.398 Intimal sarcoma. Nuclear immunoexpression of MDM2 protein in numerous tumour cells.

Interphase FISH revealed amplification of *PDGFRA* and *KIT* (*CD117*) and amplification/polysomy of *EGFR* in all and in 6 of 8 tumours, respectively {3034A}. In a recent aCGH study, 6 of 8 tumours showed 4q12 amplification, with the common region containing only *PDGFRA*. Other, less consistent alterations were gains/amplifications in 7p14-p22, 8q11-q23, 12p11, and 12q13-q15 (*GLI1* [*GLI*], *CDK4, DDIT3, HMGA2, BEST3, MDM2*) and losses in 3q12-q21, 9p21, 10q22, 12q12, and 12q23. Frequent high-level (co)amplifications/gains of *PDGFRA* (81%), *EGFR* (76%), and/or *MDM2* (65%) were confirmed in 21 tumours by FISH {808}. Recently, based on molecular analysis, intimal sarcoma was identified as the most frequent sarcoma histotype (42%) in a series of 100 cardiac sarcomas {2266}. With the use of FISH, quantitative PCR, and aCGH, *MDM2* amplification was detected in 100% of cardiac intimal sarcomas. aCGH showed a complex profile, with recurrent 12q13-q14 amplicons containing *MDM2*, 7p12 gain involving *EGFR*, 9p21 deletion targeting *CDKN2A* in all cases, and *KIT* and *PDGFRA* amplification in 2 of 5 cases {2266}.

Macroscopic appearance

By definition, intimal sarcomas are mostly intravascular masses attached to the vessel wall, grossly resembling thrombi and extending distally along the branches of the involved vessels. Occasionally, a mucoid lumen cast can be recovered intraoperatively, or harder, bony areas corresponding to osteosarcomatous differentiation are found. Some of the aortic tumours may cause thinning and aneurysmal dilatation with adherent thrombus, suggesting atherosclerosis {2258,2303}.

Histopathology

Intimal sarcomas are morphologically non-distinctive, poorly differentiated malignant mesenchymal tumours, consisting of mildly to severely atypical spindle cells with varying degrees of mitotic activity, necrosis, and nuclear polymorphism. Some tumours show myxoid areas or epithelioid morphology {1179, 2801}. Prominent spindling and bundling may resemble leiomyosarcoma. Rare cases may contain neoplastic cartilage or tumour osteoid, or show focal rhabdomyosarcomatous or angiosarcomatous features {450,1179,1419,2316}. Immunohistochemically, variable positivity for SMA is found, and some tumours exhibit positivity for desmin. Rhabdomyosarcomatous differentiation is accompanied by the expression of myogenin and MYOD1 {2266}. Nuclear expression of MDM2 can be observed in at least 70% of cases {349,808}.

Cytology

FNA specimens of intraluminal sarcomas contain obviously malignant, spindled and pleomorphic mesenchymal tumour cells.

Diagnostic molecular pathology

Demonstration of *MDM2* amplification can be helpful.

Essential and desirable diagnostic criteria

Essential: occurrence within the lumen of a large vessel of the pulmonary or systemic circulation or within the heart cavities; primary high-grade sarcoma, with or without heterologous elements.
Desirable: MDM2 amplification (in selected cases).

Staging

Not clinically relevant

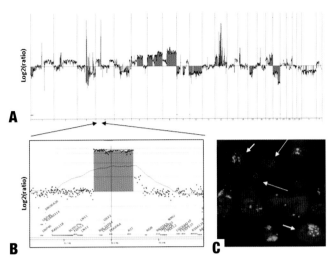

Fig. 1.399 Intimal sarcoma. **A** A representative copy-number alteration profile (Agilent 244K array comparative genomic hybridization) showing high-level amplification of the *PDGFRA*/4q12 and *MDM2*/12q14-q15 regions; gain of 6q, 7, 8q, 12p, and 17q; and partial/total losses of 1p, 3q, 5q, 9p, 10, 15q, 18, and X. The individual probes are arranged according to their genomic location (*x* axis) and their respective tumour/reference log$_2$ ratios (*y* axis). **B** Array comparative genomic hybridization profile of a selected region of chromosome band 4q12, showing high-level amplification of the genes *CHIC2*, *PDGFRA*, and *KIT*. **C** A representative example of dual-colour interphase FISH images of intimal sarcoma, showing exclusive high-level amplification of *PDGFRA* (red signals; long arrows) or *MDM2* (green signals; short arrows), intermingled with cells showing separate amplicons for both genes.

Prognosis and prediction

The prognosis for patients with intimal sarcomas is poor, with a mean survival time of 5–9 months in patients with aortic sarcomas and 13–18 months in patients with pulmonary sarcomas {349,450,2316,2485}.

Undifferentiated sarcoma

Dei Tos AP
Mertens F
Pillay N

Definition
Undifferentiated soft tissue sarcoma (USTS) shows no identifiable line of differentiation when analysed by presently available technology. At present, this is a heterogeneous group and a diagnosis of exclusion, although genetic subgroups (particularly in the round cell group) have emerged. Not included are dedifferentiated types of specific soft tissue sarcomas (e.g. dedifferentiated liposarcoma), in which the high-grade component is commonly undifferentiated.

ICD-O coding
8805/3 Undifferentiated sarcoma

ICD-11 coding
2B5F.2 & XH73J4 Sarcoma, not elsewhere classified of other specified sites & Giant cell sarcoma
2B5F.2 & XH0947 Sarcoma, not elsewhere classified of other specified sites & Malignant fibrous histiocytoma
2B5F.2 & XH6HY6 Sarcoma, not elsewhere classified of other specified sites & Undifferentiated sarcoma
2B5F.2 & XH85G7 Sarcoma, not elsewhere classified of other specified sites & Small cell sarcoma

Related terminology
None

Subtype(s)
Spindle cell sarcoma, undifferentiated; pleomorphic sarcoma, undifferentiated; round cell sarcoma, undifferentiated

Localization
USTS may be found at any location. Published data are limited, but overall it seems that these lesions are most common in somatic soft tissue.

Clinical features
USTS has no characteristic clinical features that distinguish it from other types of sarcoma, other than a frequently rapid growth rate.

Epidemiology
USTSs are uncommon mesenchymal neoplasms that are anatomically ubiquitous and occur at all ages and with no difference between the sexes. USTSs account for as many as 20% of all soft tissue sarcomas. Those with round cell morphology are most frequent in young patients and are currently in large part labelled according to their main driving genetic anomaly, if known (see Chapter 2: *Undifferentiated small round cell sarcomas of bone and soft tissue*, p. 321). Those that are pleomorphic (often known as pleomorphic malignant fibrous histiocytomas in the past) occur mostly in older adults.

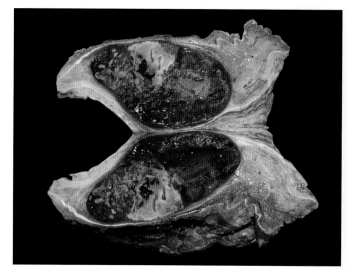

Fig. 1.400 Undifferentiated pleomorphic sarcoma. Grossly, undifferentiated pleomorphic sarcomas most often feature a fleshy appearance with areas of necrosis and haemorrhage.

Etiology
The etiology of most USTSs is unknown. However, at least 25% of radiation-associated soft tissue sarcomas are undifferentiated {1163,1761}.

Pathogenesis
Undifferentiated pleomorphic sarcomas (UPSs) typically display extensive genomic rearrangements. Cytogenetic data from > 100 cases have, with few exceptions, revealed complex karyotypes with chromosome numbers ranging from near-haploid to hyperoctaploid {1021,1390}. The extensive reshuffling of chromosomal material indicated by tumour karyotypes is corroborated by array-based genomic studies, showing structural rearrangements and copy-number shifts involving most if not all chromosomes {482,1699}, as well as by massively parallel sequencing studies {472,2935}. UPSs demonstrate substantial copy-number heterogeneity compared with other sarcoma subtypes and do not form distinct methylation subgroups {472, 2935}. Whole-genome sequencing has revealed that punctuated evolutionary events such as whole-genome duplications and chromothripsis accompanied by telomere dysfunction underpin the genomic complexity of UPS {2935}. The aberrations in telomere biology are achieved either through activation of telomerase through deregulation of *TERT* or through the alternative lengthening of telomeres pathway {472,2935}. There are no tumour-specific amplicons, but some 10–15% of cases show amplification of *VGLL3* or *YAP1*, and 10% have amplification of *CCNE1* {1344,472}. Targets of frequent deletions and disruptive rearrangements include *CDKN2A* and *CDKN2B* in 9p, *PTEN* in 10q, *RB1* in 13q, and *TP53* in 17p, each affected in 10–20% of cases {2865,576,2492,1150,472,2935}. *RB1* and *TP53*, as

well as *ATRX*, are among the few genes that recurrently show pathogenetic variants at the nucleotide level {472}. At the transcriptomic level, UPS cannot be distinguished from high-grade myxofibrosarcoma, and it is possible that these two entities may lie on a spectrum of differentiation {472}. A small subset of UPSs with low mitotic counts show gene fusions involving the *PRDM10* gene, with either *MED12* or *CITED2* as the 5' partner {1390}. Otherwise, driver gene fusions have not been found in UPS {472}.

Macroscopic appearance

USTSs are a heterogeneous group and thus have no distinctive macroscopic features, other than the frequent presence of necrosis and haemorrhage.

Histopathology

USTSs may be broadly divided into pleomorphic, spindle cell, round cell, and epithelioid subsets, but none have specific defining features other than their lack of an identifiable line of differentiation {1018}. Pleomorphic USTSs, which represent the largest group, closely resemble other specific types of pleomorphic sarcomas and are often patternless, with frequent bizarre multinucleated tumour giant cells. Spindle cell USTSs most often show a fascicular architecture with variably amphophilic or palely eosinophilic cytoplasm and tapering nuclei. Round cell USTSs consist of relatively uniform rounded or ovoid cells with a high N:C ratio, and they most often closely resemble

other specific types of round cell sarcomas, especially Ewing sarcoma. However, many cases can now probably be more precisely classified within specific molecular subsets, such as *CIC*-rearranged and *BCOR*-rearranged sarcomas, as well as within the group of round cell sarcomas associated with *EWSR1* fusions involving partners unrelated to the ETS family of genes (e.g. *PATZ1*, *NFATC2*, *SP3*, *SMARCA5*, and *POU5F1*) – see Chapter 2: *Undifferentiated small round cell sarcomas of bone and soft tissue* (p. 321). USTSs with epithelioid morphology have been little studied as yet {2716}, but they are probably not rare. Morphologically, these lesions closely resemble metastatic carcinoma or melanoma, but they generally lack nesting and have amphophilic or palely eosinophilic cytoplasm and large vesicular nuclei. Some appear to show *SMARCA4* inactivation {1789,2493}. Importantly, genomic profiling may reveal that some seemingly undifferentiated sarcomas can be classified more specifically {482,639,641,2150}.

Cytology

Not clinically relevant

Diagnostic molecular pathology

Undifferentiated pleomorphic and epithelioid sarcomas are characterized by complex genetic aberrations not suitable for diagnostic purposes. However, molecular genetics plays a major role in excluding specific molecular entities, particularly when dealing with undifferentiated round cell sarcomas. UPS must be

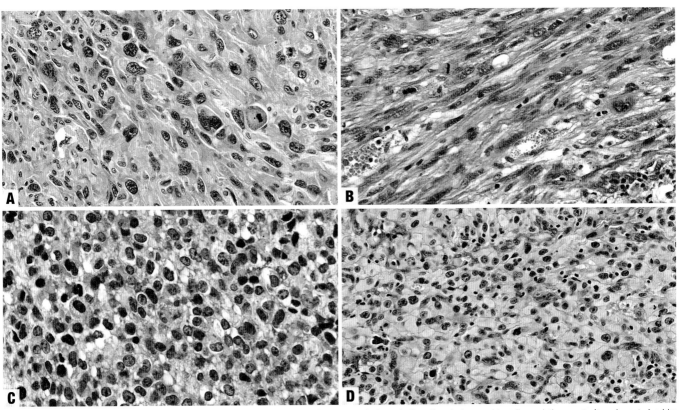

Fig. 1.401 Undifferentiated sarcoma. **A** Undifferentiated pleomorphic sarcoma is composed of a spindle cell and pleomorphic cell population most often characterized by high mitotic activity. Atypical mitoses are very common. **B** Undifferentiated spindle cell sarcoma features a highly atypical spindle cell proliferation. Mitotic activity is most often high. **C** Currently, undifferentiated round cell sarcoma can be diagnosed only if distinctive gene fusions have been ruled out. **D** Undifferentiated epithelioid sarcoma is most often composed of a high-grade epithelioid cell population lacking any specific line of differentiation.

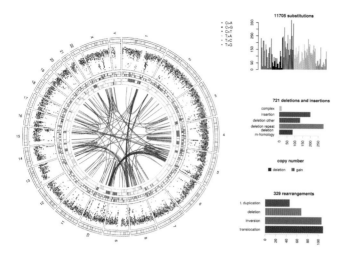

Fig. 1.402 Undifferentiated pleomorphic sarcoma. Circos plot illustrating the complex copy-number and rearrangement patterns seen in a typical undifferentiated pleomorphic sarcoma genome. The outer ring denotes chromosomal location, with subsequent rings representing single-nucleotide variants, insertions, deletions, and copy-number gains and losses. The arcs represent interchromosomal and intrachromosomal rearrangements.

separated from dedifferentiated liposarcoma, a lesion characterized molecularly by *MDM2* and *CDK4* gene amplification {575, 641}.

Essential and desirable diagnostic criteria
Essential: spindle, pleomorphic, epithelioid, and round cell (most often high-grade) morphology; absence of any morphological or immunohistochemical feature of specific differentiation; demonstrated absence of distinctive molecular aberration.

Staging
The American Joint Committee on Cancer (AJCC) or Union for International Cancer Control (UICC) TNM system may be used.

Prognosis and prediction
Because of the lack of substantive studies, data are limited. The majority of USTSs are morphologically high-grade. Among pleomorphic sarcomas in adults, those that are undifferentiated and arise in the limbs or trunk have a reported 5-year metastasis-free survival rate of 83% {1023}. USTS with epithelioid morphology seems to be more aggressive {2716}. In children, reported survival rates for USTS, whether of round cell or spindle cell / pleomorphic type, are 70–75% {59,2468,2905}.

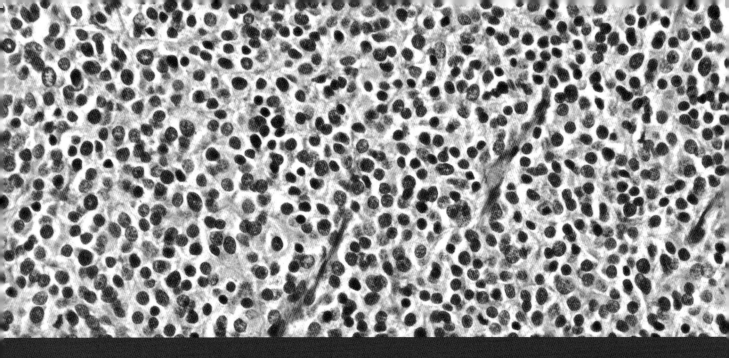

2

Undifferentiated small round cell sarcomas of bone and soft tissue

Edited by: Bridge JA

Ewing sarcoma
Round cell sarcoma with *EWSR1*–non-ETS fusions
CIC-rearranged sarcoma
Sarcoma with *BCOR* genetic alterations

WHO classification of undifferentiated small round cell sarcomas of bone and soft tissue

9364/3   Ewing sarcoma
9366/3*   Round cell sarcoma with *EWSR1*–non-ETS fusions
9367/3*   *CIC*-rearranged sarcoma
9368/3*   Sarcoma with *BCOR* genetic alterations

These morphology codes are from the International Classification of Diseases for Oncology, third edition, second revision (ICD-O-3.2) {1471}. Behaviour is coded /0 for benign tumours; /1 for unspecified, borderline, or uncertain behaviour; /2 for carcinoma in situ and grade III intraepithelial neoplasia; /3 for malignant tumours, primary site; and /6 for malignant tumours, metastatic site. Behaviour code /6 is not generally used by cancer registries.

This classification is modified from the previous WHO classification, taking into account changes in our understanding of these lesions.

* Codes marked with an asterisk were approved by the IARC/WHO Committee for ICD-O at its meeting in January 2020.

Ewing sarcoma

de Álava E
Lessnick SL
Stamenkovic I

Definition
Ewing sarcoma is a small round cell sarcoma showing gene fusions involving one member of the FET family of genes (usually *EWSR1*) and a member of the ETS family of transcription factors.

ICD-O coding
9364/3 Ewing sarcoma

ICD-11 coding
2B52.3 Ewing sarcoma of soft tissue
2B52.Y Ewing sarcoma of bone and articular cartilage of other specified sites

Related terminology
Not recommended: Askin tumour (for Ewing sarcoma arising in the chest wall); primitive neuroectodermal tumour.
Note: Some small round cell sarcomas previously considered subtypes of Ewing sarcoma (Ewing-like sarcomas) are genetically and clinically distinct entities and include *CIC*-rearranged sarcoma and sarcoma with *BCOR* genetic alterations, described in separate sections.

Subtype(s)
None

Localization
Ewing sarcoma arises in the diaphysis and diaphyseal-metaphyseal portions of long bones, pelvis, and ribs, although any bone can be affected. Extraskeletal Ewing sarcoma occurs in about 12% of patients {1238} and has a wide anatomical distribution.

Clinical features
Ewing sarcoma often presents with locoregional pain and a palpable mass, sometimes associated with pathological fracture and fever (particularly with advanced and/or metastatic disease). Plain radiographs often demonstrate poorly defined osteolytic-permeative lesions with a classic multilayered periosteal reaction (onion-skin appearance). Additional studies including CT, MRI, and/or PET imaging are used to fully define primary lesions and soft tissue extension, as well as to evaluate for metastatic disease (present in ~25% of patients).

Epidemiology
Ewing sarcoma is the second most common malignant bone tumour in children and young adults, after osteosarcoma {1260}, and it shows an M:F ratio of 1.4:1. Nearly 80% of patients are aged < 20 years, and the peak incidence occurs during the second decade of life. Cases in patients aged > 30 years are less common, and these tumours more often arise in the soft tissue. The rarity of Ewing sarcoma among individuals of African

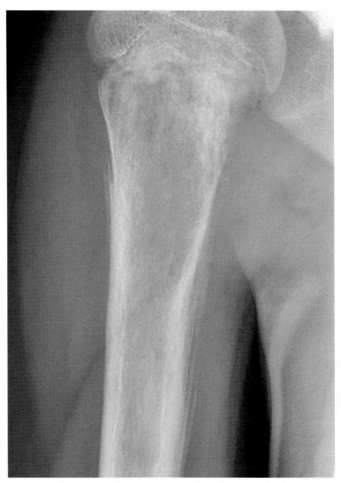

Fig. 2.01 Ewing sarcoma of bone. Anteroposterior radiograph of the right humerus shows an aggressive lesion in the proximal metadiaphysis, with permeative bone destruction, cortical lysis, and a multilamellated periosteal reaction, which is interrupted medially and laterally.

ancestry as compared to individuals of European ancestry is probably caused by genetic rather than environmental or lifestyle factors {3311}.

Etiology
The majority of cases are sporadic, but germline mutations have been detected {3394}.

Pathogenesis
All cases of Ewing sarcoma are associated with structural rearrangements that generate FET-ETS fusion genes (see below). Additional mutations may occur in *STAG2* (15–22%), *CDKN2A* (12%), and *TP53* (7%) {432,686,3077,3394}. FET-ETS fusion genes encode chimeric transcription factors that serve as master regulators to activate and repress thousands

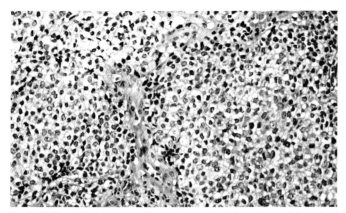

Fig. 2.02 Classic Ewing sarcoma. Notice the vaguely lobular pattern and cleared-out cytoplasm, due to glycogen deposits.

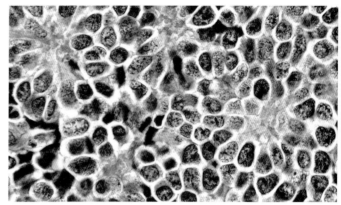

Fig. 2.03 Ewing sarcoma. Ewing sarcoma with extensive neuroectodermal differentiation (formerly called primitive neuroectodermal tumour) showing well-formed pseudorosettes, absence of nucleoli, and finely granular chromatin.

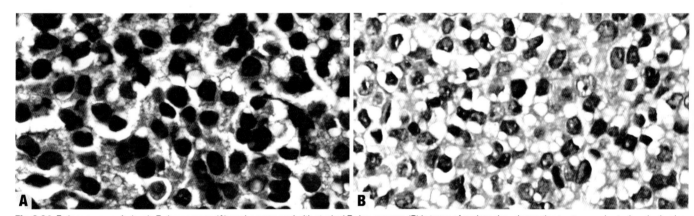

Fig. 2.04 Ewing sarcoma. A classic Ewing sarcoma (**A**) can be compared with atypical Ewing sarcoma (**B**) in terms of nuclear size, chromatin structure, and cytoplasmic clearing.

of genes. Expression of these aberrant transcription factors, presumably in the correct cellular and developmental context, is required for the development of Ewing sarcoma. Proteins bind both GGAA microsatellites and canonical ETS binding sites in the genome and recruit chromatin regulators. Binding of the fusion proteins to GGAA microsatellites results in the transition from a closed to an open chromatin state that establishes de novo enhancers, which activate genes. Conversely, binding to canonical ETS binding sites displaces wildtype ETS factors and represses gene expression. Together, these events establish an oncogenic gene expression programme that underlies transformation and subsequent tumour initiation.

Macroscopic appearance

The cut surface of untreated Ewing sarcoma specimens is greyish-white and soft, and it frequently includes areas of haemorrhage and necrosis

Histopathology

Most cases are composed of uniform small round cells with round nuclei containing finely stippled chromatin and inconspicuous nucleoli, scant clear or eosinophilic cytoplasm, and indistinct cytoplasmic membranes (classic Ewing sarcoma) {1887}. In others, the tumour cells are larger, with prominent nucleoli and irregular contours (atypical Ewing sarcoma) {1930}. Sometimes, a higher degree of neuroectodermal differentiation

(ill-defined groups of as many as 10 cells oriented towards a central space and/or with a consistent immunophenotype) is present (historically termed primitive neuroectodermal tumour) {1887}. After induction chemotherapy, Ewing sarcoma cells show a variable degree of necrosis and are replaced by loose connective tissue.

Immunohistochemically, CD99 is a cell-surface glycoprotein and a relevant diagnostic marker for Ewing sarcoma. Strong,

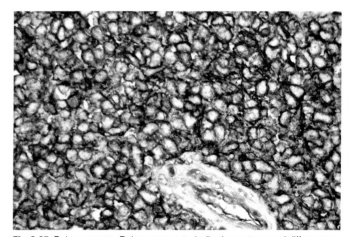

Fig. 2.05 Ewing sarcoma. Ewing sarcoma typically shows strong and diffuse membrane staining for CD99.

diffuse membranous expression of CD99 is evident in about 95% of Ewing sarcomas. NKX2-2 {1931} has a higher specificity than CD99. Keratin expression is present in approximately 25% of cases {1051}. FLI1 and ERG are often expressed in the cases with the corresponding gene fusions {3243}. Some cases express neuroendocrine antigens and/or S100.

A distinct subset of lesions carrying the same fusions has been described, predominantly in the head and neck region, as adamantinoma-like Ewing sarcoma. This subset often expresses markers of squamous differentiation. The relationship of this tumour type to classic Ewing sarcoma is uncertain {412,332}.

Cytology
Not clinically relevant

Diagnostic molecular pathology
Genetic confirmation is often required for Ewing sarcoma diagnosis. The most common Ewing sarcoma translocation (present in ~85% of cases) is t(11;22)(q24;q12), which results in the *EWSR1-FLI1* fusion transcript and protein. The second most common is t(21;22)(q22;q12), which results in *EWSR1-ERG* in about 10% of cases. The remaining cases have alternative translocations that join either *EWSR1* or *FUS* (which, along with *TAF15*, form the FET family) to other ETS family members. All cases of Ewing sarcoma harbour a FET-ETS fusion.

Essential and desirable diagnostic criteria
Essential: small round cell morphology; CD99 membranous expression.
Desirable: FET-ETS fusion detection (in selected cases).

Staging
The American Joint Committee on Cancer (AJCC) and Union for International Cancer Control (UICC) TNM systems can be applied.

Prognosis and prediction
The prognosis of Ewing sarcoma has improved considerably with current multimodal therapy, with a 65–70% cure rate for localized disease. However, metastatic and early-relapsing tumours have a poor prognosis, with a 5-year survival rate of < 30%. The presence of metastases appears to be the main prognostic factor. Other negative prognostic factors include the anatomical location of the tumour, such as the pelvis. Complete pathological response to neoadjuvant chemotherapy is a favourable prognostic factor {64}. There are currently no other prognostic markers in widespread use.

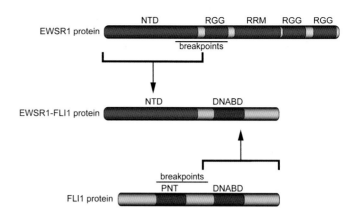

Fig. 2.06 The EWSR1-FLI1 fusion. The most common Ewing sarcoma translocation is between the *EWSR1* gene on chromosome 22 and the *FLI1* gene on chromosome 11. The EWSR1 protein has an N-terminal domain (NTD) that is an intrinsically disordered domain and a C-terminal region that contains RGG domains and an RNA-recognition motif (RRM). The FLI1 protein has an N-terminal domain with a pointed protein–protein interaction domain (PNT) and an ETS-type DNA-binding domain (DNABD) in its C-terminus. The resulting EWSR1-FLI1 protein retains the EWSR1 NTD and the FLI1 DNABD.

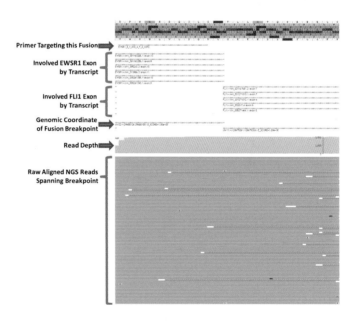

Fig. 2.07 Next-generation sequencing of *EWSR1-FLI1*. Next-generation RNA sequencing of Ewing sarcoma demonstrates in-frame fusion between *EWSR1* and *FLI1* gene products. Next-generation sequencing is more specific than *EWSR1* break-apart FISH because it provides detailed information about both translocation partners.

Round cell sarcoma with *EWSR1*–non-ETS fusions

Le Loarer F
Szuhai K
Tirode F

Definition
Round cell sarcomas with *EWSR1*–non-ETS fusions are round and spindle cell sarcomas with *EWSR1* or *FUS* fusions involving partners unrelated to the ETS gene family.

ICD-O coding
9366/3 Round cell sarcoma with *EWSR1*–non-ETS fusions

ICD-11 coding
None

Related terminology
Not recommended: Ewing-like sarcoma.

Subtype(s)
None

Localization
EWSR1-NFATC2 sarcomas are dominantly located in bones, with a 4:1 ratio over soft tissues {820}. The metaphysis or diaphysis of long bones is involved in the following sites in decreasing order of frequency: femur, humerus, radius, and tibia. Soft tissue cases involve extremities, head and neck, and chest wall {3014,633,2704}. *FUS-NFATC2* tumours have been reported exclusively in long bones {3253,348,820}. *EWSR1-PATZ1* sarcomas arise in the deep soft tissue and show a predilection for the chest wall and abdomen; however, extremity and head/neck locations have also been described {589,418}. *EWSR1-PATZ1* fusions have also been identified in CNS tumours {2556,1540, 418}.

Clinical features
EWSR1-NFATC2 and *FUS-NFATC2* sarcomas manifest as frequently painful, locally destructive bone lesions that may invade surrounding soft tissue, or less commonly, as well-circumscribed or locally invasive primary soft tissue tumours {633,820}. A subset of patients experience symptoms including a slow-growing mass for years before diagnosis {633,820}. Patients with *EWSR1-PATZ1* sarcomas may present with a palpable soft tissue mass and/or pain related to tumour location

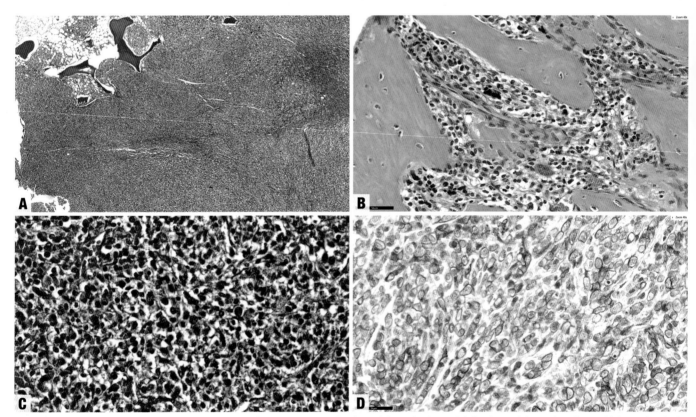

Fig. 2.08 *EWSR1-NFATC2* sarcoma. **A** Sarcomas with *NFATC2* rearrangement infiltrating and destroying bone. **B** Infiltration and destruction of bone with intertrabecular infiltration. **C** The tumour is composed of an undifferentiated round cell proliferation without admixed stroma and cytological features reminiscent of Ewing sarcoma. **D** Diffuse expression of CD99.

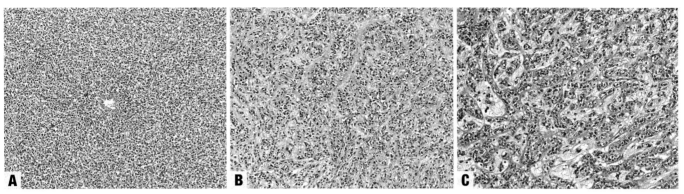

Fig. 2.09 *EWSR1-NFATC2* sarcoma. **A** Spindled to rounded tumour cells separated by scant stroma. **B** Tumour cells embedded in fibrohyaline stroma. **C** Myxohyaline stromal changes defining a nested appearance.

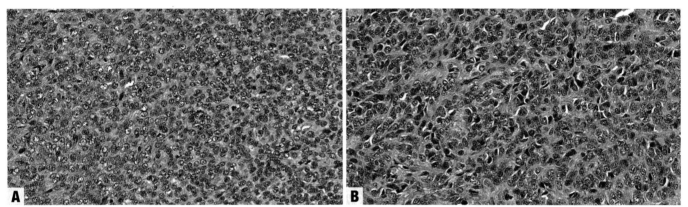

Fig. 2.10 *EWSR1-PATZ1* sarcoma. **A** Small to medium-sized tumour nuclei are round to ovoid, with fine granular chromatin. **B** Tumour nuclei may exhibit mild atypia with size/shape variation and coarse chromatin.

and size or extent of disease (a subset exhibit distant or locoregional metastases at time of diagnosis) {589,418}.

Epidemiology

These tumours are rare. *EWSR1-NFATC2* and *FUS-NFATC2* sarcomas feature a strong male predominance (M:F ratio: 5:1), with presentation in children and adults (age range: 12–67 years; median age: 32.3 years) {1931,348,3227}. The age range of patients diagnosed with *EWSR1-PATZ1* sarcoma in published cases is broad (1–81 years), with a mean of 42 years; sex distribution is near-equivalent {418}.

Etiology

Unknown

Pathogenesis

At the cytogenetic level, the translocation event resulting in fusion of the *EWSR1* (22q12.2) and *NFATC2* (20q13.2) genes typically arises within a derivative 22 ring chromosome as unbalanced and amplified {3014,3013}. The *EWSR1-NFATC2* fusion induces activation of the NFATC2 transcription factor consequent to the loss of the N-terminal regulatory domain, leading to the relocation in the nucleus of the chimeric transcription factor. Expression and methylome profiling has shown that *EWSR1-NFATC2* and *FUS-NFATC2* sarcomas differ from Ewing sarcomas, *EWSR1-PATZ1* sarcomas, and *CIC*-fused and *BCOR*-rearranged sarcomas {3253,1666,432,210}. In contrast

to *EWSR1-NFATC2*, the *FUS-NFATC2* fusion gene has not demonstrated amplification. Clustering analyses also suggest that *FUS-NFATC2* sarcomas are transcriptionally distinct from *EWSR1-NFATC2* sarcomas {3253}.

PATZ1 encodes a zinc finger protein with a Cys2-His2 motif with tumour suppressive functions involved in transcriptional regulation {977,2007}. *PATZ1* resides in close proximity (~2 Mb distance) to *EWSR1* on chromosome 22. The *EWSR1-PATZ1* fusion event is most likely the result of a submicroscopic intrachromosomal paracentric inversion (as the genes are normally transcribed in opposite directions), although genesis of this fusion via more-complex structural alterations at least for some cases cannot be fully excluded {2007,589,418}. An in-frame fusion between exon 8 or 9 of *EWSR1* and exon 1 of *PATZ1* results in removal of the putative transcriptional repressor domain and the AT-hook domain at the N-terminus of PATZ1 and converts a transcriptional repressor into a transcriptional activator. *EWSR1-PATZ1* sarcomas possess a unique expression signature, but they have not been compared with the CNS cases {3253}. In one study, comprehensive DNA and RNA sequencing revealed loss/deletion of *CDKN2A/CDKN2B* in 5 of 7 *EWSR1-PATZ1* sarcomas, with concurrent *MDM2* amplification in one (representing alterations that may have prognostic significance, because these events were evidenced in the clinically most aggressive tumours for which follow-up data was available and contrasted with absence of these alterations in a surgically resected, well-encapsulated *EWSR1-PATZ1* sarcoma

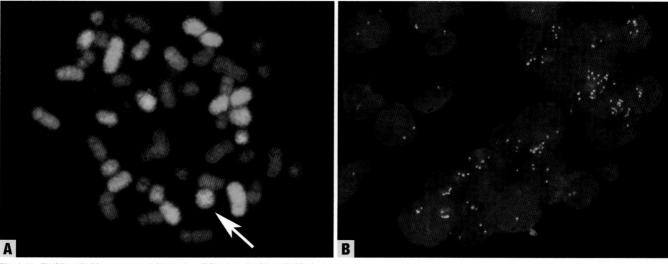

Fig. 2.11 *EWSR1-NFATC2* sarcoma. **A** Multicolour FISH of an *EWSR1-NFATC2* fusion–positive case exhibiting a ring chromosome derived from multiple alternating segments of chromosomes 20 and 22 (arrow). **B** *EWSR1* break-apart FISH demonstrates split signals with amplification of the telomeric probe (green); normal cells with colocalized signals are seen on the left.

that demonstrated no evidence of disease at 19 months after resection) {418}.

Macroscopic appearance

Gross examination of primary soft tissue or bone *EWSR1-NFATC2* sarcoma reveals a solid mass with a wide size range (4–18 cm in greatest dimension) and a yellowish-tan, firm or fleshy cut surface. Most of these sarcomas are ill defined and are locally destructive or infiltrate into adjacent tissues; however, a few primary soft tissue and bone lesions have been described as being well circumscribed or confined to the intramedullary cavity, respectively {3227,633,820}. *EWSR1-PATZ1* sarcoma is a solid-cystic mass with reported tumour sizes of 3.5 to > 10 cm in greatest dimension {589,418}.

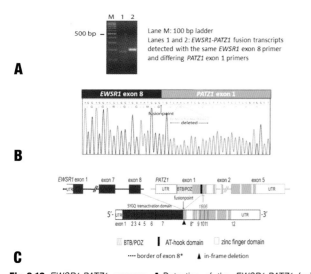

Fig. 2.12 *EWSR1-PATZ1* sarcoma. **A** Detection of the *EWSR1-PATZ1* fusion by RT-PCR. **B** Direct sequencing demonstrates the nucleotide sequence and deduced amino acid sequence around the *EWSR1-PATZ1* fusion point. **C** Schematic representation of the *EWSR1* and *PATZ1* genomic organization and fusion transcript.

Histopathology

EWSR1-NFATC2 and *FUS-NFATC2* sarcomas are composed of small to medium-sized round and/or spindled cells with limited eosinophilic or clear cytoplasm, predominantly arranged in cords, small nests, trabeculae, and pseudoacinar structures in a fibrohyaline or myxohyaline stromal background. Less commonly, matrix-poor sheets of cells are encountered focally or diffusely {125,3359,3227}. Small round monotonous to markedly pleomorphic nuclei featuring smooth or irregular nuclear contours, dense hyperchromatic or vesicular chromatin, and small or prominent nucleoli represent the morphological spectrum reported {125,3227,3359}. Tumour necrosis and mitotic activity are variable. Tumour cells diffusely express CD99 in half of cases; PAX7 and NKX2-2 may be expressed {3082,543}. Focal dot-like staining for keratin AE1/AE3 is possible, as is focal staining for CD138. Cases have been mainly misdiagnosed as myoepithelial tumour, plasmacytoma, and lymphoma {633, 2704,3359,2651,3191,1640,125}.

The histopathological and immunophenotypic features described for *EWSR1-PATZ1* sarcomas are fairly diverse {2007, 3253,589,418}. Tumour cells are small, round, and/or spindled and are often accompanied by a fibrous stroma. Necrosis and mitotic activity may or may not be evident. Coexpression of myogenic markers (desmin, myogenin, MYOD1) and neurogenic markers (S100P, SOX10, MITF, GFAP) is seen at variable levels. CD34 can be positive. CD99 is not consistently expressed.

Cytology

Not clinically relevant

Diagnostic molecular pathology

Identification of the *EWSR1-NFATC2*, *FUS-NFATC2*, and *EWSR1-PATZ1* fusions can be attained via diverse molecular approaches {3013,3227,348,2007,589,2985,3230,418}. However, for the *EWSR1-PATZ1* fusion, the sensitivity of an *EWSR1* break-apart probe may be compromised by the short genomic distance between *PATZ1* and *EWSR1* on 22q12.2 and corresponding interpretive challenges in visualizing the subtle dissociation or breaking apart of signals in balanced alterations; additional studies would be required for identification of the *PATZ1* partnership {418}.

Essential and desirable diagnostic criteria
Essential: spindled to rounded cytomorphology; mostly low-grade features, but high-grade cases are reported; fibro-hyaline stromal changes are common; *EWSR1* break-apart FISH shows amplification of the 5' probe in *EWSR1-NFATC2*–rearranged sarcomas; identification of the fusion transcript remains the gold standard.
Desirable: most *NFATC2*-rearranged tumours are located in long bone; *PATZ1*-rearranged sarcomas: round to spindled cells with divergent phenotype, both myogenic and neurogenic.

Staging
Round cell sarcoma with *EWSR1*–non-ETS fusions is staged under the Union for International Cancer Control (UICC) and American Joint Committee on Cancer (AJCC) TNM systems.

Prognosis and prediction
The clinical course may include local recurrences and/or metastatic disease. Disease control was achieved in 11 of the 14 *EWSR1-NFATC2* patients managed with surgical resection with a median follow-up of 45 months. Lung, cutaneous, and bone metastases have been reported as long as 10.5 years after initial diagnosis and clinical indolence; two patients died of disease, at 4 and 94 months {3227}. Little to no histological response has been observed in patients treated with neo-adjuvant chemotherapy {820}. Outcome data of *FUS-NFATC2* sarcomas are limited, with one unfavourable outcome at 15 months reported in a congenital case that displayed high-grade features, whereas other patients were free of disease after surgical management {348}. Evidence of metastatic disease at the time of diagnosis, of development of metastatic disease 5–24 months after diagnosis, and of patient death due to disease within 5–32 months of initial diagnosis underscores the aggressive behaviour characterizing a subset of *EWSR1-PATZ1* sarcomas for which follow-up data are available {2007, 589,418}. Responses to conventional systemic chemotherapies have been negligible to modest.

CIC-rearranged sarcoma

Antonescu CR
Yoshida A

Definition

CIC-rearranged sarcoma is a high-grade round cell undifferentiated sarcoma defined by CIC-related gene fusions, most often CIC-DUX4.

ICD-O coding

9367/3 CIC-rearranged sarcoma

ICD-11 coding

None

Related terminology

Acceptable: CIC-DUX4 sarcoma.

Subtype(s)

None

Localization

Most CIC sarcomas occur in the deep soft tissues of the limbs or trunk, and less commonly in the head and neck, retroperitoneum, or pelvis. About 10% of cases have a visceral presentation, including kidney, gastrointestinal tract, and brain {134,3370,2968}. Primary osseous involvement is rare (< 5%) {134,1109}.

Clinical features

CIC sarcoma presents as a mass with or without pain. Some of the patients (16–50%) present with symptoms from their metastatic disease {134,3370}.

Epidemiology

There is a wide age range at presentation, from children to elderly adults {134,3370}; however, there is a striking predilection for young adults (median age: 25–35 years), and < 25% of cases present in the paediatric age group {134,3370}. There is slight male predominance.

Etiology

Unknown

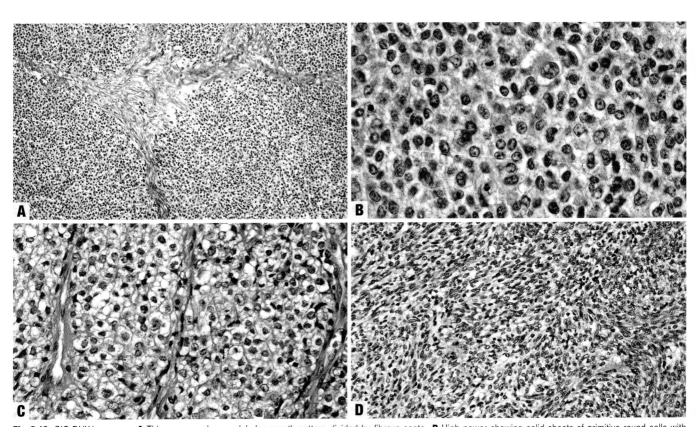

Fig. 2.13 CIC-DUX4 sarcoma. **A** This sarcoma shows a lobular growth pattern divided by fibrous septa. **B** High power showing solid sheets of primitive round cells with scattered larger cells and mild nuclear pleomorphism. **C** Solid sheets composed of relatively monomorphic epithelioid cells with moderate amount of light eosinophilic to clear cytoplasm. **D** Focal areas of short spindle cells arranged in a storiform pattern.

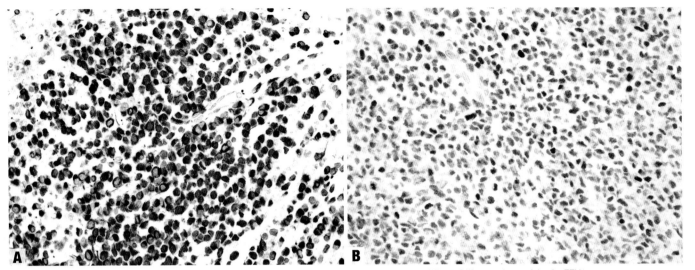

Fig. 2.14 *CIC-DUX4* sarcoma. **A** Immunohistochemical studies show consistent strong nuclear staining for WT1. **B** Diffuse nuclear staining for ETV4.

Pathogenesis

A *CIC-DUX4* fusion is present in 95% of cases, resulting from either a t(4;19)(q35;q13) or a t(10;19)(q26;q13) translocation {1597,1492}; however, rare examples are associated with non-*DUX4* partner genes, including *FOXO4*, *LEUTX*, *NUTM1*, and *NUTM2A* {1788,2974,2975,1433}. *CIC* encodes a high-mobility group (HMG) box transcriptional repressor. Most *CIC* break-points are located within *CIC* exon 20 {1578}. The *DUX4* gene, encoding for a double homeobox transcription factor, is located within the D4Z4 macrosatellite repeat region of the chromosomes 4 and 10 subtelomeric regions (4q35 or 10q26.3). DUX4 is normally expressed in germ cells, but it is epigenetically silenced in somatic differentiated tissues. The predicted CIC-DUX4 chimeric protein retains the HMG box, with a large part of the N-terminal DUX4 being lost. In a subset of cases, the *CIC-DUX4* fusion leads to a stop codon right after the breakpoint; thus, the resulting chimeric protein lacks any DUX4 sequence, suggesting that a truncated CIC protein may be sufficient to trigger oncogenesis {1578,3368}. Trisomy 8 and *MYC* amplification are some of the other common genetic changes {2896}. Concurrent *CIC* mutations have been described in the context of tumours with *CIC-LEUTX* fusion {1433}. The gene expression profile of *CIC* sarcoma is distinct from that of Ewing sarcoma {2917}. The *CIC-DUX4* fusion markedly enhances the CIC transcriptional activity, upregulating its targets, including *CCND2*, *MUC5AC*, and PEA3 family genes (e.g. *ETV1*, *ETV4*, and *ETV5*) {2917,1597,3377}.

Macroscopic appearance

The tumours are generally large, well-circumscribed, white or tan, soft masses, with frequent haemorrhage and necrosis.

Histopathology

Tumours are composed of diffuse sheets of undifferentiated round cells, displaying at least in part a lobulated growth pattern, delineated by fibrotic stroma. A minor component of spindle or epithelioid cells may be seen in many cases. The tumour

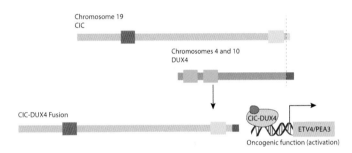

Fig. 2.15 *CIC-DUX4* sarcoma. Diagrammatic representation of *CIC-DUX4* fusions, which result from either a t(4;19) or a t(10;19) translocation. The interrupted red line highlights the common breakpoints, which include most of the coding sequence of *CIC* and a small portion of the 3′ end of *DUX4*. The resulting fusion protein drives the oncogenic activation of target genes, such as the PEA3 family of transcription factors (*ETV1*, *ETV4*).

cells have relatively uniform cytomorphology but often reveal a mild degree of nuclear pleomorphism, with vesicular chromatin and prominent nucleoli. The cytoplasm is lightly eosinophilic, with occasional clearing. Necrosis is common and mitotic activity is brisk. In one third of the cases, focal myxoid stromal changes are present, in which tumour cells exhibit reticular or pseudoacinar arrangements {1492,134,3370,2896}. Tumours with *CIC*–non-*DUX4* fusion variants are associated with histological features similar to those of tumours with the canonical *CIC-DUX4* {1788,2974,2975}. By immunohistochemistry, *CIC* sarcomas often express CD99, mostly in a patchy pattern and less commonly being diffuse and membranous (20%) {134}. WT1 (90–95%) and ETV4 (95–100%) are frequently positive and represent useful ancillary markers {1439,1786,2917}. NKX2-2 is typically negative {3370}. Sarcomas with *CIC-NUTM1* fusions express NUT protein {2968,1788}. Keratin, S100, and myogenic markers are rarely expressed. Calretinin and ERG can be positive {3370,2896,2917}.

Cytology
Not clinically relevant

Diagnostic molecular pathology
CIC gene rearrangements can be detected by a variety of techniques {1492,1578}. However, none of these methods are highly sensitive {1578,3368}.

Essential and desirable diagnostic criteria
Essential: predominant round cell phenotype; mild nuclear pleomorphism; epithelioid and/or spindle cell components; variably myxoid stroma; immunoprofile shows variable CD99 staining, with frequent WT1 and ETV4 positivity.
Desirable: *CIC* gene rearrangement (in selected cases).

Staging
CIC-rearranged sarcoma is presumably staged under Union for International Cancer Control (UICC) and American Joint Committee on Cancer (AJCC) TNM principles.

Prognosis and prediction
Most tumours follow a highly aggressive course with frequent metastases, most commonly to the lung. The estimated 5-year overall survival rate is 17–43%, significantly worse than that of Ewing sarcoma {134,3370}. The chemotherapy response to Ewing sarcoma regimens has been dismal {134}.

Sarcoma with *BCOR* genetic alterations

Antonescu CR
Puls F
Tirode F

Definition
Several groups of primitive round cell sarcomas show *BCOR* genetic alterations, resulting in oncogenic activation and BCOR overexpression. Although these pathological entities show distinct clinical presentations, there is overlap with regard to morphology, immunoprofile, and gene expression, suggesting a shared pathogenesis. The first group is characterized by sarcomas with *BCOR*-related gene fusions, most frequently *BCOR-CCNB3*. The second group shows internal tandem duplication (*BCOR*-ITD), which has been described in infantile undifferentiated round cell sarcomas and primitive myxoid mesenchymal tumours of infancy.

ICD-O coding
9368/3 Sarcoma with *BCOR* genetic alterations

ICD-11 coding
None

Related terminology
Acceptable: BCOR-CCNB3 sarcoma; *BCOR*-rearranged sarcoma; infantile undifferentiated round cell sarcoma; primitive myxoid mesenchymal tumour of infancy.

Subtype(s)
None

Localization
BCOR-CCNB3 sarcoma occurs slightly more often in bone than in soft tissue (ratio: 1.5:1), with a predilection for pelvis, lower extremity, and paraspinal region {2510,2552}. Rare locations include the head and neck region, lung, and kidney {1576,159, 2019}. Sarcomas with *BCOR*-ITD and primitive myxoid mesenchymal tumour of infancy occur mainly in the soft tissues of the trunk, retroperitoneum, and head and neck, typically sparing extremities {1582}.

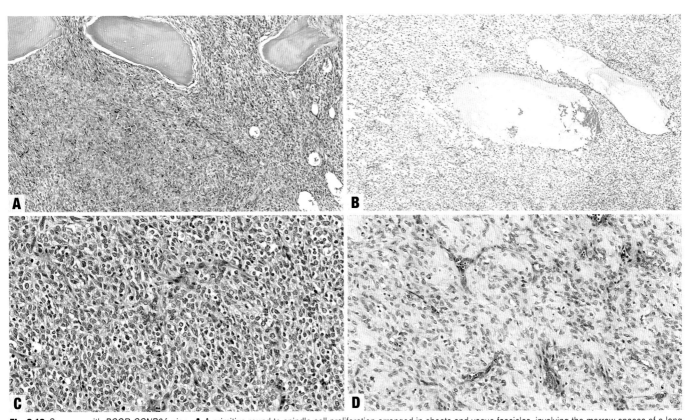

Fig. 2.16 Sarcoma with *BCOR-CCNB3* fusion. **A** A primitive round to spindle cell proliferation arranged in sheets and vague fascicles, involving the marrow spaces of a long bone. **B** Tumour of lower cellularity embedded in a loose fibromyxoid stroma and microcystic changes. **C** Solid sheets of undifferentiated round to ovoid cells with light eosinophilic to clear cytoplasm and round nuclei with fine chromatin and scattered mitotic figures. **D** Deceptively bland ovoid to short spindle cells arranged in a streaming pattern in a fibrotic background with a rich vascular network.

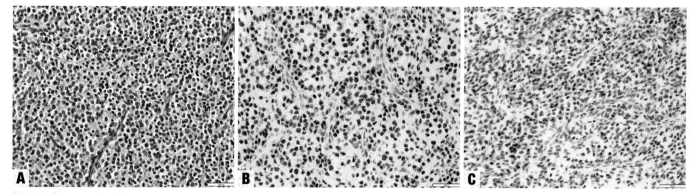

Fig. 2.17 Sarcoma with *BCOR* internal tandem duplication (*BCOR*-ITD). **A** Solid sheets of monomorphic round cells with scant eosinophilic cytoplasm and round nuclei, separated by thin septa with delicate capillaries, from an infant patient. **B** Strong and diffuse nuclear staining for BCOR with immunohistochemistry. **C** Strong nuclear reactivity for SATB2.

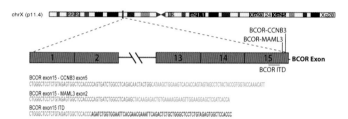

Fig. 2.18 Sarcomas with *BCOR* genetic alterations. Diagrammatic representation of *BCOR* genetic abnormalities, including the more common *BCOR-CCNB3* intrachromosomal inversion, the rare *BCOR-MAML2* interchromosomal fusion, and the *BCOR* internal tandem duplication (*BCOR*-ITD). All three of these genetic events involve the last exon (exon 15) of *BCOR* and result in consistent upregulation of *BCOR* mRNA and BCOR overexpression at the protein level.

Clinical features

Pain and swelling are the most common symptoms {636}.

Epidemiology

BCOR family tumours are uncommon, with a much lower incidence than Ewing sarcoma {2552,1582}. *BCOR-CCNB3* sarcomas have a striking predilection for children, with > 90% of patients aged < 20 years {1576,2019}, and show a male sex predominance (M:F ratio: 4.5:1) {1909,3329,2552}. Soft tissue sarcomas with alternative *BCOR* gene rearrangements are seen in a wider age range {2918}. Sarcoma with *BCOR*-ITD and primitive myxoid mesenchymal tumour of infancy occur within the first year of life or may be present at birth {60,1582}.

Etiology

Unknown

Pathogenesis

Similar to clear cell sarcoma of kidney and high-grade endometrial stromal sarcoma {3124,1982,1799}, infantile undifferentiated round cell sarcomas are characterized either by *BCOR*-ITD or in rare cases by *YWHAE-NUTM2B* fusions {1582}; both genotypes result in oncogenic upregulation of BCOR. *BCOR* family tumours share a similar gene expression signature, with strong overexpression of HOX family genes {2918,1576,3253}.

The molecular consequences of the *BCOR* genetic abnormalities remain largely unknown. BCOR is both an interactor of BCL6 and a repressor of its expression {1455}. BCOR was later shown to be part of the non-canonical polycomb repressive complex 1.1 (PRC1.1) {1125}. In high-grade neuroepithelial tumour with *BCOR* alteration, BCOR-ITD activates both sonic hedgehog and WNT/β-catenin signalling pathways {2968}. Cyclin B3 (CCNB3) expression, which in normal tissues is restricted to testis, was also shown to be sufficient to increase cellular proliferation in ectopic models {2510}.

Macroscopic appearance

Tumours are typically large (> 5–10 cm), tan-grey, soft to fleshy lesions, with areas of necrosis. Osseous lesions often show cortical destruction and extension into the soft tissues {636,2552}.

Histopathology

BCOR family tumours show substantial morphological overlap. *BCOR-CCNB3* sarcomas are typically composed of a uniform proliferation of primitive small round to ovoid cells arranged in solid sheets or a vague nesting pattern, surrounded by a rich capillary network {2019,1576,2552}. Other morphological patterns can occur, including less cellular areas of short spindle cells within a myxoid matrix {1576,2552} or solid areas of predominantly plump spindle cells arranged in short fascicles, reminiscent of poorly differentiated synovial sarcoma {1846,2499}. The nuclei have finely dispersed chromatin and nucleoli are generally inconspicuous. The mitotic activity is variable {1576, 636}. Metastatic/recurrent lesions occasionally display pleomorphic nuclei and osteoid deposition {1576,2552}. Rare tumours reported in the kidney show substantial overlap with clear cell sarcoma of the kidney {159,186}. The spectrum of tumours with *BCOR*-ITD abnormalities shows variable degrees of cellularity, ranging from solid sheets of small primitive cells to hypocellular areas of dispersed spindle cells, within a myxoid matrix and delicate vessels {60,2737,1582}. Immunohistochemically, all tumours with various *BCOR* gene alterations show strong and diffuse nuclear BCOR positivity and in most cases also express SATB2, TLE1, and cyclin D1. CD99 is positive in approximately 50% of cases {1576}. However, BCOR expression is not specific and, for example, is often observed in synovial sarcoma {1579,

2019}. *BCOR-CCNB3* sarcomas also express cyclin B3, which is not seen in other *BCOR* family tumours {2552,2019,2840}.

Cytology
Not clinically relevant

Diagnostic molecular pathology
The *BCOR* gene rearrangements and *BCOR*-ITD can be detected by various molecular approaches.

Essential and desirable diagnostic criteria
Essential: primitive round to spindle cells arranged in nests, sheets, or fascicular growth; variably myxoid stroma with delicate vasculature; immunohistochemical positivity for BCOR, SATB2, and cyclin D1.
Desirable (in selected cases): molecular confirmation of *BCOR* genetic abnormality (*BCOR* fusion, *BCOR*-ITD).

Staging
Sarcoma with *BCOR* genetic alterations is presumably staged under Union for International Cancer Control (UICC) and American Joint Committee on Cancer (AJCC) TNM principles.

Prognosis and prediction
Emerging data suggest that patients with *BCOR-CCNB3* sarcoma show 5-year survival rates similar to those of patients with Ewing sarcoma (72–80%) and show histological response to Ewing sarcoma–based treatment regimens {636,1576,2552}. A substantial proportion of patients present with metastatic disease; the most common metastatic site is the lung, followed by bone, soft tissue, and visceral locations {636,1576,2552}. The outcomes of the other *BCOR* family tumours are not well defined.

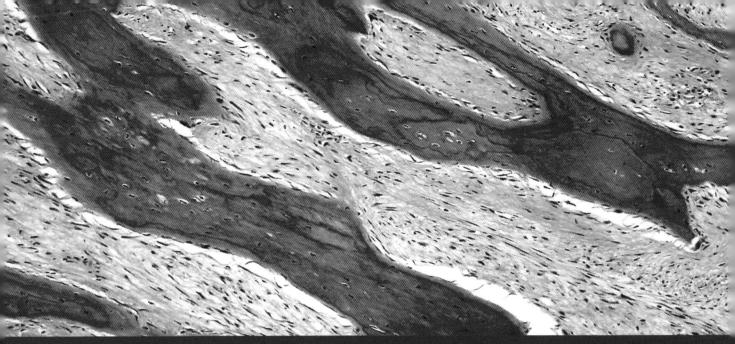

3

Bone tumours

Edited by: Bovée JVMG, Flanagan AM, Lazar AJ, Nielsen GP, Yoshida A

Chondrogenic tumours
Osteogenic tumours
Fibrogenic tumours
Vascular tumours of bone
Osteoclastic giant cell–rich tumours
Notochordal tumours
Other mesenchymal tumours of bone
Haematopoietic neoplasms of bone

WHO classification of bone tumours

Chondrogenic tumours

Benign
9213/0   Subungual exostosis
9212/0   Bizarre parosteal osteochondromatous proliferation
9221/0   Periosteal chondroma
9220/0   Enchondroma
9210/0   Osteochondroma
9230/0   Chondroblastoma NOS
9241/0   Chondromyxoid fibroma
9211/0   Osteochondromyxoma

Intermediate (locally aggressive)
9220/1   Chondromatosis NOS
9222/1   Atypical cartilaginous tumour

Malignant
9222/3* Chondrosarcoma, grade 1
9220/3   Chondrosarcoma, grade 2
9220/3   Chondrosarcoma, grade 3
9221/3   Periosteal chondrosarcoma
9242/3   Clear cell chondrosarcoma
9240/3   Mesenchymal chondrosarcoma
9243/3   Dedifferentiated chondrosarcoma

Osteogenic tumours

Benign
9180/0   Osteoma NOS
9191/0   Osteoid osteoma NOS

Intermediate (locally aggressive)
9200/1* Osteoblastoma NOS

Malignant
9187/3   Low-grade central osteosarcoma
9180/3   Osteosarcoma NOS
         Conventional osteosarcoma
         Telangiectatic osteosarcoma
         Small cell osteosarcoma
9192/3   Parosteal osteosarcoma
9193/3   Periosteal osteosarcoma
9194/3   High-grade surface osteosarcoma
9184/3   Secondary osteosarcoma

Fibrogenic tumours

Intermediate (locally aggressive)
8823/1   Desmoplastic fibroma

Malignant
8810/3   Fibrosarcoma NOS

Vascular tumours of bone

Benign
9120/0   Haemangioma NOS

Intermediate (locally aggressive)
9125/0   Epithelioid haemangioma

Malignant
9133/3   Epithelioid haemangioendothelioma NOS
9120/3   Angiosarcoma

Osteoclastic giant cell–rich tumours

Benign
9260/0   Aneurysmal bone cyst
8830/0   Non-ossifying fibroma

Intermediate (locally aggressive, rarely metastasizing)
9250/1   Giant cell tumour of bone NOS

Malignant
9250/3   Giant cell tumour of bone, malignant

Notochordal tumours

Benign
9370/0   Benign notochordal tumour

Malignant
9370/3   Chordoma NOS
         Chondroid chordoma
9370/3   Poorly differentiated chordoma
9372/3   Dedifferentiated chordoma

Other mesenchymal tumours of bone

Benign
         Chondromesenchymal hamartoma of chest wall
         Simple bone cyst
8818/0   Fibrous dysplasia
         Osteofibrous dysplasia
8850/0   Lipoma NOS
8880/0   Hibernoma

Intermediate (locally aggressive)
9261/1* Osteofibrous dysplasia–like adamantinoma
8990/1   Mesenchymoma NOS

Malignant
9261/3   Adamantinoma of long bones
         Dedifferentiated adamantinoma
8890/3   Leiomyosarcoma NOS
8802/3   Pleomorphic sarcoma, undifferentiated
         Bone metastases

Haematopoietic neoplasms of bone

9731/3   Plasmacytoma of bone
9591/3   Malignant lymphoma, non-Hodgkin, NOS
9650/3   Hodgkin disease NOS
9680/3   Diffuse large B-cell lymphoma NOS
9690/3   Follicular lymphoma NOS
9699/3   Marginal zone B-cell lymphoma NOS
9702/3   T-cell lymphoma NOS
9714/3   Anaplastic large cell lymphoma NOS
9727/3   Malignant lymphoma, lymphoblastic, NOS
9687/3   Burkitt lymphoma NOS
9751/1   Langerhans cell histiocytosis NOS
9751/3   Langerhans cell histiocytosis, disseminated
9749/3   Erdheim–Chester disease
         Rosai–Dorfman disease

These morphology codes are from the International Classification of Diseases for Oncology, third edition, second revision (ICD-O-3.2) [1471]. Behaviour is coded /0 for benign tumours; /1 for unspecified, borderline, or uncertain behaviour; /2 for carcinoma in situ and grade III intraepithelial neoplasia; /3 for malignant tumours, primary site; and /6 for malignant tumours, metastatic site. Behaviour code /6 is not generally used by cancer registries.

This classification is modified from the previous WHO classification, taking into account changes in our understanding of these lesions.

* Codes marked with an asterisk were approved by the IARC/WHO Committee for ICD-O at its meeting in January 2020.

TMN staging of tumours of bone

Bone
(ICD-O-3 C40, 41)

Rules for Classification
The classification applies to all primary malignant bone tumours except malignant lymphoma, multiple myeloma, surface/juxtacortical osteosarcoma, and juxtacortical chondrosarcoma. There should be histological confirmation of the disease and division of cases by histological type and grade.

The following are the procedures for assessing T, N, and M categories:

T categories	Physical examination and imaging
N categories	Physical examination and imaging
M categories	Physical examination and imaging

Regional Lymph Nodes
The regional lymph nodes are those appropriate to the site of the primary tumour. Regional node involvement is rare and cases in which nodal status is not assessed either clinically or pathologically could be considered N0 instead of NX or pNX.

TNM Clinical Classification
T – Primary Tumour
TX   Primary tumour cannot be assessed
T0   No evidence of primary tumour

Appendicular Skeleton, Trunk, Skull and Facial Bones
T1   Tumour 8 cm or less in greatest dimension
T2   Tumour more than 8 cm in greatest dimension
T3   Discontinuous tumours in the primary bone site

Spine
T1   Tumour confined to a single vertebral segment or two adjacent vertebral segments
T2   Tumour confined to three adjacent vertebral segments
T3   Tumour confined to four adjacent vertebral segments
T4a   Tumour invades into the spinal canal
T4b   Tumour invades the adjacent vessels or tumour thrombosis within the adjacent vessels

Note
The five vertebral segments are the:
  Right pedicle
  Right body
  Left body
  Left pedicle
  Posterior element

Pelvis
T1a   A tumour 8 cm or less in size and confined to a single pelvic segment with no extraosseous extension
T1b   A tumour greater than 8 cm in size and confined to a single pelvic segment with no extraosseous extension
T2a   A tumour 8 cm or less in size and confined to a single pelvic segment with extraosseous extension or confined to two adjacent pelvic segments without extraosseous extension
T2b   A tumour greater than 8 cm in size and confined to a single pelvic segment with extraosseous extension or confined to two adjacent pelvic segments without extraosseous extension
T3a   A tumour 8 cm or less in size and confined to two pelvic segments with extraosseous extension
T3b   A tumour greater than 8 cm in size and confined to two pelvic segments with extraosseous extension
T4a   Tumour involving three adjacent pelvic segments or crossing the sacroiliac joint to the sacral neuroforamen
T4b   Tumour encasing the external iliac vessels or gross tumour thrombus in major pelvic vessels

Note
The four pelvic segments are the:
  Sacrum lateral to the sacral foramen,
  Iliac wing,
  Acetabulum/periacetabulum and
  Pelvic rami, symphysis and ischium

N – Regional Lymph Nodes
NX   Regional lymph nodes cannot be assessed
N0   No regional lymph node metastasis
N1   Regional lymph node metastasis

M – Distant Metastasis
M0   No distant metastasis
M1   Distant metastasis
      M1a   Lung
      M1b   Other distant sites

pTNM Pathological Classification
The pT and pN categories correspond to the T and N categories.

pM – Distant Metastasis*
pM1   Distant metastasis microscopically confirmed

Note
* pM0 and pMX are not valid categories.

Stage – Appendicular Skeleton, Trunk, Skull and Facial Bones

Stage IA	T1	N0	M0	G1,GX Low Grade
Stage IB	T2,T3	N0	M0	G1,GX Low Grade
Stage IIA	T1	N0	M0	G2,G3 High Grade
Stage IIB	T2	N0	M0	G2,G3 High Grade
Stage III	T3	N0	M0	G2,G3 High Grade
Stage IVA	Any T	N0	M1a	Any G
Stage IVB	Any T	N1	Any M	Any G
	Any T	Any N	M1b	Any G

Stage – Spine and Pelvis
There is no stage for bone sarcomas of the spine or pelvis.

Chapter 3

Bone tumours: Introduction

Flanagan AM
Blay JY
Bovée JVMG
Bredella MA

Cool P
Nielsen GP
Yoshida A

The ICD-O topographical coding for the anatomical sites covered in this chapter is presented in Box 3.01.

Epidemiology and etiology

Among the wide array of human neoplasms, primary tumours of bone are relatively common; however, clinically significant bone neoplasms are infrequent.

Incidence

The true incidence of benign bone tumours is unknown, although older radiographic studies have suggested that a substantial proportion of the population has an indolent lesion. Non-ossifying fibroma is the most common bone tumour. Cartilaginous lesions are relatively common incidental findings on knee MRI and have an estimated prevalence of 2.8% {2957}. As a result of the improved sensitivity of radiological scans, the reported incidence of benign and low-grade cartilaginous tumours (atypical cartilaginous tumour / chondrosarcoma, grade 1 [ACT/CS1]) has increased over the past decade {3167}. In contrast, bone sarcomas are rare and accounted for only 0.2% of all neoplasms in one large series {1423}. Comparison of the incidence of bone sarcomas to that of soft tissue sarcomas indicates that clinically significant osseous neoplasms occur at a rate approximately one tenth that of their soft tissue counterparts. The overall annual reported incidence of bone sarcomas in both sexes in North America and Europe is about 0.75 cases per 100 000 population. Somewhat higher incidence rates have been reported by local cancer registries in China (1.7–2.0) {401A}. The incidence rates of specific bone sarcomas are age-related. Osteosarcoma, which is the most common malignant primary bone tumour excluding malignant myeloma, has a bimodal distribution. The first well-defined peak occurs during the second decade of life and the second peak occurs in people aged > 60 years. This second peak is related to other risk factors such as radiation treatment and Paget disease. Ewing sarcoma is less common than osteosarcoma, and most patients are < 30 years old. The incidence of chondrosarcoma and chordoma increases from adolescence onwards {2213}.

Predisposing lesions

Although most primary bone malignancies appear to arise de novo, it is increasingly apparent that some develop in association with benign precursor lesions or in diseased bone. Paget disease of bone, radiation injury, bone infarction, chronic osteomyelitis, and certain pre-existing benign tumours are the most clearly established precancerous conditions {53,645,1162, 1272,1447,3284,226,1073,1108,2154,3090}. There are reported cases of bone sarcoma arising in association with implanted metallic hardware, but a causal association has not been proven {1155,1281,1604,2486,1458}.

C40 Bones, joints, and articular cartilage of limbs
  C40.0 Long bones of upper limb, scapula, and associated joints
  C40.1 Short bones of upper limb and associated joints
  C40.2 Long bones of lower limb and associated joints
  C40.3 Short bones of lower limb and associated joints
  C40.8 Overlapping lesion of bones, joints, and articular cartilage of limbs
  C40.9 Bone of limb NOS

C41 Bones, joints, and articular cartilage of other and unspecified sites
  C41.0 Bones of skull and face and associated joints
  C41.1 Mandible
  C41.2 Vertebral column
  C41.3 Rib, sternum, clavicle, and associated joints
  C41.4 Pelvic bones, sacrum, coccyx, and associated joints
  C41.8 Overlapping lesion of bones, joints, and articular cartilage
  C41.9 Bone NOS

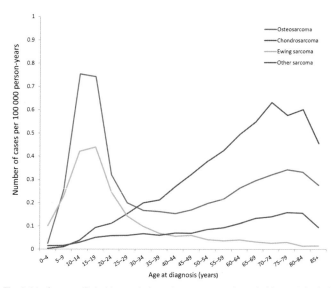

Fig. 3.01 Age-specific incidence of primary bone sarcomas by major histopathological type, world data, both sexes, from *Cancer Incidence in Five Continents*, Volume XI {401A}.

Genetic predisposition

Constitutional genetic variants affecting the risk for bone tumour development range from mutations with high penetrance, causing disorders that typically follow traditional Mendelian patterns of inheritance, to SNPs that only mildly influence the function of the proteins encoded by the genes involved. SNPs are by definition present in > 1% of the population, and their collective influence may account for a substantial proportion of bone tumours {268}. Individual genetic variants with high penetrance for bone tumour development are rare (see Table 4.02, p. 503), but they are important to identify because they may affect response to treatment or predict an increased risk for

Table 3.01 Most-common locations of presentation for primary malignant bone tumours and overall risk of a pathological fracture at time of diagnosis, based on data from 3000 primary malignant bone tumours seen at the Royal Orthopaedic Hospital in Birmingham, United Kingdom

Diagnosis	Knee[a]	Hip and pelvis[b]	Shoulder girdle[c]	Lower leg	Upper limb	Trunk[d]	Risk of pathological fracture
Osteosarcoma	66%	15%	10%	5%	3%	1%	9%
Chondrosarcoma	17%	48%	15%	4%	9%	7%	12%
Ewing sarcoma	22%	44%	11%	13%	7%	3%	6%
UPS	41%	29%	9%	5%	14%	2%	16%
All diagnoses	43%	31%	11%	7%	5%	3%	10%

UPS, undifferentiated pleomorphic sarcoma.

[a]Knee includes distal femur, proximal tibia, and proximal fibula. [b]Hip and pelvis include pelvis and proximal femur. [c]Shoulder girdle includes proximal humerus, scapula, and clavicle. [d]Trunk includes spine, ribs, etc.

developing other tumours. Such information can be used to provide genetic counselling or screening of at-risk individuals {3394}. Important examples include mutations in *TP53* (see *Li–Fraumeni syndrome*, p. 510) and *RB1* {793,1925}, both of which predispose to osteosarcoma. Non-inherited, postzygotic mutations result in mosaicism and can increase the risk of tumour development in the affected parts of the body, as exemplified by *IDH1* and *IDH2* mutations causing enchondromatosis (see *Enchondromatosis*, p. 506) and *GNAS* mutations in polyostotic fibrous dysplasia, McCune–Albright syndrome, and Mazabraud syndrome (see *McCune–Albright syndrome*, p. 514).

Clinical features

Bone tumours present in a number of different ways, including with pain, swelling, pathological fracture, and neurovascular compromise, or as an incidental finding. The most common presenting symptom of a benign bone tumour is aching pain that can be intermittent. However, a previously asymptomatic individual may present with a pathological fracture (e.g. fracture through a simple bone cyst). Osteoid osteomas typically present with night pain that is relieved by anti-inflammatory agents. Less frequently, osteoid osteomas are in a periarticular location and present clinically as a monoarthritis. Osteochondromas typically present as a painless lump, whereas chondroblastomas commonly present with severe pain. Clinical signs are often nonspecific. Swelling and tenderness over the affected bone are the most common findings. Periarticular lesions (e.g. chondroblastoma and juxta-articular osteoid osteoma) can irritate the joint, with resulting joint effusion and stiffness.

Malignant tumours typically present with worsening pain that is non-mechanical in nature {3287}. At the time of diagnosis, many patients experience night pain that interrupts sleep. Swelling usually becomes apparent once the cortex is breached and the tumour starts to grow beneath the periosteum or extend through it. Most malignant bone tumours arise in a metaphyseal location. However, Ewing sarcoma and adamantinoma are usually diaphyseal. The presence of swelling in a limb (in particular around the knee) associated with pain (in particular non-mechanical or night pain) should always lead to further investigation. There is a wide differential diagnosis for patients presenting in this manner, with the most common diagnoses being metastases, malignant bone tumour, benign bone tumour, infection, and haematological disorder. A simple algorithm based on the most likely diagnosis for a patient of a

particular age has been advocated {1223}. This is based on the fact that metastatic carcinoma is uncommon in individuals aged < 35 years, whereas the likelihood of a bone tumour being a metastasis from a known or undiagnosed carcinoma increases after that age {1954}.

As many as 43% of malignant bone tumours arise around the knee, but in patients aged < 20 years this rises to 56% (see Table 3.01). Therefore, for any child or adolescent presenting with pain and/or swelling around the knee that does not resolve, a diagnosis of a primary bone tumour should be considered and investigated. The second most common site is the pelvis, which is the most common site for both Ewing sarcoma and chondrosarcoma. Delays in diagnosis of pelvic tumours are frequent, because symptoms are nonspecific and often of considerable duration {3319}. Referred pain to the leg or knee is not infrequent and it is not unusual for patients to have been investigated before diagnosis without the possibility of a bone tumour being considered. Night pain, again, is often the key that should alert the clinician to the possibility of a bone tumour being present.

Pathological fractures in malignant bone tumours are often associated with pre-existing pain or discomfort in the limb. The fracture is often caused by minimal force. Awareness of the possibility of a neoplastic cause for the fracture is essential to prevent inadvertent internal fixation that jeopardizes clinical outcome {16}. Usually the imaging manifestations combined with the history are sufficient to raise suspicion for an underlying malignant primary bone tumour. Blood tests are usually not helpful in diagnosing bone tumours. An elevated alkaline phosphatase level is seen in about 46% of patients with osteosarcoma and is a poor prognostic sign {196}. Raised LDH, ESR, and C-reactive protein may be seen in Ewing sarcoma, also being poor prognostic indicators {194}.

Biopsy specimens

Obtaining a diagnosis for a symptomatic patient as quickly as possible is essential, but delays in diagnosis are frequent {2893}. All patients with suspected bone tumours should be discussed at a multidisciplinary team meeting that includes the radiologist and pathologist involved in the diagnosis, as well as the orthopaedic surgeon and oncologist involved in the patient's treatment {504,1221}. Local staging investigations should be completed before a biopsy. A biopsy can alter the imaging features, making interpretation and diagnosis more difficult. A reliable histological diagnosis often cannot be made without prior correlation with radiographic imaging {749}. The biopsy of a suspected tumour should be performed at a reference centre for bone sarcomas. Planning of the surgical approach to the biopsy site, tract, and diagnosis should involve the orthopaedic surgeon who will perform the surgery {504}. There is evidence that treatment in centres with a high volume of bone tumours and the presence of an experienced multidisciplinary team positively affects outcome {111,340}. The pathologist must be informed of the patient's age and the exact anatomical site and size of the tumour. This information should be correlated with the imaging. Additionally, it is important to know about the presence of other lesions, possible underlying bone disease, and family history to provide an informed diagnostic opinion.

Tissue processing

All tissue, whether from a biopsy, curettage, or resection of a suspected bone tumour should be processed in a manner that allows molecular studies to be undertaken successfully. Decalcification can be detrimental to nucleic acid; therefore, freezing samples and/or fixing non-calcified portions of the tumour in buffered formalin alone before paraffin embedding is encouraged, to facilitate modern technologies (e.g. next-generation sequencing) that facilitate diagnosis. As recommended by the European Society for Medical Oncology (ESMO) guidelines, an alternative is to decalcify material in ethylenediaminetetraacetic acid (EDTA) instead of harsher acidic reagents {504}.

Use of clinical imaging
Diagnosis

Radiographs (of the whole bone in two planes) are the initial imaging examination in the work-up of bone tumours and are usually the most specific for establishing a diagnosis {667}. CT can be helpful in complex anatomical regions, such as the spine and pelvis, showing matrix mineralization, periosteal reaction, and cortical destruction. CT is usually used for percutaneous biopsy guidance {2000}. MRI is the imaging modality of choice for local staging, treatment evaluation, and detection of recurrences. Marrow replacement typically demonstrates T1-hypointense signal (lower than surrounding muscle or disc) and hyperintense signal on fluid-sensitive sequences with avid enhancement after intravenous contrast administration {1295}. Intravenous contrast is also useful for distinguishing cystic from solid areas within tumour tissue and peritumoural oedema from viable tumour {2474}. Whole-body MRI can be used to screen the entire body for metastases or multifocal bone tumours {724, 2000}. Bone scintigraphy using methylene diphosphonate (MDP) labelled with a technetium radioisotope is used for staging and for evaluation of skip lesions, metastases, or tumour recurrence {655}. FDG PET in combination with CT (PET-CT) or MRI (PET-MRI) is primarily used for staging and has been found to be more accurate than bone scintigraphy in detecting skeletal metastases {402,537}.

Important parameters in imaging evaluation of bone tumours include tumour location, matrix, margins, and periosteal reaction. Certain tumours occur in a characteristic location in the skeleton. Adamantinoma and osteofibrous dysplasia have a strong predilection for the anterior cortex of the tibia. In long bones, epiphyseal lesions include chondroblastoma, giant cell tumour, and clear cell chondrosarcoma. Several tumours have a predilection for sites of rapid growth and involve the metaphyseal regions, often around the knee joints, such as osteosarcoma, chondrosarcoma, osteochondroma, and enchondroma. Some tumours have a predilection for the bone surface or cortex, such as osteoid osteoma, fibrous cortical defect, osteochondroma, periosteal chondroma, and parosteal and periosteal osteosarcomas {2148,2276}. Bone tumours usually produce an internal matrix that can be classified as bone, cartilaginous, or fibrous. The term "mineralization" refers to calcification of the matrix {2276,2148}. Margins and periosteal reaction of a bone tumour reflect the growth rate and biological behaviour of the tumour. Slow-growing tumours have circumscribed margins with a narrow zone of transition and solid or thick periosteal reaction. Aggressive and rapidly growing tumours have indistinct margins with a wide zone of transition and aggressive periosteal reaction, such as onion-skin, spiculated, sunburst, or hair-on-end periosteal reaction, or a Codman triangle. Radiographs are most useful in evaluating margins and periosteal reaction {1888, 2148,2276}.

Posttreatment imaging

Radiographs can be used to assess tumour recurrence and posttreatment complications, such as fracture, prosthetic loosening, or non-union. MRI provides an accurate evaluation of treatment response and tumour recurrence, and facilitates differentiation of tumour recurrence from posttreatment changes. PET-CT can be used to determine treatment response, to identify both local recurrence and metastatic disease, and to provide information on prognosis {1118,666}.

Terminology used to reflect biological potential

Bone tumours are now divided into four categories: benign, intermediate (locally aggressive), intermediate (rarely metastasizing), and malignant, which were defined in the third and fourth editions of the WHO Classification of Tumours series. The division between these categories can be somewhat arbitrary and the subject of debate, especially in regard to tumours that belong to a histological and biological spectrum of disease (e.g. conventional central and peripheral cartilaginous tumours). The intent of the classification is to specify which lesions would be best managed by regular surveillance without surgical removal, which need local treatment such as curettage, and which require wide en bloc resection. The division into these categories is maintained and further defined or revised for certain tumours in the current edition. The four categories are defined along the same lines as the soft tissue tumour counterparts.

Benign: Most benign bone tumours have a limited capacity for local recurrence. Those that do recur do so in a non-destructive fashion and are almost always readily cured by complete local excision/curettage. In the current classification, chondroblastoma is no longer in the intermediate (rarely metastasizing) category. The reported rate of metastases is < 1% and consequently chondroblastoma is better classified as benign. Likewise, chondromyxoid fibroma and aneurysmal bone cyst are now classified as benign (previously locally aggressive). Hibernoma of bone, which has been recently well characterized {362}, is a new addition to this category.

Intermediate (locally aggressive): Bone tumours in this category often recur locally and may be associated with an infiltrative and locally destructive growth pattern. They do not appear

Table 3.02 Bone sarcomas in which grade is determined by histotype

Grade	Sarcoma type
Grade 1 (low-grade)	Low-grade central osteosarcoma
	Parosteal osteosarcoma
	Clear cell chondrosarcoma
Grade 2 (intermediate-grade)	Periosteal osteosarcoma
Grade 3 (high-grade)	Osteosarcoma (conventional, telangiectatic, small cell, secondary, high-grade surface)
	Undifferentiated high-grade pleomorphic sarcoma
	Ewing sarcoma
	Dedifferentiated chondrosarcoma
	Mesenchymal chondrosarcoma
	Dedifferentiated chordoma
	Poorly differentiated chordoma
	Angiosarcoma
Variable grading	Conventional chondrosarcoma (grade 1–3 according to Evans et al. {947})
	Leiomyosarcoma of bone (grade 1–3, no established grading system)
	Low- and high-grade malignancy may occur in giant cell tumour of bone

to have the potential to metastasize but typically require wide excision with a margin of normal tissue or application of a local adjuvant to ensure local control. In the 2013 WHO classification, the term "chondrosarcoma, grade 1" was replaced with the term "atypical cartilaginous tumour" – in the intermediate (locally aggressive) category – in order to reflect the clinical behaviour of well-differentiated/low-grade lesions. The argument is made that such lesions, especially in the long bones, behave in a locally aggressive manner and do not metastasize; therefore they should not be classified as having full malignant potential. In this edition, we propose to define the use of the terminology "atypical cartilaginous tumour" and "chondrosarcoma, grade 1". Analogous to the concept of atypical lipomatous tumour (extremities) / well-differentiated liposarcoma (retroperitoneum), cartilaginous tumours in the appendicular skeleton (long and short tubular bones) should be termed atypical cartilaginous tumours, and the term "chondrosarcoma, grade 1" is reserved for tumours of the axial skeleton, including the pelvis, scapula, and skull base (flat bones) – reflecting the poorer clinical outcome of these tumours at these sites {452,3167}. Using different terminology for tumours with identical histomorphology could be considered counterintuitive and therefore controversial. However, this terminology has the dual benefit of being simple in application and reflecting the worse outcome for tumours at these sites, where there is a need for more-extensive surgery {452}. Synovial chondromatosis has now been placed in the intermediate (locally aggressive) category (previously benign) on the basis of the locally aggressive behaviour of this tumour, which has a high incidence of local recurrence {92}. Osteofibrous dysplasia–like adamantinoma is also now classified as an intermediate (locally aggressive) lesion, although it is acknowledged that exceptional cases may transform into a classic form of adamantinoma. Unlike osteofibrous dysplasia–like adamantinoma, classic adamantinoma is unequivocally a malignant disease. Fibrocartilaginous mesenchymoma, which has been newly added to this current classification, represents another example of a tumour in this disease category. Although it was originally described in 1984 {713}, there has been debate

as to its relationship with other tumours. Nonetheless, it has a characteristic morphology, and recent evidence (albeit from a small series) suggests that it lacks *GNAS* mutations, *IDH1* and *IDH2* mutations, and *MDM2* amplification {1113}, supporting the notion that it is a distinct entity. Of note, tumours may behave differently depending on their localization; for example, epithelioid haemangioma of bone is considered to be locally aggressive, whereas epithelioid haemangioma of soft tissue is considered a benign tumour.

Intermediate (rarely metastasizing): Bone tumours categorized as intermediate are often locally aggressive (see above). However, there is well-documented evidence of such lesions occasionally giving rise to distant metastases. Such metastases occur in < 2% of cases and are not predictable morphologically. These lesions usually metastasize to the lung. The prototypical example in this category is giant cell tumour of bone.

Malignant: In addition to the potential for locally destructive growth and recurrence, bone sarcomas have a substantial risk of distant metastasis, ranging in most instances from 20% to almost 100%, depending on histological type and, if applicable, histological grade. Some (but not all) histologically low-grade sarcomas have a metastatic risk of only 2–10%, but such lesions may advance in grade with local recurrence and thereby acquire a higher risk of distant spread. Examples in which progression to high-grade sarcoma can be seen include parosteal osteosarcoma and low-grade central osteosarcoma. It is important to note that in this new biological grouping, the intermediate categories do not correspond to intermediate histological grade (grade 2) in a bone sarcoma (see below). Poorly differentiated chordoma is included as a new entity in this book; it is characterized by immunoreactivity for brachyury (encoded by *TBXT*) and loss of SMARCB1 (INI1) expression representing a genetic event. Making this specific diagnosis is warranted in view of this tumour's aggressive behaviour and poor outcome. New information is now known about malignancy in giant cell tumours of bone. A small percentage (probably no more than 5%) of giant cell tumours of bone transform into a high-grade neoplasm, the morphology of which may be unrecognizable as being derived from a giant cell tumour of bone. The H3.3 p.Gly34 mutation, which is present in approximately 96% of the conventional subtype, may also be present in the frankly histologically malignant tumour. Therefore, this mutation is not helpful in making a diagnosis of malignancy. Complicating matters further, it has recently been demonstrated that absence of immunoreactivity for the mutant histone protein may be seen in some cases of malignant transformation {3376}. In such cases, a diagnosis can only be provided when the conventional component of a giant cell tumour is also available. The underlying genetic changes that account for the transformation have not been described.

Principles of grading and staging

Grading

Bone tumours vary widely in their biological behaviour. Histological grading is an attempt to predict the behaviour of a malignant tumour based on histological features. There is no generally accepted grading system for bone sarcomas, and the French Fédération Nationale des Centres de Lutte Contre le Cancer (FNCLCC) grading system used in soft tissue sarcomas has never been validated for bone tumours {642,2265}. In bone sarcomas, the histological subtype often determines clinical behaviour and therefore also the grade (see Table 3.02, p. 343). For example, Ewing sarcoma, mesenchymal chondrosarcoma, and dedifferentiated chondrosarcoma are always considered high-grade, whereas clear cell chondrosarcoma and parosteal osteosarcoma are considered low-grade. The exception to this includes conventional chondrosarcoma and leiomyosarcoma of bone; in the former, the grading system as proposed by Evans et al. {947} is widely used. Adamantinoma and conventional chordoma are malignant neoplasms but are not graded. The clinical significance of histological grading is limited by interobserver variability {883,2886}. Guidelines for reporting and grading of bone tumours are available from both US and European perspectives {504,2680,1969}.

Staging

Enneking and coauthors {910,909} described a staging system for musculoskeletal tumours that has been adopted by the Musculoskeletal Tumor Society (MSTS). It is mainly the staging for malignant tumours that has gained acceptance by orthopaedic

Table 3.03 Enneking staging for malignant bone tumours {910,909}

Stage	Grade	Site	Metastases
IA	Low	Intracompartmental	–
IB	Low	Extracompartmental	–
IIA	High	Intracompartmental	–
IIB	High	Extracompartmental	–
III	Any	Any	Regional or distant

surgeons because it helps to determine the surgical treatment. The system has not been changed since its introduction in 1980 (see Table 3.03). The Enneking stage is determined by tumour grade, extent beyond the surgical compartment, and the presence of metastases. However, there are some drawbacks to the Enneking staging system. In reality, most tumours are stage IIB, limiting the system's usefulness. Furthermore, the size of the primary tumour is an important prognostic factor. However, tumour size is not part of the Enneking staging system. In addition, there is no special consideration for tumours involving the spine or pelvis {1517,2938}.

The TNM staging system, as described by the American Joint Committee on Cancer (AJCC) and the Union for International Cancer Control (UICC), is based on evolving prognostic evidence and is now in its eighth edition {101,423}. An 8 cm cut-off point distinguishes between T1 and T2 tumours. Skip lesions are defined as T3. Most bone tumours primarily metastasize to lung and are classed as M1a (stage IVA). Metastases to bone or other sites (M1b) have a worse prognosis (stage IVB). Metastases to regional lymph nodes, which are uncommon, are also stage IVB. Bone tumours of the axial skeleton have a worse prognosis than those of the appendicular skeleton. Consequently, the eighth edition of the TNM system includes a special T classification for spine and pelvic tumours. In the spine, the classification is based on five segments (see *TNM staging of tumours of bone*, p. 339). However, in the pelvis the T classification is determined by tumour size (cut-off point: 8 cm) and tumour extent into four defined segments. There is no defined stage for malignant bone tumours of the spine or pelvis.

Subungual exostosis

Yoshida A
Bloem JL
Mertens F

Definition
Subungual exostosis is a benign osteocartilaginous surface lesion of the distal phalangeal bone underlying the nail bed.

ICD-O coding
9213/0 Subungual exostosis

ICD-11 coding
EE13.Y & XH1XL9 Other specified nail disorder & Subungual exostosis

2E83.5 & XH1XL9 Osseous and chondromatous neoplasm, benign & Subungual exostosis

Related terminology
Not recommended: Dupuytren exostosis.

Subtype(s)
None

Localization
Nearly 80% of cases affect the dorsal or medial surface of the distal phalanx of the big toe. The remaining cases involve distal phalangeal bones of other toes or fingers.

Clinical features
Signs and symptoms
Many patients present with painful swelling in the nail bed that lifts and deforms the nail plate. Ulceration and infection may occur. The preoperative period ranges from months to years.

Imaging
On radiographs, a small bony protuberance is attached to the dorsum or side of the phalangeal bone surface. There is no continuity between the lesion and the medullary cavity of native bone. The small fibrocartilaginous cap appears hyperintense on T2-weighted images {2214}.

Epidemiology
Subungual exostosis often occurs in young patients, with > 50% aged < 18 years (average: 25.7 years). There is no sex predilection {702}.

Etiology
Preceding trauma and infection are reported in 29% and 14% of cases, respectively {702}, although their causal relationship to the tumour is unknown. The clonal cytogenetic findings suggest a true neoplastic process.

Pathogenesis
Cytogenetically analysed cases of subungual exostosis consistently feature a t(X;6)(q24-q26;q15-q25), often as the sole change {717,3384,2960}. The breakpoints are located in the

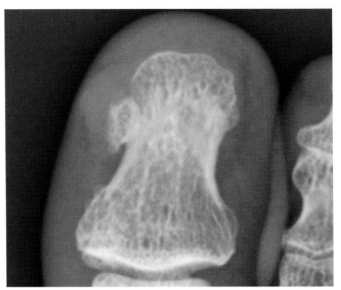

Fig. 3.02 Subungual exostosis. A mature osseous mass, with a soft tissue mass surrounding it, is attached on the cortex of the distal phalanx.

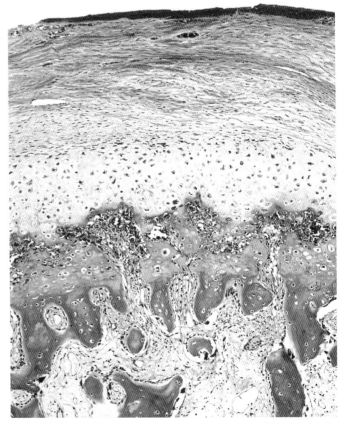

Fig. 3.03 Subungual exostosis. Low-power view showing fibrocartilaginous cap and osseous stalk involving the nail bed.

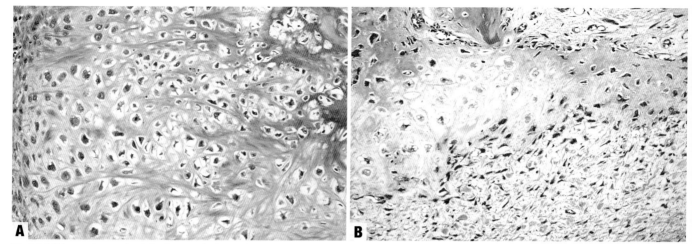

Fig. 3.04 Subungual exostosis. **A** Cartilage can be hypercellular and atypical. Note the fibrous nature of the cartilaginous matrix. **B** Cartilage can blend with spindle cell proliferation.

COL12A1 gene on chromosome 6 and near the *IRS4* gene, encoding an insulin receptor substrate, on the X chromosome. The translocation does not result in any fusion transcript; instead, it leads to increased expression of IRS4 at the mRNA and protein levels {2097}. This translocation has not been found in bizarre parosteal osteochondromatous proliferation (BPOP), supporting the existence of subungual exostosis as a distinct disease entity.

Macroscopic appearance
The lesion consists of small bony and cartilaginous fragments.

Histopathology
Subungual exostosis is composed of fibrocartilaginous tissue at the lesional periphery and bone trabeculae in the stalk. Cartilage can look atypical with hypercellularity and nuclear enlargement, and it can blend with spindle cell proliferation in the nail bed. Mitoses can be seen. The cartilaginous cap can be tenuous or even absent. Bone forms through enchondral ossification or directly from spindle cells, and intertrabecular tissue is hypervascular and fibrous. Early lesions may lack attachment to the subjacent bone {2149}. Subungual exostosis should be distinguished from osteochondroma, which is rare in the small bones of the hands and feet. Unlike in osteochondroma, a fibrillary

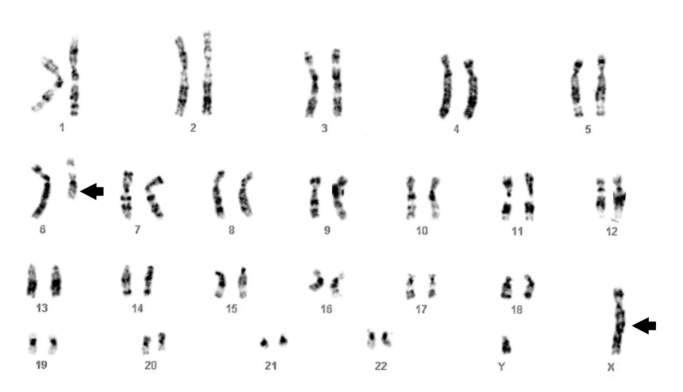

Fig. 3.05 Cytogenetic findings of subungual exostosis. Karyogram showing the characteristic t(X;6) that juxtaposes *COL12A1* with *IRS4*. Arrows indicate breakpoints.

cartilaginous matrix with marked proliferative activity and an irregular bone–cartilage interface, as well as enlarged, bizarre, and binucleated chondrocytes may be seen in subungual exostosis, and continuity with the underlying medulla is lacking. Subungual exostosis is also different from BPOP because it affects the distal phalanx by definition, whereas BPOP has a wider anatomical distribution, often involving more-proximal bones. BPOP is characterized by at least focal presence of distinct blue bone, which is generally absent in subungual exostosis.

Cytology
Not clinically relevant

Diagnostic molecular pathology
Not clinically relevant

Essential and desirable diagnostic criteria
Essential: a small osteocartilaginous lesion on the distal phalangeal bone; no continuity between the lesion and the medullary cavity of native bone.

Staging
Not clinically relevant

Prognosis and prediction
Subungual exostosis is benign and is adequately treated with simple excision. Local rapid recurrence has been reported {2149}. Rare recurrences can be managed by re-excision.

Bizarre parosteal osteochondromatous proliferation

Yoshida A
McCarthy EF

Definition

Bizarre parosteal osteochondromatous proliferation (BPOP) is a benign surface lesion of bone, composed of an admixture of spindle cells, cartilage, and bone.

ICD-O coding

9212/0 Bizarre parosteal osteochondromatous proliferation

ICD-11 coding

2E82.Z & XH23J5 Benign chondrogenic tumours, site unspecified & Bizarre parosteal osteochondromatous proliferation

Related terminology

Not recommended: Nora lesion.

Subtype(s)

None

Localization

BPOP typically affects small bones in the hands and feet, most commonly phalanges of the hand. Long tubular bones are also affected in as many as 27% of cases {2074}. BPOP has been rarely reported on the craniofacial bones.

Clinical features

Signs and symptoms

BPOP typically presents as a painless mass, which is present for a few months to several years. Some examples grow rapidly.

Imaging

Radiologically, BPOP is a well-circumscribed calcified mass plastered onto the cortical surface. The underlying cortex is intact, with no continuity between the lesion and the medullary cavity of affected bone. Exceptional cases are reported to display medullary continuity {2695,2710}.

Epidemiology

BPOP has a wide age range, with a peak in the third to fourth decades of life. There is no sex predilection.

Etiology

BPOP is viewed by some as part of a spectrum encompassing florid reactive periostitis and turret exostosis {815}, and by others as a neoplasm. A minority of the patients report preceding trauma.

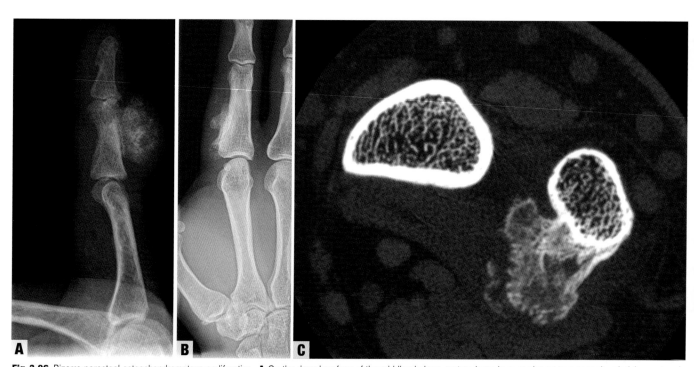

Fig. 3.06 Bizarre parosteal osteochondromatous proliferation. **A** On the dorsal surface of the middle phalanx, mature bone is seen closest to a normal underlying cortex. In the periphery, more fluffy calcifications are present. A lucent demarcation line projects between cortex and the bizarre parosteal osteochondromatous proliferation. **B** On the radial side of the proximal phalanx, a soft tissue swelling with some calcifications and mature bone is seen superficial and contiguous to an intact cortex. There are no signs of osteochondroma. **C** CT shows a calcified mass attached to the intact cortex of the ulna.

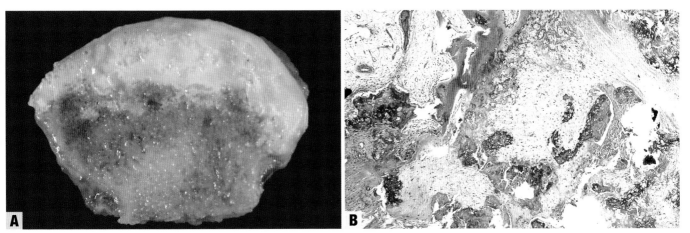

Fig. 3.07 Bizarre parosteal osteochondromatous proliferation. **A** Gross specimen showing a bony stalk with cartilaginous surface. **B** Bizarre parosteal osteochondromatous proliferation with a more disorganized mixture of mainly bone and cartilage.

Pathogenesis

Recurrent cytogenetic abnormalities of BPOP include t(1;17) (q32;q21), inv(7), and inv(6) {2300,431}. These are different from the translocations associated with subungual exostosis {2097}, supporting the notion that BPOP is a distinct entity.

Macroscopic appearance

BPOP is an exophytic bony lesion with a cartilaginous surface. Most tumours measure 1–3 cm.

Histopathology

BPOP is composed of a variable mixture of cartilage, bone, and fibrous tissue. The outermost part of the lesion can be covered by hyaline cartilage. Myxoid and fibrocartilaginous tissue may also be seen. The cartilage has an increased number of chondrocytes with enlarged nuclei and binucleation, and it therefore often looks atypical (bizarre). Marked hyperchromasia or atypical mitoses are not seen. The cartilage transitions to trabeculae of bone via enchondral ossification,

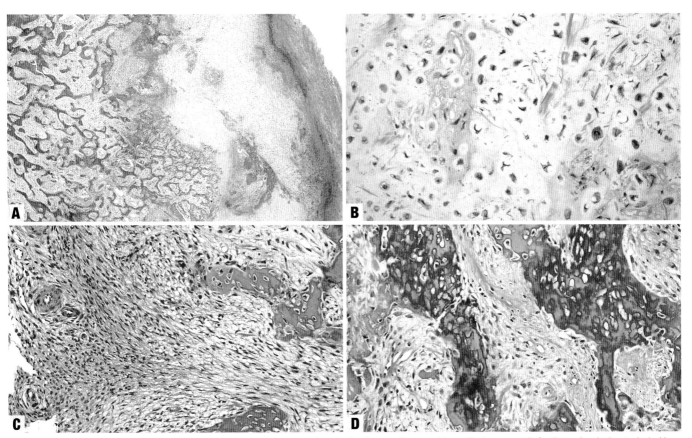

Fig. 3.08 Bizarre parosteal osteochondromatous proliferation. **A** Low-power view showing bony stalk covered by cartilaginous cap. **B** Cartilage often looks atypical with an increased number of chondrocytes with enlarged nuclei. **C** Spindle cell proliferation with osteoid formation. **D** So-called blue bone is characteristic.

with an irregular interface. Between the cartilage and bone, characteristic stroma can be seen, with a basophilic tinctorial quality (so-called blue bone), even after decalcification {2074, 622}. The intertrabecular space is filled with hypervascular tissue without a marrow component and is populated by a non-atypical spindle cell proliferation.

Differential diagnosis
The differential diagnosis includes subungual exostosis, which exclusively affects the distal phalangeal bone and lacks blue bone. Osteochondroma shows medullary continuity, cortical flaring, and fatty intertrabecular spaces, generally without cartilaginous atypia. Parosteal osteosarcoma is large and harbours intertrabecular fascicles of mildly atypical spindle cells, which are often positive for *MDM2* amplification. Periosteal osteosarcoma shows characteristic radiological findings, with prominent periosteal reaction and more atypical tumour cartilage and bone. Fibro-osseous pseudotumour of digits, which may harbour a *USP6* rearrangement {1036}, shows a fasciitis-like background and disorganized bone {2187}.

Cytology
Not clinically relevant

Diagnostic molecular pathology
Not clinically relevant

Essential and desirable diagnostic criteria
Essential: an exophytic bony growth with intact cortex; a disorganized cellular lesion comprising spindle cells, atypical chondrocytes, and bone; the presence of blue bone is characteristic.

Staging
Not clinically relevant

Prognosis and prediction
BPOP is treated with simple excision. Recurrences occur in as many as half of the cases, sometimes multiple times, but they are non-destructive and managed by re-excision. BPOP has no capacity to metastasize.

Periosteal chondroma

Bridge JA
Cleven AHG
Tirabosco R

Definition
Periosteal chondroma is a benign cartilaginous neoplasm that arises on the bone surface beneath the periosteum.

ICD-O coding
9221/0 Periosteal chondroma

ICD-11 coding
2E82 & XH3BC3 Benign chondrogenic tumours & Periosteal chondroma

Related terminology
Not recommended: juxtacortical chondroma.

Subtype(s)
None

Localization
Periosteal chondroma occurs most commonly in the small bones of the hands and the long bones of the appendicular skeleton {236,421,1834}. The proximal humerus is the most frequent location.

Clinical features
Signs and symptoms
Periosteal chondroma presents as a small palpable swelling, causing pain or local discomfort, especially if arising close to a joint. It is a sporadic tumour and usually solitary.

Imaging
Radiographically, it appears as a well-demarcated metaphyseal and juxtacortical radiolucent neoplasm, with a variable degree of internal mineralization, ranging from punctate to diffuse. The underlying cortex is scalloped and sclerotic, and the lateral borders of the tumour are typically buttressed {236,421,1834}.

Epidemiology
Periosteal chondromas most frequently affect children and young adults, with an M:F ratio of 1.5:1. They are much less common than enchondromas {236,421,1834}.

Etiology
Unknown

Pathogenesis
A subset of periosteal chondromas, similar to enchondromas, are caused by mutations in one of the IDH genes. These mutations were shown to promote chondrogenic differentiation in favour of osteogenic differentiation in preclinical models {1528, 2979}. Chromosomal aberrations described in periosteal chondroma include loss of chromosome 6 material rearrangements of 2q37, 4q21-q24, 11q13-q15, and 12q13-q15 {2421,710}.

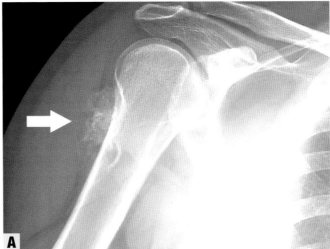

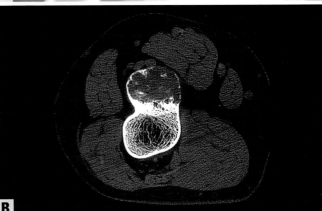

Fig. 3.09 Periosteal chondroma. **A** This radiograph depicts a mineralized tumour (arrow) with underlying cortical sclerosis. **B** CT of a periosteal chondroma of the posterior femur illustrates characteristic radiographic findings. The tumour is well demarcated, partially mineralized, and contained by a discontinuous thin layer of periosteal bone. The underlying cortex is thickened and sclerotic and there is peripheral buttressing around the base of the tumour.

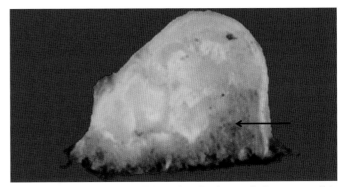

Fig. 3.10 Periosteal chondroma. Well-marginated surface cartilaginous tumour. Note the hyaline, lobulated appearance and the cortical buttressing (arrow), but no invasion.

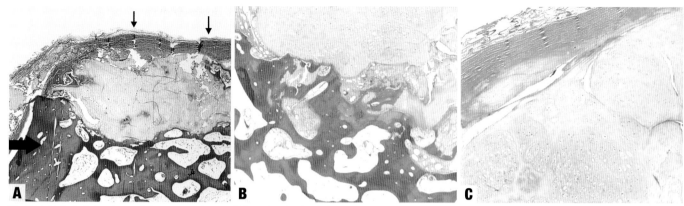

Fig. 3.11 Periosteal chondroma. **A** Low-power micrograph illustrating the classic features of periosteal chondroma. The tumour is situated beneath the periosteum (small arrows) and erodes the underlying sclerotic cortex. Thick periosteal buttressing is present at the periphery (large arrow). **B** Classic features of periosteal chondroma. Note the cortical buttressing. **C** The tumour is arranged in hyaline lobules composed of bland chondrocytes. Note the thick periosteal layer on top, covering the tumour.

Macroscopic appearance

The typical periosteal chondroma is a small lobulated tumour, < 5 cm in size, with a hyaline appearance, sited on the bone surface and covered by periosteum. The tumour induces a crisp cortical osteosclerosis with formation of the characteristic bone buttressing at the lateral edges of the tumour.

Histopathology

Periosteal chondromas are well demarcated from the underlying sclerotic cortex, which may be focally eroded but never permeated. The tumour has a lobulated arrangement and is covered by a continuous layer of attenuated periosteum. Invasion of surrounding soft tissue or medullary canal is not a feature seen in periosteal chondromas. The cellularity is variable but generally low, and the chondrocytes do not show cytological atypia. Occasionally, however, in comparison with enchondromas, periosteal chondromas are more cellular and may exhibit a greater degree of nuclear pleomorphism, including cell spindling and binucleation. Focal myxoid change of the matrix, which is typically hyaline, may also occur.

Differential diagnosis

Size > 5 cm favours the diagnosis of periosteal chondrosarcoma {1453}. The presence of invasion into the haversian system allows a definitive diagnosis of periosteal chondrosarcoma.

Cytology

Not clinically relevant

Diagnostic molecular pathology

Periosteal chondroma frequently harbours heterozygous mutations in *IDH1*, with p.Arg132Cys appearing to represent the most common amino acid alteration {93,726,2421}. IDH mutation testing will not distinguish this entity from periosteal chondrosarcoma {93}.

Essential and desirable diagnostic criteria

Essential: well-marginated, lobulated cartilaginous tumour arising on the bone surface, with elevation of periosteum; erosion but no invasion of the underlying cortex; low to moderate cellularity, with relatively uniform chondrocytes.
Desirable: size usually < 5 cm.

Staging

Not clinically relevant

Prognosis and prediction

Periosteal chondromas are treated by curettage or simple excision. Recurrence is rare regardless of surgery type {236,1834}.

Enchondroma

Bovée JVMG
Bloem JL
Flanagan AM
Nielsen GP
Yoshida A

Definition
Enchondroma is a benign hyaline cartilaginous neoplasm that arises within the medullary cavity of bone.

ICD-O coding
9220/0 Enchondroma

ICD-11 coding
2E83.Y & XH9SY5 Other specified benign osteogenic tumours & Enchondroma

Related terminology
Not recommended: chondroma.

Subtype(s)
None

Localization
Enchondromas most commonly affect the short tubular bones of the hands {2509}. The long tubular bones are less frequently affected, and location in flat bones is very uncommon (< 1%).

Clinical features
Signs and symptoms
Most enchondromas are solitary; occasionally they are multifocal affecting one or multiple bones, a syndrome referred to as enchondromatosis. The size of the enchondroma is usually < 3 cm. Typically an enchondroma does not cause pain. Enchondromas in the short tubular bones of the hands and feet may cause palpable swellings, pain, and pathological fracture, whereas long bone lesions are more often asymptomatic.

Imaging
Enchondromas are located in the medullary cavity, typically in the metadiaphysis {2530}. The ring and arcs matrix mineralization, seen on radiographs and CT, is typical for cartilaginous tumours but may be absent, especially in young patients and in tumours involving small bones of the hands and feet. In mature enchondroma, these may coalesce into solid areas of calcification. The lobulated, non-sclerotic margin is well depicted on MRI but not on radiographs. Superficial scalloping (seen on CT and MRI) of the cortex, cortical thinning, and bone expansion (especially in phalanges) are frequently present. Unless the tumour is completely calcified, additional MRI features are septonodular enhancement of the fibrovascular septations that enhance on late gadolinium chelate–enhanced images, small mucoid areas (high signal on T2), and fat {1128}. Over the years, enchondromas may change in size {598}. Radiological differentiation between enchondroma, atypical cartilaginous tumour, and high-grade chondrosarcoma is described in the section *Central atypical cartilaginous tumour / chondrosarcoma, grade 1* (p. 370).

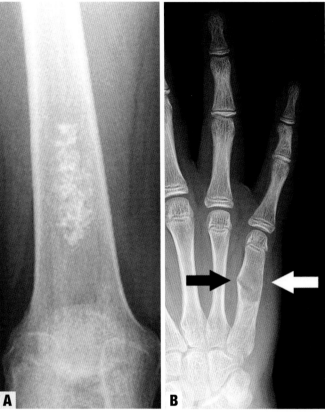

Fig. 3.12 Enchondroma. **A** Note the popcorn-like calcifications. **B** Symptomatic enchondromas in small tubular bones frequently present with pathological fractures. Note cortical attenuation (white arrow) and fracture (black arrow) in this expansile enchondroma, extending proximally.

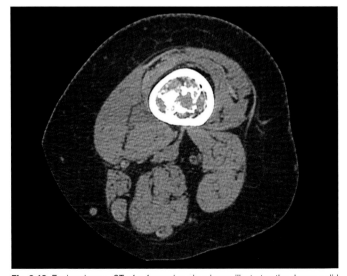

Fig. 3.13 Enchondroma. CT of a femoral enchondroma illustrates the dense, solid calcifications.

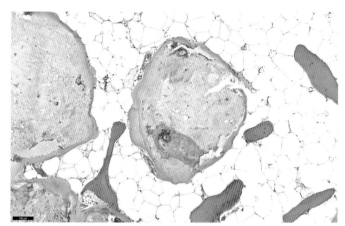

Fig. 3.14 Enchondroma. Enchondroma showing encasement: the separate nodules are surrounded by bone, which is a sign of slow growth.

Epidemiology

Enchondromas are relatively common, accounting for 10–25% of all surgically removed benign bone tumours. The exact incidence is unknown because many are discovered incidentally on radiographic images taken for other reasons. The prevalence of enchondroma as an incidental finding on knee MRI is approximately 2%; 84% measure < 2 cm {2957}. Enchondromas that come to clinical attention are usually found in the third to fourth decades of life (range: 1–86 years; median: 36 years) {2509}. On average, patients with an enchondroma are younger than those with a chondrosarcoma. The sexes are equally affected.

Etiology

Enchondromas may be caused by heterozygous somatic mutations in the isocitrate dehydrogenase genes *IDH1* and *IDH2*. Mutations are found in 52% of sporadic enchondromas and in about 90% of enchondromas in patients with enchondromatosis (see *Enchondromatosis*, p. 506), indicating that these represent an early driver event for enchondroma formation {93,2430,96}. Patients with enchondromatosis are somatic mosaic for *IDH1* or *IDH2*.

Pathogenesis

Isocitrate dehydrogenases are enzymes involved in the conversion of isocitrate to α-ketoglutarate in the tricarboxylic acid cycle, producing energy for the cell. The gain-of-function mutations give the mutant enzyme the activity to convert α-ketoglutarate into the oncometabolite D-2-HG. Indeed, increased levels of D-2-HG can be detected in cartilage tumours with an *IDH1* or *IDH2* mutation {96}. This causes epigenetic changes (i.e. altered histone methylation and hypermethylation) {2430,1242}. Indeed, D-2-HG has been shown to promote chondrogenic and inhibit osteogenic differentiation of mesenchymal stem cells, the presumed precursor cells of enchondroma {2979,1528}.

Macroscopic appearance

If treated, the specimen is usually received in fragments (curettage). These tissue fragments contain bluish-white glistening cartilage tissue admixed with medullary bone. Gritty, yellow foci are seen as a result of calcification, and red areas represent ossification or surrounding bone marrow. Resection specimens are uncommon and demonstrate a well-marginated, often

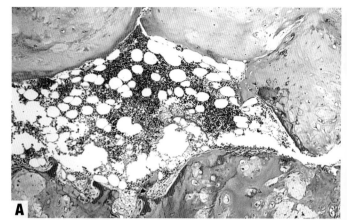

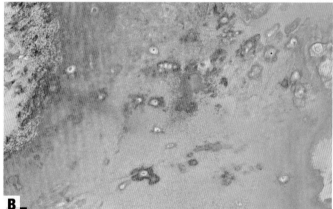

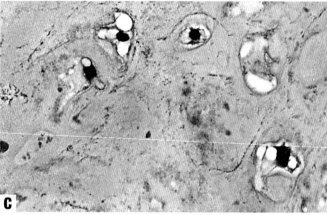

Fig. 3.15 Enchondroma. **A** Enchondromas commonly have a multinodular architectural pattern characterized by islands of cartilage encased by thin mantles of bone that are often separated by marrow. This pattern is more common in larger tumours. Enchondromas in small tubular bones tend to have a more confluent architecture. **B** Some enchondromas become heavily calcified, as shown by densely stippled and solid areas of deeply basophilic staining. The chondrocytes are often necrotic in these areas, reduced to eosinophilic bodies within lacunae. **C** The chondrocytes are typically situated within sharp-edged lacunar spaces. The cytoplasm is frequently retracted to form vacuoles and spider-like eosinophilic extensions. Nuclei are small, round, and hyperchromatic, although larger, vesicular nuclei can also be present. Mitotic figures are usually non-existent and binucleation is uncommon. Finely stippled calcifications within the hyaline matrix are common.

multinodular, whitish-blue glistening tumour in the medullary cavity of the bone, with intact cortex. In the short tubular bones, the lesions are less multinodular and have a more confluent growth pattern.

Histopathology

Histologically, enchondromas are hypocellular, with an abundance of hyaline cartilage matrix. The tumour cells are embedded within sharp-edged lacunar spaces and evenly dispersed. When the cytoplasm is visible, it is usually eosinophilic. The nuclei are typically small and round, with condensed chromatin (lymphocyte-like). Cytological atypia and mitoses are absent. The architecture can be multinodular or confluent. In cases with multinodular growth, the lobules can be separated by delicate fibrous septa with small-calibre vessels. The separate nodules can be surrounded by bone, which is referred to as encasement and is a sign of slow growth {2155}. Normal bone marrow can be present between the nodules. Enchondromas do not invade and destroy the cortex, entrap pre-existing lamellar bone, or extend into soft tissue. Degenerative features, such as ischaemic necrosis or calcification, can be prominent.

In the small phalangeal bones, as well as in patients with enchondromatosis, enchondromas can be much more cellular; in such cases, the tumour cells occasionally have more-open chromatin and small nucleoli. Binucleated cells can be seen. The matrix composition can be more myxoid, and then cells become more elongated or stellate in shape. Cortical destruction, soft tissue extension {387,768}, and entrapment of host lamellar bone (see *Central atypical cartilaginous tumour / chondrosarcoma, grade 1*, p. 370) are not allowed even under these circumstances, and often a diagnosis cannot be established without proper radiological correlation.

Immunohistochemistry

Immunohistochemistry is usually not helpful in the diagnosis. The tumour cells are positive for S100. Approximately 24% are positive for the p.Arg132His mutation–specific IDH1 antibody, limiting its usefulness because this represents only a small percentage of the IDH mutations that can be found in cartilage tumours {93,2430,96}.

Differential diagnosis

The distinction between enchondroma and central atypical cartilaginous tumour / chondrosarcoma, grade 1 (ACT/CS1) can be difficult {1130,2155} and is subject to interobserver variability, even among experts {883,2886}. A combination of five parameters (high cellularity, host bone entrapment, open chromatin, mucoid matrix degeneration > 20%, and patient age > 45 years) is helpful in differentiating between enchondromas and central ACT/CS1s {883}, with mucomyxoid matrix degeneration and host bone entrapment being most discriminating. In the phalanges, enchondromas are more cellular and can have worrisome histological features that do not predict the clinical behaviour. The main discriminating factors in distinguishing enchondroma from chondrosarcoma in the phalanges are the presence of mitoses, cortical breakthrough, soft tissue involvement {387}, and host lamellar bone entrapment.

Cytology
Not clinically relevant

Diagnostic molecular pathology
Molecular pathology is rarely used for diagnosis. Hotspot mutations are exclusively found at the *IDH1* p.Arg132 and the *IDH2* p.Arg172 positions. These mutations are specific for enchondromas, periosteal chondromas, and conventional and periosteal chondrosarcomas, and they are absent in other mesenchymal tumours of bone. Mutation analysis cannot be used to distinguish enchondroma from ACT/CS1.

Essential and desirable diagnostic criteria
Essential: abundance of cartilaginous matrix; absence of cytological atypia, mitoses, cortical invasion, and soft tissue extension; tumours arising in small bones and/or in patients with enchondromatosis may show more cellularity and atypia.

Staging
Not clinically relevant

Prognosis and prediction
Asymptomatic enchondromas can be followed clinically and do not need to be treated. In case of symptoms, curettage is usually curative. Longstanding enchondromas identified radiologically have been shown to progress. However, malignant transformation of enchondromas is thought to be rare (< 1%) in a non-syndromic setting. Pain without the presence of a fracture and radiological changes should raise the possibility of progression.

Osteochondroma

Bovée JVMG
Bloem JL
Heymann D
Wuyts W

Definition
Osteochondroma is a benign cartilaginous neoplasm consisting of a bony projection covered by a cartilage cap, arising at the external surface of bone and containing a marrow cavity that is continuous with that of the underlying bone.

ICD-O coding
9210/0 Osteochondroma

ICD-11 coding
2E83.Y & XH5Y87 Other specified benign osteogenic tumours & Osteochondroma

Related terminology
Not recommended: (osteo)cartilaginous exostosis.

Subtype(s)
None

Localization
Osteochondromas arise in bones that are formed by endochondral ossification during skeletal development, explaining their localization. The most common sites include the metaphyseal regions of the distal femur, proximal tibia, proximal humerus, and less frequently flat bones. The craniofacial bones are generally not affected, except for the mandibular condyle.

Clinical features
Signs and symptoms
Many osteochondromas, whether solitary or multiple, are asymptomatic and found incidentally. Osteochondromas develop and increase in size during the first decade of life, and they stop growing around puberty, when the growth plates close. Symptoms are often related to the size and location of the lesion. The most common presentation is that of a hard, long-standing mass. Complications include bursa formation; arthritis; and impingement on adjacent tendons, nerves, vessels, or spinal cord {3285}. Increasing pain and/or a growing mass in an adult patient may be a manifestation of progression towards a peripheral chondrosarcoma.

Imaging
Osteochondromas are typically located at the transition of diaphysis to metaphysis of the bone. The radiological hallmark of osteochondroma, best seen on CT and MRI, is the continuity of bone marrow into a pedunculated (slim base) or sessile (broad

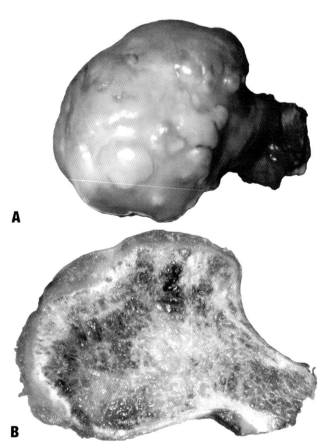

A

B

Fig. 3.17 Osteochondroma. **A** Macroscopic view showing the external cartilage cap. **B** Cut section revealing the continuity of the cortex and marrow cavity with the underlying bone.

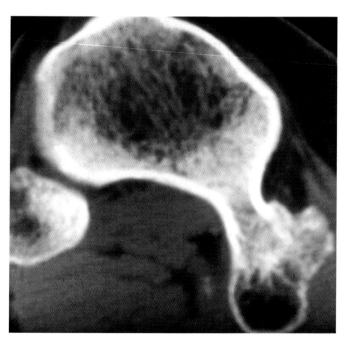

Fig. 3.16 Osteochondroma. Axial CT of an osteochondroma demonstrating continuity of both the stalk and centre of the lesion with the tibial cortex and medullary cavity, respectively.

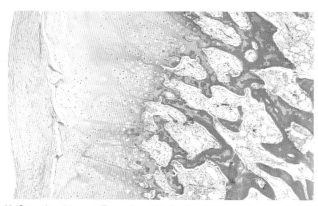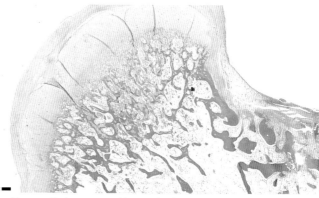

Fig. 3.18 Osteochondroma. **A** From left to right, the three layers can be recognized: perichondrium, cartilaginous cap, and bony stalk, with enchondral ossification at the interface between cartilage and bone. Note the resemblance to the growth plate with organization of hypertrophic chondrocytes in columns. **B** Low-power view of osteochondroma.

base) outgrowth combined with flaring of cortical bone into the margins of the outgrowth. Osteochondromas point away from the adjacent joint. Smooth calcifications can be seen. MRI may display the cause of symptoms based on mechanical compromise of neighbouring tendons, muscles, bones, vessels (including pseudoaneurysm), and nerves. A bursa can develop and must be differentiated from the cartilaginous cap. Bone deformity may be caused by the lesion itself, or by metaphyseal undertubulation. Fat, haematopoietic marrow, and cartilaginous nests may be seen on MRI in the base of the stalk. Septations in the lobulated lesion may enhance on MRI and/or may show mineralization on CT and MRI. The size of the cartilaginous cap is measured perpendicular to the tidemark (the bone–cartilage interface) and can be well established with T2-weighted MRI. The cap should be < 2 cm and display high homogeneous signal intensity {1131, 279}. A bulky benign cartilaginous cap may be present in the paediatric age group, but it should decrease in size with ageing. Only in young children, active enchondral ossification may cause inhomogeneity in the cap. A cartilage cap > 2 cm in the skeletally mature is suggestive of progressive disease {2220,279}.

Epidemiology
Osteochondroma is one of the most common benign bone tumours. The average age at diagnosis of solitary osteochondroma is 18 years (median: 15 years; range: 2–77 years), with a male predominance (65% vs 35%) {2509}. The reported incidence, 35% of benign and 8% of all bone tumours, may be an underestimate because many osteochondromas are asymptomatic. Approximately 15% of osteochondroma patients have multiple lesions characteristic of the autosomal dominant hereditary multiple osteochondromas syndrome (see *Multiple osteochondromas*, p. 517).

Etiology
Osteochondromas are caused by biallelic inactivation of the *EXT1* or *EXT2* gene. In patients with multiple osteochondromas, heterozygous germline alterations are found in the *EXT1* or *EXT2* gene (see *Multiple osteochondromas*, p. 517), combined with somatic loss of the remaining wildtype allele within the cartilage cap of the osteochondromas {381,1545,278,2593,3411}. In solitary sporadic osteochondromas, homozygous deletions of *EXT1* can be found in about 80% of tumours {1285,3411}. Osteochondromas have been reported to occur after total body irradiation in childhood {1639}.

Pathogenesis
The finding of biallelic inactivation of the *EXT1* or *EXT2* gene within the cartilage cap supports the neoplastic nature of these tumours. The cell of origin is considered to be either a chondrocyte within the growth plate {1545} or a mesenchymal progenitor cell from the perichondrium {1436}. Most of the mutations found in the *EXT1* or *EXT2* gene are predicted to result in a truncated or non-functional protein {1522}. The EXT gene products, EXT1 and EXT2, are glycosyltransferases involved in heparan sulfate biosynthesis. The cartilage cap of osteochondroma is composed of a mixture of wildtype (normal heparan sulfate) and mutated (heparan sulfate–deficient) cells {2012,1545,750}. Heparan sulfate proteoglycans serve as key modulators of endochondral ossification by forming an osmotic gradient around chondrocytes and by controlling signal transduction {1268}. Loss of heparan sulfate may give a proliferative advantage to the mutated chondroprogenitor cells and leads to loss of polarity {612,752}. Because defective heparan sulfate mainly affects multiple signalling pathways, including those involving hedgehog {1692}, BMP {2408}, FGFR3 {2514}, and WNT/β-catenin {2514}, disturbed signalling causes EXT-mutated cells to grow out of the bone and recruit normal cells to form an osteochondroma.

Macroscopic appearance
Osteochondroma may be cauliflower-like, sessile, or pedunculated {959}. Within the underlying stalk, a cortex and medullary cavity can be recognized. The size of the overlying glassy bluish-white cartilaginous cap is important and should be well documented. It should be measured perpendicular to the bone–cartilage interface, at its thickest portion. The cartilage cap is usually thin (and thickness decreases with age). A thick and irregular cap (> 2 cm) may be indicative of progression.

Histopathology
The lesion has three layers: perichondrium, cartilage, and bone. The outer layer is a fibrous perichondrium that is continuous with the periosteum of the underlying bone. Below this is a cartilage cap that mimics disorganized growth plate cartilage, with endochondral ossification: the superficial chondrocytes are clustered, whereas the ones close to the transition to bone become larger, similar to the hypertrophic cells of the growth plate. With age, the cellularity is progressively reduced, sometimes with extensive coarse and irregular calcification. Binucleated cells,

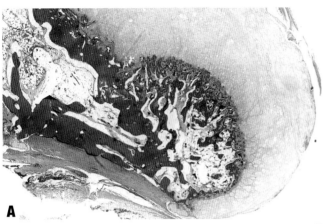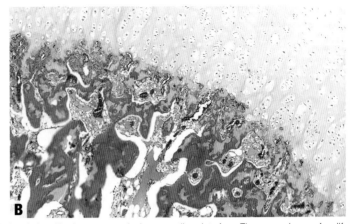

Fig. 3.19 Osteochondroma. **A** The cartilage cap centred by trabecular bone. **B** Endochondral ossification occurs at the bone–cartilage interface. There are columns of proliferative chondrocytes surrounded by cartilaginous hyaline matrix, resembling the normal growth plate.

calcification, focal necrosis, nodularity, and degenerative cystic/mucoid changes can be seen and do not indicate malignancy {749}. Nuclear atypia and mitoses are absent.

Differential diagnosis
The distinction between osteochondroma and secondary peripheral atypical cartilaginous tumour / chondrosarcoma, grade 1 (ACT/CS1) is histologically difficult and should be made in a multidisciplinary team taking the radiology, especially the size of the cartilage cap, and the patient's age into account. Loss of architecture, nodularity, wide fibrous bands, myxoid change, binucleated cells, and increased chondrocyte cellularity should be considered with caution. Fractures within a stalk may elicit a focal fibroblastic response. Periosteal chondrosarcoma differs from osteochondroma by the absence of a stalk. Subungual exostosis can be very cellular but has a

characteristic fibrillary cartilaginous matrix, which is not seen in osteochondroma. Dysplasia epiphysealis hemimelica (Trevor disease), a non-hereditary skeletal dysplasia, demonstrates cartilaginous overgrowth at the epiphysis, strongly resembling an osteochondroma, although there is clumping of chondrocytes within a more fibrillary chondroid matrix {382}.

Immunohistochemistry
Immunohistochemistry is not of help in the diagnosis of osteochondroma.

Cytology
Not clinically relevant

Diagnostic molecular pathology
Molecular testing is not required for the diagnosis of osteochondroma. Chromosomal aberrations involve 8q22-q24.1, where the *EXT1* gene is located {416,2099,979}, or 11p11.2, where the *EXT2* gene is located {1521}. Mutations in *IDH1* or *IDH2* are absent in osteochondromas {93,2430}.

Essential and desirable diagnostic criteria
Essential: cartilaginous cap, with growth plate–like architecture (in children) or extensive calcification (with increasing age); underlying stalk, with medullary and cortical bone that is continuous with that of the underlying bone; the size of the cartilaginous cap should be well documented and should be < 2 cm in the skeletally mature.

Staging
Not clinically relevant

Prognosis and prediction
Excision of the osteochondroma is usually curative, although recurrence is seen after incomplete removal. Multiple recurrences or recurrence of a well-excised lesion should raise suspicion for progression. The risk of progression to secondary peripheral chondrosarcoma is estimated at about 1% for solitary and as high as 5% for multiple osteochondromas {3285, 1823,2767}. In very rare instances, osteosarcomas, spindle cell sarcomas, and dedifferentiated chondrosarcomas can develop in osteochondroma {1741,385,2930}.

Fig. 3.20 Osteochondroma formation. A second hit in EXT in a proliferating cell of the growth plate near the bony collar underlies osteochondroma formation in patients with multiple osteochondromas. The cells lose polarity and grow out of the bone through a defective bony collar. In the cartilaginous cap, EXT–/– cells are intermingled with EXT+/– cells (mosaicism). In solitary osteochondromas, two somatic hits are required in a single chondrocyte.

Chondroblastoma

Amary F
Bloem JL
Cleven AHG
Konishi E

Definition

Chondroblastoma is a benign tumour of bone that has a predilection for epiphyseal or apophyseal regions, composed of chondroblastic cells and islands of eosinophilic chondroid matrix.

ICD-O coding

9230/0 Chondroblastoma NOS

ICD-11 coding

2E82.Z & XH4NK2 Benign chondrogenic tumours, site unspecified & Chondroblastoma NOS

Related terminology

None

Subtype(s)

None

Localization

Approximately 75% of chondroblastomas involve the epiphyseal (subchondral) region of long bones, with the femur being the most commonly affected site, followed by the proximal tibia and proximal humerus {1718,343}. Other sites include the talus, calcaneus, patella, and pelvic bones (especially the acetabulum). Less frequently, the ribs, vertebrae, and small bones of the hands and feet are affected. Involvement of craniofacial bones is exceptional. In adult patients aged > 30 years, short tubular bones and flat bones, rather than long bones, are more commonly affected {714,1718}.

Clinical features

Signs and symptoms

The clinical presentation varies with the site of disease. The most common symptom is pain. Local tenderness, joint effusion, impaired movement, and muscle atrophy may be found as presenting symptoms.

Imaging

Radiographically, a well-defined, often sclerotically marginated lucent lesion is present, showing geographical bone destruction. Chondroblastoma is typically located adjacent to a growth plate, usually in the epiphysis or in the epiphysis and metaphysis, and rarely in the metaphysis or apophysis only {2039, 343,714}. The lesions are usually < 5 cm {1718}. Mineralization, trabeculation, cortical erosion, and expansion are frequently present; expansion is more common in flat and small bones {343}. MRI characteristically exhibits reactive changes outside the tumour, which are reflected by synovitis and periosteal reaction also distant from the tumour, as well as increased signal intensity in bone and surrounding soft tissues on fluid-sensitive and gadolinium chelate–enhanced images {343,714,1718}. The

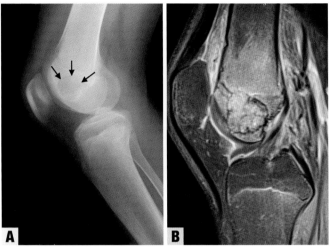

Fig. 3.21 Chondroblastoma. A Lateral radiograph showing a lytic lesion in the distal femoral epiphysis (arrows). B Sagittal short-tau inversion recovery (STIR) MRI showing a well-defined lesion of increased signal in the epiphysis, with similar, oedema-like, high signal in the adjacent marrow and soft tissues.

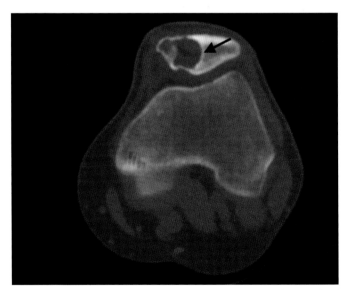

Fig. 3.22 Chondroblastoma. Axial CT of patella showing an eccentric well-defined lytic lesion (arrow).

tumour itself is inhomogeneous and has areas of low signal intensity on fluid-sensitive sequences due to mineralization and trabeculation, which are also well seen on CT {2562}. Aneurysmal bone cyst–like changes can be seen as fluid-fluid levels on MRI in areas of marked expansion {1630,1519}.

Epidemiology

Chondroblastomas account for < 1% of all bone tumours. Most occur in patients with an immature skeleton in the second to

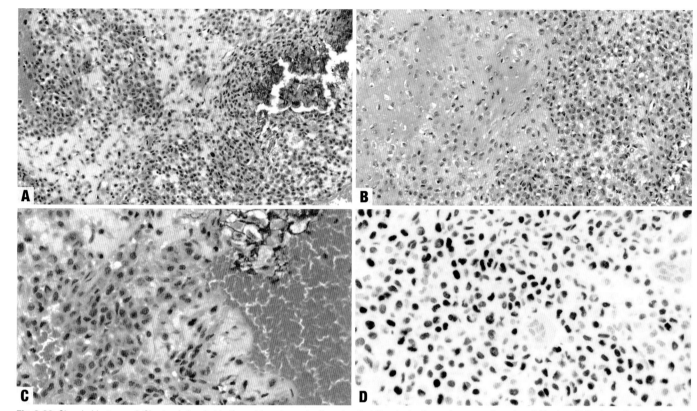

Fig. 3.23 Chondroblastoma. **A** Sheets of chondroblastic oval to polygonal cells, osteoclast-like giant cells, and an area of matrix calcification. **B** Oval to polygonal chondroblasts with well-defined cytoplasmic borders, merging with an area of eosinophilic cartilaginous matrix. **C** Chondroblastic cells with nuclear indentation and grooves. The top-right corner shows chicken-wire pericellular calcification. **D** H3.3 p.Lys36Met (K36M) diffuse nuclear expression in the chondroblastic cells. Note that the osteoclast-like giant cells show no expression.

early third decades of life (10–25 years of age), although it may present at any age {343,114,1718}. It is twice as prevalent in males {3119,343,1718}.

Etiology
Unknown

Pathogenesis
H3.3 alterations are seen in various tumour types including bone tumours like chondroblastoma and giant cell tumour of bone. Specific substitutions are associated with different tumour types: p.Lys36Met with chondroblastoma and p.Gly34Trp with giant cell tumours of bone, suggesting that specific substitutions provide a growth advantage to specific cell types {257, 237}. p.Lys36Met substitutions in chondroblastoma are more frequent in the *H3-3B (H3F3B)* gene on chromosome 17 {257, 2538}.

The p.Lys36Met mutations inhibit the H3K36 methyltransferases NSD2 (MMSET) and SETD2, which results in reduced global H3K36 methylation {971,3352}. These epigenetic pathway alterations probably block mesenchymal differentiation and influence tumorigenesis in chondroblastoma {1897,1742,3225}.

Macroscopic appearance
Macroscopically, chondroblastomas are usually well-defined eccentric lesions with a thin sclerotic rim. The features vary from soft to rubbery with gritty and haemorrhagic areas. Chondroid matrix may be prominent. Blood-filled spaces may be seen in some cases with aneurysmal bone cyst change {714,2759}.

Histopathology
Histologically, chondroblastomas are composed of sheets of ovoid to polygonal cells with small singular grooved nuclei and eosinophilic cytoplasm {3146,714}. The cytoplasmic border is usually distinct. Epithelioid cells may be present. There are interspersed osteoclast-like giant cells and islands of eosinophilic chondroid matrix. Basophilic hyaline cartilage is infrequent. Pericellular lace-like or chicken-wire calcification is characteristic and usually noted among degenerative cells. Nuclear atypia and/or mitotic figures may be found. Aneurysmal bone cyst–like change is common.

Immunohistochemistry
Immunohistochemistry using an antibody against H3.3B (H3F3B) p.Lys36Met (K36M) shows diffuse nuclear expression in > 96% of the cases and is helpful in small biopsies or cases with extensive aneurysmal bone cyst–like change {95,615}. SOX9, S100, cytokeratin, and DOG1, although not specific, may be focally positive {1681,2174,2814,614}.

Differential diagnosis
The differential diagnosis includes primary aneurysmal bone cyst, giant cell tumour of bone, clear cell chondrosarcoma, chondromyxoid fibroma, Langerhans cell histiocytosis, and an

extremely rare subtype of osteosarcoma: chondroblastoma-like osteosarcoma {192}.

Cytology
Not clinically relevant

Diagnostic molecular pathology
The vast majority of chondroblastomas harbour a p.Lys36Met substitution in one of the genes that encode H3.3: *H3-3B (H3F3B)* (> 95%) on chromosome 17 or, less frequently, *H3-3A (H3F3A)* on chromosome 1 {257,95,615}. Among bone tumours, this is highly specific for chondroblastoma, although one case of clear cell chondrosarcoma was reported to harbour an *H3-3B (H3F3B)* p.Lys36Met mutation {257}. *IDH1* and *IDH2* substitutions are not seen in chondroblastomas {726,93,615}.

Essential and desirable diagnostic criteria
Essential: epiphyseal/apophyseal location; sheets of chondroblastic cells, island of eosinophilic chondroid matrix and osteoclast-like giant cells.

Desirable: a fine network of pericellular chicken-wire calcification; presence of H3.3 mutation demonstrated by p.Lys36Met (K36M) expression or *H3-3A (H3F3A)* / *H3-3B (H3F3B)* mutation analysis.

Staging
Not clinically relevant

Prognosis and prediction
Chondroblastomas are benign tumours that in > 80% of the cases are successfully treated with surgical curettage with or without adjuvant treatment of the surgical bed {878,2994}. Radiofrequency ablation may be used {2696}. The recurrence rates vary with site of disease, being lower in long bones and higher in flat bones and craniofacial bones, ranging from 10% to 18% {878,2994,295,3119}. There are no reliable histological parameters predicting local recurrence {3119,801,1682}. In exceptional cases, so-called benign lung metastasis may develop {2406}.

Chondromyxoid fibroma

Hogendoorn PCW
Bloem JL
Bridge JA

Definition
Chondromyxoid fibroma is a benign lobulated cartilaginous neoplasm with a zonal architecture composed of chondroid, myxoid, and myofibroblastic areas.

ICD-O coding
9241/0 Chondromyxoid fibroma

ICD-11 coding
2E82.Z & XH89S0 Benign chondrogenic tumours, site unspecified & Chondromyxoid fibroma

Related terminology
None

Subtype(s)
None

Localization
Chondromyxoid fibroma can occur at almost any osseous site. It is most frequent in the long bones, most often the proximal tibia and distal femur. Approximately 25% of cases occur in the flat bones, mainly the ilium. When involving bones of the feet, chondromyxoid fibroma often involves metatarsals. Other sites of involvement include the ribs, vertebrae, skull and facial bones, and tubular bones of the hand.

Clinical features
Signs and symptoms
Pain, which is the most common symptom, is usually mild and sometimes present for several years {3313}. Swelling is infrequent, most commonly observed in the bones of the hands and feet.

Imaging
Radiographically, chondromyxoid fibroma in a long bone is typically a well-demarcated, oval-shaped, lobulated osteolytic, eccentric, and metaphyseally located lesion, with attenuation and expansion of the cortex. Lesions of the rib or ilium may be discovered as incidental radiological findings {3313}. Less frequently, the tumour is juxtacortical {207}. The longitudinal axis of the lesion corresponds to that of the involved bone, and the average size is 3 cm (range: 1–10 cm). In the small bones, fusiform expansion of the entire bone is typical. Approximately 10% of cases may show focal calcified matrix, more often detectable with CT. There may be cortical destruction, but this is contained by the periosteum {2653,3313}. On MRI, chondromyxoid fibroma has an intermediate to high signal intensity on fluid-sensitive sequences, with a strong homogeneous or peripheral contrast enhancement {477}. Reactive high signal intensity changes may be present on fluid-sensitive sequences.

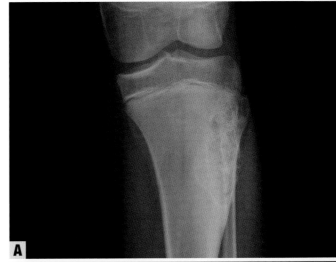

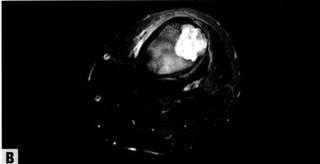

Fig. 3.24 Chondromyxoid fibroma. **A** Radiograph shows an eccentrically localized, expansile mixed osteolytic-sclerotic tumour with a well-defined sclerotic margin in the metaphysis and proximal diaphysis of the tibia. The combination of these morphological characteristics with the location is indicative of chondromyxoid fibroma. **B** The myxoid components have a high signal intensity on the T2-weighted fat-suppressed images. Note the reactive high signal surrounding the tumour in the bone marrow and in the periosteum medially.

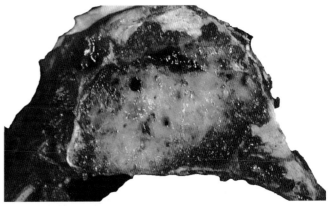

Fig. 3.25 Chondromyxoid fibroma of the ilium. Note the yellowish-grey, relatively uniform lesion, with sharply demarcated borders and expansion of the bone.

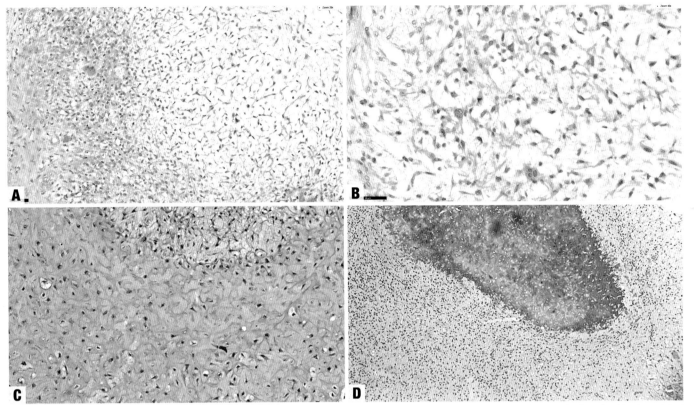

Fig. 3.26 Chondromyxoid fibroma. **A** Stellate cells embedded in a myxoid matrix are seen on the right, with more-cellular areas containing round cells and multinucleated giant cells on the left. **B** Moderate nuclear enlargement may be present. The eosinophilic cytoplasmic processes are evident. **C** Lobular architecture. In addition to myxoid areas, areas with more hyaline cartilaginous matrix can be seen in a subset of cases. **D** Focal coarse calcification.

Epidemiology

Chondromyxoid fibroma is a rare tumour {2653,3151}. Although it may affect a wide age range (first to seventh decades of life), it occurs most often in the second and third decades of life and more frequently in males {1138,3313}.

Etiology

Unknown

Pathogenesis

Recombination of the glutamate receptor gene *GRM1* with several 5′ partner genes through promoter swapping and gene fusion events leading to upregulated expression of transcripts encompassing the entire *GRM1* coding region, with or without non-coding 5′ partner remnants, is considered the driver event for chondromyxoid fibroma development {2318}. These canonical gene fusions were shown to be caused by complex rearrangement processes, predominantly chromoplexy, but also chromothripsis {107}. GRM1 expression is absent or very low in other cartilaginous neoplasms, emphasizing the high level of specificity of this finding in chondromyxoid fibroma {2318}. However, approximately 10% of chondromyxoid fibromas do not exhibit upregulation of GRM1 expression, suggesting that this small subset may develop via a different genetic pathway.

Macroscopic appearance

The gross features of chondromyxoid fibroma include well-defined margins, grey or white tumour, lack of obvious necrosis, cystic change, and liquefaction. The tumour is multilobulated and well demarcated from the surrounding bone. Typically, there are scalloped margins.

Histopathology

Typically, chondromyxoid fibroma is sharply demarcated from the surrounding bone. Lobules of tumour may be separate from the main lesion. A lobular pattern with stellate or spindle-shaped cells in a myxoid background is evident {3313}. Lobules demonstrate hypocellular centres with hypercellular peripheries. The centre of the lobules shows morphological features more similar to those of hyaline cartilage, in terms of both extracellular matrix and cell composition {2650,2901}. Microscopic cystic or liquefactive change is uncommon and usually focal when present. Hyaline cartilage is present in 19% of cases {3313}. Calcification, when present, is usually coarse, and it occurs more frequently in older patients and in flat-bone tumours {3331}. Individual cells within lobules have oval to spindled nuclei and indistinct to densely eosinophilic cytoplasm. Cytoplasmic extensions, often bipolar or multipolar, are frequent. Enlarged, hyperchromatic and pleomorphic nuclei are noted in 20–30% of cases. Mitoses are uncommon, although atypical mitoses have been noted {3313}. Entrapment of surrounding bone trabeculae by tumour is very rare. Because of these features, differential diagnosis with high-grade central chondrosarcoma is considered. However, clinicoradiological features and histology are quite distinct; chondrosarcomas more often affect older patients and the diaphysis of long bones, with more frank atypia and mitoses. Moreover, osteoclast-like giant cells are often present at the periphery of the lobules. There may also be haemosiderin

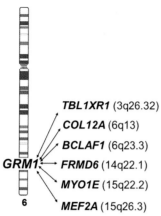

Fig. 3.27 Chondromyxoid fibroma. *GRM1* recombines with or has been predicted to recombine with one of the following 5′ gene partners: *TBL1XR1*, *COL12A1*, *BCLAF1*, *FRMD6*, *MYO1E*, and *MEF2A*.

deposition and inflammatory cells, usually lymphocytes. Aneurysmal bone cyst–like areas are noted in approximately 10% of long- and flat-bone lesions {3313}.

Immunohistochemistry

Immunohistochemistry is not required for routine clinical practice. The cartilaginous nature of this tumour is reflected by immunopositivity for S100 {342,727,1681,3406}.

Electron microscopy

Ultrastructurally, the stellate cells have irregular cell processes, scalloped cell membranes, cytoplasmic fibrils, and glycogen,

features of both chondroblastic and fibroblastic differentiation {2652,2283}. Cells with the classic features of chondrocytes, those with myofibroblastic features, and intermediate forms have been described in chondromyxoid fibroma {2652,2283}.

Cytology

Not clinically relevant

Diagnostic molecular pathology

Molecular analysis is generally not needed for diagnosis. In selected cases, identification of the exceedingly specific upregulation of GRM1 expression in chondromyxoid fibroma could be a strong diagnostic adjunct in distinguishing this entity from its mimics {2318}.

Essential and desirable diagnostic criteria

Essential: lytic metaphyseal eccentric appearance on conventional radiograph with sharp margins; lobulated lesion with zonal architecture; chondroid and stellate cells embedded in chondroid and/or myxoid matrix in the centre of the lobules; spindle-shaped myofibroblast-like cells at the periphery of the lobules admixed with osteoclast-like giant cells.

Staging

Not clinically relevant

Prognosis and prediction

The prognosis is excellent, even for recurrent tumours. Recurrence has been reported in approximately 9–15% of cases treated locally {303}.

Osteochondromyxoma

Bovée JVMG

Definition
Osteochondromyxoma is an extremely rare, benign, sometimes locally aggressive, chondroid and osteoid matrix-producing tumour, with extensive myxoid changes, predominantly occurring in patients with Carney complex.

ICD-O coding
9211/0 Osteochondromyxoma

ICD-11 coding
2E82.Z & XH6KR3 Benign chondrogenic tumours, site unspecified & Osteochondromyxoma

Related terminology
Not recommended: Carney bone tumour.

Subtype(s)
None

Localization
Tumours are found in the nasal region and the diaphysis of the tibia and radius. Individual cases have been reported in rib, chest wall, and spine {1180}.

Clinical features
Signs and symptoms
Patients present with a painless mass, usually found on screening for skeletal involvement in cases of Carney complex. Carney complex is a rare, autosomal dominant, multiple endocrine neoplasia and lentiginosis syndrome. In Carney complex, at least two of the following are found: spotty pigmentation, endocrine overactivity, osteochondromyxomas, recurrent cardiac myxomas, cutaneous and bilateral breast myxomas, multiple endocrine neoplasms, psammomatous melanotic schwannomas,

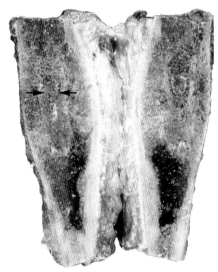

Fig. 3.28 Tibial osteochondromyxoma. The longitudinally sectioned tibia showed a heterogeneous, elongated, oval tumour. Inferiorly, the lesion was demarcated by a zone of haemorrhage (probably biopsy-related). Superiorly, the lesion was poorly delineated. A vague cylindrical zone (arrows) had a cartilaginous appearance and contained a small cyst with mucoid content.

pigmented mucosal and skin lesions, large cell calcifying Sertoli cell tumours, growth hormone–secreting pituitary adenomas, and breast ductal adenomas {1180}.

Imaging
Osteochondromyxomas do not have a uniform radiographic appearance and can manifest as a permeative lytic periosteal lesion with aggressive new bone formation or as an expansile bone area with sclerotic and lucent regions {668,669,485}. On MRI, increased T2-weighted signalling is seen {1180}.

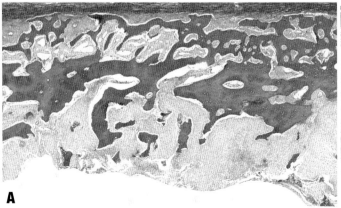

A

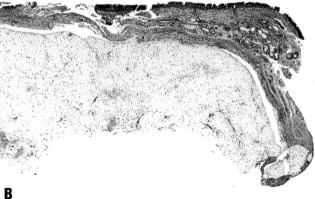

B

Fig. 3.29 Osteochondromyxoma. **A** A sheet of tumour cells with overall clear appearance and vague lobular pattern (right) erodes the bony cortex of the tibial lesion. The hypocellular tumour with dilated sinusoids penetrates between narrow reactive bony trabeculae just beneath the periosteum (top). **B** The circumscribed but unencapsulated hypocellular myxochondroid tumour abuts the nasal submucosa.

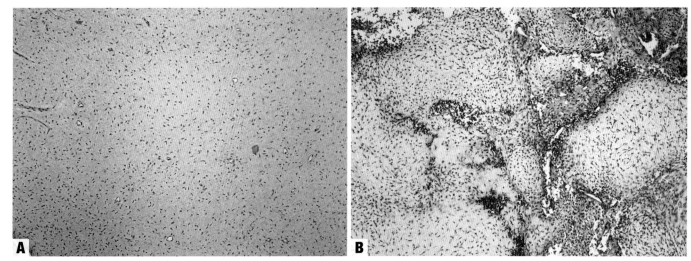

Fig. 3.30 Osteochondromyxoma. **A** The tumour is composed of a patternless sheet of cells separated by abundant basophilic mucopolysaccharide ground substance. **B** Polygonal, elongated, and stellate-shaped cells are arranged in moderate-sized lobules.

Epidemiology

Osteochondromyxoma is extremely rare, occurring in about 1% of patients with Carney complex {486,487}. The tumour can occur over a wide age range, but it typically presents early and can be congenital {485}. In adults, osteochondromyxoma can occur as an isolated entity {485,2208}.

Etiology

Osteochondromyxoma is part of the Carney complex, a genetically heterogeneous syndrome in which the majority of patients carry inactivating mutations in *PRKAR1A*, the gene encoding the type IA regulatory subunit of PKA.

Pathogenesis

Karyotypes were normal {485}. Carney complex is genetically heterogeneous, with two genetic loci: *PRKAR1A* (*CNC1*) at chromosome 17 and *CNC2* at chromosome 2. Most often, inactivating mutations are found in the tumour suppressor gene *PRKAR1A* at chromosome 17. *PRKAR1A* encodes the type IA regulatory subunit of PKA, an important regulator of cAMP signalling. *PRKAR1A* inactivation causes hyperstimulation of PKA, which results in incomplete osteoblastic differentiation when

occurring in osteoblasts {2467}. *Prkar1a* (+/–) mice develop bone tumours with a high frequency {1643,1180,2467}.

Macroscopic appearance

The lesions are circumscribed and unencapsulated and show a lobulated growth pattern with a white and light-yellow gelatinous, cartilaginous, and haemorrhagic gross appearance. Usually there is erosion of the cortex without penetration.

Histopathology

Tumour cells are embedded in an abundant clear and basophilic myxoid matrix in a moderately cellular to hypocellular, loose mesenchyme. The cells form sheets, with or without a poorly or well-defined microlobular or macrolobular pattern. The cells are polygonal, stellate, round, and bipolar in shape; a minority are spindle-shaped. In limited areas, the cells are packed together. The nuclei are medium-sized, pale, and vesicular, with a small nucleolus. They have a uniform and bland appearance. There are occasional mitotic figures. Binucleation is very rare. Chondroblast-like cells and osteoblast-like cells are found. The matrix varies from stringy, clear, and lightly basophilic to gel-like, solid, and cartilage-like. These zones blend with areas of

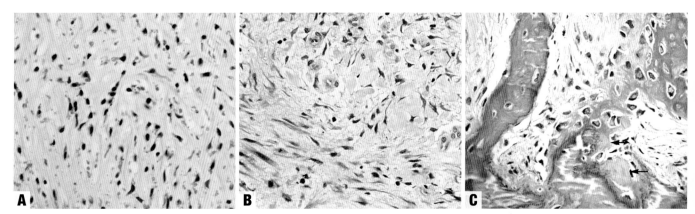

Fig. 3.31 Osteochondromyxoma. **A** Polygonal and bipolar tumour cells in a barely perceptible, weakly basophilic matrix. Nuclei are hyperchromatic as a result of decalcification. **B** Spindle cells and polygonal cells in a loose matrix with round eosinophilic hyaline areas. **C** Osteoid formation present in an area of polygonal cells with lightly eosinophilic cytoplasm. The nuclei are round and regular, with occasional lobulation and grooving (arrows).

mature cartilage, where well-outlined round cells occupy evenly disposed spaces. Acidophilic hyaline fibrous nodules and bands may be present, which can coalesce, trap cells, become calcified, and form osteoid and bone. Some of the mature bony trabeculae are bordered by plump osteoblasts. The cells are PAS-positive, diastase sensitive. Colloidal iron staining is positive.

Immunohistochemistry
Tumour cells are occasionally S100-positive.

Cytology
Not clinically relevant

Diagnostic molecular pathology
Not clinically relevant

Essential and desirable diagnostic criteria
Essential: variably cellular chondroid and osteoid matrix-producing tumour with extensive myxoid changes; patient has other symptoms of Carney complex.

Staging
Not clinically relevant

Prognosis and prediction
Complete excision is curative; however, local recurrence is common with incomplete resection {485,1180}. No metastases have been reported.

Synovial chondromatosis

Flanagan AM
Bloem JL
Cates JMM
O'Donnell PG

Definition

Synovial chondromatosis is a locally aggressive neoplasm consisting of multiple hyaline cartilaginous nodules involving the joint space, subsynovial tissue, or tenosynovium (extra-articular subtype). A small subset of cases are malignant.

ICD-O coding

9220/1 Chondromatosis NOS

ICD-11 coding

2E82.Z & XH5BT0 Benign chondrogenic tumours, site unspecified & Chondromatosis NOS

Related terminology

Not recommended: synovial osteochondromatosis; synovial chondrosis; Reichel syndrome; synovial chondrometaplasia.

Subtype(s)

Extra-articular synovial chondromatosis (tenosynovial chondromatosis)

Localization

Most cases involve the large joints, with approximately 60–70% of cases affecting the knee. Any joint can be affected, including the temporomandibular and intervertebral joints. Some cases are entirely extra-articular and termed tenosynovial chondromatosis, typically arising in the hands and feet {1002}.

Clinical features

Signs and symptoms

Symptoms include pain, swelling, and mechanical symptoms (including locking, crepitus, and reduced range of movement) {2264}. Palpable nodules can be detected on examination. Malignant change is associated with persistent and increased pain.

Imaging

Radiographs show a calcified mass in 75–90% of cases {2225}, showing either chondroid mineralization (punctate, ring and arc, so-called feathery calcification) {3300} or ossified nodules, typically of similar size and shape {2225}. The joint space is usually maintained, but pre-existent or resultant osteoarthritis may be present {2225}. Pressure erosion occurs where joint capacity is restricted, for example the hip {2323}. Although CT shows subtle calcification that can be missed on radiographs, approximately one third of patients lack calcifications on CT. Other imaging features common to well-differentiated cartilaginous neoplasms are shown using cross-sectional imaging {2225}. On MRI, the mass may consist of lobulated areas of low signal intensity (calcification and ossification), T2 hyperintensity (cartilage), or fatty signal (mature bone marrow) {2225}. Septal and peripheral enhancement is seen on MRI and CT after contrast administration {2225}. MRI also frequently shows synovial

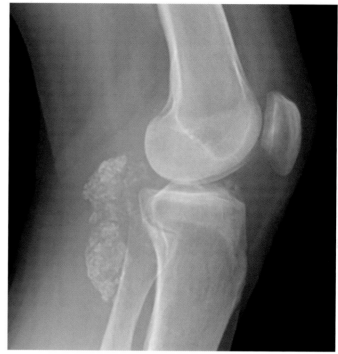

Fig. 3.32 Synovial chondromatosis. Lateral radiograph of the left knee. Lobular mass at the posterior aspect of the knee with extension into the proximal calf. The mass shows diffuse punctate calcification. Small foci of calcification are also visible at the anterior aspect of the knee.

thickening, effusions, and bone erosion. Tenosynovial chondromatosis is suggested by an elongated mineralized mass within a tendon sheath, with otherwise similar imaging appearances to intra-articular chondromatosis and eroding the adjacent bone in as many as 43% of cases {3219}. Tumours with similar imaging appearances can occur at the site of a known bursa {3219}. Multiple osteochondral loose bodies due to severe degenerative joint disease typically vary in shape and size on radiographs, but they may show similar appearances to synovial chondromatosis.

Epidemiology

Synovial chondromatosis is a rare neoplasm, with an estimated incidence of about 1.8 cases per 1 million person-years {2264}. It typically occurs in the third to fifth decades of life and is twice as common in males as in females {745,2264}.

Etiology

Unknown

Pathogenesis

FN1-ACVR2A and *ACVR2A-FN1* fusions, as assessed by FISH, are found in at least 50% of benign synovial chondromatosis, as well as in cases of malignant synovial chondromatosis {3094,

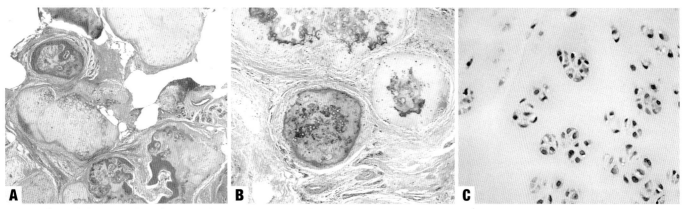

Fig. 3.33 Synovial chondromatosis. **A** Composed of multiple cartilaginous nodules. The lesions are cellular and the maturity of the ossification of the nodules is variable, from osteoid deposition to mature bone. **B** A low-power view showing multiple cartilaginous nodules embedded in synovium. There is peripheral ossification of the nodules. **C** Clustered chondrocytes in a hyaline matrix with little atypia.

92}. It is not clear whether it is the *FN1* or *ACVR2A* altered gene that drives tumour development, because both *FN1-ACVR2A* and *ACVR2A-FN1* are predicted to be in-frame. Both genes have been implicated in the development of other neoplasms {2420,2550,1881}.

Macroscopic appearance

Synovial chondromatosis appears as multiple greyish-white, smooth or irregular, uniform or variably sized nodules, usually in the form of intra-articular loose bodies but sometimes embedded within or attached to synovium.

Histopathology

Nodules consist of hypercellular hyaline cartilage, in which chondrocytes are typically clustered. Nodules are often surrounded by a rim of residual synovial tissue. Calcification and/or endochondral ossification may be seen in longstanding lesions {745}.

Differential diagnosis

Primary synovial chondromatosis must be distinguished from multiple osteochondral loose bodies within the synovium seen in severe degenerative joint disease, as well as from soft tissue

chondromas {92}. Formation of concentric layers of cartilage and a uniform, more orderly distribution of chondrocytes is suggestive of osteochondral loose bodies.

Benign lesions can exhibit atypia, and making a diagnosis of malignancy requires observation of unequivocal substantial nuclear enlargement, pleomorphism, hyperchromasia, and loss of chondrocyte clustering {296}. Permeative infiltration of adjacent cortical or cancellous bone, conspicuous and/or atypical mitotic figures, and merging with a high-grade non-chondroid sarcoma are strong indicators of malignancy {745,3300,2272}.

Cytology

Not clinically relevant

Diagnostic molecular pathology

FISH can be used to detect *FN1-ACVR2A* rearrangements but will not distinguish benign from malignant {237}. *IDH1* and *IDH2* mutations are absent {93,726}.

Essential and desirable diagnostic criteria

Essential: nodular cartilaginous tumour within synovium or loose in joint space; clustering of chondrocytes; minimal atypia and increased cellularity; malignancy is defined by unequivocal nuclear atypia, loss of chondrocyte clustering, bone invasion, conspicuous and/or atypical mitotic figures, or merging with a high-grade non-chondroid sarcoma.

Staging

Not clinically relevant

Prognosis and prediction

The disease recurs in 15–20% of patients, with higher rates reported for tenosynovial cases {2264,1002}. Malignant transformation is uncommon, occurring in 5–10% of cases, usually in large tumours and in longstanding cases after multiple local recurrences over several years {745,950}. However, malignant cases may present de novo. Early and rapid growth of a local recurrence after treatment should raise suspicion for malignancy {2272}.

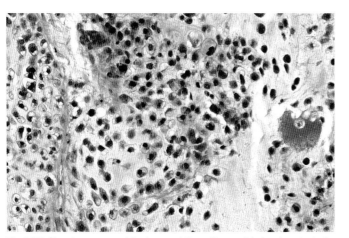

Fig. 3.34 Chondrosarcoma arising in association with synovial chondromatosis. Increased cellularity, loss of organization, nuclear aypia, and increased mitoses suggest chondrosarcoma arising in synovial chondromatosis.

Central atypical cartilaginous tumour / chondrosarcoma, grade 1

Bovée JVMG
Bloem JL
Flanagan AM
Nielsen GP
Yoshida A

Definition

Central atypical cartilaginous tumour / chondrosarcoma, grade 1 (ACT/CS1) is a locally aggressive, hyaline cartilage–producing neoplasm arising in the medulla of bone. Tumours in the appendicular skeleton (long and short tubular bones) are termed ACTs, whereas tumours of the axial skeleton (flat bones, including the pelvis, scapula, and skull base) should be called CS1s. Primary conventional central ACT/CS1s are tumours arising centrally within bone without a benign precursor; secondary conventional central ACT/CS1s are tumours arising centrally in bone in association with a pre-existing enchondroma.

ICD-O coding

9222/1 Atypical cartilaginous tumour
9222/3 Chondrosarcoma, grade 1

ICD-11 coding

2B50.Z & XH0FY0 Chondrosarcoma of bone and articular cartilage of unspecified sites & Atypical cartilaginous tumour / chondrosarcoma, grade 1

Related terminology

Acceptable: low-grade central chondrosarcoma.

Subtype(s)

None

Localization

Central ACT/CS1s arise in bones formed by endochondral ossification. The most common locations are the femur (31% of cases overall: 17% proximal, 2.5% midshaft, and 11% distal), the pelvic bones (22% overall, 18% in the ilium), the humerus (11%), the tibia (8%), and the ribs (6%). The short tubular bones of the hands and feet are rarely involved. Central ACT/CS1 is rare in the spine and the base of the skull.

Clinical features

Signs and symptoms

Patients with central ACT/CS1 can be asymptomatic or can present with pain and/or swelling. Central ACT/CS1 can also be found incidentally. Tumours in the skull base can cause neurological symptoms.

Imaging

Radiographically, ACT is a lytic lesion with geographical destruction, which is ill-defined and usually contains the typical cartilaginous popcorn calcifications. Cortical scalloping without breakthrough is often present. Approximately 50% of central ACTs are located in the metaphysis of long bones, a third in the diaphysis, and the rest in the epiphysis. In the long bones, the radiographic and MRI features of ACT are different from those of grade 2 or 3 chondrosarcoma but overlap with

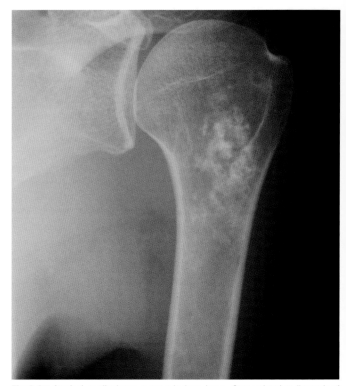

Fig. 3.35 Atypical cartilaginous tumour in long bone. Conventional radiograph of atypical cartilaginous tumour in long bone shows features identical to those of enchondroma, including popcorn-like calcifications.

those of enchondroma, and this distinction can be difficult {992, 685,1130}. As a rule of thumb, cartilaginous tumours in the phalanges are most often enchondromas, whereas cartilaginous tumours in the axial skeleton are probably chondrosarcomas.

Enchondromas are typically < 5 cm long; > 80% of enchondromas in long bones are < 2 cm and are located close to the physis {2957}. Larger tumours with cortical remodelling, deep scalloping, and enhancement seen on dynamic gadolinium chelate–enhanced MRI within 10 seconds of the start of arterial enhancement favour a diagnosis of ACT over enchondroma {2226,1130,444,1128,1131,582,758,844}. Diffusion-weighted MRI and PET-CT do not allow reliable differentiation between enchondroma and ACT {843,2971}. The distinction between central ACT and grade 2 or 3 chondrosarcoma is more clinically relevant and also more reliable. The absence of MRI features of high-grade chondrosarcoma and the presence of trapped fat allow reliable differentiation between ACT/CS1 and grade 2 or 3 chondrosarcoma {3367}.

Epidemiology

The incidence of central ACT/CS1 has increased over the years, from 1.2 cases per 1 million person-years in 1989–1996 to 6.63 cases per 1 million person-years in 2005–2013, which can be explained by ageing and increased use of diagnostic imaging {3167}. The estimated population prevalence of enchondroma and ACT/CS1 is 2.8% {2957}. Conventional central ACT/CS1 is seen mainly in adults in the third to sixth decades of life, with equal sex distribution. Of the central cartilage tumours, 75% are found in patients aged 21–75 years (median: 49 years). Patients with tumours arising in enchondromatosis are generally younger than patients with primary tumours. Central cartilaginous tumours have also been found to occur in association with the development of ER-positive breast cancer at a relatively early age {2351,613}. Central ACT/CS1s (85–90%) are much more common than peripheral ACT/CS1s (10–15%).

Etiology

Patients with enchondromatosis (see *Enchondromatosis*, p. 506), carrying a somatic mosaic mutation in *IDH1* or *IDH2* {96, 2430}, are at increased risk of progression towards central ACT/CS1, depending on the localization of the tumours. Although the overall risk is about 40%, patients with multiple enchondromas in the hands and feet have a risk of only 15%, whereas patients with multiple enchondromas affecting both small and long/flat bones have a risk of 46% {3193}. The risk of developing chondrosarcoma is especially increased when enchondromas are located in the pelvis {3193}.

Pathogenesis

Similar to enchondromas, about 50% of primary central ACT/CS1s and as many as 78% of secondary central ACT/CS1s (in enchondromatosis) harbour somatic mutations in the isocitrate dehydrogenase genes *IDH1* and *IDH2* {93,2430,96}.

Macroscopic appearance

Tissue fragments obtained from curettage are composed of translucent, bluish-grey or greyish-white tissue, usually admixed with red fragments of bone marrow. Yellowish-white chalky areas of calcification are often present. In resection specimens, the tumour is usually sharply demarcated and may demonstrate erosion of the surrounding cortex, which corresponds to the cortical scalloping seen in imaging studies. Soft tissue extension is usually not seen in central ACT/CS1. Extensive sampling is required to rule out areas of dedifferentiation.

Histopathology

Central ACT/CS1 has abundant hyaline cartilage matrix. A lobulated growth pattern is often recognized, and lobules can be irregularly shaped and vary in size. The lobules may be separated by fibrous bands containing small vessels. The lobular growth pattern can cause typical cortical thinning represented in radiographs by cortical scalloping. The typical encasement pattern (deposition of bone surrounding the tumour lobules, a sign of indolent growth as seen in slow-growing enchondromas) is highly uncommon {2155}. Instead, as a sign of more-rapid growth, the tumour lobules usually permeate and entrap the pre-existing lamellar bone trabeculae, although this may be difficult to appreciate in fragmented curettage specimens {2155, 883}. Entrapment is defined as the presence of tumour around three sides of a normal spicule of medullary trabecular bone. The cellularity in central ACT/CS1 is low, but slightly higher than in enchondroma. The nuclei can be small and condensed

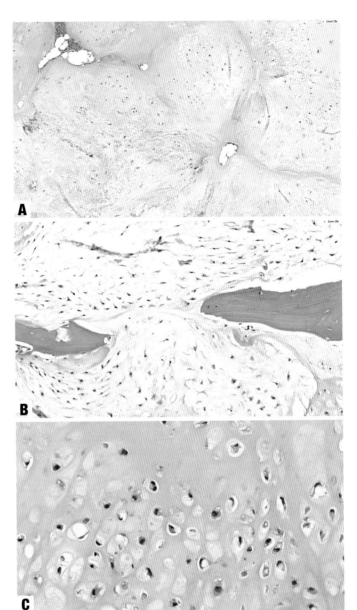

Fig. 3.36 Atypical cartilaginous tumour / chondrosarcoma, grade 1 (ACT/CS1). **A** ACT/CS1 showing a lobular growth pattern, abundance of predominantly hyaline cartilaginous matrix, and low cellularity. **B** ACT/CS1 demonstrating entrapment of pre-existing lamellar host bone, as well as myxoid matrix changes. These two criteria distinguish ACT/CS1 from enchondroma. **C** Tumours show moderate cellularity, with cells embedded in hyaline cartilaginous matrix. Nuclei usually show condensed chromatin. Note the presence of binucleated cells, whereas mitoses are absent.

(lymphocyte-like), although they sometimes have more-open chromatin with a visible nucleolus. The nuclei are generally uniform in size. Binucleation is frequently seen, but mitoses are absent. The surrounding matrix is predominantly hyaline, sometimes with more mucoid or myxoid changes. Necrosis may be present. Areas of a pre-existing enchondroma, with extensive calcifications, may be recognized in central ACT/CS1.

Immunohistochemistry

The tumour cells strongly express S100 and are negative for brachyury. Because the p.Arg132His mutation–specific IDH1 antibody only recognizes a small percentage of the IDH mutations in central ACT/CS1, its usefulness is limited {93,2430,96}.

Differential diagnosis

There is overlap between the histological features of enchondroma and those of central ACT/CS1, and the distinction is made by the higher cellularity, irregular distribution of the cells, and occurrence of binucleated cells in central ACT/CS1. A very important criterion is the growth pattern, in which the presence of entrapment (of pre-existing lamellar bone) and the absence of encasement are indicative of central ACT/CS1 {2155,883}. The presence of > 20% myxoid changes of the matrix also favours the diagnosis of ACT/CS1 over enchondroma {883}. The distinction can be extremely difficult on small biopsy specimens, and clinicoradiological correlation is essential. When these criteria are used, the localization of the lesion and the age of the patient are important {768}. With regard to localization, if the tumour is located in the medullary cavity of a long tubular bone, then increased cellularity with irregular distribution, more-open chromatin with visible nucleoli, and the presence of binucleated cells are indicative of central ACT/CS1, whereas if the tumour is located in the phalangeal bone, these histological features are accepted in an enchondroma because they are not indicative of more-aggressive behaviour {387}. Similarly, in patients with enchondromatosis and for tumours arising in patients before puberty (before growth plate fusion), increased cellularity, more-open chromatin, and the presence of binucleated cells do not exclude the diagnosis of enchondroma {749}. Thus, a multidisciplinary approach with clinicoradiological correlation is often indispensable. Grade 2 conventional central chondrosarcoma is distinguished from ACT/CS1 on the basis of its increased cellularity, the presence of mitoses, myxoid matrix degeneration, spindle cell changes at the periphery of the lobules, increased vascularization, and increased nuclear pleomorphism.

Cytology

Not clinically relevant

Diagnostic molecular pathology

Hotspot mutations are exclusively found at the *IDH1* p.Arg132 and the *IDH2* p.Arg172 positions; the *IDH1* p.Arg132Cys mutation is the most frequently found mutation. About 50% of primary central ACT/CS1s and as many as 78% of central ACT/

CS1s occurring in enchondromatosis have *IDH1* or *IDH2* mutations {93,2430,96}. Mutations at the *IDH1* p.Arg140 position are extremely rare {1910}. In the rare occurrence in the skull base, the mutation frequency is very high (85.7%), whereas mutations are rare to absent in the laryngeal and tracheal tumours (11.8%) {3032}.

Essential and desirable diagnostic criteria

Essential: location in the medulla of bone; abundance of cartilaginous matrix, often hyaline, sometimes with myxoid changes; lobular growth pattern with entrapment of pre-existing lamellar bone trabeculae; increased cellularity, with small condensed nuclei; binucleated cells are common; absence of mitoses, severe nuclear atypia, and encasement.

Staging

Staging is according to bone sarcoma protocols (see *TNM staging of tumours of bone*, p. 339). See also the information on staging in *Bone tumours: Introduction* (p. 340).

Prognosis and prediction

Central ACT/CS1 has a locally aggressive behaviour. Local recurrence is seen in 7.5–11% of the cases, compared with 0% in enchondroma {930,436,113}. In about 10% of recurring central ACT/CS1s, progression to a higher grade is seen {420,1701,947}. Reported 5-year overall survival rates for ACT/CS1 are 87–99%, and 10-year overall survival rates are 88–95% {864,113,1161,1079,947,3167}. Patients die from locally recurrent tumours that are sometimes difficult to manage surgically, depending on the location {947,1132}. In the long bones, central ACT is treated with curettage and local adjuvants, giving a good prognosis {1132}. Overall, tumours located in the axial skeleton have a worse outcome {325,1079,3167}. Therefore, CS1s of the pelvis and spine are treated with surgical excision and negative margins. For skull base CS1, the mortality rate is 5%. A large proportion of the mortality of ACT/CS1 is probably caused by intracranial or axial tumours that are difficult to treat because of their location. Therefore, the location determines whether to diagnose ACT (in the appendicular skeleton) or CS1 (in the axial skeleton and pelvis), to better reflect outcome {768}. It is at present unclear whether the presence of an IDH mutation is associated with prognosis {93,1910,2430,618}.

Secondary peripheral atypical cartilaginous tumour / chondrosarcoma, grade 1

Bovée JVMG
Bloem JL
Flanagan AM
Nielsen GP
Yoshida A

Definition

Secondary peripheral atypical cartilaginous tumour / chondrosarcoma, grade 1 (ACT/CS1) is a locally aggressive, hyaline cartilage–producing neoplasm arising within the cartilaginous cap of a pre-existing osteochondroma. Tumours in the appendicular skeleton can be called peripheral ACTs, whereas tumours of the axial skeleton (including the pelvis, scapula, and skull base) can be called peripheral CS1s.

ICD-O coding

9222/1 Atypical cartilaginous tumour
9222/3 Chondrosarcoma, grade 1

ICD-11 coding

2B50.Z & XH0FY0 Chondrosarcoma of bone and articular cartilage of unspecified sites & Atypical cartilaginous tumour / chondrosarcoma, grade 1

Related terminology

Acceptable: low-grade peripheral chondrosarcoma.

Subtype(s)

None

Localization

Localization in the flat bones (CS1) includes the ilium (19%), followed by the scapula (15%), pubic bone (10%), and ribs (10%). In the appendicular skeleton (ACT), the tibia (12%) and femur (11%) are most often affected.

Clinical features

Signs and symptoms

Patients usually present with a longstanding mass with recent rapid enlargement or pain {45}. Tumour growth after puberty and pain should raise suspicion for malignant progression.

Imaging

The radiological features of secondary peripheral ACT/CS1 largely overlap with those of osteochondroma. MRI is the best-validated method to detect ACT/CS1 arising in an osteochondroma. In the literature, 1.5 and 2 cm cut-off points for cartilage cap thickness are used to indicate the presence of ACT/CS1 {2220,279}. The use of a 2 cm cut-off point seems the best: 18% of osteochondromas have a cap > 1 cm and 7% have a cap > 1.5 cm, whereas a cap of > 2 cm is extremely rare for osteochondroma (seen in < 1.5% of cases), and none of the chondrosarcomas have a cap < 2 cm {279}. The 2 cm cut-off point has a sensitivity of 100%, specificity of 98%, positive predictive value of 96%, and negative predictive value of 100% {279}.

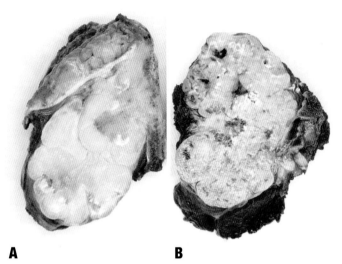

A **B**

Fig. 3.37 Secondary peripheral atypical cartilaginous tumour / chondrosarcoma, grade 1 (ACT/CS1), two resection specimens. **A** Secondary peripheral ACT/CS1 arising juxtaposed to a pre-existing osteochondroma. The size of the cartilaginous cap, which should be measured perpendicular to the tidemark, exceeds 2 cm. **B** Large secondary peripheral ACT/CS1. Note the remnants of the stalk on the right, as well as the abundant nodular proliferation of cartilage, with areas of calcification.

Epidemiology

Progression towards secondary peripheral ACT/CS1 occurs predominantly in patients aged 20–40 years (in 75.2%), and 56.2% of cases occur at the pelvis and proximal femur {980}. Thus, patients with secondary peripheral chondrosarcoma are 1–2 decades younger than those with primary chondrosarcoma {45}. After progression in osteochondroma, > 90% of these neoplasms are ACT/CS1, whereas only 9% are grade 2 or 3 {45}.

Etiology

Patients with multiple osteochondromas, carrying germline mutations in *EXT1* or *EXT2*, are at increased risk of developing ACT/CS1 within the cartilaginous cap of an osteochondroma (see *Multiple osteochondromas*, p. 517). The risk is estimated to be as high as about 5% for patients with multiple osteochondromas, compared with about 1% for those with solitary osteochondromas {3285,1823,2767,980}.

Pathogenesis

Unlike in secondary peripheral chondrosarcoma's precursor osteochondroma, in which *EXT1* or *EXT2* is biallelically inactivated in at least a subset of the tumour cells {381,1545,278,2593, 3411,1285}, upon progression the cartilaginous cap of secondary peripheral chondrosarcoma becomes gradually populated by cells that retain at least one functional copy of *EXT1* or *EXT2* {751,2229}. In secondary peripheral ACT/CS1, the proportion of *EXT1*- or *EXT2*-mutated alleles among all EXT alleles is about 40%, showing that EXT-mutant alleles and EXT-wildtype alleles coexist {3094}. This suggests that the wildtype cells in osteochondroma are prone to undergoing progression, and that (genetic) factors other than *EXT1* or *EXT2* mutations are also involved. These other factors probably involve mutations in cell-cycle regulatory genes such as *CDKN2A* {754}.

Macroscopic appearance
Secondary peripheral ACT/CS1s show a thick (> 2 cm), lobulated cartilaginous cap (mean cap thickness: 3.9 cm) {45}. Careful gross macroscopic documentation of the thickness of the cartilaginous cap is crucial, and the cap should be measured perpendicular to the bone–cartilage interface, at its thickest portion, because the thickness is one of the most important determinants for progression in an osteochondroma {749}.

Histopathology
There are no generally accepted histological criteria that indicate progression from osteochondroma towards secondary peripheral ACT/CS1 {749}. Coarse and irregular calcifications are usually prominent, and evidence of a pre-existing osteochondroma can often be seen. A lobular pattern is common, and sometimes nodules are separated from the main mass lying in the surrounding soft tissue {45}. Binucleated cells, cystic changes (areas of cystic spaces containing mucoid material), and necrosis can be seen within the cartilaginous cap and should not be interpreted as evidence of progression, because these features can also be seen in osteochondroma {749}. Increased vascularization can also be seen {753}. Correlation between clinical and radiological features combined with the thickness of the cartilaginous cap is crucial to establish a diagnosis of secondary peripheral ACT/CS1 {749}. Mitoses and nuclear pleomorphism are absent. Invasion in the stalk is rare and indicative of progression.

Immunohistochemistry
The tumour cells strongly express S100.

Differential diagnosis
The distinction between osteochondroma and secondary peripheral ACT/CS1 solely based on the morphology is not possible. It has been shown that cystic degeneration, nodularity, or necrosis does not indicate progression {749}. The distinction should be made in a multidisciplinary setting in which the thickness of the cartilaginous cap is most important. In grade 2 and 3 secondary peripheral chondrosarcoma, mitoses and nuclear pleomorphism are seen, both of which should be absent in secondary peripheral ACT/CS1.

Cytology
Not clinically relevant

Diagnostic molecular pathology
Not clinically relevant

Essential and desirable diagnostic criteria
Essential: location at the surface of the bone; presence of a pre-existing osteochondroma; size of the cartilaginous cap exceeds 2 cm, measured perpendicular to the bone–cartilage interface; absence of nuclear pleomorphism and mitoses.

Staging
Staging is according to bone sarcoma protocols (see *TNM staging of tumours of bone*, p. 339). See also the information on staging in *Bone tumours: Introduction* (p. 340).

Prognosis and prediction
The clinical course can be variable and is dependent on localization and operability. The 5-year and 10-year local recurrence rates for secondary peripheral chondrosarcoma are 15.9% and 17.5%, respectively, and the 5-year and 10-year mortality rates are 1.6% and 4.8% {45}. Local recurrences can occur and are usually related to incomplete excision in difficult locations. In the pelvis, peripheral CS1 can become very large and thereby difficult to excise completely, eventually becoming inoperable and fatal in some cases {1132,45}.

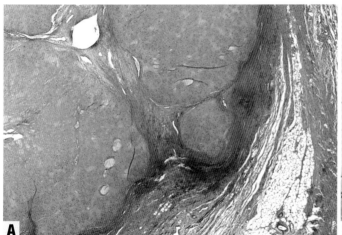
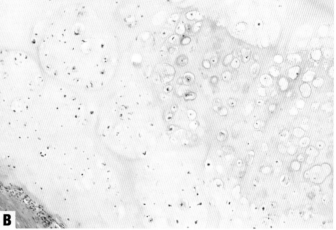

Fig. 3.38 Secondary peripheral atypical cartilaginous tumour / chondrosarcoma, grade 1 (ACT/CS1). **A** A lobular hyaline cartilaginous tumour is seen with nodular extension into the surrounding soft tissues. **B** Tumours show moderate cellularity and an abundance of hyaline cartilaginous matrix. Areas of hypertrophic differentiation and calcification (right) can be seen.

Central chondrosarcoma, grades 2 and 3

Bovée JVMG
Bloem JL
Flanagan AM
Nielsen GP
Yoshida A

Definition
Grade 2 and 3 central chondrosarcomas are central (intramedullary), intermediate-grade (grade 2) and high-grade (grade 3) malignant cartilaginous matrix-producing neoplasms.

ICD-O coding
9220/3 Chondrosarcoma, grade 2
9220/3 Chondrosarcoma, grade 3

ICD-11 coding
2B50.Z & XH6LT5 Chondrosarcoma of bone and articular cartilage of unspecified sites & Chondrosarcoma, grade 2
2B50.Z & XH0Y34 Chondrosarcoma of bone and articular cartilage of unspecified sites & Chondrosarcoma, grade 3

Related terminology
None

Subtype(s)
None

Localization
The localization is similar to that of central atypical cartilaginous tumour / chondrosarcoma, grade 1 (ACT/CS1), and all parts of the skeleton arising from endochondral ossification can be affected: the long tubular bones (especially proximal femur, proximal humerus, and distal femur), the flat bones (especially pelvis [most frequently the ilium] and ribs), and occasionally the spine or base of the skull.

Clinical features
Signs and symptoms
Patients present with pain and/or swelling. Occasionally the lesion is found as a consequence of a pathological fracture. Especially when arising in the pelvis, but also in the ribs, chondrosarcomas can grow to a large size before becoming symptomatic.

Imaging
In long bones and pelvis, these tumours are normally > 5 cm and show large osteolytic areas on radiographs, with moth-eaten or permeative bone destruction, and often cortical destruction and soft tissue extension. MRI is the method of choice to show areas similar to that of ACT/CS1, as well as features of intermediate- to high-grade chondrosarcoma. Features include abundant (> 50%) mucoid areas with high signal intensity on fluid-sensitive MRI sequences and an osteolytic appearance on CT and radiographs, cortical thickening (also well seen on radiographs and CT), bone expansion with cortical thinning, cortical destruction, soft tissue extension, perilesional inflammatory reaction in bone and soft tissue, and periostitis {3367,844}. On PET-CT, there is a significant difference

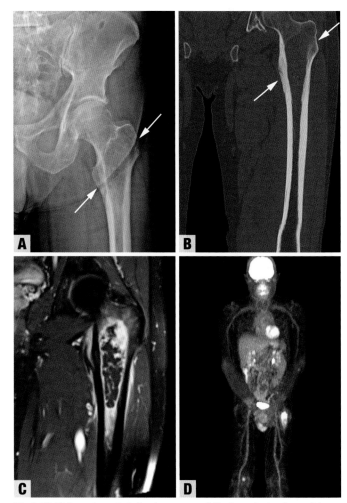

Fig. 3.39 High-grade central chondrosarcoma. **A** Radiograph showing mainly osteolytic, ill-defined lesion in the proximal femur (arrows). There are small calcifications centrally. **B** Coronal reconstruction of CT showing an osteolytic, ill-defined lesion in the proximal femur (arrows). Tunnelling is depicted in the cortex at the minor trochanter. **C** Coronal gadolinium chelate–enhanced fat-suppressed MRI. Centrally septonodular enhancement typical for cartilaginous tumour is seen. Apart from size (> 5 cm), there are several features indicating the presence of high-grade chondrosarcoma rather than atypical cartilaginous tumour. In the periphery, enhancement is more homogeneous. Peripheral to the tumour, intraosseous and extraosseous ill-defined reactive changes are enhancing. Also, high signal in cortical bone medially and circumferential periostitis are visualized. **D** Whole-body maximum intensity projection of FDG PET shows markedly increased FDG uptake in the lesion, consistent with high-grade sarcoma and not atypical cartilaginous tumour.

in the FDG uptake of grade 2 or 3 chondrosarcoma (with a maximum standardized uptake value of > 4.4 with specificity of 99%) versus that of enchondroma and ACT (with a standardized uptake value of < 2); however, 46% of tumours are in the indeterminate range, with standardized uptake values of 2–4.5 {1802}.

Chapter 3

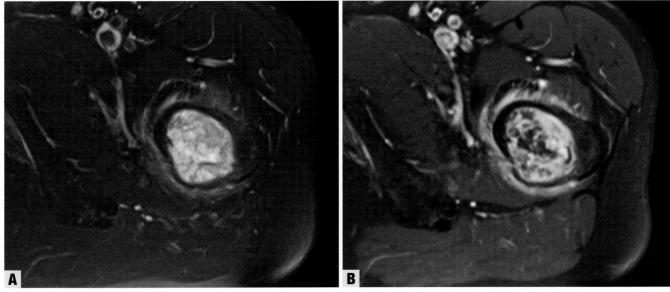

Fig. 3.40 High-grade central chondrosarcoma. **A** Axial T2-weighted fat-suppressed image shows the cortical involvement and the periosteal and soft tissue reactive changes as high signal intensity. The intraosseous tumour component has an inhomogeneous mainly high signal intensity, consistent with mucoid areas (non-enhancing on gadolinium chelate images) and cellular areas (enhancing on gadolinium chelate images). **B** Axial gadolinium chelate–enhanced fat-suppressed MRI. Centrally septonodular enhancement typical for cartilaginous tumour is seen. Apart from size (> 5 cm), there are several features indicating the presence of high-grade chondrosarcoma rather than atypical cartilaginous tumour. In the periphery, enhancement is more homogeneous. Peripheral to the tumour, intraosseous and extraosseous ill-defined reactive changes are enhancing. High signal in cortical bone medially and circumferential periostitis are also visualized.

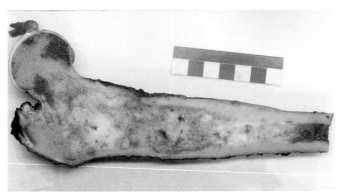

Fig. 3.41 High-grade central chondrosarcoma. This tumour involves the proximal femur. Note the haemorrhagic and necrotic areas, and the cortical scalloping.

Epidemiology

The incidence of grade 2 and 3 central chondrosarcoma was 0.95 cases per 1 million person-years in 1989–1996 and 1.81 cases per 1 million person-years in 2005–2013 {3167}. Adults in the third to sixth decades of life are predominantly affected, with an equal sex distribution. Patients with central chondrosarcoma in enchondromatosis are generally younger than patients with primary chondrosarcoma. In patients with enchondromatosis, the overall risk of developing chondrosarcoma is about 40%, which is less when enchondromas are confined to the hands and feet, and increases when the long bones or bones of the pelvis are also involved {3193}.

Etiology

Patients with enchondromatosis, carrying a somatic mosaic mutation in *IDH1* or *IDH2* {93,96,2430}, are at increased risk of progression towards chondrosarcoma, depending on the localization of the tumours (see *Enchondromatosis*, p. 506).

Pathogenesis

About half of these tumours carry *IDH1* or *IDH2* mutations, suggesting that they have progressed from enchondroma and ACT/CS1. Grade 2 and 3 central chondrosarcomas are characterized by aneuploidy and complex karyotypes {410,1963,3033}. Polyploidization of an initially hyperhaploid/hypodiploid cell population is a common mechanism of progression in a subset {1280,2382}. Alterations in the p53 and RB1 signalling pathways are involved in tumour progression; the RB1 pathway is affected in 86% of high-grade chondrosarcomas {2782,3148}, including by loss of p16 and overexpression and/or amplification of *CDK4* {179,2782,2401,3051}. *TP53* is mutated in 20–49% of the cases, whereas mutations in *CDKN2A* (encoding p16) are infrequent {179,378,1910}. For central chondrosarcoma, several active signalling pathways have been identified {384,2920}, which might provide novel treatment options, such as hedgehog signalling {386,2676,3074,1284}, mTOR signalling {17}, SRC and AKT {2781}, and metabolic pathways {350,2677,2500,2501}. Members of the BCL2 family seem to play an important role in the chemoresistance of chondrosarcoma {3165,759}.

Mutations in the *COL2A1* gene were found in about 45% of central chondrosarcomas {3051,3094}. The *COL2A1* gene encodes the alpha chain of type II collagen fibres, which are a major component of the cartilaginous matrix. *CDKN2A* copy-number variation occurs in about 75% of high-grade central chondrosarcomas and not in enchondroma or central ACT/CS1 {99}. Additional recurrent mutations involve *YEATS2* (12.3%), *EGFR* (19%), *NRAS* (p.Gln61Lys and p.Gln61His; up to 12%), and IHH signalling (18%) {3051,3094,3398,1910}.

Macroscopic appearance

Resection specimens reveal a translucent, often lobular, bluish-grey or white cut surface. Cystic changes can be seen, as well as areas of myxoid material. Calcification can be visible as yellowish-white chalky areas. Erosion and destruction of the cortex with soft tissue extension are frequently present. Extensive sampling is needed to rule out areas of dedifferentiation and chondroblastic osteosarcoma.

Histopathology

The tumours are cellular with an overall lobular configuration in which the tumour lobules permeate and entrap the pre-existing bone trabeculae {2155}. The tumour cells are embedded within the cartilaginous matrix, which can still be hyaline but most often shows myxoid changes to a variable extent. The cellularity is higher than in ACT/CS1 and mitoses are present. The nuclei can still be small and condensed, and severe condensation of the nuclei may hamper the detection of mitoses. More often the nuclei vary in size, with open chromatin and a visible nucleolus. Nuclear atypia can be present but is usually not severe. Binucleation can be seen and necrosis can be present. In grade 3 chondrosarcomas, mitoses are more easily found, and the cells at the periphery of the mostly myxoid, highly cellular tumour lobules are spindled and less differentiated. These spindled cells gradually merge with the fibrous cells in the fibrous septations surrounding the lobules that contain numerous small vascular channels and immune cells. The tumours often destroy and grow through the cortex.

Immunohistochemistry

Tumours can be positive for S100 {2853} and are negative for brachyury {3210}. The p.Arg132His mutation–specific IDH1 antibody only recognizes a small percentage of the IDH mutations in chondrosarcoma, and its usefulness is therefore limited {93,2430,96}.

Grading

The tumour must be graded on the areas demonstrating the highest grade. It should be noted that histological grading is subject to interobserver variability {883,2886}. Histological grading does not appear to be useful for central chondrosarcomas located in the phalanx {387}. Grade 2 chondrosarcoma is separated from ACT/CS1 predominantly on the basis of its increased cellularity, a greater degree of nuclear atypia,

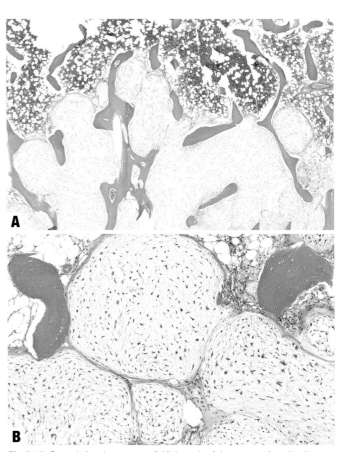

Fig. 3.42 Central chondrosarcoma. **A** High-grade. A low-power view showing permeative growth pattern, in which the pre-existing bone trabeculae are entrapped by the tumour, filling the marrow cavities. **B** Grade 2. This low-power view demonstrates the typical lobular growth pattern. There are extensive myxoid matrix changes.

hyperchromasia, nuclear size, myxoid matrix changes, and the presence of mitoses. Grade 3 chondrosarcoma is highly cellular and more pleomorphic, mitoses are more easily found, and the cells at the periphery of the mostly myxoid tumour lobules are spindled and less differentiated.

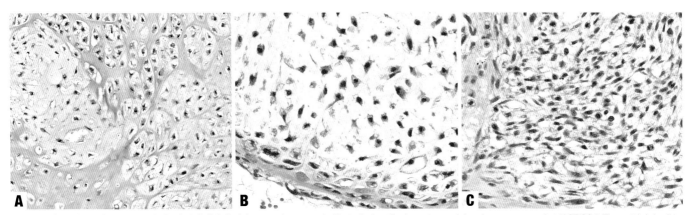

Fig. 3.43 Central chondrosarcoma. **A** Grade 2. Cellularity is increased compared with atypical cartilaginous tumour / chondrosarcoma, grade 1 (ACT/CS1). The matrix is hyaline, with focal myxoid changes. **B** Grade 2. This high-power view shows extensive myxoid matrix, increased cellularity, and more nuclear atypia compared with ACT/CS1. **C** Grade 3. High cellularity, myxoid matrix changes, and spindle cell changes. Mitoses are easily seen.

Differential diagnosis

Chondrosarcoma in the skull base should be distinguished from chordoma, including the chondroid subtype. Grade 3 chondrosarcoma can resemble chondroblastic osteosarcoma.

Cytology

Not clinically relevant

Diagnostic molecular pathology

Molecular analysis is not needed for diagnosis in most cases. Detection of mutations in the isocitrate dehydrogenase genes *IDH1* and *IDH2* may be helpful in distinguishing these tumours from chondroblastic osteosarcoma {93}.

Essential and desirable diagnostic criteria

Essential: origin in the medulla of the bone; lobulated cartilaginous tumour with entrapment of pre-existing host bone; increased cellularity, myxoid matrix, and presence of mitoses; absence of osteoid deposition associated with malignant cells.

Staging

Staging is according to bone sarcoma protocols (see *TNM staging of tumours of bone*, p. 339). See also the information on staging in *Bone tumours: Introduction* (p. 340).

Prognosis and prediction

Patients are usually treated with en bloc resection to obtain negative margins {1132}. The reported 5-year overall survival rate for grade 2 chondrosarcoma is 74–99% and for grade 3 tumours 31–77% {113,1161,1079,947,3167,864,2328}. The 10-year overall survival rate for grade 2 is 58–86% and for grade 3 tumours 26–55%. Even after 10 years, deaths due to disease can still occur {864}. Local recurrence rates are 19% for grade 2 and 26% for grade 3 chondrosarcoma {113}; 10–30% of the grade 2 tumours and 32–71% of the grade 3 tumours metastasize {113, 1079,947,334}. Chondrosarcomas with axial localization have a significantly lower survival than extremity chondrosarcoma {864,325,1079,3167}. It is unclear at present whether the IDH mutation is associated with outcome {1910,2430,618}.

Secondary peripheral chondrosarcoma, grades 2 and 3

Bovée JVMG
Bloem JL
Flanagan AM
Nielsen GP
Yoshida A

Definition

Grade 2 and 3 secondary peripheral chondrosarcomas are intermediate-grade to high-grade malignant cartilaginous matrix–producing neoplasms originating at the surface of the bone in a pre-existing osteochondroma.

ICD-O coding

9220/3 Chondrosarcoma, grade 2
9220/3 Chondrosarcoma, grade 3

ICD-11 coding

2B50.Z & XH6LT5 Chondrosarcoma of bone and articular cartilage of unspecified sites & Chondrosarcoma, grade 2
2B50.Z & XH0Y34 Chondrosarcoma of bone and articular cartilage of unspecified sites & Chondrosarcoma, grade 3

Related terminology

Not recommended: chondrosarcoma secondary to osteochondroma.

Subtype(s)

None

Localization

These tumours most commonly arise in osteochondromas of the pelvis, trunk, and proximal femur {45}.

Clinical features

Signs and symptoms

Enlargement or pain in a longstanding mass, especially after puberty, should raise suspicion for malignancy {45}. Neurological symptoms and limited joint motion can be present.

Imaging

Because grade 2 and 3 peripheral chondrosarcomas are very rare compared with peripheral atypical cartilaginous tumour / chondrosarcoma, grade 1 (ACT/CS1), no specific radiological criteria have been validated. Radiological features in the adult population that favour the presence of a higher-grade peripheral chondrosarcoma are solid enhancing areas, mucoid degeneration, irregular ossification, and cartilaginous cap thickness largely exceeding 2 cm.

Epidemiology

Grade 2 or 3 secondary peripheral chondrosarcomas are very rare (accounting for only ~9% of chondrosarcomas arising in osteochondroma) {45} and arise mainly in patients aged 20–40 years {980}.

Etiology

Patients with the multiple osteochondromas syndrome are at increased risk (~5%) of developing secondary peripheral chondrosarcoma within an osteochondroma {3285,1823,2767,980}. See *Multiple osteochondromas* (p. 517).

Pathogenesis

Whereas in secondary peripheral ACT/CS1, EXT-mutant cells and EXT-wildtype cells coexist, in high-grade secondary peripheral chondrosarcoma, the EXT-wildtype cells predominate {751}. Similar to grade 2 and 3 central chondrosarcoma, these chondrosarcomas display chromosomal instability and a complex karyotype that increases with increasing histological grade {378,1280}, probably caused by alterations in the p53 and RB1 pathways {1280,754,3051}.

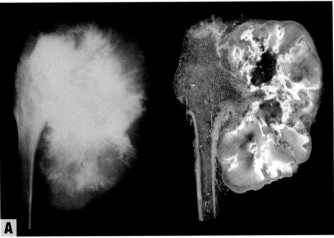
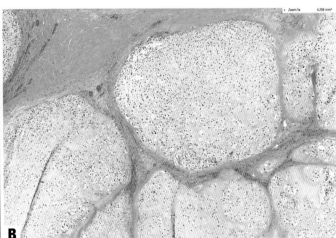

Fig. 3.44 Secondary peripheral chondrosarcoma arising in a patient with multiple osteochondromas. **A** Conventional radiograph (**left**) and surgical specimen (**right**) of the right proximal fibula. Note the thickness of the cartilaginous cap (> 2 cm), flaring of the cortex (macro), and indistinct margins with irregular mineralization (radiograph). **B** Discrete peripheral nodules of cartilage are embedded in the soft tissue at the periphery of the lesion. These features explain the irregular margins and the possibility of local recurrence when the lesion is resected with inadequate surgical margins.

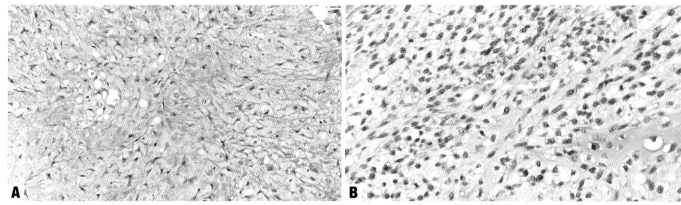

Fig. 3.45 Secondary peripheral chondrosarcoma. **A** Grade 2 chondrosarcoma with increased cellularity and myxoid matrix changes. **B** Grade 3 chondrosarcoma with increased cellularity, myxoid matrix changes, and spindled cells. Mitoses are easily found.

Macroscopic appearance

These lesions are translucent lobular bluish-white tumours in which there may be areas with myxoid material and cystic changes. The stalk of the pre-existing osteochondroma might still be recognized; the cap size exceeds 2 cm.

Histopathology

Grade 2 and 3 secondary peripheral chondrosarcomas are lobular cartilaginous matrix–producing tumours that are morphologically identical to grade 2 and 3 central chondrosarcomas. Sometimes areas of endochondral ossification suggestive of pre-existing osteochondroma can be seen. Nuclear pleomorphism and mitoses are often easily seen. At the periphery of the neoplastic cartilaginous lobules, spindle cell changes may occur. Coarse and irregular calcification, binucleated cells, cystic change, and necrosis can be observed.

Immunohistochemistry

These tumours can be positive for S100 {2853}.

Grading

Criteria for histological grading are identical to those for grade 2 and 3 central chondrosarcoma {947}.

Differential diagnosis

Periosteal osteosarcoma is included in the differential diagnosis. Peripheral chondrosarcoma is separated from central chondrosarcoma based on its location at the surface of the bone.

Cytology

Not clinically relevant

Diagnostic molecular pathology

Molecular analysis is rarely needed for diagnosis. Mutations in *IDH1*, *IDH2*, and *NRAS* are absent {93,2430,3398}.

Essential and desirable diagnostic criteria

Essential: chondrosarcoma arising in a pre-existing osteochondroma or with evidence of the stalk of a precursor osteochondroma; cartilage cap exceeds 2 cm; mitoses and nuclear pleomorphism are present.

Staging

Staging is according to bone sarcoma protocols (see *TNM staging of tumours of bone*, p. 339). See also the information on staging in *Bone tumours: Introduction* (p. 340).

Prognosis and prediction

Local recurrences can occur, generally related to incomplete excision. The majority of patients who die of their disease have local recurrence {45}.

Periosteal chondrosarcoma

Cleven AHG
Bloem JL
Tirabosco R

Definition

Periosteal chondrosarcoma is a malignant cartilaginous neoplasm that occurs on the surface of bone in close association with the periosteum and invades the underlying cortex or is > 5 cm.

ICD-O coding

9221/3 Periosteal chondrosarcoma

ICD-11 coding

2B50.Z & XH1S32 Chondrosarcoma of bone and articular cartilage of unspecified sites & Periosteal chondrosarcoma

Related terminology

Not recommended: juxtacortical chondrosarcoma.

Subtype(s)

None

Localization

Periosteal chondrosarcoma predominantly affects the metaphysis of long tubular bones, most commonly the distal femur, followed by the humerus {1172}.

Clinical features

Signs and symptoms

Patients with periosteal chondrosarcoma frequently present with pain, with or without swelling or limitation of movement {1172}.

Imaging

Periosteal chondrosarcoma is usually located in the metaphysis, and it often shows a large lobulated mass (> 5 cm) located on the cortex {528,1172,2314}. The cortex may be thickened or thinned, but bone marrow involvement is rare. A calcified shell may be seen.

Epidemiology

Periosteal chondrosarcoma is a rare chondrosarcoma subtype, representing about 2.5% of all chondrosarcomas {2509}. Periosteal chondrosarcoma has a peak incidence in the third decade of life, with a wide age range (9–79 years) and a male predominance {616}.

Etiology

Unknown

Pathogenesis

A subset of periosteal chondrosarcomas bear the same *IDH1* and *IDH2* mutations as enchondroma and conventional central chondrosarcoma {93,616,2430}.

Macroscopic appearance

A large (often > 5 cm) lobulated mass is located on the surface of the bone {2314}. On cut section, the tumour is grey and glistening and is often associated with gritty white areas of calcification. The tumour erodes or invades the cortex; the medullary canal is usually not involved.

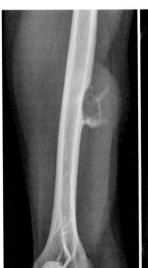
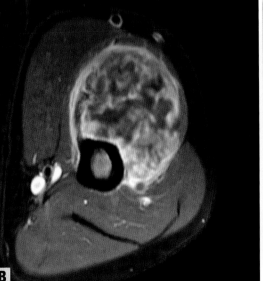
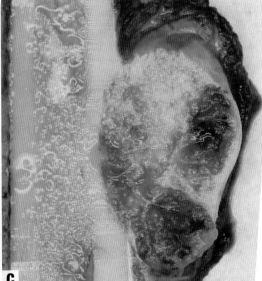

Fig. 3.46 Periosteal chondrosarcoma. **A** Conventional radiograph of the left humerus, with a periosteal tumour extending into the soft tissue. **B** Axial T1-weighted MRI (with fat suppression after intravenous contrast administration) showing a periosteal tumour (diameter: 5.5 cm) with septonodular enhancement typical for a cartilaginous tumour. **C** Gross features of the same periosteal chondrosarcoma show a large lobulated cartilaginous tumour (diameter: 5.5 cm) at the surface of bone, with growth into the cortex.

Histopathology

A lobular, moderately cellular cartilaginous tumour is seen with myxoid matrix. Calcification and endochondral ossification can be present {528,2314,616}. Osteoid or bone directly formed by the tumour cells is absent, although formation of metaplastic bone at the periphery of the cartilage lobules and the tumour (formation of a so-called neocortex) can be found {528,2314, 616}. The features resemble those of atypical cartilaginous tumour / chondrosarcoma, grade 1 (ACT/CS1) or grade 2 central chondrosarcoma {528,2314,616}. There is often invasion of the underlying cortex. Intramedullary extension and subsequent host bone entrapment are seen in a subset of cases. Demarcation with the soft tissue is usually sharp {528,2314, 616}.

Differential diagnosis

The differential diagnosis also includes periosteal chondroma, periosteal osteosarcoma, and parosteal osteosarcoma. The distinction between periosteal chondroma and chondrosarcoma is based on cortical invasion. In periosteal chondrosarcoma, the tumour is often > 5 cm {528,2314,616,1453}.

Grading

Histological grading is not applicable {616}.

Cytology

Not clinically relevant

Diagnostic molecular pathology

Although *IDH1* and *IDH2* mutations are found in a subset of periosteal chondrosarcomas {93,616,2430}, mutation analysis is rarely used in the diagnostic work-up for periosteal chondrosarcoma. It might be used to distinguish periosteal chondrosarcoma and periosteal osteosarcoma, the latter being negative. The EXT1 protein is normally expressed, whereas RB1 signalling can be deregulated by loss of p16 expression, and WNT/β-catenin signalling is lost in the majority of cases. Amplification of *CDK4* or *MDM2* is absent, unlike in parosteal osteosarcoma {616}.

Essential and desirable diagnostic criteria

Essential: cartilaginous tumour arising on the surface of bone in close association with periosteum; invasion of the underlying cortex or size > 5.0 cm.

Staging

The Union for International Cancer Control (UICC) *TNM classification of malignant tumours* {423} does not recommend that the TNM staging system for bone tumours be applied to surface/juxtacortical osteosarcoma or juxtacortical chondrosarcoma. However, other staging systems, such as the American Joint Committee on Cancer (AJCC) TNM system {101}, do include these tumours in the bone staging system. See also the information on staging in *Bone tumours: Introduction* (p. 340).

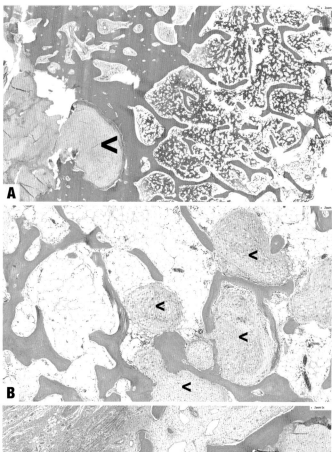

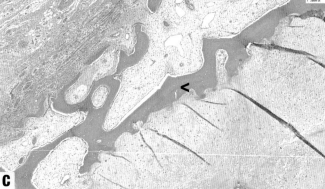

Fig. 3.47 Periosteal chondrosarcoma. **A** Cortical extension (arrowhead) of the cartilaginous tumour. **B** Occasionally, cartilage tumour lobules may be observed in the medullary bone (arrowheads). **C** Formation of metaplastic bone (arrowhead) on the edges of the cartilaginous lobules.

Prognosis and prediction

Periosteal chondrosarcomas have a relatively low metastatic rate (5–12.2%), and metastases especially involve the lungs and rarely the lymph nodes {1172}. Histological grading does not predict outcome {616}.

Clear cell chondrosarcoma

Baumhoer D
Bloem JL
Oda Y

Definition
Clear cell chondrosarcoma is a low-grade malignant cartilaginous epiphyseal neoplasm characterized by lobules of cells with abundant clear cytoplasm.

ICD-O coding
9242/3 Clear cell chondrosarcoma

ICD-11 coding
2B50.Z & XH7XB9 Chondrosarcoma of bone and articular cartilage of unspecified sites & Clear cell chondrosarcoma

Related terminology
None

Subtype(s)
None

Localization
Approximately two thirds of clear cell chondrosarcomas develop in the femoral and humeral head. However, tumours have been reported in most bones of the skeleton, including in the ribs, skull, spine, hands, and feet.

Clinical features
Signs and symptoms
Pain is the most common presenting symptom: 55% of patients experienced pain for > 1 year; 18% had symptoms for > 5 years {335}.

Imaging
Radiographically, clear cell chondrosarcoma presents as a well-defined, purely lytic lesion in the epiphysis of a long bone that may extend into the metaphysis. A sclerotic rim may be present. Some lesions may contain stippled radiodensities, characteristic of cartilage. On MRI, clear cell chondrosarcoma shows a specific low signal intensity on T1-weighted images and moderate or marked high signal on fluid-sensitive images {647}. Clear cell chondrosarcoma and chondroblastoma can be difficult to distinguish radiologically {1562}.

Epidemiology
Clear cell chondrosarcomas account for approximately 2% of all chondrosarcomas {2537}. Men are almost three times as likely to develop clear cell chondrosarcoma as women. The reported age range is 12–84 years {335,1481}, but most patients present in their third to fifth decades of life. Rarely, synchronous tumours have been reported {1967}.

Etiology
Unknown

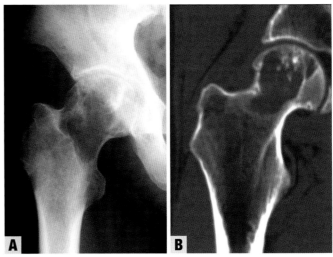

Fig. 3.48 Clear cell chondrosarcoma. **A** Plain radiography shows a well-defined lytic lesion with calcification in the femoral head and neck. **B** Coronal reformatted CT highlights the intramedullary tumour with spotty mineralization.

Pathogenesis
Cytogenetic analyses of small series have revealed clonal abnormalities, with diploid or near-diploid complements predominating and loss or structural aberrations of chromosome 9 and gain of chromosome 20 {2925,2405,1963,2880,2309}. *CDKN2A* alterations appear to be infrequent, although all clear cell chondrosarcomas examined lacked expression of p16 (CDKN2A) {2447,2055}. p53 overexpression is frequently found in the absence of detectable mutations {2448}. Neither *IDH1* nor *IDH2* mutations are present {93,2054}. One of 15 clear cell chondrosarcomas investigated for H3.3 mutations to date has shown an *H3-3B (H3F3B)* p.Lys36Met mutation, a highly specific driver mutation of chondroblastoma, suggesting a pathogenetic relation in at least a small subset of tumours {257}.

Macroscopic appearance
Lesions range from 2 to 13 cm in maximum diameter. They contain soft but gritty material, sometimes with cystic areas. Gross features characteristic of hyaline cartilage can be focal or absent.

Histopathology
The tumours consist of lobules of cells with abundant pale, clear or slightly eosinophilic cytoplasm, which resemble hypertrophic cells of the growth plate {48,380}. The cells have distinct cytoplasmic membranes and large round nuclei with only minor atypia and central nucleoli. Mitotic figures are rare. Further characteristics frequently observed include regularly distributed woven bone formation with intermingled osteoclast-like giant cells. Areas of conventional low-grade chondrosarcoma with minimally atypical nuclei can be observed in about half of

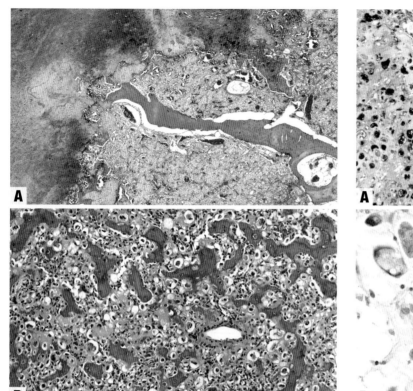

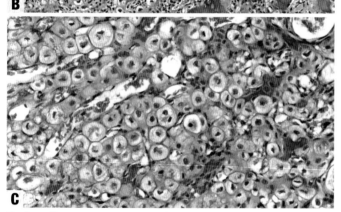

Fig. 3.49 Clear cell chondrosarcoma. **A** Low-power view of the transition to low-grade clear cell chondrosarcomatous areas. **B** Round or polygonal cells with slightly eosinophilic cytoplasm are arranged in lobules and sheets, admixed with trabeculae of woven bone. **C** High-power view of clear cell chondrosarcoma; note the abundant cytoplasm, with the centrally placed nucleus with central nucleolus.

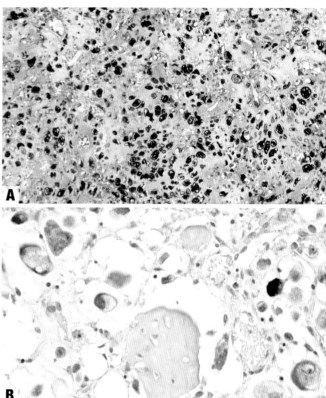

Fig. 3.50 Clear cell chondrosarcoma. **A** Tumour cells stain strongly with antibodies against S100. **B** Tumour cells focally show positivity for pancytokeratin AE1/AE3.

Differential diagnosis
The differential diagnosis includes metastatic clear cell renal cell carcinoma, chondroblastoma, and osteosarcoma, as well as (depending on localization) a notochordal tumour.

Cytology
Not clinically relevant

Diagnostic molecular pathology
Not clinically relevant

Essential and desirable diagnostic criteria
Essential: clear cells with abundant cytoplasm and a centrally placed nucleus; presence of woven bone and osteoclast-like giant cells.
Desirable: epiphyseal location.

Staging
Staging is according to bone sarcoma protocols (see *TNM staging of tumours of bone*, p. 339). See also the information on staging in *Bone tumours: Introduction* (p. 340).

Prognosis and prediction
En bloc resection with clear margins is usually curative. Marginal excision or curettage results in high recurrence rates of up to 86% {2537,335}. Metastases, usually to the lungs and other skeletal sites, develop in 15–20% of cases. The overall mortality rate is 15% {1484}. Dedifferentiation to high-grade sarcoma has been reported in 3 cases {1563}.

cases {3129}. The hyaline cartilage can become calcified and/or ossified, which can be detected radiologically as a cartilage-type pattern of mineralization. Areas of cystic degeneration resembling aneurysmal bone cyst can also occur. Infiltrative growth can be seen.

Immunohistochemistry
Immunohistochemically, the clear cells are strongly positive for S100, as well as for collagen types II and X {48}. They also show occasional immunoreactivity for cytokeratins (AE1/AE3 and CK18) {2016}.

Mesenchymal chondrosarcoma

Fanburg-Smith JC
de Pinieux G
Ladanyi M

Definition
Mesenchymal chondrosarcoma is a high-grade, malignant, biphasic, primitive mesenchymal tumour with a well-differentiated, organized hyaline cartilage component.

ICD-O coding
9240/3 Mesenchymal chondrosarcoma

ICD-11 coding
2B50.Z & XH8X47 Chondrosarcoma of bone and articular cartilage of unspecified sites & Mesenchymal chondrosarcoma

Related terminology
None

Subtype(s)
None

Localization
These tumours have widespread anatomical distribution in bone, soft tissue, and intracranial sites {962}. Intraosseous lesions are mainly in the craniofacial region (50% jaw) {3186, 525}, ribs or chest wall, ilium, vertebrae (sacral/spinal), or lower extremities (especially femur) {962}. Within bone the tumour usually presents in the medulla; location on the bone surface is less common {1711}. Overall, approximately 40% of cases affect the somatic soft tissue {1240}. The meninges are one of the most common extraskeletal sites {962}. Visceral location is unusual and includes the kidney {963,2822,2772,1071,988}.

Clinical features
Signs and symptoms
The cardinal symptoms are pain and swelling {3110}. About 15% of patients present with metastasis {1071}.

Imaging
On radiological imaging, skeletal lesions are primarily lytic and destructive, with poor margins {2226}. Mottled calcification can be prominent. Some have well-defined margins with a sclerotic rim. Expansion of the bone is frequent, and cortical destruction or cortical breakthrough with extraosseous extension into the soft tissue is common. Bone sclerosis, cortical thickening, and superficial involvement of the bone surface may be observed. Imaging features of extraskeletal tumours are also nonspecific, demonstrating chondroid-type calcifications and foci of low signal intensity within enhancing lobules. This tumour takes up contrast medium on CT or MRI.

Epidemiology
Mesenchymal chondrosarcomas account for 2–4% of all chondrosarcomas. The peak incidence is in the second and third decades of life, with a wide age range and a median age of

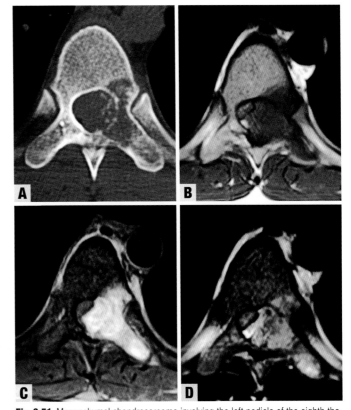

Fig. 3.51 Mesenchymal chondrosarcoma involving the left pedicle of the eighth thoracic vertebra. **A** CT showing an osteolytic and destructive lesion with irregular calcification accompanied by extraosseous extension into the soft tissue in the vertebral foramen and spinal canal. **B** T1-weighted MRI. **C** T1-weighted MRI with gadolinium enhancement. **D** T2-weighted MRI.

30 years {962,963}. There is a minimal male predilection (M:F ratio: 1.3:1) {962,963,1071,2772,3325}.

Etiology
Unknown

Pathogenesis
A highly specific recurrent gene fusion between *HEY1* and *NCOA2* occurs in almost all mesenchymal chondrosarcomas {3231}. Mesenchymal chondrosarcomas are thought to arise from early, immature cartilage cells (chondroblasts), which differentiate into well-differentiated hyaline cartilage and then often undergo endochondral ossification to bone {963}. The cartilage to bone production in this region involves the WNT/β-catenin pathway {963}.

Macroscopic appearance
The tumours are variably grey/white/pink, firm to soft, and usually circumscribed masses, 0.9–30 cm in maximum diameter.

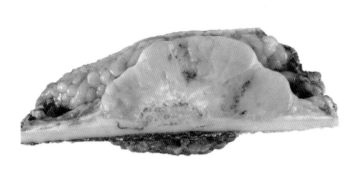

Fig. 3.52 Mesenchymal chondrosarcoma. This gross pathology picture of a bone surface tumour demonstrates a well-delineated and circumscribed tumour with zonal white cartilaginous (closer to bone surface) and tan-pink solid components.

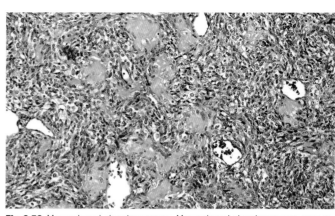

Fig. 3.53 Mesenchymal chondrosarcoma. Mesenchymal chondrosarcoma may uncommonly show spindle cell morphology and eosinophilic matrix resembling osteoid.

Most lesions contain hard mineralized deposits that vary from dispersed foci to prominent areas; often either the cartilaginous component or the sheeted round cell component with necrosis and haemorrhage may predominate {962,963,1450}.

Histopathology

Mesenchymal chondrosarcoma is composed of small to medium-sized, poorly differentiated round cells with a high N:C ratio and a characteristic staghorn or pericytoid vascular pattern, admixed with various proportions of islands of

well-differentiated hyaline cartilage. Spindle cell morphology can be present. In areas, the matrix may mimic osteoid deposition.

Immunohistochemistry

Tumour cells can be positive for S100, CD99, and SOX9 {963}. FLI1 is negative {1795}. Aberrant expression of EMA, desmin, myogenin (MYF4), and MYOD1 may be identified, whereas SMARCB1 (INI1) is retained {962,1053}. SMA, GFAP, and keratins are negative {962}.

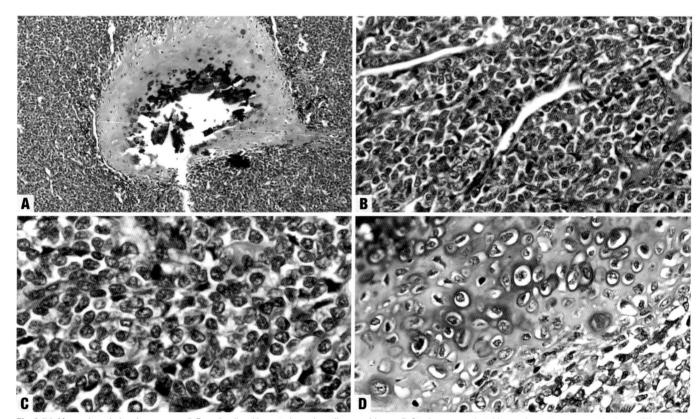

Fig. 3.54 Mesenchymal chondrosarcoma. **A** Round cells with central zonal cartilage and bone. **B** Staghorn or pericytoid vascular pattern present in the undifferentiated area. **C** A round cell tumour of undifferentiated tumour cells, which may be seen in small biopsies. **D** Linear progression from resting chondrocytes to proliferating to hypertrophic to endochondral ossification to bone.

Differential diagnosis

When the undifferentiated component is biopsied alone, there may be confusion with other small cell neoplasms.

Cytology

There is a biphasic appearance of medium-sized cells, oval to spindled in CNS tumours, that have a high N:C ratio and basophilic extracellular matrix {3100,962,963}.

Diagnostic molecular pathology

Mesenchymal chondrosarcoma harbours a recurrent *HEY1-NCOA2* rearrangement {3231}, representing an in-frame fusion of *HEY1* exon 4 to *NCOA2* exon 13 at the mRNA level. This fusion is detected in almost all well-characterized mesenchymal chondrosarcomas tested, and it is absent in other subtypes of chondrosarcomas. Given that *HEY1* and *NCOA2* are only approximately 10 Mb apart on chromosome 8, mapping to 8q21.13 and 8q13.3, respectively, and that both are in the same orientation, this fusion may arise via a small interstitial deletion, del(8)(q13.3q21.1), which is difficult to detect in most conventional cytogenetic preparations. The consistent molecular detection of the *HEY1-NCOA2* fusion in this sarcoma establishes it as a defining molecular diagnostic marker {891}.

A recent study using genome-wide array-based methylation profiling found that mesenchymal chondrosarcomas form a very distinct methylation cluster {1665}. Finally, although > 90% have the highly recurrent *HEY1-NCOA2* fusion, there has been a single case report of a mesenchymal chondrosarcoma bearing an *IRF2BP2-CDX1* fusion gene generated by a t(1;5)(q42;q32) {2337}. Downregulation of the RB1 pathway has been reported {2054}, and *IDH1* and *IDH2* mutations, characteristic of conventional chondrosarcoma, are absent {93,2054}.

Essential and desirable diagnostic criteria

Essential: undifferentiated tumour cells with a high N:C ratio; islands of cartilage.
Desirable: staghorn vascular pattern; *HEY1-NCOA2* fusion.

Staging

Staging is according to bone sarcoma protocols (see *TNM staging of tumours of bone*, p. 339). See also the information on staging in *Bone tumours: Introduction* (p. 340).

Prognosis and prediction

Mesenchymal chondrosarcoma is an aggressive neoplasm, with estimated overall 5-year and 10-year survival rates (which range from study to study) as high as 60% and 40%, respectively. Distant metastases are occasionally observed even after a delay of > 20 years. The clinical course is frequently protracted and relentless, requiring long-term follow-up. There are no histological features correlative with prognosis. The presence of metastatic disease at initial presentation, tumour size, and (to a lesser degree) original site of the tumour, have been demonstrated to have an impact on survival in mesenchymal chondrosarcoma {1071,2772,3325,3110,891}. Children, adolescents, and young adults tend to have a slightly better outcome {1102,962,963}. Craniofacial origin appears to be associated with a more indolent course and favourable prognosis, whereas axial origin has worse outcome. Complete resection combined with chemotherapy should be considered the standard of care {1071,2772,3325,3110,891,2196}.

Dedifferentiated chondrosarcoma

Inwards CY
Bloem JL
Hogendoorn PCW

Definition

Dedifferentiated chondrosarcoma is a high-grade subtype of chondrosarcoma with the bimorphic histological appearance of a conventional chondrosarcoma component with abrupt transition to a high-grade, non-cartilaginous sarcoma.

ICD-O coding

9243/3 Dedifferentiated chondrosarcoma

ICD-11 coding

2B50.Z & XH6E77 Chondrosarcoma of bone and articular cartilage of unspecified sites & Dedifferentiated chondrosarcoma

Related terminology

None

Subtype(s)

None

Localization

The most common sites of involvement are the femur (46%), pelvis (28%), humerus (11%), and scapula (5%) {1224}. In dedifferentiated peripheral chondrosarcoma, the preferred site of involvement follows that of conventional chondrosarcoma, i.e. pelvis, scapula, and ribs {2675,2930}.

Clinical features

Signs and symptoms

The most common clinical presentations include pain and a palpable mass. Pathological fracture is found in about 20% of patients {1224}.

Imaging

Imaging findings are usually indicative of an aggressive, destructive tumour, often with a heterogeneous radiological presentation of both conventional chondrosarcoma (the presence of ring-like densities) and lytic, permeable, destructive areas. Bimorphic features, suggesting dedifferentiation, are seen on CT in approximately 50% of histologically proven cases and on MRI and radiographs in 30%. These features include a dominant lytic area within, or adjacent to, a mineralized tumour on radiographs and a large unmineralized soft tissue mass {1874}. Rarely, dedifferentiation occurs in secondary peripheral chondrosarcoma {2675}. The imaging characteristics of central and peripheral dedifferentiated chondrosarcomas are similar {1347}.

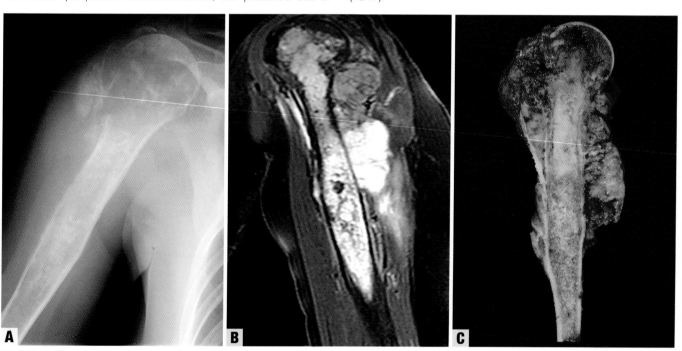

Fig. 3.55 Dedifferentiated chondrosarcoma. Anteroposterior radiograph (**A**) and sagittal fat-suppressed T2-weighted MRI of the humerus (**B**) demonstrate imaging features of a high-grade chondrosarcoma. The radiograph and MRI show, in the intramedullary portion of the mid- and proximal humeral diaphysis, chondroid matrix with homogeneous high signal, associated expansion, cortical permeation, irregular periosteal reaction, and soft tissue reactive oedema or even tumour extension. More proximally, the more aggressive part of the tumour shows an area with more lytic destruction with an associated pathological fracture and an adjacent soft tissue mass containing amorphous osteoid matrix. **C** Corresponding resection specimen of the dedifferentiated chondrosarcoma. The greyish-white hyaline cartilage component fills the medullary cavity, whereas the fleshy, tan and reddish-brown high-grade sarcoma component involves surrounding soft tissue.

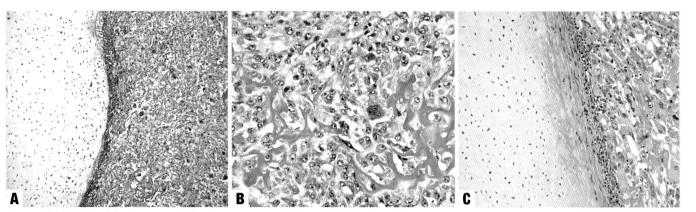

Fig. 3.56 Dedifferentiated chondrosarcoma. **A** There is an abrupt transition between the low-grade chondrosarcoma and high-grade sarcoma components. **B** The high-grade sarcoma in this dedifferentiated chondrosarcoma shows deposition of osteoid. **C** The high-grade sarcoma in this dedifferentiated chondrosarcoma is undifferentiated pleomorphic sarcoma.

Epidemiology

Dedifferentiation develops in 10–15% of central chondrosarcomas {1068,2928}. The median age of patients with dedifferentiated chondrosarcoma is 59 years (range: 15–89 years), and there is a slight male predominance {1224}. On very rare occasions, dedifferentiation of peripheral chondrosarcoma has been reported {2675}, and these patients are slightly younger (average: 46 years; range: 22–74 years) {2930}.

Etiology

Unknown

Pathogenesis

The finding of identical *TP53* and IDH mutations in the conventional and dedifferentiated components indicates a common origin of the components {93,379}. Potential genetic targets for treatment are under study and could be BCL2 family members and TGFB genes {3166}.

Macroscopic appearance

The cartilaginous and non-cartilaginous components of the tumour are grossly evident in varying proportions. The bluish-grey, lobulated cartilage component is usually located centrally, whereas the fleshy, pale-yellow or tan-brown high-grade sarcoma component is predominantly extraosseous or near the site of pathological fracture.

Histopathology

There is an abrupt transition between the conventional hyaline cartilage and high-grade sarcoma components of dedifferentiated chondrosarcoma {712}. The cartilaginous portion can range from enchondroma-like appearance to grade 1 or grade 2 chondrosarcoma. The high-grade dedifferentiated component usually has the appearance of a high-grade undifferentiated pleomorphic sarcoma or osteosarcoma. Less frequently, it demonstrates features of a high-grade angiosarcoma, leiomyosarcoma, or rhabdomyosarcoma {2941}. Rare cases of dedifferentiated chondrosarcoma with epithelial differentiation, including squamous, epithelial, and adamantinoma-like, have been reported {3397,1552,1111}. The ratio of conventional to dedifferentiated is highly variable, and the percentage of dedifferentiated component ranges from 2% to 98% (median: 60%) {2928}. Dedifferentiated chondrosarcomas usually show a poor histological response to preoperative chemotherapy.

Immunohistochemistry

The immunophenotype of the non-cartilaginous component follows its histological line of differentiation, and keratin and desmin expression can be observed. A small subset of H3K27me3-deficient dedifferentiated chondrosarcomas histologically resembling malignant peripheral nerve sheath tumour has also been described {1951}. Immunohistochemistry to detect an IDH mutation is of limited use because only a small percentage of the *IDH1* mutations (< 20%) can be identified using the p.Arg132His mutation–specific IDH1 antibody {93}. p53 overexpression may be present, especially in the dedifferentiated component (59%), whereas MDM2 is overexpressed in 16% of the tumours in the dedifferentiated component {2054}. PDL1 expression has been reported in approximately 50% of dedifferentiated chondrosarcomas, a finding that may play a role in future immunotherapeutic strategies {1686}.

Differential diagnosis

It can be impossible to make a histological diagnosis of dedifferentiated chondrosarcoma on a limited amount of biopsy tissue if only the high-grade sarcoma component is sampled. Correlation with imaging findings is crucial to come to the correct diagnosis. Because the characteristic IDH mutation is present in both components, mutation analysis can be helpful, although these heterozygous mutations are found in only 50–87% of cases {2054,558,93}. Cytokeratin positivity can be seen in the high-grade undifferentiated sarcoma component, making it difficult to distinguish from metastatic sarcomatoid carcinoma. Careful review of radiological images and thorough sampling of resected tissue are helpful in identifying the low-grade cartilaginous component. Molecular studies revealing H3-3 (H3F3) mutations in dedifferentiated chondrosarcoma mimicking giant cell tumour of bone support the notion that some cases represent giant cell tumours of bone with cartilaginous differentiation {1615}.

Cytology

Not clinically relevant

Diagnostic molecular pathology

Dedifferentiated chondrosarcomas harbour complex karyotypes {2054}. About 50–87% of dedifferentiated chondrosarcomas carry mutations in *IDH1* or *IDH2*, which can be found in both the conventional chondrosarcoma and the dedifferentiated component {93,2430,558,2054,3397}. Because the two components share identical genetic aberrations, including the early IDH mutation, a common precursor cell for the components is presumed {379,3397,2655,2054}. Additional genetic changes occur in the anaplastic component {379,2655}, indicating early diversion of the two components during the development of dedifferentiated chondrosarcoma. Mutations in *TP53* are also frequently found {2054}.

Essential and desirable diagnostic criteria

Essential: conventional chondrosarcoma juxtaposed to a high-grade sarcoma, with a sharp interface.
Desirable: IDH mutations present.

Staging

Staging is according to bone sarcoma protocols (see *TNM staging of tumours of bone*, p. 339). See also the information on staging in *Bone tumours: Introduction* (p. 340).

Prognosis and prediction

Patients with dedifferentiated chondrosarcoma have a dismal prognosis, most often as a result of widespread lung metastases. Overall 5-year survival rates of 7–24% have been reported {821,1068,1224}. Treatment consists of surgery with wide or radical margins. Poor prognostic factors include size > 8 cm, presence of a pathological fracture, metastatic disease at diagnosis, pelvic location, and inadequate surgical margin or treatment without surgery {1224,1835,1875,2965}. Chemotherapy and radiation therapy have not been shown to improve prognosis {821,1224,2317}.

Osteoma

Baumhoer D
Bredella MA
Sumathi VP

Definition

Osteoma is a benign tumour arising on the surface of bone and composed primarily of lamellar/cortical-type bone. When osteoma develops within the medullary cavity, the term "bone island" is used.

ICD-O coding

9180/0 Osteoma NOS

ICD-11 coding

2E83.Z & XH4818 Benign osteogenic tumours, unspecified & Osteoma NOS

Related terminology

Osteoma
Not recommended: ivory exostosis; parosteal osteoma; torus palatinus/mandibularis.

Bone island
Not recommended: enostosis.

Subtype(s)

None

Localization

Osteomas predominantly affect bone formed by membranous ossification, i.e. calvarial, facial, and jaw bones {1752}. They rarely occur outside the skull {298}. Intramedullary lesions generally originate in the epiphysis and metaphysis of long bones, the pelvic bones, and vertebral bodies.

Clinical features

Signs and symptoms
Osteomas are usually slow-growing and asymptomatic, but they can cause pain and headache, obstruction of the paranasal sinuses, and/or local swellings {1752}.

Imaging
Osteomas are round, dense, well-defined ivory-like lesions, which are attached to the underlying bone without cortical invasion. The presence of multiple osteomas suggests the diagnosis of Gardner syndrome {2991}. Bone islands are intramedullary lesions typically measuring < 1 cm, although larger lesions can occur (sometimes referred to as giant bone islands). Both osteomas and bone islands can grow slowly {1678}. Osteomas and bone islands may show mild radionuclide uptake on bone scan, mimicking a sclerotic metastasis. CT density measurements can be used to distinguish these lesions from sclerotic metastases, using a cut-off point of > 885 Hounsfield units {3127}. Bone islands in osteopoikilosis are usually bilateral and symmetrical in distribution, typically involving the metaphyseal and epiphyseal regions of tubular bone, although any bone

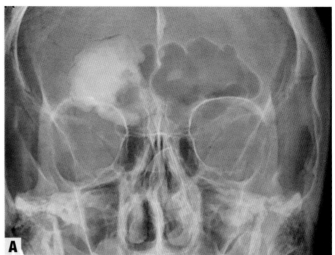
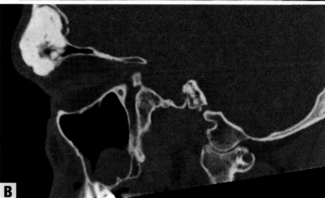

Fig. 3.57 Osteoma of the right frontal sinus. **A** Frontal radiograph. **B** Sagittal reformatted CT demonstrating an ossified mass arising on the surface of bone.

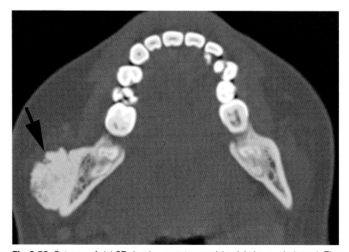

Fig. 3.58 Osteoma. Axial CT showing an osteoma of the right jaw angle (arrow). The tumour is arising on the surface of the bone and is homogeneously dense.

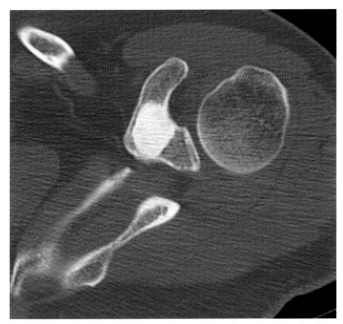

Fig. 3.59 Bone island. Axial CT shows an intramedullary dense bone island involving the coracoid process.

may be affected {267}. On MRI, osteomas and bone islands are hypointense on T1- and T2-weighted images.

Epidemiology

Due to their high amount of inorganic matrix, osteomas are among the best-preserved and best-documented tumours in human history, dating back to the Late Period of ancient Egypt (664–332 BCE) {2807}. They affect men and women equally, whereas bone islands seem to be more common in males. Since osteomas commonly represent incidental findings, their actual prevalence is difficult to determine but has been reported to reach 6.4% in selected case series {1800}.

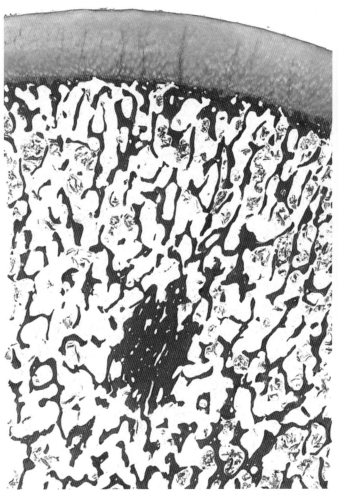

Fig. 3.61 Bone island / enostosis. Low-power image of a bone island involving the medullary cavity of the proximal femur. The lesion is composed of lamellar/cortical-type bone that merges with the surrounding trabecular bone.

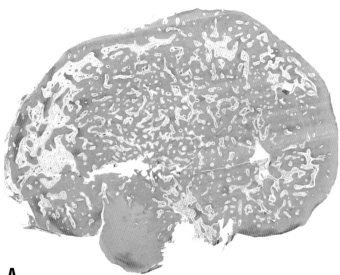

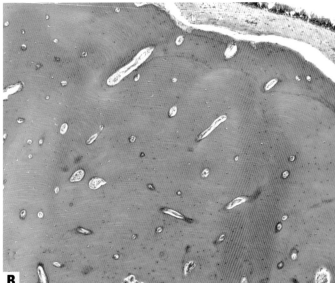

Fig. 3.60 Osteoma. **A** Well-demarcated tumour composed of trabecular bone. **B** Osteoma of the frontal sinus. The tumour is composed of lamellar/cortical-type bone adjacent to sinus epithelium.

Etiology

The etiology of sporadic cases is unknown. The presence of multiple osteomas is suggestive of Gardner syndrome, a subtype of familial adenomatous polyposis {2991}; familial adenomatous polyposis is an autosomal dominant disorder caused by mutations in the *APC* gene. Multiple bone islands are observed in osteopoikilosis (spotted bone disease), an autosomal dominant disorder caused by loss-of-function mutations of the *LEMD3* gene, with or without melorheostosis and/or dermatofibrosis (dermato-osteopoikilosis, Buschke–Ollendorff syndrome) {446,2269,1685,2526,1345}. However, most cases of bone islands seem to represent hamartomatous lesions.

Pathogenesis

LEMD3 encodes for an inner nuclear membrane protein that interacts with both the BMP and TGF-β signalling pathways and antagonizes both pathways in humans {446,2269,1685, 2526}.

Macroscopic appearance

Osteomas arise on the surface of the bone and are typically well-circumscribed tumours with a broad attachment to the underlying bone. Bone islands are intramedullary and composed of compact bone that merges with the surrounding trabecular bone. Bone islands are usually small, although rare giant bone islands do occur.

Histopathology

Osteomas are predominantly composed of mature lamellar/cortical-type bone and can be divided histologically into compact and (less frequent) spongious subtypes. In cancellous areas, a well-vascularized and moderately cellular and fibrous stroma fills the marrow spaces. Osteoblasts and osteocytes are generally inconspicuous; inflammatory infiltrates are typically absent. However, in the frontoethmoid region, conspicuous osteoblastic and osteoclastic activity may be present, mimicking osteoblastoma {2037,2023}.

Cytology

Not clinically relevant

Diagnostic molecular pathology

Not clinically relevant

Essential and desirable diagnostic criteria

Essential: bone tumour with compatible imaging; tumour arises on the surface of bone or within the medullary cavity; tumour composed of lamellar/cortical-type bone.

Staging

Not clinically relevant

Prognosis and prediction

Asymptomatic cases generally do not require treatment and follow an indolent clinical course; symptomatic cases can be conservatively excised.

Osteoid osteoma

Amary F
Bredella MA
Horvai AE
Mahar AM

Definition
Osteoid osteoma is a benign bone-forming tumour characterized by small size (< 2 cm) and limited growth potential.

ICD-O coding
9191/0 Osteoid osteoma NOS

ICD-11 coding
2E83.Z & XH61J9 Benign osteogenic tumours, unspecified &
   Osteoid osteoma NOS

Related terminology
None

Subtype(s)
None

Localization
Long bones are affected in 50% of patients, particularly femur
and tibia. Other typical locations include the small bones of the
hands and feet and the spine, where the neural arch (posterior
elements) are most commonly affected. Uncommon locations
include flat bones; it is rare in the craniofacial bones. Osteoid
osteoma preferentially involves the cortex (75% of cases) and
less frequently the medulla (25%); subperiosteal/surface lesions
are rare.

Clinical features
Signs and symptoms
The usual presenting symptom is pain. The pain, at first intermittent and mild with nocturnal exacerbation, eventually becomes
relentless to the point of interfering with sleep. In about 80% of
patients, NSAIDs, even in small doses, completely, albeit tem-
porarily, relieve the pain {1336}. On physical examination, there
is often an area of exquisite localized tenderness, redness, and
swelling. Less common manifestations are site-dependent.
For example, osteoid osteomas at the ends of long bones may
present with swelling and effusion of the nearest joint, and
intra-articular osteoid osteomas can result in osteoarthritis and
ectopic ossification {1999,2322}. Patients with osteoid osteomas
in the spine may present with painful scoliosis due to spasm of
the paraspinal muscles {1644}. In the fingers, the persistent soft
tissue swelling and periosteal reactions may result in functional
loss that leads to numerous surgeries and large en bloc excisions {2902}.

Imaging
Radiographs often show only periosteal reaction with cortical thickening, with or without central lucency (nidus). CT is
the imaging modality of choice to detect the nidus, an ovoid
lucency, < 2 cm, which can have central areas of mineralization. Lucent channels representing vessels may be seen

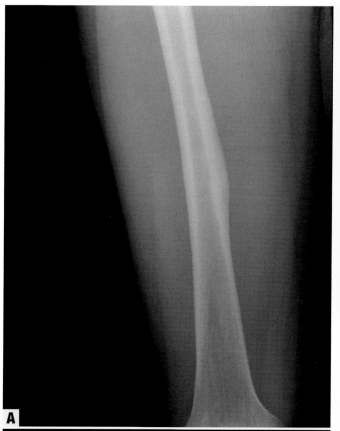

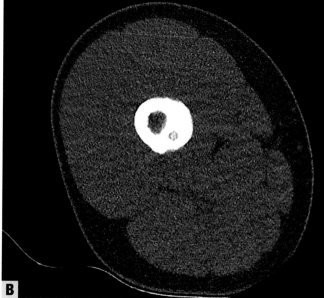

Fig. 3.62 Osteoid osteoma. **A** Frontal radiograph of the femur demonstrates cortical thickening and sclerosis of the medial femoral shaft. **B** Axial CT showing a small
nidus with central calcification, surrounded by diffuse sclerosis and cortical thickening.

in the thickened cortex {1880,180}. MRI can be misleading, showing reactive oedema-like signal within the bone marrow and surrounding soft tissues, without demonstration of the nidus. Technetium scintigraphy shows intense uptake at the site of the nidus and less-marked activity in the surrounding reactive bone (the double-density sign). Intramedullary lesions may incite little reactive cortical thickening but usually show surrounding medullary sclerosis. Subperiosteal lesions show little reactive sclerosis but can cause erosion of the underlying cortex. Intra-articular lesions can mimic a monoarthropathy, with joint space narrowing, joint effusion, and synovitis {2923}.

Epidemiology
Osteoid osteoma represents 10–12% of primary bone tumours. It usually affects children and adolescents, although it is occasionally seen in older individuals. There is a male predominance (M:F ratio: 2:1).

Etiology
Unknown

Pathogenesis
Rearrangement of *FOS* has been identified in both osteoblastomas and osteoid osteomas, further strengthening the link between these two lesions {1012,91A}. The rearrangement is present in 91% of the cases and may be detected at the protein level using anti–FOS (c-FOS) N-terminus immunohistochemistry, resulting in nuclear immunoreactivity in the osteoblastic cells {1012,91A,1739A}. Prostaglandins, especially PGE2, PGI2, and COX-2, have been implicated in the characteristic pain syndrome of osteoid osteoma and may explain the exquisite sensitivity to NSAIDs {1952,2215}.

Macroscopic appearance
Osteoid osteoma is a small, round, often cortically based red gritty or granular lesion surrounded by (and sharply circumscribed from) ivory-white sclerotic bone. The lesion seldom exceeds 1 cm in greatest diameter.

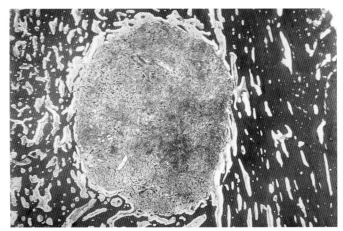

Fig. 3.64 Osteoid osteoma. A very sharp circumscription of nidus near the cortical surface showing dense cortex to the right and reactive neocortex to the left of the lesion.

Histopathology
The central portion of the lesion (nidus) contains differentiated plump osteoblasts present as a single layer around trabeculae of unmineralized or mineralized woven bone {1505}. Vascularized connective tissue, within which there are fibroblast-like stromal cells and cells differentiating into osteoblasts, separates the trabeculae. The osteoid may be microscopically disposed in a sheet-like configuration, but it is often organized into microtrabecular arrays. Osteoclasts may be conspicuous. Substantial nuclear pleomorphism and cartilage are absent. Hypervascular sclerotic bone with enlarged haversian canals surrounds the nidus and tends to be more pronounced as lesions become closer to the bone surface. The interface between the nidus and the surrounding reactive bone is abrupt and circumscribed, a finding that supports the indolent local behaviour of osteoid osteoma. The central area of the nidus may display intense mineralization. The nidus can be histologically indistinguishable from osteoblastoma, and the two lesions are separated by size: lesions < 2 cm are osteoid osteomas.

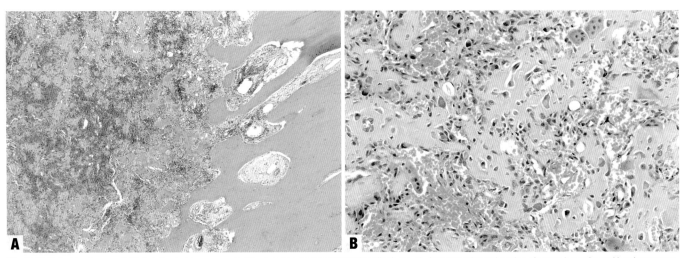

Fig. 3.63 Osteoid osteoma. **A** Well-defined nidus surrounded by dense cortical / compact lamellar bone. **B** Anastomosing trabeculae of woven bone rimmed by plump osteoblasts in a highly vascular background with numerous osteoclast-like giant cells.

The pathological evaluation of osteoid osteoma has undergone changes because of the increasing use of minimally invasive techniques to ablate these tumours. If the diagnosis of osteoid osteoma can be made clinically and radiographically, the tumour is sometimes ablated without prior biopsy, although a core biopsy may be obtained immediately before ablation. In other cases, fragments obtained from a drill procedure are sent for histological examination. Not only is the scant yield of diagnostic tissue in these cases lower than with resection specimens, but the histopathology may be obscured by heat or crush artefact {54,1651}.

Cytology
Not clinically relevant

Diagnostic molecular pathology
FOS gene rearrangement (not necessary for diagnosis) may be found in osteoid osteoma, but it can also be found in osteoblastomas and epithelioid haemangiomas {1012}.

Essential and desirable diagnostic criteria
Essential: bone tumour with compatible imaging; radiographic demonstration of small (< 2 cm) central nidus, often surrounded by sclerosis; bone-forming tumour composed of microtrabeculae of woven bone rimmed by plump osteoblasts in a vascularized stroma.

Desirable: nocturnal pain relieved by NSAIDs; abrupt transition between central nidus and peripheral sclerotic bone.

Staging
Not clinically relevant

Prognosis and prediction
The prognosis is excellent. Recurrences are uncommon. Some lesions have been reported to disappear without therapy {1117}. Although traditional surgical excision is curative, it is sometimes challenging to resect small lesions, particularly when there is a great deal of reactive sclerosis. Consequently, less invasive techniques including CT-guided core drill excision, image-guided percutaneous radiofrequency ablation, cryoablation, high-intensity focused ultrasound, and laser photocoagulation have largely replaced the traditional approach {474,1117,1997,2234}. Arthroscopic excision is used for intra-articular tumours {2921}.

Osteoblastoma

Amary F
Bredella MA
Horvai AE
Mahar AM

Definition
Osteoblastoma is a locally aggressive bone-forming tumour, morphologically similar to osteoid osteoma but with growth potential and generally > 2 cm in dimension.

ICD-O coding
9200/1 Osteoblastoma NOS

ICD-11 coding
2E83.Z & XH4316 Benign osteogenic tumours, unspecified & Osteoblastoma NOS

Related terminology
Acceptable: epithelioid osteoblastoma.
Not recommended: pseudomalignant osteoblastoma; aggressive osteoblastoma.

Subtype(s)
None

Localization
The spine, in particular the neural arch (posterior elements), is the most frequent site, affected in more than one third of cases. Although the tumours may extend into the vertebral body, they are very rarely seen in isolation in the vertebral body {1907}. Other sites include the pelvis, the limbs (particularly the femur and tibia), the jaws, and other craniofacial bones {1542A}. However, any bone may be involved {1907}.

Clinical features
Signs and symptoms
The presenting symptom is frequently pain, but unlike with osteoid osteoma, NSAIDs usually do not provide relief {1907}. Neurological symptoms may be present with spinal lesions. Rarely, there may be systemic symptoms including fever, weight loss, and hyperdynamic circulation {725}. Systemic symptoms have been attributed to an exaggerated immune response to the tumour. Exceptionally, cases can be associated with oncogenic phosphaturic syndrome {596}.

Imaging
On radiographs and CT, osteoblastomas present as lytic lesions > 2 cm in size, with surrounding reactive sclerosis. Internal mineralization can be present, which may be ossified or chondral-type {1105}. Medullary lesions are associated with surrounding sclerosis and non-aggressive periosteal reaction. In the spine, osteoblastomas typically involve the posterior elements and can have aneurysmal bone cyst–like changes. Bone scintigraphy shows nonspecific increased radiotracer uptake. On MRI, osteoblastomas can demonstrate low signal intensity on T1- and T2-weighted images, corresponding to heavily

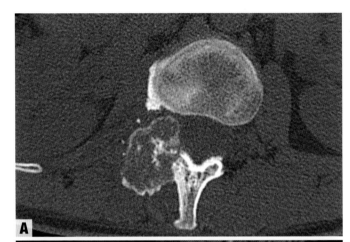

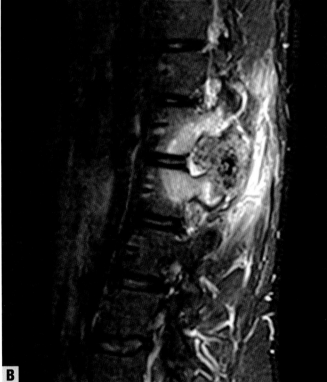

Fig. 3.65 Osteoblastoma. **A** Axial CT shows an expansile tumour in the posterior elements, with matrix mineralization. **B** Sagittal short-tau inversion recovery (STIR) MRI showing a well-defined lesion with hyperintense oedema-like signal in the adjacent marrow and soft tissue.

mineralized lesions with variable adjacent oedema-like signal and enhancement in the marrow and surrounding soft tissues {284}. Fluid-fluid levels can be seen in lesions with aneurysmal bone cyst–like changes.

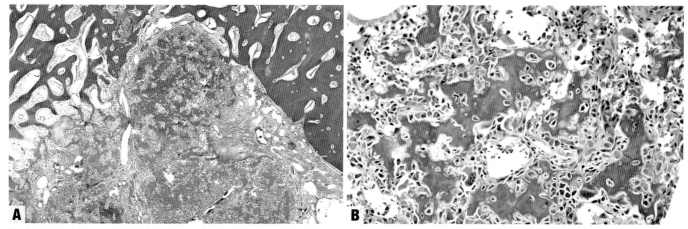

Fig. 3.66 Osteoblastoma. **A** Well-defined tumour borders. The tumour is focally merging with remodelled bone at the periphery (maturation). **B** Woven bone trabeculae lined by one or more layers of plump osteoblasts, scattered osteoclast-type giant cells, and intervening vascular stroma. Anaplasia and atypical mitotic figures are absent.

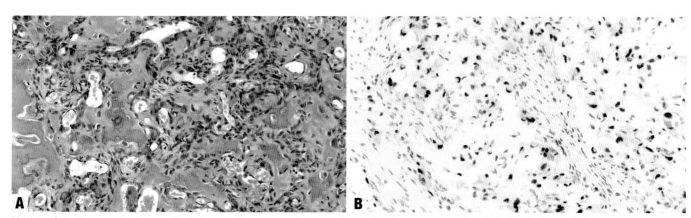

Fig. 3.67 Osteoblastoma. **A** Interconnecting trabeculae of woven bone rimmed by plump osteoblasts. Richly vascularized fibroblastic stroma. **B** Nuclear expression of FOS (c-FOS), highlighting the osteoblastic cells.

Epidemiology

Osteoblastomas are rarer than osteoid osteomas, representing < 1% of primary bone tumours {284,1907}. The peak incidence is between the second and third decades of life. Osteoblastoma is twice as frequent in males as females {284,1907}.

Etiology

Unknown

Pathogenesis

Rearrangement of *FOS* has been identified in both osteoblastomas and osteoid osteomas, further strengthening the link between these two lesions {1012,237}. The rearrangement is present in 87% of the cases. The breakpoints in *FOS* cluster to exon 4, which is fused to introns of other genes or intergenic regions. The resulting transcript lacks regulatory elements, similar to the *v-Fos* retroviral oncogene {1012}. FOS is a member of the AP-1 family of transcription factors, increased levels of which can promote cell growth. *FOS* rearrangements can be detected at the protein level using an antibody against the FOS N-terminus, which results in nuclear immunoreactivity in the osteoblastic cells {237,91A,1739A}. In a smaller percentage of cases, *FOSB* rearrangement has been detected {1012}. Whole-genome DNA sequencing analysis performed in osteoblastomas shows diploid tumour cells with few other somatic alterations {1012}. Previously, karyotypic abnormalities such as rearrangement of chromosome 13 {1146} and deletions on chromosome 22 have been reported {2320}; these activate the WNT/β-catenin signalling pathway {2320,2625}.

Macroscopic appearance

Macroscopically, osteoblastomas are usually red to tan lesions, reflecting their intense vascularity {1907}. Bone expansion with marked cortical thinning or surrounding areas of sclerosis may be seen. The borders are usually well defined. Blood-filled cystic spaces (aneurysmal bone cyst change) may be present.

Histopathology

Osteoblastomas are microscopically similar to osteoid osteomas. Osteoblastomas are characterized by interconnecting, delicate, woven bone trabeculae, usually rimmed by a single layer of polygonal osteoblasts {1907}. The trabeculae may show different levels of mineralization, from osteoid to densely mineralized woven bone that shows multiple cement lines (pagetoid appearance) {1907}. The stroma is loose and usually richly vascularized, with dilated capillary-type blood vessels. Osteoclast-like giant cells are scattered throughout the tumour. Lace-like osteoid deposition, although uncommon, can be present, as can cartilaginous differentiation. The borders are usually well defined, often showing peripheral bone maturation towards lamellar bone {1907}. Destructive host bone permeation should not be seen, and it is possibly the most reliable histological feature in differentiating osteoblastoma from osteoblastoma-like osteosarcoma {1110}. Atypical mitotic figures should be absent. The diagnosis of so-called aggressive osteoblastoma is controversial and not recommended. This entity was initially reported with a more aggressive clinical course and morphologically characterized by the presence of large, epithelioid osteoblasts (twice the size of normal osteoblasts) that are frequently mitotically active {841,1907}. However, the presence of epithelioid osteoblasts does not seem to predict an aggressive clinical course in osteoblastoma {1907,782}; therefore, the term "epithelioid osteoblastoma" is preferred. Rarely osteoblastomas may show degenerative atypia, which should not be mistaken for malignancy.

Cytology
Not clinically relevant

Diagnostic molecular pathology
FOS gene rearrangement or rarely *FOSB* gene rearrangement is found in the majority of osteoblastomas {1012}.

Essential and desirable diagnostic criteria
Essential: bone tumour with compatible imaging; radiological demonstration of a > 2 cm lesion; well-defined tumour borders, absence of host bone permeation; bone-forming tumour composed of trabeculae of woven bone rimmed by plump osteoblasts in a vascularized stroma.

Staging
Not clinically relevant

Prognosis and prediction
The prognosis is good, but recurrences are described in as many as 23% of the cases {284}, more frequently in patients treated with curettage than with en bloc resection, with which a 14% recurrence rate is reported {284}. Although osteoid osteoma and osteoblastoma may be morphologically indistinguishable, and they may in fact be different clinical manifestations of the same disease, an attempt to differentiate these tumour types is justified by the tendency for clinical progression and recurrence seen in the latter.

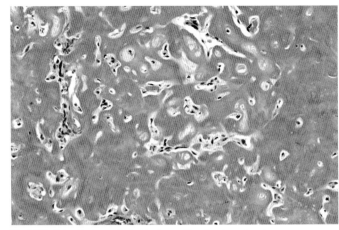

Fig. 3.68 Osteoblastoma. Osteoblastoma with extensive sclerosis.

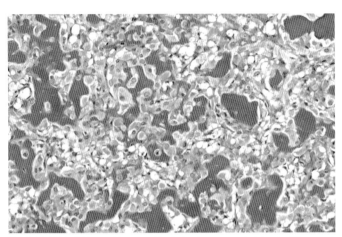

Fig. 3.69 Epithelioid osteoblastoma. The lesion is composed of sheets of large, epithelioid osteoblasts associated with bone formation.

Epithelioid osteoblastoma was initially reported with a more aggressive clinical course and morphologically characterized by the presence of large, epithelioid osteoblasts that are frequently mitotically active {841,1907}. The presence of epithelioid osteoblasts does not consistently predict an aggressive clinical course in osteoblastoma {1907,782}. Conversely, some osteoblastomas > 4 cm with locally destructive features and repeated recurrences may lack epithelioid cytomorphology. Rare cases of malignant transformation are described {840,1715}.

Low-grade central osteosarcoma

Yoshida A
Bredella MA
Gambarotti M
Sumathi VP

Definition
Low-grade central osteosarcoma (LGCOS) is a low-grade malignant bone-forming neoplasm that originates within the intramedullary cavity and consists of fibroblastic tumour cells with low-grade nuclear atypia and well-formed neoplastic bony trabeculae.

ICD-O coding
9187/3 Low-grade central osteosarcoma

ICD-11 coding
2B51.Z & XH7N84 Osteosarcoma of bone and articular cartilage of unspecified sites & Low-grade central osteosarcoma

Related terminology
Acceptable: well-differentiated intramedullary osteosarcoma.

Subtype(s)
None

Localization
LGCOS most often affects the metaphysis of long bones, predominantly the femur and tibia. Jaw bones, small tubular bones, and axial bones are rarely involved {786,1955,2785}.

Clinical features
Signs and symptoms
The tumour often presents with swelling or pain. The preoperative period tends to be longer than with conventional osteosarcoma

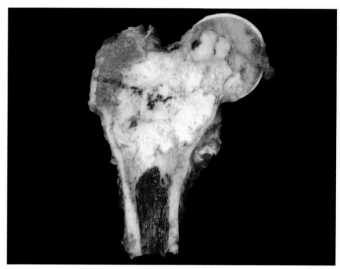

Fig. 3.72 Low-grade central osteosarcoma. Bisected resection specimen of the proximal femur showing a fibrous tumour with focal gritty areas and cortical expansion.

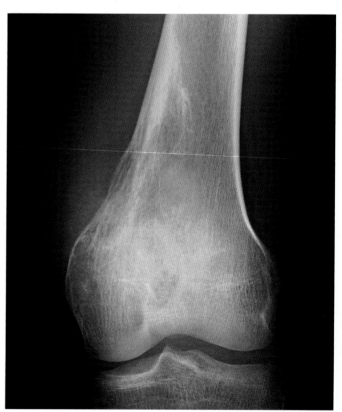

Fig. 3.71 Low-grade central osteosarcoma with focal dedifferentiation. A large lytic and sclerotic lesion with trabeculation in the distal femoral metaphysis, extending to the end of the bone. The tumour margin is partly well defined, and bone cortex is mildly expanded. Cloud-like soft tissue density represents a dedifferentiated component.

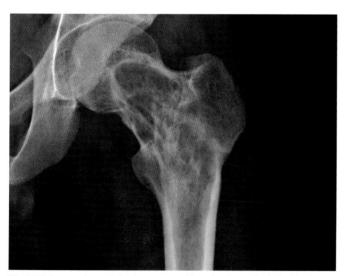

Fig. 3.70 Low-grade central osteosarcoma. Frontal radiograph of the hip demonstrates an ill-defined lytic and sclerotic lesion with coarsened trabeculations in the proximal femoral metaphysis.

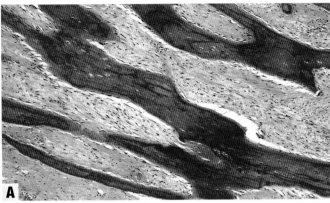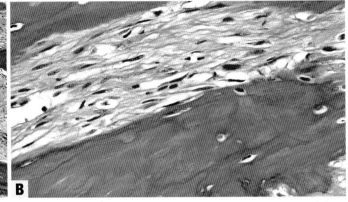

Fig. 3.73 Low-grade central osteosarcoma. **A** Low-power view showing a mildly cellular fascicular proliferation of spindle cells, admixed with well-formed neoplastic bone trabeculae in a parallel distribution. **B** Tumour spindle cells display mild nuclear atypia.

(COS) and can exceed 10 years (average: > 2 years) {1955, 587}.

Imaging

On radiographs, LGCOSs typically present as large intramedullary expansile lytic and/or sclerotic lesions with coarsened incomplete trabeculations. Dense sclerotic lesions are less likely. LGCOS usually involves the metaphysis or metadiaphysis of long bones, often extending to the end of the bone {112}. The tumour border may be circumscribed but often shows at least focal areas of cortical destruction {112}. Cortical disruption and/or soft tissue extension is commonly seen on MRI and CT.

Epidemiology

LGCOS is rare, accounting for 1–2% of all osteosarcomas. It most commonly affects young adults, with a peak incidence in the third decade of life {1717}. There is a mild female predilection {2785,112,3372}.

Etiology

Unknown

Pathogenesis

Amplification of 12q13-q15 involving *MDM2* and *CDK4* is common {1335,3050,867}. *MDM2* amplification is maintained in high-grade progression. A subset of LGCOSs lack *MDM2* amplification.

Macroscopic appearance

LGCOS is a large, relatively well-circumscribed, white rubbery fibrous tissue mass with gritty calcification, located in the medullary cavity.

Histopathology

LGCOS is composed of mildly to moderately cellular fascicles of spindle cells with mild nuclear atypia in a fibrosclerotic stroma. These are admixed with a neoplastic bone component, which typically consists of long and thick bony trabeculae, often with parallel arrangement, resembling parosteal osteosarcoma. Bone can be thinner and more irregular. Bone is typically woven, but it may be lamellar. Pagetoid bone with irregular cement lines may be present {1067}. Permeation of host bone is invariably present. Cortical destruction with soft tissue infiltration may also

be present. Mitotic activity is low. Cartilage formation may be focally present {1717}. Some tumours focally lack bone matrix. In 10–36% of cases, LGCOS progresses to high-grade sarcoma. This phenomenon, known as dedifferentiation, may occur at presentation or in a recurrence. High-grade areas often show high-grade osteosarcoma histology indistinguishable from that of COS, with lace-like immature osteoid formation and higher cellularity, nuclear grade, and mitotic activity. High-grade areas

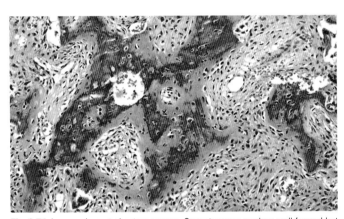

Fig. 3.74 Low-grade central osteosarcoma. Some tumours produce well-formed but irregular bone trabeculae, reminiscent of fibrous dysplasia.

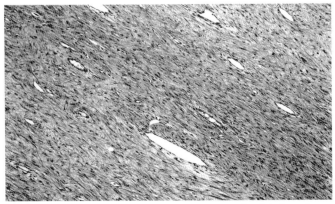

Fig. 3.75 Low-grade central osteosarcoma. Some tumours focally lack matrix production, resembling desmoplastic fibroma.

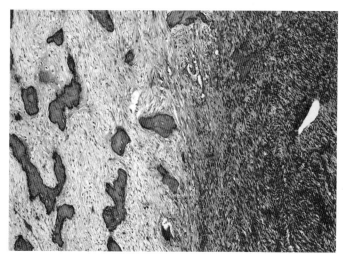

Fig. 3.76 Dedifferentiated low-grade central osteosarcoma. Low-grade central osteosarcoma (left half) progresses (dedifferentiates) to high-grade sarcoma (right half) with greater degrees of cellularity and nuclear atypia.

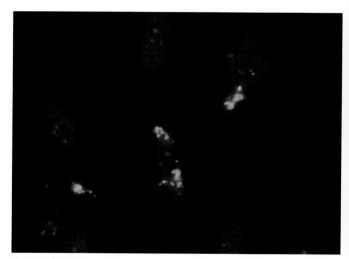

Fig. 3.77 Low-grade central osteosarcoma. FISH shows *MDM2* amplification in tumour cells. Green, *MDM2*; red, CEN12.

may lack osteoid formation and resemble undifferentiated pleomorphic sarcoma or fibrosarcoma.

Immunohistochemistry
LGCOSs and the high-grade sarcomas that result from their progression express MDM2 and/or CDK4 in a high proportion of cases, and this feature can be used as a surrogate when access to *MDM2* molecular testing is limited {3372,867}.

Differential diagnosis
LGCOS should be distinguished from benign fibro-osseous lesions such as fibrous dysplasia. When bone formation is inapparent, LGCOS can mimic desmoplastic fibroma or low-grade fibrosarcoma.

Cytology
Not clinically relevant

Diagnostic molecular pathology
Testing for *MDM2* amplification is helpful to differentiate LGCOS from benign mimics. Because *MDM2* amplification is rare in COS {866}, it may help separate dedifferentiated LGCOS from COS in the appropriate histological context {867,3373}. Unlike fibrous dysplasia, LGCOS lacks *GNAS* mutation {2724}. The lack of *MDM2* amplification cannot exclude the diagnosis of LGCOS.

Essential and desirable diagnostic criteria
Essential: bone tumour with compatible imaging; intramedullary location; predominantly fibroblastic osteosarcoma with mild nuclear atypia and well-formed neoplastic bony trabeculae.
Desirable: MDM2 amplification.

Staging
Staging is according to bone sarcoma protocols (see *TNM staging of tumours of bone*, p. 339). See also the information on staging in *Bone tumours: Introduction* (p. 340).

Prognosis and prediction
LGCOS has a good prognosis when widely resected, with a metastatic rate of < 5% and 5-year and 10-year overall survival rates of 90% and > 80%, respectively {1955,587,1717}. The tumour invariably recurs after curettage and incomplete excision. The presence of dedifferentiation confers a worse prognosis, and detecting such areas is therefore critical. It remains to be determined whether the volume of the dedifferentiated component may be prognostically significant {2785,2631}. Chemotherapy is reserved for dedifferentiated tumours.

Osteosarcoma

Baumhoer D
Böhling TO
Cates JMM
Cleton-Jansen AM
Hogendoorn PCW
O'Donnell PG
Rosenberg AE

Definition
Osteosarcoma is an intramedullary high-grade sarcoma in which the tumour cells produce bone.

ICD-O coding
9180/3 Osteosarcoma NOS

ICD-11 coding
2B51.Z & XH1XF3 Osteosarcoma of bone and articular cartilage of unspecified sites & Osteosarcoma NOS
2B51.Z & XH5CL5 Osteosarcoma of bone and articular cartilage of unspecified sites & Telangiectatic osteosarcoma
2B51.Z & XH4EZ4 Osteosarcoma of bone and articular cartilage of unspecified sites & Small cell osteosarcoma

Related terminology
None

Subtype(s)
Conventional osteosarcoma; telangiectatic osteosarcoma; small cell osteosarcoma

Localization
Conventional osteosarcomas (COSs) can arise in any bone, but the vast majority originate in the long bones of the extremities, most commonly in the distal femur (30%), followed by the proximal tibia (15%) and the proximal humerus (15%), i.e. sites of the most proliferative growth plates. In long bones, the tumour is usually metaphyseal (90%) and only infrequently develops in the diaphysis (9%) or rarely in the epiphysis. The jaws are the fourth most common site of origin {2747,238}. Involvement of the small bones of the extremities and multifocal osteosarcoma, either synchronous or metachronous, are rare, the latter representing metastatic spread rather than multiple independent primary tumours {193}. Telangiectatic osteosarcomas (TAEOSs) also frequently develop around the knee (~60%) and in the proximal humerus (~20%) {116}. They occur in the metaphysis, commonly with direct extension into the adjacent epiphysis and diaphysis. Small cell osteosarcoma (SCOS) has a similar distribution but more commonly develops in the diaphysis of long bones (10–15%) {188,2627}.

Clinical features
Signs and symptoms
There is usually a short history (weeks to months) of a painful, enlarging mass and occasionally restricted movement at the adjacent joint. The skin overlying the tumour may be warm and

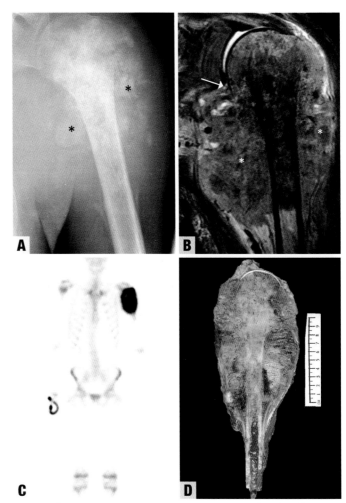

Fig. 3.78 Conventional osteosarcoma. **A** Anteroposterior radiograph shows sclerosis of proximal humerus and ossification within a large extraosseous mass (asterisks). **B** Coronal T2-weighted MRI shows hypointense tumour within the humerus and a heterogeneous circumferential mass (asterisks). Tumour extends to the humeral head and involves the shoulder joint (arrow). **C** Technetium radioisotope bone scan showing markedly increased uptake in the tumour in the proximal humerus but no other lesions. **D** Macroscopic appearance of a resected tumour of the proximal humerus.

erythematous {1652}. A minority of patients (10–15%) present with pathological fracture, most commonly seen in tumours of the femur and humerus {1507}. The clinical presentation of TAEOS and SCOS is similar to that of COS, although pathological fracture is more common in TAEOS (seen in ~30% of cases) {2101,2240,116}.

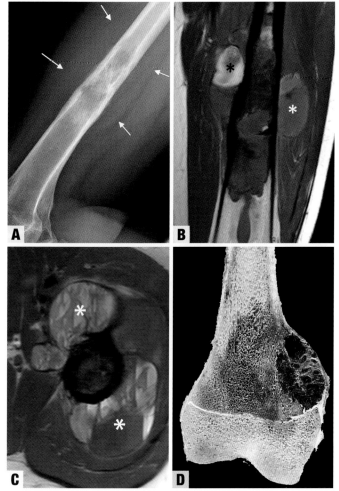

Fig.3.79 Telangiectatic osteosarcoma. **A** Lateral radiograph of the distal femur shows a predominantly lytic lesion with a striated appearance, cortical destruction, mild expansile remodelling, and an extraosseous mass (arrows). **B,C** Coronal T1-weighted MRI (**B**) and axial proton density MRI (**C**) show an elongated intramedullary tumour and a cystic, haemorrhagic extraosseous mass (asterisks) containing multiple fluid levels. **D** Gross appearance of telangiectatic osteosarcoma with dominant cystic architecture, incompletely filled with blood clots (a bag of blood). There is no fleshy or sclerotic tumour bone formation. The tumour permeates the surrounding medullary canal.

Imaging

Imaging of COS typically shows permeative bone destruction in conjunction with tumour mineralization – a mixed lytic/sclerotic appearance – with ill-defined, immature (fluffy, cloud-like) tumour ossifications {2999}. There is usually non-expansile cortical destruction and mechanical displacement of the periosteum that produces reactive new bone, which is classically oriented perpendicular to the tumour but may be parallel (onion skin–like) or divergent (sunburst-like). The periosteal response may be interrupted centrally and results in Codman triangles peripherally {1652}. An extraosseous extension is common and usually large, often eccentric and mineralized. Isotope bone scans show increased activity on all phases within osteoblastic tumour areas (in primary and metastatic sites), as well as an extended uptake in adjacent bone, which is thought to reflect peritumoural hyperaemia {574}. CT demonstrates cortical destruction and extraosseous extension and helps to identify ossification in poorly mineralized tumours or those involving complex anatomical sites (e.g. spine and pelvis). COS shows a heterogeneous intermediate signal on T1-weighted MRI and hyperintensity on fluid-sensitive sequences, with hyperintense haemorrhagic and hypointense mineralized areas {2999}. Perpendicular periosteal ossification may be seen as radiating low-signal strands; the outer periosteum may form a low-signal capsule, which is often focally breached. After administration of contrast medium, viable tumour enhances, whereas ossified tumour areas may remain hypointense and there may be septal/nodular enhancement in chondroblastic areas {1129}.

The diagnosis can often be predicted from radiographic appearances {1979}, but histological subtypes cannot be reliably identified. Atypical appearances are common {2662,2993}. A predominantly lytic tumour suggests certain osteosarcoma subtypes (fibroblastic, small cell, telangiectatic, and secondary tumours) but may nevertheless be osteoblastic with immature and still-uncalcified matrix deposition {797}. SCOS frequently resembles COS but occasionally also shows a predominantly lytic, non-mineralized appearance that can mimic Ewing sarcoma, particularly when occurring in the diaphysis of a long bone {293,2240}. TAEOS is typically associated with aggressive bone destruction, expansile remodelling, extraosseous extension, and pathological fracture {2227}. Sclerosis is rare and tumour ossification is frequently subtle, requiring CT for visualization {2227}. Cortical striations suggesting hypertrophied intraosseous veins may be seen adjacent to the tumour {3174}. MRI reveals a multicystic tumour consisting largely of blood-filled spaces and often revealing fluid-fluid levels. TAEOS can resemble aneurysmal bone cyst, but it usually presents more aggressively, with thickened septa and nodular/solid components {2227}.

Epidemiology

Osteosarcoma is the most common primary high-grade sarcoma of the skeleton. It has a bimodal age distribution, with most cases developing between the ages of 14 and 18 years and a second smaller peak in older adults (30% of cases occur in individuals aged > 40 years) {2152,2398,3143}. The annual incidence rate is about 4.4 cases per 1 million population for people aged 0–24 years, about 1.7 cases per 1 million population for people aged 25–59 years, and about 4.2 cases per 1 million population for people aged ≥ 60 years {119}. Males are affected more frequently (M:F ratio: 1.3:1) {3143}. Tumours of the jaws primarily occur in the third to fourth decades of life {238}. TAEOS is a rare subtype, accounting for 2–12% of all high-grade osteosarcomas. It also commonly develops in the second decade of life and has a male predominance similar to that of COS {116}. SCOSs account for only 1.5% of all osteosarcomas and have been observed in patients aged 5–83 years. However, they occur most frequently during the pubertal growth spurt {293,188,2240}. There is a slight female predominance (M:F ratio: 0.9:1) {293,188,1991,2240}.

Etiology

Although the etiology is unknown, there is an increased incidence of primary osteosarcoma associated with several genetic syndromes. Inactivation of the *TP53* gene due to mutations or loss of heterozygosity / deletions occurs in individuals with Li–Fraumeni

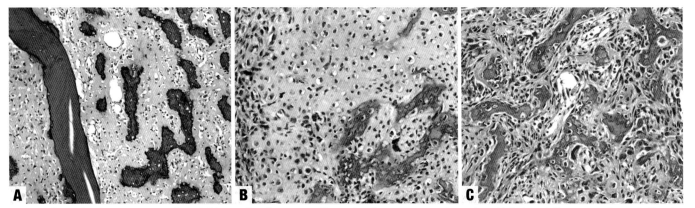

Fig. 3.80 Conventional osteosarcoma. **A** Pre-existing cancellous bone encased by a sclerosing osteosarcoma in a patient with Rothmund–Thomson syndrome. **B** Chondroblastic osteosarcoma with high-grade cartilaginous component. **C** Highly atypical spindle cells producing immature and lace-like bone.

syndrome, who have an increased incidence of osteosarcoma {1957,2354}. Patients with hereditary retinoblastoma also have a high risk of developing osteosarcoma {856}, in particular after receiving ionizing radiation therapy. The genes causing these syndromes are also the most commonly mutated genes in sporadic osteosarcoma (*TP53* in > 90% and *RB1* in as many as 56% of cases) {562,2495,1690}. Germline mutations in various RECQ helicases underlie another group of rare syndromes associated with COS, including Bloom syndrome (*BLM* [*RECQL3*]), Werner syndrome (*WRN*), and Rothmund–Thomson syndrome (*RECQL4*) {592}. Acquiring chromosomal instability is also the hallmark of sporadic COS and probably the most crucial step for initiating and driving tumour development. Syndrome-related COSs have been recognized for a long time, but the increasing use of DNA sequencing for genotyping neoplasms and also the germline of individuals has identified pathogenic germline mutations in as many as 17.9% of COSs in larger studies {3394}, a figure that is likely to increase in sequencing studies to come.

Pathogenesis

The pathogenesis and cell of origin of COS are unknown. Many potential driver genes in osteosarcoma have been identified; the largest sequencing study to date found 67 different driver genes in a series of 112 COSs {256}. Although these mutations certainly occur early in the course of the disease, it seems likely that chromothripsis/chromoplexy caused by an unknown trigger initiates chromosomal instability and subsequent tumour development {256}.

Somatic genetics

COS is characterized by highly complex chromosomal aneuploidy and both intertumoural and intratumoural heterogeneity due to chromosomal instability. Somatic alterations involve various numerical and structural alterations, whereas specific point mutations are rather infrequent {256}. Specific translocations have not been identified so far.

There is general consensus about recurring amplifications for some regions, such as gains of chromosome arms 6p (40–50% of cases, harbouring *RUNX2*, *VEGFA*, *E2F3*, and *CDC5L* [*CDC5*]), 8q (45–55% of cases, harbouring *MYC*), and 17p, which have been detected by classic karyotyping and conventional comparative genomic hybridization, as well as deep sequencing. However, studies are difficult to compare because the definition of a recurrent alteration varies {2924,1768,1960, 2889,562,2495,1690,256}. The *TP53* antagonist *MDM2* is amplified in about 10% of cases, suggesting a pre-existing central low-grade osteosarcoma that underwent dedifferentiation in at least a subset of cases {2067,2724}. *FGFR1* amplifications have been demonstrated in 18.5% of cases; alterations in the IGF1R signalling pathway were observed 14% of COSs {985, 256}. Homozygous loss of *CDKN2A* occurs in 10% of COSs, is associated with an adverse outcome, and has been implicated

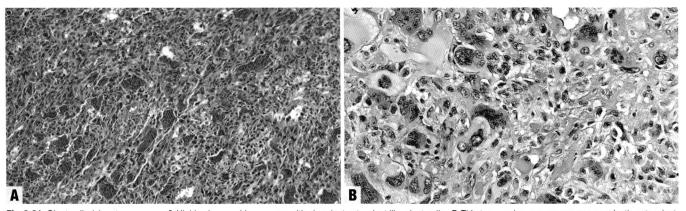

Fig. 3.81 Giant cell–rich osteosarcoma. **A** Highly pleomorphic sarcoma with abundant osteoclast-like giant cells. **B** This tumour shows numerous non-neoplastic osteoclast-type giant cells admixed with malignant tumour giant cells and filigree-pattern neoplastic bone.

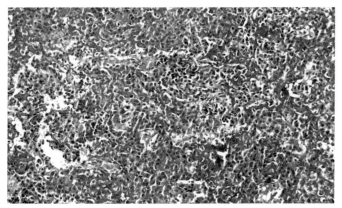

Fig. 3.82 Small cell osteosarcoma. Densely packed small blue round cells showing a delicate and immature bone formation.

in osteosarcoma development from a mesenchymal progenitor {2169}. *RB1* is deleted in about 50% of osteosarcomas {2495}. Other recurrently deleted genes include *LSAMP*, *DLG2*, and *WWOX* {2890}. Distinct patterns of large-scale transitions and loss of heterozygosity reminiscent of that seen in *BRCA1/ BRCA2*-deficient tumours have been identified in COS, suggesting a deficiency in homologous recombination repair (so-called BRCAness) {1690}. These findings indicate a potential sensitivity to poly (ADP-ribose) polymerase (PARP) inhibitors {907}.

Chromothripsis and chromoplexy, subsumed under the term "chromoanagenesis", cause massive, chaotic, and complex chromosomal alterations through a single catastrophic event {2478}. Sequencing studies found evidence that chromoanagenesis is the molecular mechanism initiating the chromosomal complexity of COS in > 90% of cases {1690,256}; however, the trigger of the process itself remains unclear. Inactivating mutations of *TP53* with subsequent inability to mediate cell-cycle arrest, apoptosis, and cellular senescence have been proposed as the trigger, but errors in mitotic chromosome segregation producing whole chromosome–containing micronuclei might better explain the spatial distribution of chromosomal regions affected {674,2478}. A specific pattern of chromothripsis and amplification has been observed recently, which might result in

the generation of distinct cancer driver events, i.e. *CDK4/MDM2* amplification {256}.

Kataegis, a phenomenon of localized hypermutations, has been demonstrated in 50% of COSs {562}, but recurrent single-nucleotide variants are rare. Inactivation of *TP53* is the most common mutation in COS (> 90%) and can occur through chromosomal deletion, single-nucleotide variants, and rearrangements affecting the first intron of the gene, with rearrangements appearing to be relatively specific for COS {562,2620}. Mutations of *IDH1* and *IDH2* have not been detected in COS and can be helpful in distinguishing between chondroblastic osteosarcoma and chondrosarcoma {93}. Other recurrent somatic point mutations have been identified in *RB1*, *ATRX*, and *NF2* {256}.

Gene expression

Gene expression profiling demonstrated an association between macrophage expression profiles and lack of metastases, suggesting a beneficial effect of macrophage infiltration. These findings have also been confirmed by immunohistochemical analysis {443}. A number of genes have been demonstrated to be hypermethylated in COS, affecting transcriptional activity: *HIC1*, *WIF1*, *PHLDA2* (*TSSC3*), *RASSF1* (*RASSF1A*), *GADD45*, and *RUNX2* {1571}. Methylation of ER (*ESR1*) seems particularly interesting, because this steroid receptor is involved in osteoblastic differentiation. Relieving *ESR1* hypermethylation by DNA methyltransferases resulted in growth inhibition of tumour cells {1859}.

Tumour markers

Tumour mutation burden has been shown to be relatively low, at 0.3–1.2 mutations per megabase {2495}, thereby designating osteosarcoma as a so-called cold tumour, with limited potential for immunotherapy. Indeed, only 1 of 22 COSs treated with the checkpoint inhibitor pembrolizumab (directed against PD1) showed a partial response to treatment {3055}.

Macroscopic appearance

COS usually presents as a large (> 5–10 cm) intramedullary mass centred in the metaphyseal region with variable extension into the adjacent diaphysis and epiphysis. The cut surface is heterogeneous, depending on the type and degree of mineralization of the predominant matrix. Heavily mineralized tumours

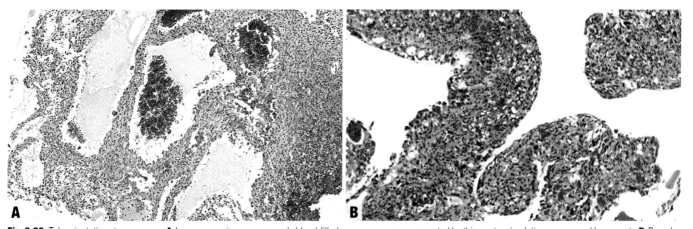

Fig. 3.83 Telangiectatic osteosarcoma. **A** Low-power microscopy reveals blood-filled spaces or spaces separated by thin septa, simulating aneurysmal bone cyst. **B** Pseudocystic septa filled with highly atypical spindle cells and intermingled multinucleated giant cells.

are tan-white/yellow and densely solid (resembling cortical bone), whereas non-mineralized cartilaginous components are either grey and rubbery (if hyaline in nature) or mucoid (if the matrix has undergone myxoid degeneration). Areas of haemorrhage, tumour necrosis, and cystic change are common. Intramedullary involvement is often considerable. When extraosseous infiltration occurs, the tumour usually forms an eccentric or circumferential soft tissue mass that displaces the periosteum peripherally. TAEOS shows a haemorrhagic multicystic lesion filled with blood clots, classically described as a bag of blood {2014}. Solid fleshy or sclerotic areas are usually not seen. Extensive cortical erosion or destruction associated with nearby soft tissue involvement may be seen. The gross features of SCOS are indistinguishable from those of COS.

Histopathology

COS has a broad histomorphological spectrum. Essential to the diagnosis is the identification of neoplastic bone formation. The tumour grows with a permeative pattern; replacing the marrow space and encasing and eroding pre-existing trabeculae, it fills and expands haversian systems within cortical bone. The neoplastic cells typically demonstrate severe anaplasia and pleomorphism, and they may be fusiform, plasmacytoid, or epithelioid. Neoplastic cells often become small and normalized in appearance (mimicking benign osteocytes) when surrounded by bone matrix. Mitotic activity is usually brisk, and abundant atypical mitotic figures are often present, which are useful in the differential diagnosis of benign mimics of osteosarcoma. No minimum quantity of bone formation is required; any amount is sufficient to render the diagnosis. Characteristically, the bone is intimately associated with the tumour cells; varies in quantity; is woven in architecture; and is deposited as primitive, disorganized trabeculae that may produce fine (filigree) or coarse lace-like patterns, or as broad, large sheets of compact bone formed by coalescing trabeculae.

Bone matrix is eosinophilic on H&E-stained sections if unmineralized and basophilic/purple if mineralized, and it may have a pagetoid appearance imparted by haphazardly deposited cement lines. Distinguishing unmineralized matrix (osteoid) from other eosinophilic extracellular materials such as collagen or compacted fibrin matrices may be difficult and subjective. Collagen tends to be less glassy and more fibrillar, and it is frequently deposited in broad aggregates or elongated fibrils compressed between lesional cells.

COS may have different histological patterns. Currently, however, there is no relationship between histological patterns, treatment, and prognosis {1322}. COS commonly contains varying amounts of neoplastic cartilage and/or fibroblastic components; on the basis of the predominant matrix, they are subdivided into osteoblastic (76–80%), chondroblastic (10–13%), and fibroblastic (10%) types {1322,197}. In osteoblastic osteosarcoma, neoplastic bone is the principal matrix and varies from thin, lace-like trabeculae to compact bone. When the latter is pronounced, the tumour is designated as a sclerosing type.

In chondroblastic osteosarcoma, the predominant component is hyaline cartilage with severe cytological atypia, but the chondroid matrix may also appear myxoid with single cells or delicate cords of cells displaying more-subtle atypia, particularly in tumours arising in gnathic bones. Neoplastic cartilage usually merges with areas containing neoplastic bone, often

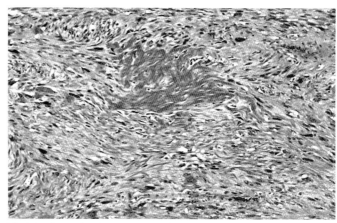

Fig. 3.84 Conventional osteosarcoma. Fibroblastic osteosarcoma composed of intersecting fascicles of pleomorphic spindle cells with central focus of neoplastic bone.

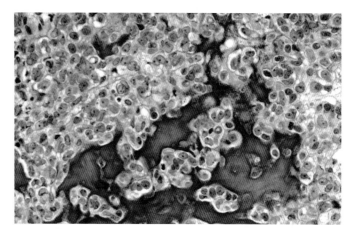

Fig. 3.85 Small cell osteosarcoma. High-power image.

with condensation and spindling of tumour cells at the periphery of the chondroid nodules. In the appropriate context, a biopsy containing only high-grade malignant cartilage should strongly raise the suspicion of chondroblastic osteosarcoma, especially in younger patients (in whom chondrosarcoma is much less common) and in the jaws, where chondrosarcoma practically does not occur. In fibroblastic osteosarcoma, the malignant cells are usually spindled and less frequently epithelioid; they often, but not always, demonstrate severe cytological atypia. The tumour cells are associated with extracellular collagen, which can be extensive, and they are often arranged in a storiform pattern. Non-neoplastic, osteoclast-type giant cells scattered throughout the tumour are the hallmark of the giant cell–rich subtype {288}. Some bone sarcomas without associated giant cell tumour of bone histology harbour an *H3-3A* (*H3F3A*) or *H3-3B* (*H3F3B*) p.Gly34 mutation; these are usually sited in the epiphysis in young people, suggesting a relationship with a giant cell tumour of bone. Therefore, there is a move to expand the definition of primary malignant giant cell tumour of bone on the basis of an *H3-3A* (*H3F3A*) or *H3-3B* (*H3F3B*) p.Gly34 mutation {91}. Large polyhedral tumour cells characterize the epithelioid osteosarcoma subtype {1693}. In the osteoblastoma-like subtype, the tumour cells usually show less-pronounced atypia and rim the neoplastic bony trabeculae as typically observed in osteoblastoma. However, the tumour

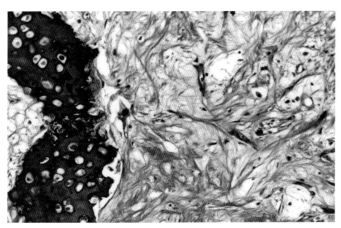
Fig. 3.86 Conventional osteosarcoma. Chemotherapy-induced change in osteosarcoma. There is neoplastic woven bone and the area previously inhabited by tumour cells is composed of reactive fibrous tissue.

infiltrates and encases pre-existing bone trabeculae as a sign of osteodestructive growth {287,192,1110}.

In TAEOS, the tumour is composed of blood-filled or empty cystic spaces closely simulating aneurysmal bone cyst. The septa show variable thickness and are populated by pleomorphic cells showing substantial nuclear hyperchromasia. Some malignant cells can be seen floating in the haemorrhagic areas. Atypical mitoses are easily identified. Osteoid formation is usually focal and confluent but may be absent in a biopsy. The septa also contain osteoclast-type giant cells. At the edges of the lesion, tumour permeation into pre-existing bone trabeculae is often observed.

SCOS is composed of small cells with scant cytoplasm, associated with osteoid production. Nuclei are round to oval and the chromatin may be fine to coarse; mitoses can easily be found. In the less frequent spindle cell type, nuclei are short and oval to spindle, with granular chromatin and inconspicuous nucleoli. A focal haemangiopericytoma-like pattern may be seen. Lace-like osteoid production is always present. Particular care must be taken to distinguish osteoid from fibrin deposits that may be seen among Ewing sarcoma cells.

Immunohistochemistry
COS has a broad immunoprofile that lacks diagnostic specificity. Commonly expressed antigens include SATB2, osteocalcin (*BGLAP*), osteonectin (*SPARC*), osteoprotegerin (*TNFRSF11B*), RUNX2, S100, actins, and CD99 {1311,961,742}. Importantly (because it is a diagnostic pitfall), osteosarcomas may also express keratin and EMA {2364,1779}. Tumour cells are generally negative for CD31, CD45, and FOS, with FOS representing a relatively recent surrogate marker for the *FOS* gene rearrangements typically observed in osteoid osteoma and osteoblastoma {1012,91A,1739A}. FOS immunohistochemistry might also be helpful in differentiating osteoblastoma and osteoblastoma-like osteosarcoma. TAEOS and SCOS have an immunophenotype similar to that of COS. SATB2 is regarded as a very sensitive marker for osteoblastic differentiation but lacks specificity.

It can help to distinguish SCOS from Ewing sarcoma, because it has been reported only rarely in the latter {654,2627,1929}.

Ultrastructure
Ultrastructurally, osteosarcoma cells have the features of mesenchymal cells with abundant dilated rough endoplasmic reticulum. The nuclei may be eccentric and the Golgi apparatus prominent. The matrix contains collagen fibres, which may show calcium hydroxyapatite crystal deposition. These findings can be helpful in excluding Ewing sarcoma, metastatic carcinoma, melanoma, and lymphoma.

Cytology
Not clinically relevant

Diagnostic molecular pathology
No specific diagnostic molecular pathology tests are available.

Essential and desirable diagnostic criteria
Essential: bone tumour with compatible imaging; bone production by tumour cells; permeative and destructive growth pattern; TAEOS: blood-filled or empty cystic spaces separated by fibrous septa; SCOS: small blue round cell morphology with focal neoplastic bone formation.
Desirable: tumour cells with high-grade atypia; atypical mitotic figures frequently present.

Staging
The eighth edition of the Union for International Cancer Control (UICC) *TNM classification of malignant tumours* stages osteosarcoma of the appendicular skeleton, trunk, skull, and facial bones on the basis of the greatest tumour dimension (≤ 8 cm: T1; > 8 cm: T2) and discontinuous involvement of the primary bone site (T3). Staging of spinal and pelvic tumours is based on anatomical intraosseous and extraosseous extension and size {423}.

The eighth edition of the American Joint Committee on Cancer (AJCC) *AJCC cancer staging manual* stages osteosarcoma arising in the appendicular, truncal, and craniofacial bones on the basis of the presence or absence of distant metastasis, histological grade, and greatest tumour dimension (≤ 8 cm or > 8 cm) {101}. However, dichotomization of tumour size fails to contribute prognostically significant information in this staging system {516, 517}. Tumours of the pelvic or spinal skeleton are now substaged on the basis of the anatomical extent of intraosseous invasion or presence of extraosseous invasion; prognostic stage groupings for these anatomical sites have not yet been developed.

The Musculoskeletal Tumor Society (MSTS) staging system is arguably the more clinically useful staging system for planning optimal surgical therapy and is based on the presence of metastatic disease, histological grade, and local anatomical extent (defined by the presence of extraosseous extension). However, breaking through the cortex with periosteal elevation (and intact periosteum) does not appear to be associated with worse outcome per se. Instead, tumour extension beyond the periosteum has been shown to significantly correlate with an inferior prognosis {2916,513,517}.

Prognosis and prediction

Aggressive local growth and rapid haematogenous systemic dissemination characterize the clinical course of COS. Pulmonary metastases, followed by skeletal deposits (sometimes presenting as skip metastases), are the most frequent sites of systemic disease. High-grade osteosarcoma is therefore usually treated with preoperative and postoperative chemotherapy; local control is achieved via surgical resection with wide margins, often using limb-salvage techniques {1968}. Radiation can be used for unresectable tumours {2638}. The use of multiagent chemotherapy for COS has had a dramatic impact on outcome {119,703}. In the pre-chemotherapy era, > 80% of patients treated with surgery alone died of disease, whereas 70% of patients with localized osteosarcoma of the extremities are currently long-term survivors {2638,119,703}. Unfortunately, patients presenting with metastatic or recurrent disease have a survival rate of < 30% {1560,588}.

The histological response to neoadjuvant chemotherapy remains one of the most important prognosticators of overall and disease-free survival {119,703}. A good response is usually defined as ≥ 90% necrosis {2726,516}. The prognosis of osteosarcoma is also influenced by tumour stage, anatomical location, and adequacy of surgical resection margins {314}. Localized distal disease, > 90% chemotherapy-induced tumour necrosis, and complete resection are positive prognostic factors associated with a 5-year survival rate of > 80% {989}. Predictors of poor outcome include proximal extremity or axial skeleton involvement, large tumour size/volume, detectable metastases at diagnosis, and poor response to preoperative chemotherapy (< 90% tumour necrosis). TAEOS is exquisitely sensitive to chemotherapy {116}, and the overall survival for these patients is similar to that seen with COS {195,3267}. SCOS has a slightly worse prognosis than COS, but no particular histological, imaging, or genetic findings related to prognosis have been identified to date {188,2240}.

Parosteal osteosarcoma

Wang J
Nord KH
O'Donnell PG
Yoshida A

Definition

Parosteal osteosarcoma is a low-grade malignant bone-forming neoplasm that arises on the cortical surface of bone.

ICD-O coding

9192/3 Parosteal osteosarcoma

ICD-11 coding

2B51.Z & XH8HG5 Osteosarcoma of bone and articular cartilage of unspecified sites & Parosteal osteosarcoma

Related terminology

Not recommended: juxtacortical osteosarcoma.

Subtype(s)

None

Localization

Approximately 70% of parosteal osteosarcomas are located at the posterior aspect of the distal femur in the metaphyseal region {2363,1292}; the next most common sites are the proximal portions of the tibia and humerus. Other less frequently involved sites include the craniofacial bones, ribs, and small bones of the hands and feet {1358,556,3171}.

Clinical features

Signs and symptoms

Patients present with a mass, which is occasionally painful. Distal femoral lesions are associated with restricted knee flexion.

A long history, frequently over a year, is typical {2363}; the history is sometimes shorter with primary dedifferentiated tumours {2836}.

Imaging

Radiographs show a mineralized, lobular mass at the bone surface, denser centrally than peripherally. Attachment to the bone may be slender or broad, with the remainder of the lesion separated by a lucent cleavage plane, representing intact periosteum. The underlying cortex may be normal, thickened, or destroyed. CT shows cortical changes, the lucent cleavage plane, and ossified intramedullary extension (which is seen with equal frequency in low-grade and dedifferentiated tumours) {2836,1520}. The mass is usually hypointense and heterogeneous on T1- and T2-weighted MRI sequences, but appearances suggesting fatty marrow may be seen in well-differentiated tumours {2732}. Lucent areas on radiographs and CT, which are hyperintense on fluid-sensitive MRI, raise the possibility of focal dedifferentiation {1520}, particularly when they are large, located deeply, and enhancing {1099,837}. A thin, usually incomplete, hyperintense rim corresponding to cartilage is occasionally seen on the tumour surface {1520}.

Epidemiology

Parosteal osteosarcoma accounts for about 4% of all osteosarcomas, and it is the most common type of surface osteosarcoma. It occurs in young adults, with a peak incidence in the third decade of life. There is a slight female predominance {2363}.

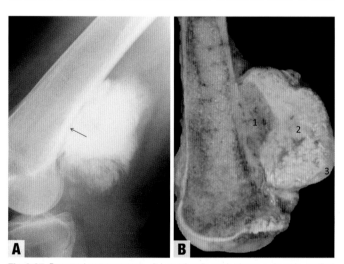

Fig. 3.87 Parosteal osteosarcoma. **A** Lateral radiograph shows a densely ossified mass attached to the posterior aspect of the distal femur superiorly, separated by a lucent plane inferiorly (arrow). **B** Gross appearance (sagittal section) showing the three tumour components: a well-differentiated deep component (1); a large, mineralized overlying mass (2); and the layer of cartilage on the tumour surface (3).

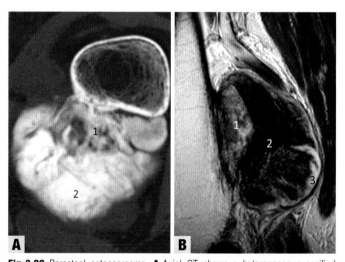

Fig. 3.88 Parosteal osteosarcoma. **A** Axial CT shows a heterogeneous ossified mass with slender attachment to the posterior cortex of the femur. A well-differentiated, relatively lucent component is seen deeply (1) and a lobular, sclerotic mass superficially (2). **B** Sagittal T2-weighted MRI shows a deep, well-differentiated (partially fatty) component (1) abutting femoral cortex, a large surrounding low-signal (ossifying) mass (2), and a thin hyperintense rim of cartilage on the surface of the tumour (3).

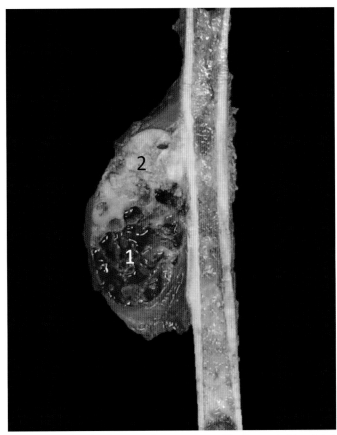

Fig. 3.89 Dedifferentiated parosteal osteosarcoma. The large dedifferentiated, haemorrhagic component is seen inferiorly (1); low-grade ossified tumour is present superiorly (2).

Etiology
Unknown

Pathogenesis
Parosteal osteosarcomas are cytogenetically characterized by one or more supernumerary ring chromosomes, often as the sole aberration. The chromosome number is typically near-diploid, and the tumours do not show the massive chromosomal rearrangements associated with high-grade osteosarcomas

{2160}. The ring chromosomes contain amplified material from chromosomal region 12q13-q15 {1160,1341,3017}. Potential target genes in these amplicons include *MDM2* and *CDK4*, which are amplified in > 85% of the cases {866,867,1341,2067,3317}. The same genes may be amplified in high-grade osteosarcoma with ring chromosomes, but the overall frequency of amplification is about 10% in conventional high-grade osteosarcomas, some of which may represent unrecognized dedifferentiated low-grade osteosarcomas {2067,562,256,866,3373}. Gene amplification is usually accompanied by increased expression of *MDM2* and *CDK4* at the RNA and protein levels {867,2067}.

Macroscopic appearance
Parosteal osteosarcoma presents as an exophytic, lobulated mass, typically attached to the underlying cortex by a broad base. Large tumours may encircle the involved bone. Satellite nodules may be noted, particularly in recurrent lesions. The cut surface shows a tan-white tumour with a hard gritty texture. Nodules of cartilage may be present. Occasionally, the cartilage may form an incomplete cartilage cap on the outer surface, simulating an osteochondroma {1866}. Penetration of the underlying cortex with or without invasion into the medullary cavity may be seen. Soft and fleshy areas, if present, suggest dedifferentiation of the tumour. Focal necrosis, haemorrhage, and fluid cavities may be present.

Histopathology
Parosteal osteosarcoma is composed of well-formed bone trabeculae with intervening fascicles of spindle cells. Typically, the tumour is hypocellular with minimal atypia and low mitotic activity. At the periphery of the tumour, the spindle cell component may show invasion into the adjacent skeletal muscle. Some tumours may resemble desmoplastic fibroma because of focal lack of bone formation. In about 20% of the cases, the tumour is more cellular and the spindle cells show moderate atypia. The bone trabeculae are arranged mostly in a parallel fashion and may or may not show osteoblastic rimming. Some tumours contain irregular anastomosing and curved bone trabeculae, simulating woven bone in fibrous dysplasia. Approximately 50% of cases display cartilaginous differentiation, in the form of small scattered nodules or a cartilaginous cap. Progression to high-grade sarcoma, which can also be referred to as

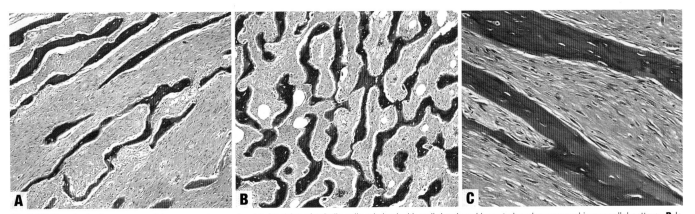

Fig. 3.90 Parosteal osteosarcoma. **A** Low-power image showing fascicles of spindle cells admixed with well-developed bone trabeculae arranged in a parallel pattern. **B** Irregular anastomosing and curved bone trabeculae in parosteal osteosarcoma simulating fibrous dysplasia. **C** Higher magnification showing spindle cells with mild atypia and bone trabeculae.

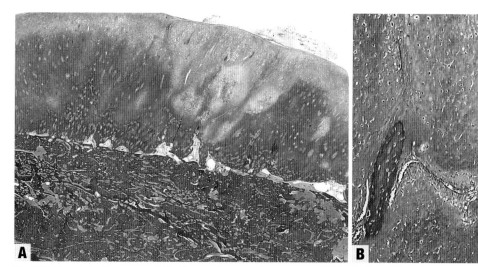

Fig. 3.91 Parosteal osteosarcoma. **A** Cartilage cap in parosteal osteosarcoma. **B** Cartilaginous differentiation in parosteal osteosarcoma.

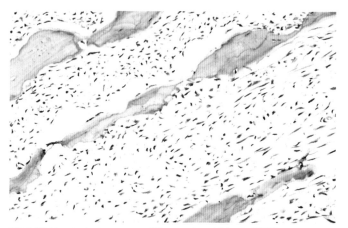

Fig. 3.92 Parosteal osteosarcoma. Diffuse nuclear staining for MDM2.

dedifferentiation, occurs in 15–43% of cases, either at presentation or (more often) at the time of recurrence {2363,2836, 3303,290}. The high-grade component can be osteosarcoma or undifferentiated spindle cell sarcoma {290,190}, or very rarely rhabdomyosarcoma {2599}.

Immunohistochemistry

Immunohistochemical study of MDM2 and CDK4 may provide a useful diagnostic tool in parosteal osteosarcoma, particularly in small biopsies and/or when molecular access is limited {3372, 867}. Analysis of MDM2 and CDK4 may also help identify dedifferentiated parosteal osteosarcoma with limited low-grade components {3373}.

Differential diagnosis

Because of its deceptively bland appearance, parosteal osteosarcoma must be differentiated from a variety of benign fibrous and fibro-osseous lesions, including florid reactive periostitis, juxtacortical myositis ossificans, desmoplastic fibroma, and fibrous dysplasia protuberans. In addition to the clinical, radiological, and pathological features, *MDM2* amplification assay or the surrogate immunostaining of MDM2 and CDK4 is helpful in the distinction, because the above-mentioned mimics are negative for *MDM2* amplification. Unlike in osteochondroma, the cartilage cap in some parosteal osteosarcomas is mildly hypercellular and the chondrocytes show mild atypia and lack the perpendicular columnar arrangement seen in osteochondromas. Parosteal osteosarcoma can be morphologically distinguished from periosteal osteosarcoma and high-grade surface

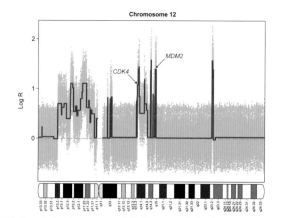

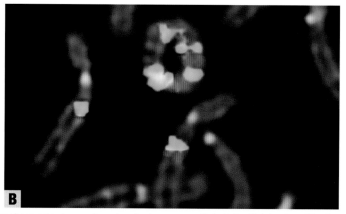

Fig. 3.93 Parosteal osteosarcoma. **A** SNP array analysis of a parosteal osteosarcoma shows gain of genomic regions in chromosome 12, including high-level amplification of *CDK4* and *MDM2*. **B** Partial metaphase spread from a parosteal osteosarcoma. FISH analysis using probes specific for *MDM2* (red) and *CDK4* (green) shows that the ring chromosome contains many copies of these genes.

osteosarcoma, the other two subtypes of surface osteosarcoma. The presence of a focal low-grade spindle cell component and/ or *MDM2* amplification suggests dedifferentiated parosteal osteosarcoma over high-grade surface osteosarcoma.

Cytology
Not clinically relevant

Diagnostic molecular pathology
FISH for *MDM2* amplification is more sensitive and specific than immunohistochemistry.

Essential and desirable diagnostic criteria
Essential: bone tumour with compatible imaging; parosteal location; low-grade spindle cell tumour with woven bone formation.
Desirable: MDM2 amplification.

Staging
The Union for International Cancer Control (UICC) *TNM classification of malignant tumours* {423} does not recommend that the TNM staging system for bone tumours be applied to surface/ juxtacortical osteosarcoma or juxtacortical chondrosarcoma. However, other staging systems, such as the American Joint Committee on Cancer (AJCC) TNM system {101}, do include these tumours in the bone staging system. See also the information on staging in *Bone tumours: Introduction* (p. 340).

Prognosis and prediction
The prognosis is excellent, with a 90% overall survival rate at 5 years {2363}. For pure low-grade tumours, wide surgical excision is curative. Incomplete resection results in local recurrence. Metastasis, usually a late phenomenon, occurs rarely in low-grade tumours, whereas dedifferentiated tumours metastasize at a high rate, leading to a poor prognosis. Chemotherapy is reserved for dedifferentiated tumours.

Periosteal osteosarcoma

Bonar SFM
Klein MJ
O'Donnell PG

Definition
Periosteal osteosarcoma is a malignant, predominantly chondroblastic, intermediate-grade bone-forming sarcoma arising on the surface of the bone, typically underneath the periosteum.

ICD-O coding
9193/3 Periosteal osteosarcoma

ICD-11 coding
2B51.Z & XH48A9 Osteosarcoma of bone and articular cartilage of unspecified sites & Periosteal osteosarcoma

Related terminology
Not recommended: juxtacortical chondroblastic osteosarcoma.

Subtype(s)
None

Localization
Periosteal osteosarcoma usually occurs in the diaphysis of the femur and tibia {524,532,1222,1943,2221,291,697,3133}. Occasionally, cases occur in other long bones and flat bones, with rare examples arising in craniofacial and acral bones {2221,532, 1222}. Rare bilateral metachronous and synchronous cases are documented {1943}, and a single case in a patient with Marfan syndrome is recorded {3324}.

Clinical features
Signs and symptoms
Swelling and/or pain of short duration (weeks to months) is characteristic {291,2221,697,3133}.

Imaging
Radiographs show a lucent, fusiform mass on the surface of bone, with variable mineralization (usually fine perpendicular (hair-on-end) ossific striations, frequently accompanied by focal clumps of calcification). The cortex is thickened, with an adjacent solid or lamellated periosteal reaction and occasionally a Codman triangle. Although the thickened cortex is eroded by the mass, the endosteal cortex typically remains intact. CT and MRI often suggest an extensive chondroblastic component, based on low attenuation, hyperintensity on fluid-sensitive MRI sequences, and typical enhancement. Axial images show that tumour encircles at most approximately 50% of the bone circumference. Marrow infiltration is rare and abnormal marrow signal usually reactive {2221}.

Epidemiology
Periosteal osteosarcoma accounts for < 2% of all osteosarcomas {3128,2221,524,532,697,3133}. Peak incidence is in the second decade of life (range: first to seventh decade) {524,532,1222,1250}. Overall, the sexes are affected equally {524,532,1250,2221}.

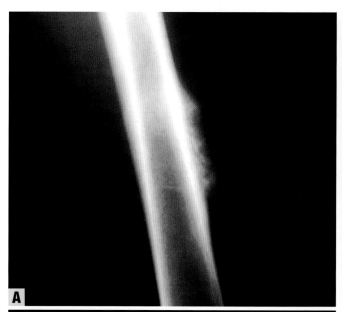

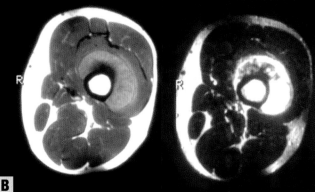

Fig. 3.94 Periosteal osteosarcoma. **A** Lateral radiograph of the left femur. There is a fusiform mass on the bone surface, showing dense calcification and lobular less-mineralized tumour superficially, within which are irregular bone spicules. The cortex of the femur appears intact. **B** Axial T1-weighted (**left**) and T2-weighted (**right**) MRI of the left femur. The surface mass incompletely surrounds the bone. It is hyperintense on both sequences, with homogeneous low signal at its base, indicating ossification, and slender hypointense strands, best seen on the T1-weighted image, due to fine bone spicules. The cortex is thinned laterally but not disrupted, and marrow signal is normal.

Etiology
Unknown

Pathogenesis
Very rare cases in large series of osteosarcomas have been genetically studied, but no consistent anomaly is documented {2404,415}. In some cases, more-complex chromosomal alterations and point mutations in *TP53*, similar to those seen in high-grade osteosarcoma, are recorded {256,1943,2404}.

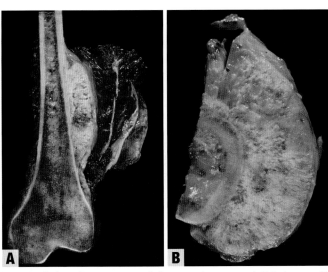

Fig. 3.95 Periosteal osteosarcoma. **A** Gross specimen, coronal. Pale tumour with visible vertical perpendicular spiculation confined to the surface of the cortex and entirely beneath the periosteum, lending a fusiform architecture. The cortex and medullary cavity are unremarkable. **B** Gross specimen, axial. In this section, much of the tumour has a translucent, chondroid appearance. Irregular cream-coloured ossification is visible near the cortex, whereas the spiculated linear appearance predominates at the perimeter. A surface rim of periosteum surrounds the tumour, and the cortex and medulla are intact.

Macroscopic appearance

The tumour, in continuity with the inner periosteum, has a demarcated lobulated broad-based ovoid appearance and is attached to the surface of the cortex, elevating the outer periosteum, producing a fusiform architecture. Cortical thickening may be conspicuous, with the mass causing cortical scalloping. The tumour comprises lobulated pale glistening cartilaginous tissue. Reactive bone spicules emanating from the cortex may be visible, and a delineated surface capsule derived from the periosteum is usual {3128,291,697,3133}.

Histopathology

The tumour comprises poorly delineated lobules of cytologically atypical cartilage with intervening bands of primitive sarcomatous cells in which bone formation is present. Atypical fibroblastic areas may occur. Perpendicular periosteal reaction may be present, corresponding to the hair-on-end reaction seen on conventional radiographs. Primitive-appearing undifferentiated mesenchymal cells with nuclear atypia and mitoses prevail at the perimeter of the tumour. In cartilaginous areas, transition to osteoid matrix occurs {3128,291,697,3133}.

Immunohistochemistry

SATB2 immunoexpression does not distinguish chondroblastic osteosarcoma from high-grade chondrosarcoma and is unhelpful in diagnosis {1929}.

Differential diagnosis

Periosteal chondrosarcomas occur in older individuals, are metaphyseal in distribution, have coarse calcification, and contain large lobules of well-differentiated hyaline cartilage. Tumour bone is absent. Parosteal osteosarcoma exhibits a protuberant mushrooming architecture arising from outer layers of the periosteum and is fibroblastic, with more mature appearing bone

formation. High-grade surface osteosarcoma has anaplastic high-grade features throughout, with distribution and demographic status similar to those of conventional osteosarcoma {2365,697}.

Cytology

Not clinically relevant

Diagnostic molecular pathology

MDM2/CDK4 amplification and IDH mutations have not been identified {2626,93}.

Essential and desirable diagnostic criteria

Essential: bone tumour with compatible imaging; surface location under the periosteum; intermediate-grade, largely chondroblastic osteosarcoma.

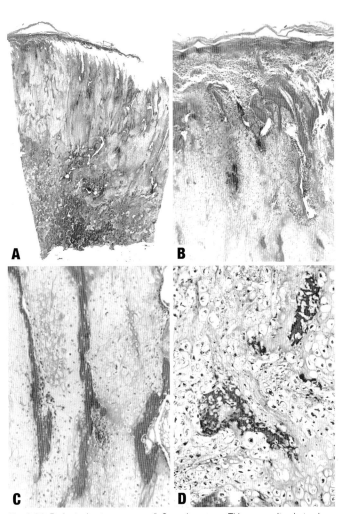

Fig. 3.96 Periosteal osteosarcoma. **A** Scanning power. This composite photomicrograph demonstrates pale cartilaginous areas with intervening linear arrays of reactive bone coursing through the matrix towards the perimeter. The base is more densely ossified and consists of tumour bone and cartilage matrix. Note the thin layer of periosteum along the surface. **B** Higher power of the tumour periphery demonstrates a tendency of the tumour cells to spindle. **C** At higher power, the linear reactive bone spicules are separated by cartilaginous tumour matrix, with focal central lace-like osteoid production. **D** Atypical nuclear morphology of the cartilaginous matrix is illustrated and central osteoid formation is present.

Staging

The Union for International Cancer Control (UICC) *TNM classification of malignant tumours* {423} does not recommend that the TNM staging system for bone tumours be applied to surface/juxtacortical osteosarcoma or juxtacortical chondrosarcoma. However, other staging systems, such as the American Joint Committee on Cancer (AJCC) TNM system {101}, do include these tumours in the bone staging system. See also the information on staging in *Bone tumours: Introduction* (p. 340).

Prognosis and prediction

Periosteal osteosarcoma has a better prognosis than conventional osteosarcoma, with disease-free survival rates of 89% at 5 years and 77–86% at 10 years. Marrow involvement, originally thought to preclude the diagnosis, is rare and may predict more-aggressive behaviour: cases without marrow involvement show a trend towards a better outcome at 5 years {524, 532,1250,2617}. Wide excision is optimal. Local recurrence, metastasis, and death usually occur within 3 years of diagnosis {1222,2657}. Chemotherapy, although frequently used, does not appear to influence prognosis or survival {524,532,1250, 2657,2617}. Assessment of postchemotherapy necrosis is not predictive of outcome {524,532,1222,697}. Occasional patients treated with chemotherapy developed a second malignancy {524,1222}.

High-grade surface osteosarcoma

Klein MJ
Bonar SFM
O'Donnell PG

Definition
High-grade surface osteosarcoma is a high-grade malignant bone-forming neoplasm arising on the surface of the bone.

ICD-O coding
9194/3 High-grade surface osteosarcoma

ICD-11 coding
2B51.Z & XH6TL0 Osteosarcoma of bone and articular cartilage of unspecified sites & High-grade surface osteosarcoma

Related terminology
None

Subtype(s)
None

Localization
The three most common sites, in descending frequency, are the femur, tibia, and humerus. In the long bones, high-grade surface osteosarcomas are most frequently diaphyseal or diametaphyseal.

Clinical features
Signs and symptoms
Swelling and pain of short duration are usual.

Imaging
A radiodense mass extends into soft tissue from the bone surface, usually showing fluffy, ill-defined immature ossification. Purely radiolucent lesions are rare {572,2365}. Dense ossification may occur {3173}, and the mass may show radiating bone spicules similar to periosteal osteosarcoma. A cleavage plane of radiolucency representing the periosteum is unusual {3173}. Cortical erosion and medullary involvement, rare in periosteal osteosarcomas, are seen in about half of patients with high-grade surface osteosarcomas and are best demonstrated using cross-sectional imaging {2929}. Soft tissue extension may be seen. A periosteal reaction is uncommon and variable {2365}. There is usually greater circumferential involvement than in other types of surface osteosarcomas {3357}.

Epidemiology
High-grade surface osteosarcomas account for < 1% of osteosarcomas. The published incidence shows a male predominance and a peak incidence in the second decade of life {2365}. However, because there are very few published cases and most of them are derived from consultation files, the statistical significance is questionable.

Etiology
Unknown

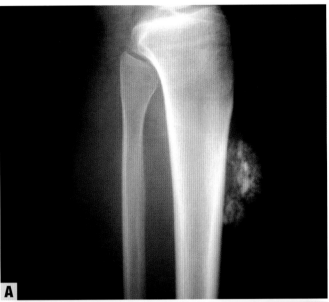

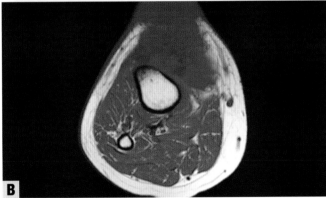

Fig. 3.97 High-grade surface osteosarcoma. **A** Lateral radiograph of the right tibia and fibula. An elliptical mass is projected adjacent to the tibial bone surface, showing fairly dense lobular and punctate mineralization. No cortical destruction is identified. **B** Axial T1-weighted MRI of the right proximal calf. A lobular mass is located on the subcutaneous surface of the tibia. It causes cortical thinning, invades adjacent muscle, extends into the subcutaneous fat, and fungates through the skin. Lobular low signal in the deep aspect of the mass is consistent with ossification.

Pathogenesis
The pathogenetic mechanisms of high-grade surface osteosarcoma are unknown. High-grade surface osteosarcomas arising in parosteal osteosarcomas (dedifferentiated parosteal osteosarcomas) display amplification of *MDM2* and *CDK4*. The single case of *TSPAN31* (*SAS*) amplification in a high-grade surface osteosarcoma heretofore described {2616} was an example of dedifferentiated parosteal osteosarcoma because it had grade 1 foci.

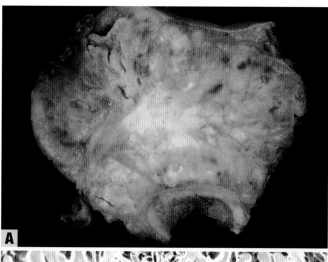

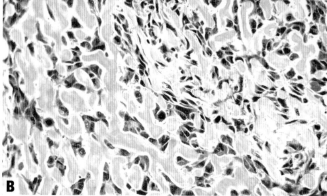

Fig. 3.98 High-grade surface osteosarcoma. **A** Gross specimen sectioned axially demonstrates a large tumour mass extending from the bone surface to the skin. The cortex and medullary cavity are not involved. The tumour has a heterogeneous appearance, ranging from densely ossified to fleshy. **B** The histology is typical of high-grade osteoblastic osteosarcoma, with malignant-appearing polyhedral and spindle cells producing an immature osteoid matrix with a lace-like pattern. Note the abundant mitoses.

Macroscopic appearance

The tumour is usually well circumscribed externally and situated on the fibrous periosteal surface. It often extends through the periosteum to attach to or even erode the underlying cortical surface. Endosteal extension may be present, but the bulk of the tumour is outside the bone. Its cut surface is variable because its appearance depends on the predominant type of

extracellular matrix produced, as well as on the cellularity of the tumour stroma.

Histopathology

These tumours are histologically identical to high-grade conventional osteosarcoma, with the same degree of matrix variability. Immunohistochemistry is not relevant to making the diagnosis.

Differential diagnosis

The degree of cytological atypia is greater than in periosteal osteosarcoma. No areas of low-grade osteosarcoma should be demonstrable {2365}.

Cytology

Not clinically relevant

Diagnostic molecular pathology

Not clinically relevant

Essential and desirable diagnostic criteria

Essential: bone tumour with compatible imaging; histologically high-grade osteosarcoma; arising on the surface of the bone without a substantial intraosseous component.

Staging

The Union for International Cancer Control (UICC) *TNM classification of malignant tumours* {423} does not recommend that the TNM staging system for bone tumours be applied to surface/juxtacortical osteosarcoma or juxtacortical chondrosarcoma. However, other staging systems, such as the American Joint Committee on Cancer (AJCC) TNM system {101}, do include these tumours in the bone staging system. See also the information on staging in *Bone tumours: Introduction* (p. 340).

Prognosis and prediction

The overall 5-year survival rate of patients with high-grade surface osteosarcoma, compiled from the two studies reporting follow-up, is 62% {2365,2929}. Factors that favour survival include good response to neoadjuvant chemotherapy {2365} and localized disease. Poor response to chemotherapy, metastatic disease at the time of presentation, and local recurrence are adverse factors {2365,2929}. The presence of medullary involvement does not seem to be an independent prognostic factor {2365}.

Secondary osteosarcoma

Flanagan AM
Bridge JA
O'Donnell PG

Definition
Secondary osteosarcoma is osteosarcoma arising in abnormal bone.

ICD-O coding
9184/3 Secondary osteosarcoma

ICD-11 coding
2B51.Z & XH06W9 Osteosarcoma of bone and articular cartilage of unspecified sites & Osteosarcoma in Paget disease of bone (encompasses secondary osteosarcoma)

Related terminology
Acceptable: Paget sarcoma; osteosarcoma in Paget disease of bone (PDB); radiation-associated osteosarcoma.
Not recommended: postirradiation sarcoma; radiation-induced sarcoma

Subtype(s)
Osteosarcoma in Paget disease of bone; radiation-associated sarcoma; infarct-related osteosarcoma; osteosarcoma due to chronic osteomyelitis; implant-related osteosarcoma; osteosarcoma secondary to early postzygotic disorders such as fibrous dysplasia

Localization
Paget sarcoma most commonly affects the femur (34%), pelvis (24%), and humerus (24%) {1893}, reflecting the distribution of uncomplicated PDB, except for a disproportionately high and low incidence in the humerus (24%) and the spine (2%) {1893}, respectively. Multifocal synchronous tumours may occur (2–17%) {3209}. Long bone lesions tend to be metaphyseal {2894}, and tumours have been noted to occur at the site of a previous fracture {2185}. Radiation-associated osteosarcoma occurs at the site of radiotherapy, most frequently in the flat bones of the chest wall and pelvis {3019}.

Osteosarcoma related to premalignant bone syndromes generally affects the same locations as non-syndromic osteosarcoma. However, tumours may be multifocal in Rothmund–Thomson syndrome and occur at unusual sites in Werner syndrome (foot and ankle, patella) {465}. Bone sarcomas outside the radiation field in hereditary retinoblastoma develop predominantly in the lower limbs {1975}.

Clinical features
Signs and symptoms
New pain and an enlarging mass in a patient with a history of predisposing bone condition suggest the diagnosis of secondary osteosarcoma; occasionally, the underlying condition is unknown. Paget sarcoma typically develops in a background of polyostotic symptomatic PDB {2185}. Tumours are frequently lytic, occasionally mineralized {2185,2833}, and

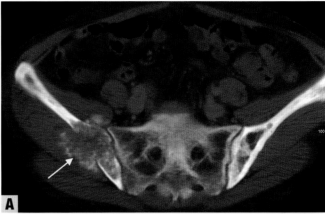
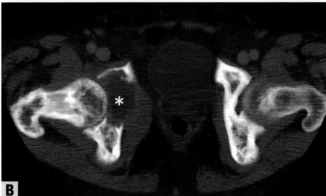

Fig. 3.99 Paget osteosarcoma. **A** Axial CT shows multifocal synchronous tumour at presentation. An osteoblastic lesion is present in the right ilium (arrow). **B** The more inferior tumour in the acetabulum is lytic (asterisk). There is background cortical thickening and trabecular coarsening in the pelvis and right proximal femur due to Paget disease.

may be multifocal {3209}. Pathological fracture is common {1893}.

Imaging
Radiographs show lytic (65%) destruction of pagetic bone {2894}, and there is typically a large extraosseous mass. Lytic tumours appear photopenic on isotope scintigraphy {1893}; mineralized lesions may be difficult to distinguish from adjacent PDB {2185}. Replacement of fatty, heterogeneous pagetic marrow, cortical destruction, and an extraosseous mass are useful MRI findings to differentiate secondary osteosarcoma from PDB. Radiation-associated osteosarcoma usually presents some years after treatment, with aggressive bone destruction and an extraosseous mass, superimposed on postradiotherapy bone changes {2833}. Syndromes predisposing individuals to secondary osteosarcoma may show evidence of a bone dysplasia (e.g. in Rothmund–Thomson syndrome {465}) but otherwise show similar presentation and imaging to non-syndromic

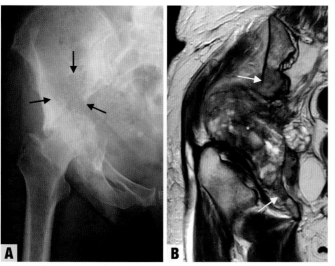

Fig. 3.100 Postirradiation osteosarcoma. **A** Anteroposterior radiograph of the right hemipelvis showing lytic destruction of the right ilium (arrows) and pathological fracture of the acetabulum, with central dislocation of the right hip. Postradiotherapy sclerosis is present in the right ilium after radiotherapy 12 years previously for a gynaecological malignancy. **B** Coronal T2-weighted MRI of the right hemipelvis. The lytic tumour corresponds to a haemorrhagic mass (asterisk), which has destroyed the acetabulum and infiltrated the ilium and ischium (arrows).

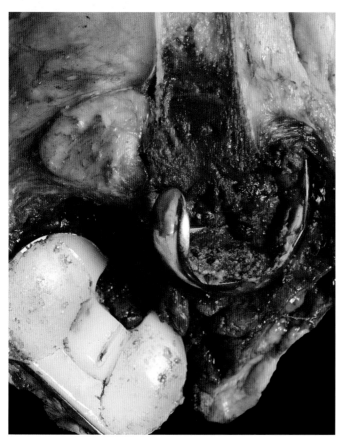

Fig. 3.101 Secondary osteosarcoma. Osteosarcoma arising in association with a total knee prosthesis. The tumour is haemorrhagic and has destroyed the bone.

osteosarcoma {465,1282,1899}. Osteosarcoma at the site of a pre-existing benign bone tumour or chronic osteomyelitis may show imaging evidence of the underlying disease, posttreatment

changes, and aggressive bone destruction. Infarct-related osteosarcoma usually occurs at the knee. The tumour usually develops in the margin {2933} but may obliterate all evidence of the infarct {2933}.

Epidemiology

Osteosarcoma is the most common sarcoma associated with PDB {1296}. PDB develops predominantly in populations of English descent: 50% of bone sarcomas in patients aged > 50 years are secondary to PDB in endemic areas {1893}. In areas where PDB is not found, there is no second, older peak in the bimodal incidence of osteosarcoma {2542,1296}. The incidence of Paget sarcoma in PDB is 0.7–6.3% {1893}, but as the incidence of PDB is declining, Paget sarcoma also appears to be less frequent {1970} and is occurring at older ages {1970}. Most patients are in the sixth to seventh decades of life {1893} (range: 32–86 years {1212}).

Radiation-associated osteosarcoma most commonly arises in bone after treatment of tumours with long survival (breast and cervical carcinomas, Hodgkin lymphoma, retinoblastoma) {2462}. Radiation-associated osteosarcoma is estimated to occur in 0.03% of patients receiving radiotherapy {2462}, with osteosarcoma accounting for 21–77% {396,2833}. The median latency period after radiotherapy is 10 years {2462} (range: 3–55 years {1451,3254}). Most patients are in the fifth decade of life, with an earlier peak in the second decade (children treated for hereditary retinoblastoma and other malignancies) {2462}. Osteosarcoma in older populations is most frequently due to Paget disease or irradiation {2815}.

Etiology

Ionizing irradiation is the strongest risk factor for developing secondary osteosarcoma. Development of a radiation-associated osteosarcoma appears to be dose-dependent, with lower, potentially mutagenic doses at the edge of the radiation field {2833}. Most patients who develop radiation-associated osteosarcoma have received a median of 50 Gy {2462}. Bone infarction is an acknowledged cause of undifferentiated sarcoma, and an association between caisson disease, sickle cell disease, other biological insults, and osteosarcoma is now recognized {1541,1094,3090}. Sarcomas, including osteosarcoma, infrequently develop adjacent to orthopaedic implants {1594}. A causal link to the constituents of implanted material, which may be carcinogenic in vitro, has been suggested but not proven {1604}.

Pathogenesis

The pathogenesis of secondary osteosarcoma is likely to be variable and determined by its etiology. Comparison of transcriptome modification identified a signature of 135 genes discriminating radiation-associated sarcomas from sporadic sarcomas; the functions of the signature genes suggest that radiation-associated osteosarcomas were subject to chronic oxidative stress, probably as a result of mitochondrial dysfunction {1269}. Two mutation signatures of ionizing radiation, an excess of small deletions and balanced inversions (both aberration types generate driver mutations), have been identified by paired tumour–normal tissue whole-genome sequencing in radiation-associated malignancies, including radiation-associated osteosarcoma {255}. Radiation-associated osteosarcomas feature complex karyotypes {2096,256,255}. Unlike in primary osteosarcoma, losses are more frequent than gains; in particular, loss at 1p is more common (57% vs 3%).

Macroscopic appearance

The macroscopic features of secondary osteosarcoma are not significantly different from those of primary osteosarcoma. The tumours occur at all sites in bone: in a series of 23 radiation-associated osteosarcomas in children/adolescents (excluding retinoblastomas), 21 were central, 1 was a high-grade surface lesion, and 1 was a periosteal osteosarcoma {3019}. When an osteosarcoma develops in association with fibrous dysplasia and is diagnosed early, the features of the fibrous dysplastic bone may be apparent, but this is rare.

Histopathology

The histological features of secondary osteosarcoma are not distinguishable from those of primary osteosarcoma.

Cytology

Not clinically relevant

Diagnostic molecular pathology

Not clinically relevant

Essential and desirable diagnostic criteria

Essential: bone tumour with compatible imaging; known history of previous radiation therapy or the presence of an underlying bone abnormality; osteosarcoma histology.
Desirable: histological evidence of underlying abnormal bone.

Staging

Staging is according to bone sarcoma protocols (see *TNM staging of tumours of bone*, p. 339). See also the information on staging in *Bone tumours: Introduction* (p. 340).

Prognosis and prediction

The prognosis of Paget sarcoma and radiation-associated osteosarcoma, which are typically high-grade tumours unresponsive to chemotherapy, is worse than that of conventional osteosarcoma. In Paget sarcoma, patient age contributes to poor prognosis: the 2-year survival rate is 25%; 29% of patients have pulmonary metastases at presentation {1893}.

The 5-year survival rate in radiation-associated osteosarcoma is 10–32% {2833}; 87% of tumours are high-grade {396}, and many patients die from metastatic disease within a few months {2641}. Prognosis is better in operable extremity lesions {1470}.

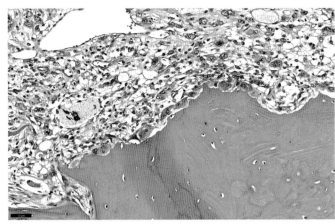

Fig. 3.102 Osteosarcoma in Paget disease of bone. The pre-existing bone shows features of Paget disease: the bone is thickened with mosaic lines of mineralization and is bordered by osteoclasts. A highly pleomorphic sarcoma is present, with bizarre nuclei and atypical mitoses, adjacent to the aberrant bone.

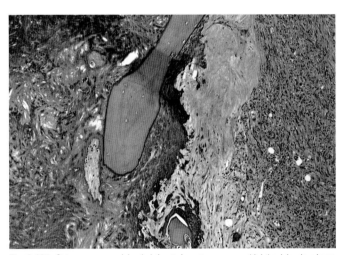

Fig. 3.103 Osteosarcoma arising in infarct. An osteosarcoma (right) arising in a bone affected by infarction (left).

The use of alkylating agents {3117} and younger age at treatment {3019} increase the risk of radiation-associated osteosarcoma and may reduce the latency period {2833}.

In the setting of cancer predisposition syndromes, the treatment and prognosis of individual tumours are similar to those of non-syndromic lesions; management is complicated and aims to maximize clinical surveillance while minimizing radiation exposure {465}.

Desmoplastic fibroma of bone

Suurmeijer AJH
Cleton-Jansen AM

Definition
Desmoplastic fibroma of bone is an extremely rare locally aggressive bone tumour composed of bland spindle cells set in abundant collagen, with histology reminiscent of desmoid-type fibromatosis.

ICD-O coding
8823/1 Desmoplastic fibroma

ICD-11 coding
2F7B & XH6YK5 Neoplasms of uncertain behaviour of bone and articular cartilage & Desmoplastic fibroma

Related terminology
Not recommended: desmoid tumour of bone.

Subtype(s)
None

Localization
Desmoplastic fibroma may involve any bone but is most frequently found in the mandible, followed by long bones (femur, radius, tibia) and pelvic bones.

Clinical features
Signs and symptoms
Some tumours are found incidentally in asymptomatic patients. However, most patients have a longstanding history of pain or bone deformity. In about 10% of cases, a pathological fracture is the presenting symptom.

Imaging
Radiographically, desmoplastic fibroma is a well-defined, lobulated, radiolucent lesion that may expand the host bone. Intralesional trabeculation is often present. Larger lesions may destroy cortical bone and extend into surrounding soft tissue, which is well appreciated by MRI. Desmoplastic fibroma has low signal intensity in both T1- and T2-weighted MRI images and may show increased uptake with bone scintigraphy or FDG PET.

Epidemiology
Desmoplastic fibroma accounts for < 0.1% of all primary bone tumours. The tumour mainly affects adolescents and young adults, with near-equal sex distribution.

Etiology
Unknown

Pathogenesis
Unknown

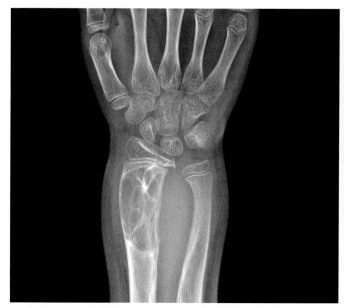

Fig. 3.104 Desmoplastic fibroma of bone with a *CTNNB1* (p.Ser45Phe) mutation. Plain radiograph showing a well-demarcated lytic tumour of the distal radius with cortical breakthrough, extension in surrounding soft tissue, and bowing of the ulna.

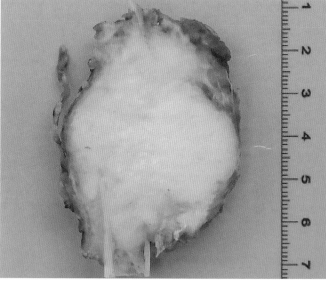

Fig. 3.105 Desmoplastic fibroma of bone. Recurrent tumour showing invasion of bone and surrounding soft tissue. The cut surface of the tumour has a fibrous appearance.

Macroscopic appearance
Due to its high collagen content, desmoplastic fibroma is a firm, creamy-white tumour with a whorled architecture. The tumour

border is well defined and has scalloped margins, even when it extends into soft tissue.

Histopathology

Desmoplastic fibroma has an infiltrative growth pattern and typically consists of a tumour of low cellularity composed of fascicles of bland nondescript spindle cells set in a collagenous matrix. Mitoses are scant. Necrosis is not present. The fibroblastic spindle cells show variable immunoreactivity for SMA; β-catenin can be present {2908}, most commonly in the cytoplasm {1321}. The differential diagnosis includes fibrous dysplasia, low-grade central osteosarcoma, low-grade myofibroblastic sarcoma, myoepithelial tumours, follicular dendritic cell tumours, and synovial sarcoma.

Cytology

Not clinically relevant

Diagnostic molecular pathology

In view of recent advances in molecular pathology allowing classification of bone tumours more objectively, the diagnosis of desmoplastic fibroma should be one of exclusion. In particular, fibrous dysplasia and low-grade central osteosarcoma should be excluded by molecular tests for *GNAS* single-nucleotide variants and *MDM2* amplification, respectively. There are reports of two cases of desmoplastic fibroma in bone revealing a *CTNNB1* mutation: one p.Thr41Ala {1038} and one p.Ser45Phe alteration {2908}. Both cases exhibited nuclear β-catenin immunostaining. Previously, *CTNNB1* mutations were not detected in a series of 13 cases {1321}.

Essential and desirable diagnostic criteria

Essential: a bland spindle cell lesion in bone; collagenous matrix.

Desirable: exclude fibrous dysplasia by showing the absence of *GNAS* mutations; exclude low-grade central osteosarcoma by showing the absence of *MDM2* amplification.

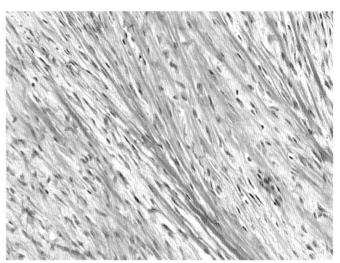

Fig. 3.106 Desmoplastic fibroma of bone. Tumour with fascicles of fibroblastic spindle cells embedded in fibrillary collagen.

Staging

Not clinically relevant

Prognosis and prediction

Prognosis and prediction are difficult to predict because so few cases have been reported. Desmoplastic fibroma is a slowly progressive and locally aggressive tumour, which may recur after curettage or intralesional excision {2261A}.

Fibrosarcoma of bone

Dei Tos AP
Czerniak B
Inwards CY

Definition
Fibrosarcoma of bone is a spindle cell malignant neoplasm of bone composed of relatively monomorphic fibroblastic tumour cells with variable collagen production and a fascicular (commonly herringbone) architecture. The diagnosis is one of exclusion.

ICD-O coding
8810/3 Fibrosarcoma NOS

ICD-11 coding
2B5J & XH4EP1 Malignant miscellaneous tumours of bone or articular cartilage of other or unspecified sites & Fibrosarcoma NOS

Related terminology
None

Subtype(s)
None

Localization
The distal femur is the most common site (21–47%), with the proximal femur (16%), distal humerus (14%), and proximal tibia (11%) also involved {1449,3021}.

Clinical features
Signs and symptoms
The most common clinical signs and symptoms are local pain, swelling, limitation of motion, and pathological fracture.

Imaging
Typical imaging findings include eccentrically located, lytic lesions with a geographical, moth-eaten, or permeative pattern of destruction and frequent extension into adjacent soft tissues.

Epidemiology
Historically, the term "fibrosarcoma of bone" has been applied to primary malignant spindle cell neoplasms of bone in which the tumour cells are typically organized in a fascicular or herringbone pattern. But a variety of primary bone tumours occupying other specific diagnostic categories may also show this histological pattern; therefore, there are no properties distinctive of or specific for fibrosarcoma of bone. This term is uncommonly used as a specific diagnostic category today, particularly due to the advent of ancillary techniques and evolving classification schemes. Therefore, the incidence is probably far less than the reported rates of as many as 5% of all primary malignant bone tumours. Tumours with a predominance of this fibrosarcomatous pattern, but probably representing a variety of tumour types, have been described with equal sex distribution and relatively uniform incidence over the second to sixth decades of

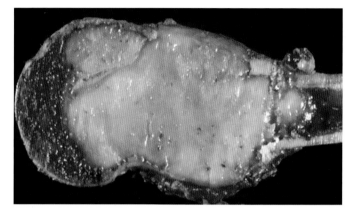

Fig. 3.107 Fibrosarcoma. Gross specimen of primary fibrosarcoma of bone. Cut surface is whitish and translucent, with more dense areas at the periphery.

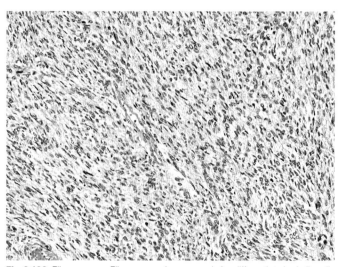

Fig. 3.108 Fibrosarcoma. Fibrosarcoma is composed of undifferentiated spindle cells organized in fascicles. No specific line of differentiation is present.

life, with occasional occurrence in infants {276,711,1449,1753, 2651}. Fibrosarcoma of bone represents a diagnosis of exclusion once specific lines of differentiation are excluded.

Etiology
Unknown

Pathogenesis
There is little information in the literature regarding genetic changes in tumours with fibrosarcomatous differentiation {1277, 1319,2296}. The average number of imbalances, detected by high-resolution array comparative genomic hybridization, is as high as 43 per tumour {2296}. The most common losses, observed by array comparative genomic hybridization, are 6q, 8p, 9p, 10, 13, and 20p; the most common gains are 1q, 4q, 5p,

8q, 12p, 15, 16q, 17q, 20q, 22, and Xp {2296}. *CDKN2A* (in 9p) is homozygously deleted in > 60% of 17 cases, and *STARD13* (in 13q) is heterozygously or homozygously deleted in 45% of cases {2296}. Recently, a novel *STRN-NTRK3* gene fusion has been reported in one case of primary fibrosarcoma of the radius {3344}. This finding, albeit rare, seems relevant considering the successful attempt to target NTRK with specific inhibitors {621}.

Macroscopic appearance
Grossly, fibrosarcomas are collagenous, resulting in a firm consistency with a trabeculated, white cut surface and circumscribed margins. High-grade lesions show a fleshy appearance.

Histopathology
Microscopically, fibrosarcoma is composed of a uniformly cellular population of spindle-shaped cells arranged in a fascicular pattern with a variable amount of collagen production. Given that these fibrosarcomatous features can be seen in a wide variety of bone tumours, the great majority of tumours previously considered to reside in this category are probably better placed in other categories, such as leiomyosarcoma, monophasic synovial sarcoma {3192,308,1416}, and solitary fibrous tumour {3192}. Thus, fibrosarcoma is a diagnosis of exclusion. The presence of osteoid and cartilaginous differentiation excludes the diagnosis of fibrosarcoma.

Differential diagnosis
The differential diagnosis includes solitary fibrous tumour, desmoplastic fibroma, synovial sarcoma, low-grade leiomyosarcoma, osteosarcoma, and dedifferentiated chondrosarcoma. Tumours with marked cytological atypia and a storiform growth pattern are best classified as undifferentiated pleomorphic sarcomas. STAT6 is of great help in excluding a diagnosis of solitary fibrous tumour, and expression of desmin and h-caldesmon is helpful in making a diagnosis of leiomyosarcoma.

Sclerosing epithelioid fibrosarcoma can occur as either a primary or a metastatic bone lesion {3302,2628}. In this context, the presence of striking epithelioid morphology combined with MUC4 immunopositivity or demonstration of a fusion between *FUS* or *EWSR1* and one of the CREB3L genes allows accurate classification. Epithelial markers (and absence of *SS18* gene rearrangements) distinguish fibrosarcoma from synovial sarcoma. The expression of SATB2 in the absence of tumour osteoid visible on routine microscopy as a marker for osteosarcoma is controversial.

Cytology
Not clinically relevant

Diagnostic molecular pathology
Molecular genetics plays a major role in excluding tumour-specific aberrations.

Essential and desirable diagnostic criteria
Essential: bone tumour with compatible imaging; monomorphic cellular spindle cells; fascicular growth pattern; diagnosis of exclusion – lack of morphological, immunohistochemical, and genetic features suggesting an alternative diagnosis.
Desirable: herringbone fascicles.

Staging
Staging is according to bone sarcoma protocols (see *TNM staging of tumours of bone*, p. 339). See also the information on staging in *Bone tumours: Introduction* (p. 340).

Prognosis and prediction
The 5-year and 10-year survival rates are as poor as 34% and 28%, respectively, depending on patient age and tumour grade, site, and stage, with metastases to the lungs and other bones commonly noted {292,2431,1449,3021}.

Haemangioma of bone

Hameed M
Bloem JL
Righi A

Definition
Haemangioma of bone is a benign tumour in bone composed of vascular channels of small or large calibre. When haemangiomas involve a large localized region, or are widespread throughout the skeleton, this is known as angiomatosis.

ICD-O coding
9120/0 Haemangioma NOS

ICD-11 coding
2E81.0Y & XH5AW4 & XA5GG8 Benign vascular neoplasms & Haemangioma NOS & Bones

Related terminology
Acceptable: Gorham–Stout syndrome; massive osteolysis; cystic angiomatosis.

Subtype(s)
Cavernous haemangioma; capillary haemangioma; angiomatosis

Localization
Vertebral bodies are the most commonly affected site, followed by the craniofacial skeleton and the long bones, where haemangiomas tend to involve the metaphysis or diaphysis {20,698, 3272}. Multifocal occurrence is frequent.

Clinical features
Signs and symptoms
The majority of haemangiomas, especially those arising in the spine, are incidental radiographic findings. However, large vertebral tumours may cause cord compression, pain, and neurological symptoms. Symptomatic tumours occurring elsewhere are painful and may cause a pathological fracture. Gorham–Stout syndrome, a rare non-hereditary disorder, is characterized by diffuse angiomatosis with massive osteolysis, frequently involving contiguous bones {3221}.

Imaging
Haemangioma often presents as a well-demarcated lucent mass containing fat and coarse primary trabeculations. These features are frequently seen as incidental findings on MRI and CT of the spine. In flat bones, such as the calvaria, the tumour is expansile and lytic, and it produces a centrally localized spoke-wheel or sunburst pattern of reactive bone formation. Some haemangiomas show absence or paucity of fat and abundant vasculature, which has a high signal on fluid-sensitive and gadolinium chelate–enhanced MRI. These tumours are usually expansile, compromise neurological structures, and cause related symptoms {698,3130,2013}.

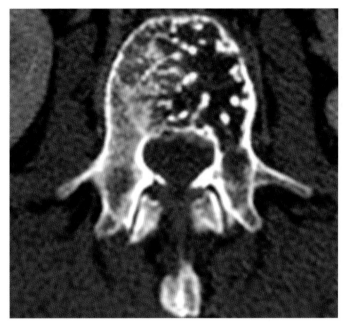

Fig. 3.109 Haemangioma of bone. CT axial image demonstrates a low-density, fat-containing lytic vertebral lesion with coarse trabeculae, known as the polka-dot pattern.

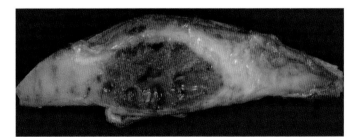

Fig. 3.110 Haemangioma of bone. Portion of tibia with a well-circumscribed tumour showing a solid component and coarse trabeculations.

Epidemiology
Haemangiomas are common lesions; autopsy studies have identified them in the vertebrae of approximately 10% of the adult population {20}. However, clinically significant symptomatic tumours are uncommon and account for < 1% of primary bone tumours {698}. Haemangiomas can occur at any age, but most are diagnosed during middle-age or late middle-age, with the peak incidence in the fifth decade of life. The M:F ratio is about 0.7:1 {20,698,3131,3272}.

Etiology
The etiology is unknown. Both developmental and neoplastic origins have been postulated.

Pathogenesis
Unknown

Macroscopic appearance
Haemangioma manifests as a soft, well-demarcated, dark-red mass. It may also have a honeycomb appearance, with intralesional sclerotic bone trabeculae and scattered blood-filled cavities.

Histopathology
Haemangiomas have variable histological features. Capillary and cavernous haemangiomas are composed of thin-walled blood-filled vessels lined by a single layer of flat, cytologically banal endothelial cells. The vessels permeate the marrow and surround pre-existing trabeculae. In angiomatosis, a lymphangiomatous component may be seen.

Immunohistochemistry
Reactive new bone formation can be prominent. The tumour cells stain for endothelial markers, such as CD31, ERG, FLI1, CD34, and factor VIII–related antigen.

Cytology
Not clinically relevant

Diagnostic molecular pathology
Not clinically relevant

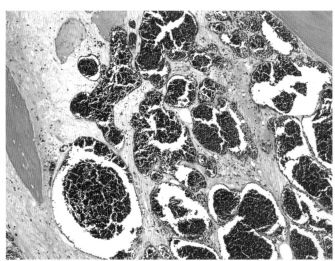

Fig. 3.111 Haemangioma of bone. Cavernous haemangioma consisting of dilated blood vessels lined by flat banal endothelial cells.

Essential and desirable diagnostic criteria
Essential: bone tumour with compatible imaging; thin-walled blood vessels lined by a single layer of non-atypical endothelial cells.

Staging
Not clinically relevant

Prognosis and prediction
Haemangiomas have an excellent prognosis and a low rate of local recurrence.

Epithelioid haemangioma of bone

Bovée JVMG
Rosenberg AE

Definition
Epithelioid haemangioma of bone is a locally aggressive vascular neoplasm arising in bone, composed of cells that have an epithelioid morphology and endothelial differentiation.

ICD-O coding
9125/0 Epithelioid haemangioma

ICD-11 coding
2E81.0Y & XH10T4 Other specified neoplastic haemangioma & Epithelioid haemangioma

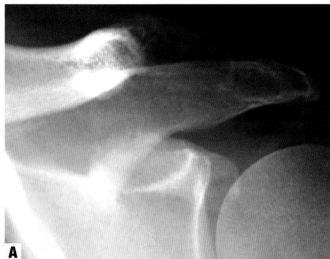

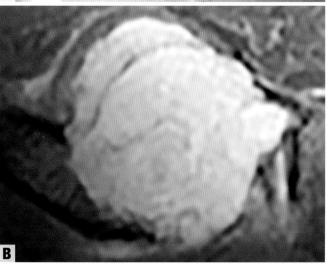

Fig. 3.112 Epithelioid haemangioma of bone. **A** Lytic and expansile mass of the distal clavicle surrounded by a thin rim of reactive bone. **B** Lobulated mass that is sharply demarcated and shows high signal intensity on axial proton density fat-saturated MRI.

Related terminology
Not recommended: histiocytoid haemangioma; haemorrhagic epithelioid and spindle cell haemangioma.

Subtype(s)
None

Localization
Tumours most commonly involve long tubular bones (~40%), followed by short tubular bones of the distal lower extremities (18%), flat bones (18%), vertebrae (16%), and small bones of the hands (8%) {2289}. Approximately 18–25% of the tumours are multifocal in a regional distribution {2289,931}.

Clinical features
Signs and symptoms
Patients usually present with pain localized to the involved anatomical site; identification as an incidental finding is rare.

Imaging
The tumour usually involves the metaphysis or diaphysis of the long tubular bones and manifests as a well-defined lytic, sometimes expansile, septated mass that may erode the cortex and extend into the soft tissue. In paediatric patients, epiphyseal involvement is common {2764}. On MRI, signal intensities are not specific {931}.

Epidemiology
Epithelioid haemangioma is uncommon; the true incidence is unknown. Patients range in age from the first to ninth decades of life, with most being adults; an average age of 35 years has been reported {2289,931}. The M:F ratio is 1.4:1 {2289}.

Etiology
Unknown

Pathogenesis
Epithelioid haemangioma of bone is characterized by fusion genes involving the *FOS* gene at 14q24.3 in 59–71% of the cases. Fusion partners for *FOS* are variable and include *MBNL1*, *VIM*, lincRNA (*RP11-326N17.1*), and *LMNA* {3162,1432}. Alternatively, the *FOSB* gene in 19q13.32 is fused to *ZFP36* or (rarely) *WWTR1* {128}. Dysregulation of the FOS family of transcription factors through chromosomal translocation is the key event in the majority of epithelioid haemangiomas of bone. The FOS family includes FOS, FOSB, FOSL1, and FOSL2, which encode leucine zipper proteins that can dimerize with proteins of the JUN family, thereby forming the transcription factor complex AP-1. In this way, the FOS proteins regulate cell proliferation, differentiation, and survival. In the FOS fusions, the various fusion partners are at the C-terminal end of the protein and cause loss of the transactivating domain {3162}. The C-terminal part

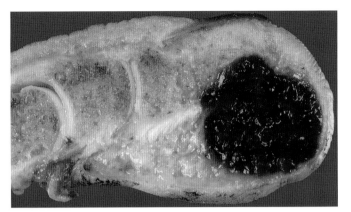

Fig. 3.114 Epithelioid haemangioma of bone. A dark-red, well-circumscribed tumour arises in the bone and extends into the soft tissue.

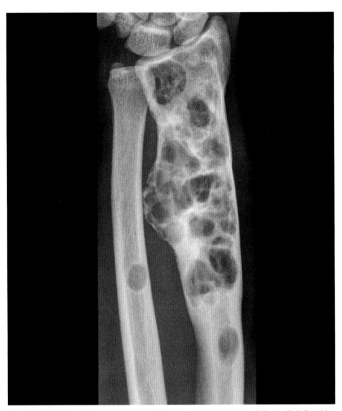

Fig. 3.113 Epithelioid haemangioma of bone. Numerous round, lytic, well-defined lesions in distal radius and ulna.

is essential for fast, ubiquitin-independent FOS degradation via the 20S proteasome. Loss of the C-terminal part prevents the normal rapid degradation of FOS, and the resulting prolonged FOS activation accounts for the abnormal vessel growth in epithelioid haemangioma {3163}. The FOSB fusions occur at the N-terminal part of the protein and are most likely activating promoter-swap events causing upregulation of FOSB {3177}.

Macroscopic appearance

The lesions range in size from several millimetres to 15 cm; most are < 7 cm and are well defined, nodular, soft, solid, red, and haemorrhagic. They may expand the bone, erode the cortex, and extend into the soft tissue.

Histopathology

The tumours have a lobular architecture, replace the marrow cavity, and often infiltrate pre-existing bony trabeculae. The centres of the lobules are the most cellular and contain epithelioid cells that form vascular lumina or grow in solid sheets {2289,931,3190}. The periphery of the lobules may contain many small arteriole-like vessels lined by flat endothelial cells. In some tumours, solid cellular sheet-like areas predominate, whereas in others they account for a small portion of the neoplasm. The large and polyhedral epithelioid cells have oval or kidney-shaped nuclei, which tend to be hyperlobated or cleaved, with fine chromatin. The cytoplasm is abundant and deeply eosinophilic, occasionally containing one or a few clear vacuoles, which may contain intact or fragmented erythrocytes {2289,931,3190}. Vacuolated cells may aggregate such that neighbouring vacuoles coalesce to form vascular lumina. Most tumours contain many well-formed vessels lined by the epithelioid cells that sometimes protrude into lumina in a tombstone-like fashion. Mitoses are relatively infrequent and are not atypical. Small foci of necrosis may be present. The stroma consists of loose connective tissue and may contain a prominent inflammatory infiltrate rich in eosinophils (angiolymphoid hyperplasia with eosinophilia–like), which may even mimic osteomyelitis. Foci of intralesional haemorrhage are present in some tumours, especially those involving the short tubular bones of the extremities. These areas may

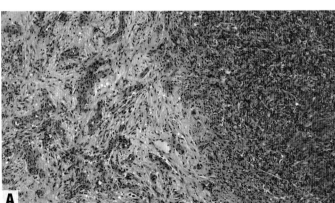
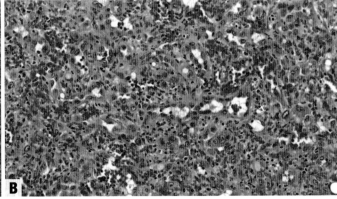

Fig. 3.115 Epithelioid haemangioma of bone. **A** Lobulated architecture with a congeries of arteriole-like structures surrounding tumour. **B** Epithelioid endothelial cells bulge into well-formed vascular lumina and also grow in solid clusters.

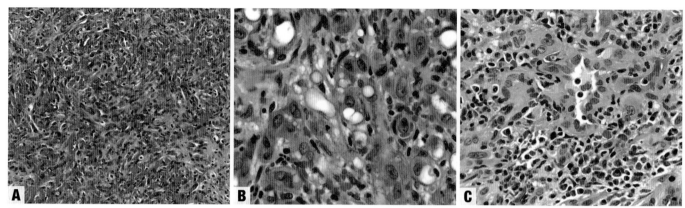

Fig. 3.116 Epithelioid haemangioma of bone. **A** Intratumoural haemorrhage with spindle-shaped neoplastic cells. **B** Epithelioid endothelial cells with vesicular nuclei and densely eosinophilic cytoplasm that contains vacuoles. **C** Numerous eosinophils are present within the tumour in a subset of cases.

also contain cytologically banal, sometimes mitotically active spindle cells that are arranged in fascicles {1605}. Infrequent findings include scattered intratumoural osteoclast-type giant cells, reactive bone formation that compartmentalizes the tumour into small nodules, and a large dilated vessel lined by epithelioid endothelial cells located within the centre of the tumour. A subset of cases, referred to as atypical epithelioid haemangiomas, display more solid growth, increased cellularity, nuclear pleomorphism, and necrosis {128}. These cases more often harbour *FOSB* fusions.

Immunohistochemistry
Tumour cells express endothelial markers, such as CD31, CD34, FLI1, ERG, and factor VIII–related antigen. Many cases are also positive for keratin and EMA {2343,3190}. SMA highlights the pericytic lining and the vasoformative architecture. FOS or FOSB can be expressed in a subset of cases {3163, 1440}.

Differential diagnosis
Epithelioid haemangioma should be distinguished from angiosarcoma, which lacks the lobular architecture, displays more nuclear atypia, and has a higher mitotic activity. It should also be separated from epithelioid haemangioendothelioma, which usually shows myxohyaline stroma and no vasoformation.

Cytology
Not clinically relevant

Diagnostic molecular pathology
Rearrangement of *FOS* or *FOSB* can be detected in the majority of cases {3162,1432,128}.

Essential and desirable diagnostic criteria
Essential: primarily located in bone; large epithelioid endothelial cells with densely eosinophilic cytoplasm.
Desirable: lobular architecture with distinct vasoformation.

Staging
Not clinically relevant

Prognosis and prediction
Epithelioid haemangioma is a locally aggressive lesion, and treatment usually consists of curettage and less frequently marginal en bloc excision. Radiation has been used for tumours in inaccessible locations. The prognosis is very good, and in the largest reported series the local recurrence rate is about 10%; regional lymph nodes can be involved and it is unclear whether this represents multicentric disease or metastatic deposits {1032,2289,931,3190,3404}. Clinicopathological features that are predictive of local recurrence or lymph node involvement have not been reported.

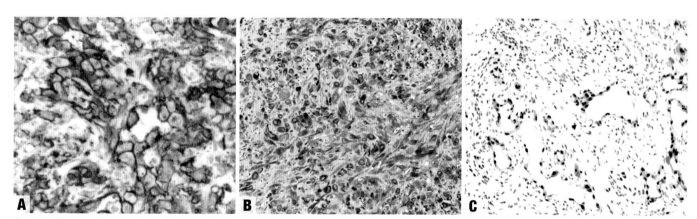

Fig. 3.117 Epithelioid haemangioma of bone. **A** The epithelioid cells stain strongly with CD31 on immunohistochemistry. **B** The epithelioid cells can stain strongly with keratin. **C** The epithelioid cells stain strongly with FOSB.

Epithelioid haemangioendothelioma of bone

Bovée JVMG
Antonescu CR
Rosenberg AE

Definition

Epithelioid haemangioendothelioma of bone is a low- to inter-mediate-grade malignant neoplasm arising from the bone, composed of epithelioid endothelial cells within a distinctive myxohyaline stroma.

ICD-O coding

9133/3 Epithelioid haemangioendothelioma NOS

ICD-11 coding

2B5Y & XH9GF8 Other specified malignant mesenchymal neo-plasms & Epithelioid haemangioendothelioma NOS

Related terminology

Not recommended: malignant epithelioid haemangioendothe-lioma.

Subtype(s)

Epithelioid haemangioendothelioma with *WWTR1-CAMTA1* fusion; epithelioid haemangioendothelioma with *YAP1-TFE3* fusion

Localization

The skeleton can be the only organ involved or a component of multiorgan (liver, lung, soft tissue) disease {1769}. Any bone can be affected; 50–60% of cases arise in long tubular bones, especially in lower extremities, followed by pelvis, ribs, and spine; 50–64% are multifocal within a single bone or involving separate bones; however, they tend to cluster in an anatomical region {1650,2344,3190}.

Clinical features

Signs and symptoms

Common symptoms are localized pain and swelling, but some-times the lesions are asymptomatic. Epithelioid haemangioen-dothelioma with *YAP1-TFE3* has a clinical presentation similar to that of classic epithelioid haemangioendothelioma.

Imaging

The tumours manifest as a lytic lesion with well-circumscribed or poorly circumscribed margins. They may be expansile and erode cortex. Transgression of the cortex with extension into the soft tissue is uncommon.

Epidemiology

Epithelioid haemangioendothelioma is rare, and the true inci-dence is unknown. The prevalence for all organ sites is < 1 case per 1 million individuals {1769}. The age range is broad (first to eighth decades of life), with most patients diagnosed during the second to third decades of life. The sexes are equally affected, although some studies have reported a male predominance {1650,2344,3190,115}.

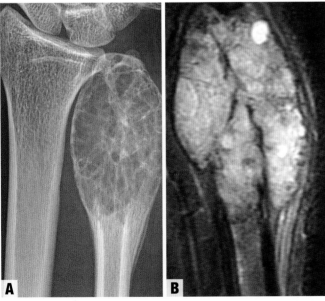
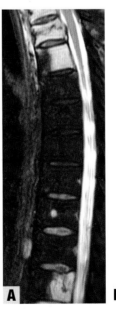

Fig. 3.118 Epithelioid haemangioendothelioma of bone. **A** Expansile lytic tumour of the distal ulna has a trabeculated pattern. **B** Tumour has multinodular growth pattern and has high signal intensity on coronal T2 fat-saturated MRI.

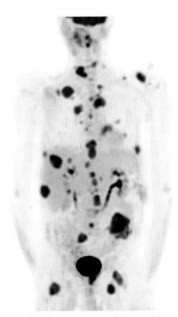

Fig. 3.119 *YAP1-TFE3*–positive epithelioid haemangioendothelioma of bone. **A** Tu-mour replaces the marrow in multiple vertebral bodies and has high signal intensity in sagittal T2 MRI. Also note vertebral fractures and epidural extension. **B** FDG PET showing multiple lesions that have avid FDG uptake.

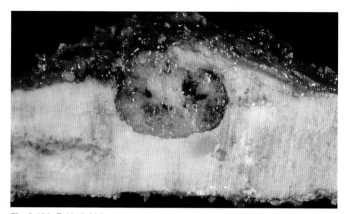

Fig. 3.120 Epithelioid haemangioendothelioma of bone. Sharply demarcated tan-white mass involving the cortex.

Etiology

Unknown

Pathogenesis

The overwhelming majority of epithelioid haemangioendotheliomas harbour a t(1;3)(p36;q25), resulting in a fusion of *WWTR1* at 3q25.1 with *CAMTA1* at 1p36.31-p36.23 {2073,932,3041}. The WWTR1 (TAZ) protein is a transcriptional coactivator and effector of the Hippo pathway. The Hippo pathway phosphorylates WWTR1 (TAZ), which leads to its cytoplasmic localization and ubiquitin-dependent degradation {3040}. Fusion of WWTR1 (TAZ) to CAMTA1 results in dysregulation of the Hippo pathway, such that WWTR1-CAMTA1 constitutively localizes in the nucleus, where it acts as a neomorphic transcription factor to activate a WWTR1 (TAZ)-like transcriptional programme {3040}. The monoclonal origin of multifocal epithelioid haemangioendothelioma has also been established using *WWTR1-CAMTA1* breakpoint analysis. This indicates that multiple lesions arise from locoregional or distant metastatic spread from a single primary as opposed to multiple independent primaries {929}. A small subset of tumours (< 5%) have a *YAP1-TFE3* fusion resulting in oncogenic activation of TFE3 {133}.

Macroscopic appearance

The tumours are ovoid, rubbery, tan or less frequently haemorrhagic masses that are < 1 cm to 10 cm in size.

Histopathology

Epithelioid haemangioendothelioma is a solid mass that lacks a lobular architecture and is composed of large epithelioid and spindle cells with round or elongated vesicular nuclei, prominent nucleoli, and abundant densely eosinophilic cytoplasm. Intracytoplasmic lumina appear as clear vacuoles that may contain intact or fragmented red blood cells (so-called blister cells or signet-ring cells). Well-formed blood vessels are not present in the classic epithelioid haemangioendothelioma; instead, the tumour cells are arranged in cords and nests, which are embedded within a myxohyaline stroma that may resemble cartilaginous matrix. Cytological atypia and mitotic activity are often limited. A small subset of epithelioid haemangioendotheliomas have atypical histological features, including nuclear pleomorphism, increased mitotic activity, solid sheet-like growth, and necrosis. Epithelioid haemangioendothelioma with *YAP1-TFE3* fusion is associated with distinct morphology. The tumour cells are large, with abundant voluminous cytoplasm that is sometimes feathery in appearance. The nuclei can exhibit mild to moderate atypia. The epithelioid cells may delineate well-formed vascular lumina or grow in solid sheets; a myxohyaline stroma is usually absent or inconspicuous {133}.

Immunohistochemistry

The tumour cells express endothelial markers, such as CD31, CD34, ERG, FLI1, factor VIII–related antigen, D2-40, and PROX1. They may be strongly positive for keratin (~40%) and EMA {1650,2344,1153,1705}. Nuclear staining for CAMTA1 is positive in 86–88% and is highly specific {2841,849}. TFE3 immunohistochemistry can be used to identify epithelioid haemangioendotheliomas with *YAP1-TFE3*, although positivity is not always correlated with *TFE3* fusion {1041}.

Differential diagnosis

Epithelioid haemangioendothelioma of bone, especially when multifocal and positive for keratin, can be easily misdiagnosed as metastatic carcinoma. Epithelioid haemangioendothelioma with atypical histological features should be distinguished from epithelioid angiosarcoma, which lacks the typical myxohyaline stroma and specific fusion genes of epithelioid haemangioendothelioma. The presence of the cord-like cellular arrangement or characteristic stroma also helps distinguish epithelioid haemangioendothelioma from epithelioid haemangioma.

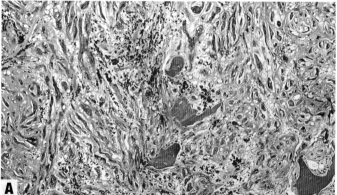 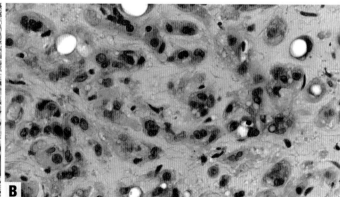

Fig. 3.121 Epithelioid haemangioendothelioma of bone. **A** Tumour infiltrates the bone. The neoplastic cells are arranged in cords within a myxohyaline stroma. **B** The tumour consists of cords of epithelioid cells with deeply eosinophilic cytoplasm, with some containing clear vacuoles, in a basophilic myxohyaline stroma.

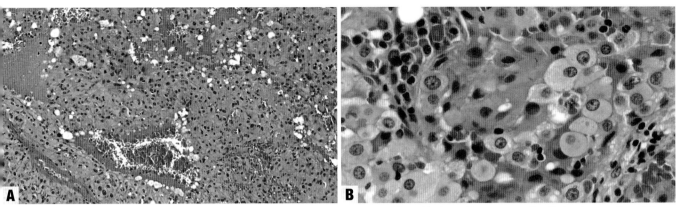

Fig. 3.122 Epithelioid haemangioendothelioma of bone with *YAP1-TFE3* fusion. **A** Tumour shows well-formed lumina and large tumour cells with abundant cytoplasm. **B** Large tumour cells have voluminous eosinophilic cytoplasm.

Cytology
Not clinically relevant

Diagnostic molecular pathology
The *WWTR1-CAMTA1* fusion can be detected in 89–100% of all epithelioid haemangioendotheliomas with classic histological features, and it is not found in epithelioid haemangioendothelioma's mimics {3041,932}. *YAP1-TFE3* fusions are found in a small subset of cases.

Essential and desirable diagnostic criteria
Essential: classic epithelioid haemangioendothelioma is composed of cords or nests of epithelioid endothelial cells within a myxohyaline stroma; epithelioid haemangioendothelioma with *YAP1-TFE3* fusion shows either solid growth or well-formed vascular channels lined by epithelioid endothelial cells with nuclear atypia and abundant pale cytoplasm.
Desirable (in selected cases): CAMTA1 expression by immunohistochemistry and/or *WWTR1-CAMTA1* fusion; TFE3 overexpression by immunohistochemistry and/or *TFE3* gene rearrangement.

Staging
Staging is according to bone sarcoma protocols (see *TNM staging of tumours of bone*, p. 339). See also the information on staging in *Bone tumours: Introduction* (p. 340).

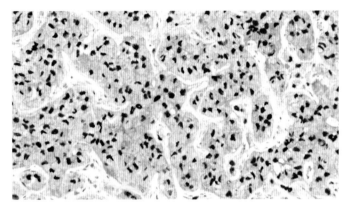

Fig. 3.123 Epithelioid haemangioendothelioma of bone. Tumour cells show strong nuclear immunohistochemical staining for CAMTA1.

Prognosis and prediction
Wide resection is the treatment of choice. The clinical course can be highly variable {2344}. The overall survival rate of patients with epithelioid haemangioendothelioma of bone is 92% at 10 years {115}. Involvement of two or more bones is associated with a worse prognosis (74% 10-year overall survival rate), regardless of the number of organs involved {1769,115}. The mortality rate is about 20% {1650,1769}. One study found no correlation between histological parameters and prognosis {1650}. Histological risk stratification systems, which were proposed for soft tissue or thoracic examples {813,108}, have not been tested for bone tumours.

Angiosarcoma of bone

Nielsen GP
Bovée JVMG

Definition
Angiosarcoma of bone is a high-grade malignant neoplasm of bone demonstrating endothelial differentiation.

ICD-O coding
9120/3 Angiosarcoma

ICD-11 coding
2B56.Y & XH6264 Angiosarcoma, other specified primary site & Haemangiosarcoma

Related terminology
None

Subtype(s)
None

Localization
Angiosarcoma shows a wide skeletal distribution with preferential involvement of long and short tubular bones (74%), especially the femur, followed by the pelvis (15%), axial skeleton (7%), and trunk (4%). Approximately one third of cases are multifocal and affect contiguous (64%) or distant bones (36%) {3189,800}.

Clinical features
Signs and symptoms
Angiosarcoma most commonly presents as a painful lesion that may be associated with a palpable mass.

Imaging
The tumour manifests as a single or regionally multifocal osteolytic tumour, with a well- to poorly defined margin and a geographical pattern of destruction. Most lesions show cortical destruction, whereas a periosteal reaction is usually absent {3197}. MRI demonstrates a heterogeneous lesion, with extensive reactive changes seen on T2-weighted images {3197}.

Epidemiology
Angiosarcoma of bone is rare, accounting for < 1% of malignant bone tumours. Patients have a broad age range, but the tumour usually arises in older individuals and is slightly more common in males {3189,800}.

Etiology
The etiology is unknown for most cases. A small number of cases are associated with previous radiation therapy {2162, 2242} or bone infarct {4,523}.

Pathogenesis
Genetic information on angiosarcoma of bone is limited. An array comparative genomic hybridization study distinguished two molecular groups: cases with few or no gross aberrations and cases with numerous genetic aberrations consisting of chromosomal losses, chromosomal gains, and high-level amplifications or complex aberrations {3191}. The most common finding was amplification of 2q and 17q, which was also found in angiosarcoma of soft tissue, suggesting overlap in tumorigenesis irrespective of their location {3191}. One angiosarcoma of bone was shown to harbour a *KDR* mutation, while *CIC* abnormalities were absent {1433}. MYC overexpression can be seen in some cases {3191}.

The RB1 pathway is involved in tumorigenesis in about 55% of angiosarcomas of bone (loss of p16 and/or overexpression of cyclin D1), whereas overexpression of p53 or MDM2 is absent, suggesting that the p53 pathway is less important {3188}. In addition, TGF-β signalling is highly active in angiosarcoma of bone when compared with angiosarcoma of soft tissue {3188}. Although the PI3K/AKT pathway is active in angiosarcomas in

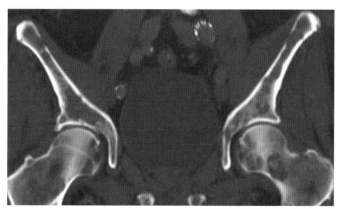

Fig. 3.124 Angiosarcoma of bone. Coronal CT of an angiosarcoma producing multiple lytic lesions involving the femur and pelvic bones.

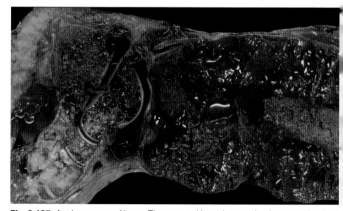

Fig. 3.125 Angiosarcoma of bone. The resected large haemorrhagic tumour involves and destroys several bones, extending into soft tissues.

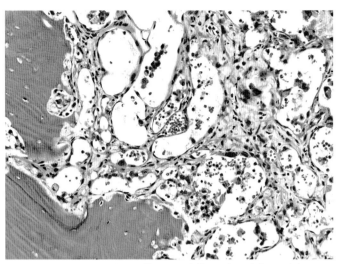

Fig. 3.126 Angiosarcoma of bone. The tumour infiltrates bone. It forms obvious vascular spaces, with some of the lumina being lined by malignant endothelial cells.

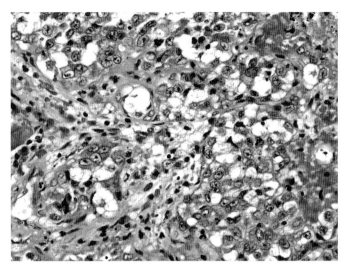

Fig. 3.127 Epithelioid angiosarcoma of bone. The tumour cells are epithelioid and form a solid growth pattern, mimicking metastatic carcinoma.

both bone and soft tissue, different mechanisms seem to be involved: 41% of angiosarcomas of bone show a decrease in expression of PTEN, whereas angiosarcomas of soft tissue overexpress KIT {3188}.

Macroscopic appearance

Angiosarcoma is usually > 5 cm in greatest dimension, friable, haemorrhagic, and tan-red. The tumour erodes and destroys the cortex and infiltrates into the soft tissues. Areas of necrosis are difficult to identify because of the haemorrhagic appearance of the tumour.

Histopathology

Angiosarcoma is characterized by cytologically malignant cells that are most often epithelioid in appearance (> 90% of cases) and less frequently spindled. The nuclei are usually vesicular and contain one or several small nucleoli or a macronucleolus. The cytoplasm is deeply eosinophilic and often contains one or more vacuoles, which may be clear and empty or may hold intact or fragmented erythrocytes {3273,2344,949}. Mitotic figures are often numerous, and atypical forms can be seen. The tumour cells usually grow in solid sheets; however, in approximately one half of cases, they line irregular vascular lumina {3189}. Extravasated erythrocytes can be numerous, and scattered deposits of haemosiderin may also be present. A variable inflammatory infiltrate is present, generally consisting of lymphocytes and neutrophilic or eosinophilic granulocytes {3189}. Reactive bone formation can sometimes be observed. In the absence of obvious vascular differentiation, abundant intratumoural haemorrhage and intratumoural neutrophils are useful morphological features that may suggest the diagnosis {800}.

Immunohistochemistry

Expression of various endothelial markers is seen; ERG, CD31, and FLI1 are usually positive, whereas positivity for CD34 and factor VIII–related antigen is less common {800,3189,2129}. In addition, tumour cells may be positive for SMA and D2-40 {3189}. Keratin and EMA are frequently positive, particularly, but not exclusively, in tumour cells that have an epithelioid morphology {2121,2361,3189}.

Differential diagnosis

The combination of multifocality, epithelioid morphology, and expression of epithelial markers can lead to confusion with metastatic carcinoma {800,2736,3197,3189}. Given its wide spectrum of morphology, angiosarcoma should be considered in the differential diagnosis of any high-grade (especially epithelioid) malignancy of bone. Epithelioid angiosarcoma will stain for endothelial markers, which should be negative in metastatic carcinoma.

Cytology
Not clinically relevant

Diagnostic molecular pathology
Not clinically relevant

Essential and desirable diagnostic criteria
Essential: primary origin in bone; vasoformative architecture and/or expression of endothelial markers; prominent nuclear atypia and readily observed mitoses.

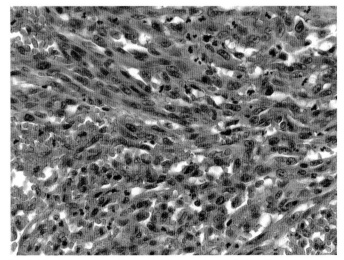

Fig. 3.128 Angiosarcoma of bone. This tumour shows spindle cell morphology and extravasation of erythrocytes.

Staging

Staging is according to bone sarcoma protocols (see *TNM staging of tumours of bone*, p. 339). See also the information on staging in *Bone tumours: Introduction* (p. 340).

Prognosis and prediction

Patients are usually treated with surgery, radiation therapy, and/or chemotherapy. The biological behaviour of individual cases is unpredictable, although as a group angiosarcomas of bone are high-grade and clinically extremely aggressive {3304,469}.

In a study of 31 patients, the 1-year, 2-year, and 5-year survival rates were 55%, 43%, and 33%, respectively {3189}. The presence of a macronucleolus, $\geq$ 3 mitoses per about 2 mm², and < 5 eosinophilic granulocytes per about 2 mm² within a tumour has been shown to be associated with a worse survival {3189}. Lymphangiogenic differentiation as evidenced by D2-40 expression also seems to predict a more aggressive course {3189}. Loss of p16 expression is also associated with a significantly worse prognosis {3188}.

Aneurysmal bone cyst

Agaram NP
Bredella MA

Definition
Aneurysmal bone cyst (ABC) is a benign neoplasm of bone containing multiloculated blood-filled cystic spaces.

ICD-O coding
9260/0 Aneurysmal bone cyst

ICD-11 coding
FB80.6 & XH23E0 Aneurysmal bone cyst & Aneurysmal bone cyst

Related terminology
Not recommended: giant cell reparative granuloma of small bone; giant cell lesion of small bones.

Subtype(s)
None

Localization
ABC can affect any bone but usually arises in the metaphysis of long bones, especially the femur, tibia, and humerus, and the posterior elements of vertebral bodies. Rare tumours occur in the soft tissues {103,2282,2907}.

Clinical features
Signs and symptoms
The most common signs and symptoms are pain and swelling, which are rarely due to fracture. In the vertebrae, ABC can compress nerves or the spinal cord and cause neurological symptoms.

Imaging
On radiographs and CT, ABC presents as a lytic, expansile lesion with well-defined margins. Most tumours contain a thin shell of subperiosteal reactive bone. On MRI, characteristic fluid-fluid levels created by the different signal intensities of the cyst contents are present. Signal intensity can be variable on T1- and T2-weighted images, depending on the age of the blood products. Contrast administration can show septal enhancement and can be helpful in detecting solid components, which suggest ABC-like changes {1695,3195}. On bone scan, ABCs show increased peripheral radiotracer uptake, with a central photopenic area.

Epidemiology
ABC affects all age groups but is most common during the first two decades of life (80%). The sexes are equally affected {1994, 3195}. The estimated annual incidence is 0.15 cases per 1 million population {1825}.

Etiology
Unknown

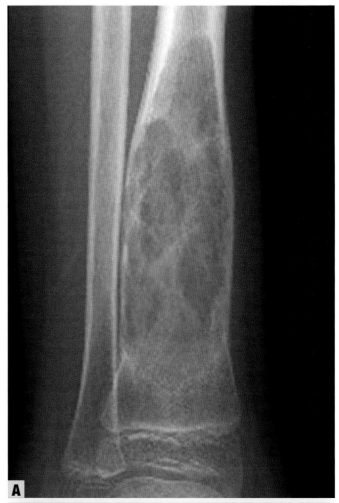

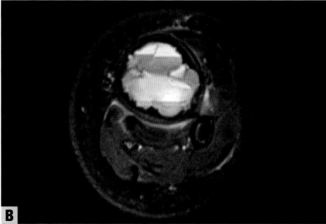

Fig. 3.129 Aneurysmal bone cyst. **A** Lateral radiograph demonstrates an expansile multiloculated lytic lesion in the distal tibia. **B** Axial fat-suppressed T2-weighted MRI of the distal tibia demonstrates multiple fluid-fluid levels.

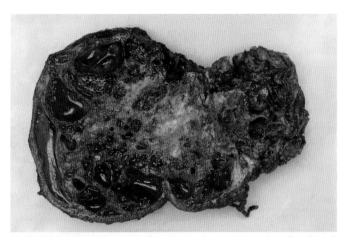

Fig. 3.130 Aneurysmal bone cyst. Gross image of a resected specimen from the pelvic bone showing multiple haemorrhagic cystic spaces with intervening septations.

Pathogenesis

ABC contains cytogenetic rearrangements of the *USP6* gene at chromosome band 17p13.2. The most common translocation, t(16;17)(q22;p13) {716,2373,2428,2506,2799}, leads to the fusion of *CDH11* with *USP6*, with resultant upregulation of USP6 transcription {2373,2374}. *USP6* rearrangements are found in approximately 70% of ABCs but not in ABC-like changes in other tumours {2375}. *USP6* rearrangements do not seem to be associated with distinct biological behaviour {2375}. The most frequent *USP6* fusion partner is *CDH11* (30% of *USP6* fusions); others include *THRAP3* (*TRAP150*), *CNBP* (*ZNF9*), *OMD*, *COL1A1*, *CTNNB1*, *STAT3*, *FOSL2*, *EIF1*, *SPARC*, *PAFAH1B1*, *USP9X*, and *RUNX2* {2374,3249,2811,1261,336}. The ABC neoplastic component, containing the *USP6* rearrangement, is a spindle cell population indistinguishable from normal fibroblasts and myofibroblasts {2375}. Other cells commonly seen in ABC, including inflammatory cells, endothelial cells, metaplastic bone-associated osteoblasts, and multinucleated osteoclast-like giant cells, do not contain a *USP6* rearrangement and are presumably reactive {2375}. *USP6* gene rearrangements occur in the cystic and solid ABCs of the small bones of the hands and feet, but not in the giant cell reparative granulomas in gnathic locations {33}.

Macroscopic appearance

Grossly, ABC is well defined, multiloculated, and composed of blood-filled, cystic spaces separated by tan-white, gritty septa (sponge-like). More-solid areas can be present, representing a solid portion of the ABC. The peripheral soft tissue component is surrounded by a thin shell of reactive bone formation.

Histopathology

ABC is well circumscribed and contains blood-filled cystic spaces separated by fibrous septa. The fibrous septa are composed of a moderately dense, cellular proliferation of bland fibroblasts, with scattered, multinucleated, osteoclast-type giant cells and reactive woven bone rimmed by osteoblasts. The woven bone frequently follows the contours of the fibrous septa. In about one third of the cases, the bone is basophilic and has been termed blue bone, although its presence is not diagnostic. Mitoses are commonly present and can be numerous; however, atypical forms are absent. Necrosis is rare unless there has been a pathological fracture. The solid subtype of ABC has the same components. What was previously considered giant cell lesion of small bones has identical morphology to the solid subtype of ABC {286,2730}.

Immunohistochemistry

Immunohistochemically, the lack of expression of H3.3 p.Gly34Trp could help to distinguish ABCs from giant cell tumours of bone with ABC-like changes.

Differential diagnosis

ABC-like areas can be seen in other benign and malignant bone tumours that have undergone haemorrhagic cystic change. The term "secondary aneurysmal bone cyst" was previously used for such areas but is no longer acceptable. The majority of ABC-like changes develop in association with benign neoplasms, most commonly giant cell tumour of bone, osteoblastoma, chondroblastoma, and fibrous dysplasia {1695,1994,3195}. However, ABC-like changes may also complicate sarcomas, especially osteosarcoma. The most

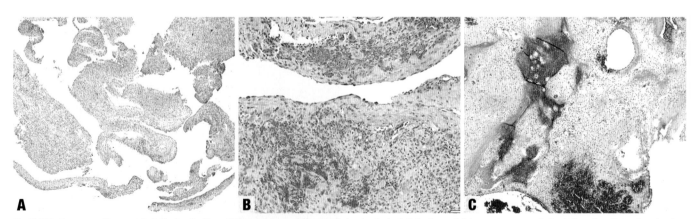

Fig. 3.131 Aneurysmal bone cyst. **A** Cyst wall with multiple septations. **B** Cyst wall showing lack of distinctive cell lining and composed of spindle cells with scattered osteoclast-like giant cells, haemorrhage, and haemosiderin pigment deposition. **C** Aneurysmal bone cyst with areas of basophilic blue bone formation.

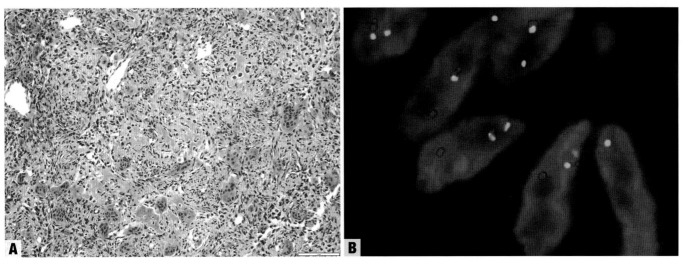

Fig. 3.132 Solid aneurysmal bone cyst. **A** Tumour composed of fibroblast-like spindle cells, osteoclast-like giant cells, and reactive new bone formation. **B** FISH for *USP6* gene using break-apart probe showing split green and red signals indicating rearrangement.

important differential diagnosis is telangiectatic osteosarcoma because both may have similar imaging characteristics and gross appearance. In telangiectatic osteosarcoma, the fibrous septa contain obvious malignant neoplastic cells, which are not seen in ABC.

Cytology
Not clinically relevant

Diagnostic molecular pathology
USP6 gene rearrangement can be detected by FISH. The percentage of lesional cells carrying the rearrangement can sometimes be low.

Essential and desirable diagnostic criteria
Essential: radiology: multicystic lesion with fluid-fluid levels; histology: cyst wall composed of fibroblasts, osteoclast-like giant cells, haemosiderin pigment, and new bone formation.
Desirable: molecular: *USP6* gene rearrangement.**Staging**
Not clinically relevant

Prognosis and prediction
ABC is a potentially locally recurrent neoplasm. The recurrence rate after curettage is variable (20–70%). Spontaneous regression after incomplete removal is very unusual. The presence or absence of *USP6* fusion does not seem to affect prognosis.

Giant cell tumour of bone

Flanagan AM
Larousserie F
O'Donnell PG
Yoshida A

Definition

Giant cell tumour of bone is a locally aggressive and rarely metastasizing neoplasm composed of neoplastic mononuclear stromal cells with a monotonous appearance admixed with macrophages and osteoclast-like giant cells. A small subset of cases are malignant.

ICD-O coding

9250/1 Giant cell tumour of bone NOS

ICD-11 coding

2F7B & XH4TC2 Neoplasms of uncertain behaviour of bone or articular cartilage & Giant cell tumour of bone NOS

Related terminology

Not recommended: benign fibrous histiocytoma; osteoclastoma.

Subtype(s)

Conventional giant cell tumour of bone; giant cell tumour of bone, malignant

Localization

Giant cell tumour of bone typically affects the ends of long bones (distal femur, proximal tibia, distal radius, and proximal humerus) in the mature skeleton and occasionally the metaphysis {91}, particularly in skeletally immature individuals. Giant cell tumours in the axial skeleton arise most commonly in the sacrum and vertebral body {2733,1990}; a tumour confined to the posterior elements only is not a giant cell tumour of bone. Flat bone involvement is rare but most frequent in the pelvis. Small numbers of giant cell tumours affect the tubular bones of the hands and feet {2377,2538}. Mutant-proven giant cell tumours are rarely reported in the gnathic bones {2538, 91}. Malignant giant cell tumours affect bones similar to those involved in conventional giant cell tumour {289,1185,91,2538}.

Clinical features

Signs and symptoms

Giant cell tumour presents with pain, swelling, and occasionally restricted joint movement. The duration of symptoms is typically weeks to months {468}. Tumours may be discovered incidentally and occasionally during pregnancy {468}. A pathological

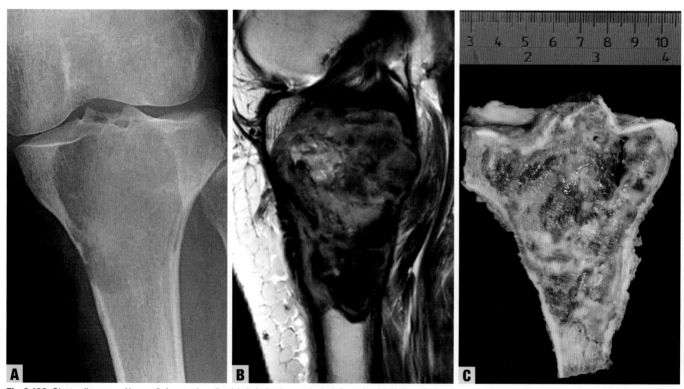

Fig. 3.133 Giant cell tumour of bone. **A** A non-mineralized, lytic lesion is seen in the left proximal tibia. No sclerosis is seen in the margin, and it extends to the articular surface. The cortex is markedly thinned inferomedially. **B** Sagittal T2 MRI. The lesion shows marked hypointensity due to haemosiderin. **C** The gross appearance of the giant cell tumour is shown in a coronal plane, filling and expanding the central marrow space. The tumour abuts the subarticular space but does not extend into the joint, reflecting what is seen in the radiograph and MRI. The features are typical of a giant cell tumour, showing variegated red and pale areas of tumour.

fracture occurs in 5–12% of patients {468,3118}, most commonly in the distal femur {879}. Vertebral and sacral lesions cause insidious onset of pain {3118} and frequently a neurological deficit {3153}.

Imaging
When arising in long bones it is typically lytic and eccentric and extends to the articular cartilage {879}. Trabeculation is common, ranging from fine to coarse, and it represents endosteal ridging {2223}. The lesion shows a narrow zone of transition, with a well-defined, non-sclerotic border and no matrix mineralization. It is unusual for there to be a periosteal reaction, and its presence may indicate a fracture {1811}. Less commonly, the tumour is centrally located {1435} and shows a poorly defined margin {1435} or incomplete marginal sclerosis {2202}. The overlying cortex may be normal, thinned to a variable degree, or breached by tumour that is contained within an attenuated periosteum; extension into soft tissue is the exception {3118}. Primary malignant giant cell tumours may show aggressive appearances but they are usually indistinguishable from conventional tumours; secondary malignant giant cell tumours resemble recurrent conventional disease but may also show postradiotherapy or postsurgical changes {289}. Giant cell tumour in the sacrum is often poorly visualized on radiographs due to its location {2403}, but it is typically located eccentrically within proximal sacral segments, causing lytic destruction {3153}, frequently involving the sacroiliac joint {3153,1990}. Vertebral lesions cause lytic destruction and kyphosis. The lytic, non-mineralized nature and lack of periosteal reaction is best shown using CT {2223}. Scintigraphy most typically shows increased activity in the periphery of the lesion, with central photopenia (donut appearance) {1435}. Intermediate to low T2 signal intensity, due to haemosiderin from chronic haemorrhage, is typical on MRI studies, but evidence of recent haemorrhage {146,90} and fluid-fluid levels {2223} may also be seen, the latter suggesting aneurysmal changes. Denosumab-treated giant cell tumours show new bone formation in > 50% of cases, predominantly at the periphery of the tumour {2359,3362}.

Epidemiology
Giant cell tumours represent 4–5% of all primary bone tumours and 20% of benign bone tumours, with an estimated incidence rate of 1.2–1.7 cases per 1 million person-years {100,1853,3198}. The peak incidence is between the ages of 20 and 45 years, with approximately 10% of cases occurring in the second decade of life {71}. Giant cell tumours, as defined by the H3.3 mutation, arise (although rarely) in the immature skeleton {1181,91,71}. A slight female predominance is reported, with the notable exception of a slight male predominance in a large series of subjects/patients from China {1863,2312}. Malignant giant cell tumours account for < 10% of all giant cell tumours, and the affected patients are generally the same age as those with conventional giant cell tumours {835,100,91}.

Etiology
The etiology of the majority of sporadic giant cell tumours is not known, whereas the phaeochromocytoma-paraganglioma and giant cell tumour syndrome is caused by an early postzygotic H3.3 mutation {3085,3084}. Synchronous or metachronous multicentric giant cell tumours are rare, most commonly

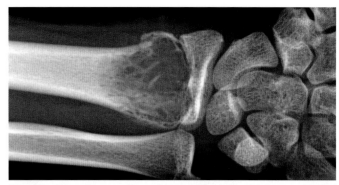

Fig. 3.134 Giant cell tumour of bone. A 14-year-old girl with a lytic lesion in the distal radial metaphysis; note that the growth plate is open. A pathological fracture is present in the lateral cortex.

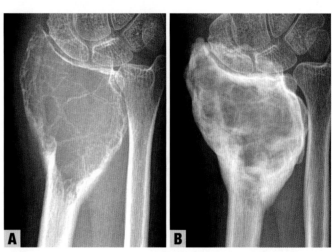

Fig. 3.135 Giant cell tumour of bone. **A** Giant cell tumour of bone before denosumab treatment. Lytic, trabeculated tumour in the distal radius showing mild expansile remodelling and marked cortical thinning. **B** Denosumab-treated giant cell tumour of bone. There is peripheral and internal sclerosis after 3 months of treatment with denosumab.

involving extremities in young patients {1142}. Multicentric giant cell tumours with early postzygotic H3.3 mutations are reported in the phaeochromocytoma-paraganglioma and giant cell tumour syndrome {3085}. However, many so-called multicentric giant cell tumours occur in a disease setting with known predisposing genetic alterations, such as Paget disease of bone {2614}, Gorlin–Goltz syndrome {368,2825}, and Jaffe–Campanacci syndrome {2947,239}. Osteoclast-rich tumours in these settings may also occur as single lesions. In most cases, it has not been determined whether such osteoclast-rich lesions harbour an H3.3 mutation, but they are not detected in osteoclast-rich lesions of the severe familial form of Paget disease of bone caused by *ZNF687* mutations {830}. Transformation to malignancy may occur after radiation therapy.

Pathogenesis
Conventional giant cell tumour
There is evidence that the neoplastic stromal cells in giant cell tumour are of osteoblastic lineage: when treated with denosumab, a RANK ligand inhibitor, the mutant cells mature and form bone, a process reversed on withdrawal of treatment. In addition, the stromal cells express (pre)osteoblast markers, including alkaline phosphatase, RUNX2, SP7 transcription

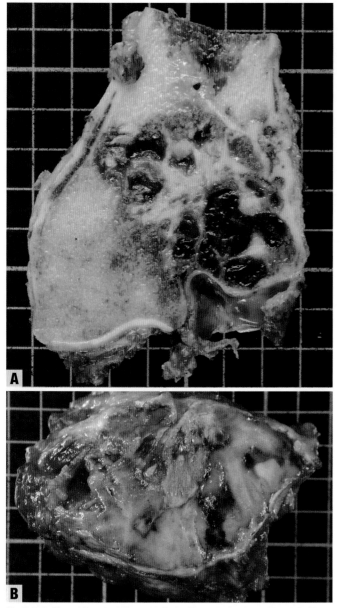

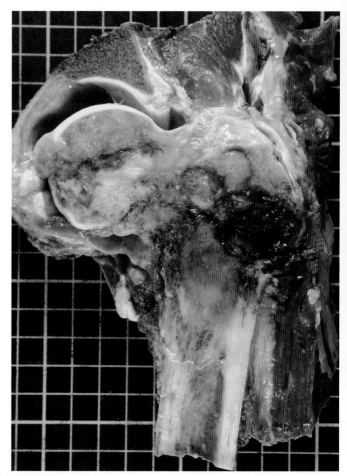

Fig. 3.137 Malignant giant cell tumour in proximal femur. A destructive tumour focally destroying the articular cartilage and the cortical bone and extending into soft tissue. The tumour is nodular, has a firm rubbery texture, and shows haemorrhage and necrosis.

Fig. 3.136 Giant cell tumour of bone. **A** Typical features of a giant cell tumour of bone in a distal femur showing extensive cystic haemorrhagic areas. **B** Typical features of a giant cell tumour in the distal radius showing homogeneous pale soft tumour with focal recent haemorrhage and cyst formation.

factor (osterix), and SATB2 {1961}. Depletion of osteoclast-like cells implies that an osteoclast-like growth factor suppresses stromal cell differentiation and results in proliferation.

At least 95% of giant cell tumours harbour pathogenic *H3-3A* (*H3F3A*) gene mutations, approximately 90% of which are H3.3 p.Gly34Trp, with the next most common being p.Gly34Leu; rarer variants (p.Gly34Met, p.Gly34Arg, and p.Gly34Val) have also been reported {257,91,2358,3337}. Copy-number and rearrangement analysis showed that tumours are diploid overall, with a paucity of structural changes {257,2358}. The mechanism by which the mutant H3.3 drives the neoplasm is not defined.

Malignancy in giant cell tumour

The mechanism by which malignant transformation occurs is

unknown. *TP53* and *HRAS* mutations have been identified in malignant giant cell tumour not associated with prior irradiation {1193}. Strong expression of p53 has been demonstrated in some (but not all) secondary malignant giant cell tumours {1185,2369}.

Macroscopic appearance

Conventional giant cell tumour is well defined and often lies eccentrically within the end of a long bone, which is typically asymmetrically expanded. The surrounding cortex is often thinned and in areas may be destroyed completely, but it is generally contained by the periosteum. The subchondral bone plate can be focally eroded, but the tumour seldom penetrates the articular cavity. Viable tumour is characterized by a soft, friable, tan-red and haemorrhagic appearance, but cream-yellow and firm white areas corresponding to xanthomatous change and fibrous tissue are commonly seen. Areas of haemorrhage and blood-filled cystic spaces corresponding to aneurysmal changes may be seen. In contrast to conventional giant cell tumour, the texture of a malignant giant cell tumour is typically firm and fleshy.

Histopathology

Giant cell tumour is a highly cellular lesion typically dominated by large numbers of non-neoplastic osteoclast-like giant cells, between which mononuclear cells are embedded. The giant cells have a variable number of nuclei, some with > 50 per cell. Mononuclear cells in giant cell tumour exhibit a variety of morphological appearances, including round to oval cells in a non-fibrotic background and spindled cells associated with fibrous matrix. The neoplastic cells have an ill-defined cell membrane with pale eosinophilic cytoplasm; their nuclei exhibit an open chromatin pattern and contain one or two small nucleoli. However, it is difficult to distinguish the neoplastic cells from macrophages (CD68-positive cells) without immunolabelling; the former show a variable (occasionally high) mitotic count {71}. The presence of atypical mitotic figures should raise suspicion for malignancy.

The typical features of a giant cell tumour can be obscured by extensive necrosis, recent haemorrhage, haemosiderin deposition, aneurysmal change, collections of foamy macrophages, and reactive/reparative non-mutant fibrous tissue. In addition, areas of stromal overgrowth of the neoplastic mononuclear cells are uncommon. The presence of substantial deposition of bone is not common, although reactive/metaplastic bone formation can occasionally be striking and can be prominent when associated with a fracture. Exceptionally, otherwise typical giant cell tumour contains benign-appearing hyaline cartilaginous nodules, and the differential diagnosis then includes dedifferentiated chondrosarcoma and chondroblastoma {1615,71}.

Small numbers of otherwise typical giant cell tumours may contain scattered mononuclear cells with marked nuclear

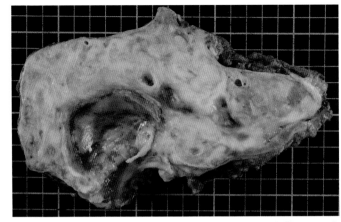

Fig. 3.138 Pelvic giant cell tumour of bone treated with denosumab. The tumour is composed of white nodules surrounded by pale-yellow fibrous-type tissue.

pleomorphism, enlarged hyperchromatic nuclei, irregular nuclear contours, smudged nuclear chromatin, and nuclear pseudoinclusions. The nature of these cells is uncertain and probably represents degenerative change {2744,201}, because their scattered distribution/pattern is not suggestive of malignancy. Nevertheless, these cases can be challenging to classify, particularly on a biopsy specimen.

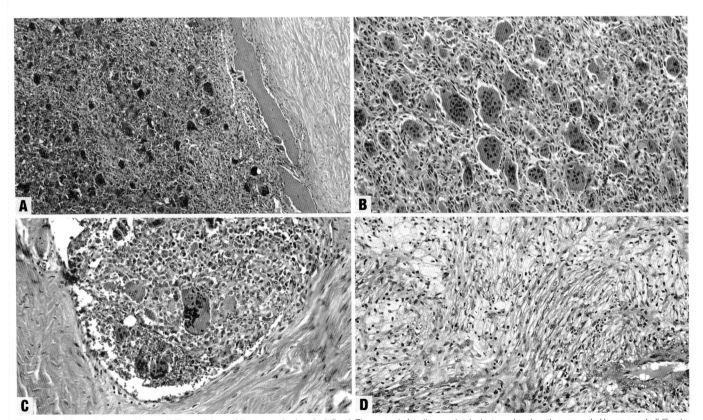

Fig. 3.139 Giant cell tumour of bone. **A** The periphery of the tumour is sharply defined. The cortex is focally completely destroyed and partly surrounded by an eggshell-like rim of reactive bone. **B** Typical features of a giant cell tumour. The osteoclast-like giant cells dominate, between which are the mononuclear neoplastic cells. **C** Vascular invasion of a giant cell tumour of bone outside the main bulk of the tumour. This is of no prognostic significance. **D** An area of foamy macrophages in a giant cell tumour of bone, which would have previously been called a benign fibrous histiocytoma. Elsewhere in the tumour there is diffuse H3.3 p.Gly34Trp immunoreactivity (not shown).

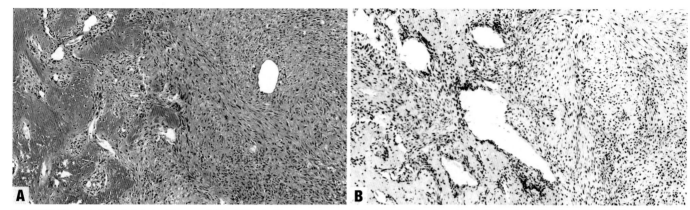

Fig. 3.144 Denosumab-treated giant cell tumour. **A** The right part of the figure shows spindle-shaped cells and no osteoclast-type giant cells, whereas the left side demonstrates the deposition of bone by the neoplastic cells. **B** H3.3 p.Gly34Trp immunohistochemistry showing numerous positive neoplastic cells and lack of osteoclast-type giant cells.

giant cell tumour is undifferentiated sarcoma of bone and giant cell–rich osteosarcoma.

Cytology
Not clinically relevant

Diagnostic molecular pathology
An *H3-3A* gene mutation is detected in the neoplastic stromal cell population in as many as 96% of giant cell tumours {91, 257,2358,615,1615,3337}; 90% of these are represented by the H3.3 p.Gly34Trp mutation. The p.Gly34Leu mutation is much less frequent and is mostly found in tumours in the small bones of the hand, patella, and axial skeleton. There have also been occasional reports of p.Gly34Val, p.Gly34Arg, and p.Gly34Met {257,2358,2538}. Detection of the mutation does not distinguish between conventional and malignant giant cell tumours. Failure to detect an H3.3 mutation should prompt testing for alterations in other osteoclast-rich lesions.

Essential and desirable diagnostic criteria
Essential: bone tumour with compatible imaging; an osteolytic circumscribed tumour involving the epiphysis, generally in a skeletally mature individual; numerous large osteoclasts together with a mononuclear cell neoplastic component without atypia.
Desirable: Detection of H3.3 p.Gly34–mutated cells.

Staging
Not clinically relevant

Prognosis and prediction
Between 15% and 50% of conventional giant cell tumours recur locally after curettage and usually within 2 years. Between 3% and 7% of patients develop metastatic lung disease with histological features of conventional giant cell tumour {63,551,2656}. Predictors of metastatic disease include local recurrence, but also possibly surgical manipulation. Vascular invasion is commonly seen in cases that metastasize to the lung.

The median interval between metastasis and local recurrence is 15 months and most occur within 36 months, but delayed metastasis (up to 10 years) has been described {2656}. Pulmonary metastases are slow-growing and are thought to represent pulmonary implants that result from embolization of intravascular growths of giant cell tumour. Some conventional pulmonary implants can regress spontaneously. A small number exhibit progressive enlargement and lead to the death of the patient as a result of reduced lung volume {551,294}. Denosumab has been used with benefit in the treatment of benign metastasizing disease {2410, 885}.

Denosumab may be used as the treatment for giant cell tumours that are unresectable or where surgical resection is likely to result in excessive morbidity. Neoadjuvant denosumab therapy can be used to facilitate surgical resection of locally advanced tumours. However, there is no consensus about optimal treatment dose, duration, or interval between treatments. Furthermore, the safety of this drug when taken over long periods remains unknown {2410}. The prognosis for patients with secondary malignant giant cell tumours is similar to that of patients with a high-grade sarcoma and is reported to be worse than that for patients with primary malignant giant cell tumour {120,289,835}.

Non-ossifying fibroma

Baumhoer D
Rogozhin DV

Definition
Non-ossifying fibroma (NOF) is a benign and generally self-limiting storiform spindle cell tumour of bone containing osteoclast-like giant cells.

ICD-O coding
8830/0 Non-ossifying fibroma

ICD-11 coding
2E85.Y & XH06N0 Benign fibrohistiocytic tumour of other specified sites & Benign fibrous histiocytoma

2E85.Y & XA5GG8 Benign fibrohistiocytic tumour of other specified sites & Bones

Related terminology
Not recommended: fibrous cortical defect (confined to the cortex); metaphyseal fibrous defect; benign fibrous histiocytoma.

Subtype(s)
None

Localization
The vast majority of NOFs arise in the metaphysis of long bones of the lower extremities, especially around the knee and in the distal tibia. Multifocal lesions may occur.

Clinical features
Signs and symptoms
NOF arises in skeletally immature individuals, with a peak incidence in the second decade of life. It is usually asymptomatic and often discovered incidentally. Larger tumours can affect the biomechanical properties of the affected bone, become painful (probably related to microfractures), and/or cause pathological fracture {149,2714}.

Imaging
The radiological features on plain radiographs are usually pathognomonic and show a well-defined, lobulated lesion centred in the cortical bone with sclerotic and scalloped borders. The tumours are aligned to the long axis of the bone. They are often eccentric and generally appear radiolucent. Sectional images are usually not required; however, CT confirms a well-demarcated and purely lytic appearance; MRI shows low T1-weighted and heterogeneous T2-weighted signal intensity. Remarkably, (residual) NOFs are rarely seen in adults, suggesting spontaneous regression and resolution over time, the cause of which is still unclear. Multiple NOFs can develop sporadically but also in patients with neurofibromatosis type 1, Jaffe–Campanacci syndrome, and the rare oculoectodermal syndrome {470,149,2470,239}.

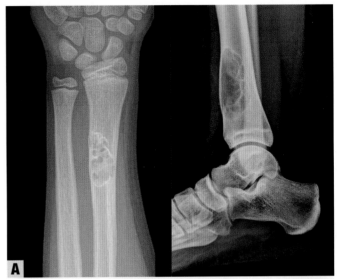

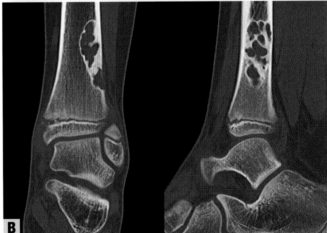

Fig. 3.145 Non-ossifying fibroma. **A** Plain radiographs of non-ossifying fibromas of the distal radius (**left**) and the distal tibia (**right**). Both lesions are lobulated and well demarcated, with a sclerotic rim. **B** Coronal (**left**) and sagittal (**right**) formatted CT of a non-ossifying fibroma of the distal tibia.

Epidemiology
The incidence of NOF is unknown, because most lesions will not come to clinical attention due to lack of specific symptoms. However, it has been estimated that approximately 30–40% of children have one or more occult NOFs, rendering NOF the most common tumour of bone {1958}. Radiographic studies have shown that 54% of boys and 22% of girls have NOF at the age of 4 years {1506,2909}.

Etiology
The cause of sporadic NOFs is not known. However, NOFs (single or multiple) may also occur on a background of germline

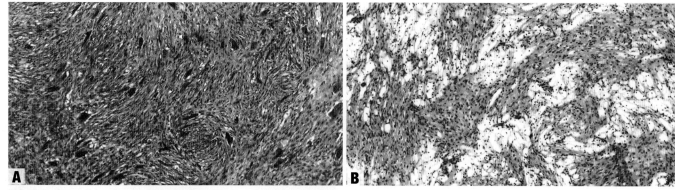

Fig. 3.146 Non-ossifying fibroma. **A** Non-ossifying fibroma composed of spindle-shaped cells arranged in a storiform growth pattern, with scattered osteoclast-type giant cells. **B** Non-ossifying fibroma with large collections of foamy histiocytes.

or postzygotic mosaic mutations in *NF1*, causing neurofibromatosis type 1 and Jaffe–Campanacci syndrome, and in *KRAS* (oculoectodermal syndrome). Notably, in Jaffe–Campanacci syndrome and oculoectodermal syndrome, patients may develop multifocal NOFs and giant cell lesions of the jaws.

Pathogenesis

In sporadic NOFs, mutually exclusive hotspot mutations in *KRAS* and *FGFR1* have been identified in > 80% of cases, indicating that NOFs represent true neoplasms driven by activated MAPK signalling {239,383}. NOFs appear to be related to giant cell lesions of the jaws, as they share histological and genetic alterations {1183}.

Macroscopic appearance

Grossly, NOFs are rarely seen; they are well circumscribed, appear reddish-brown with areas of yellow discolouration, and have sclerotic borders. Cystic changes may be present, and haemorrhage and necrosis can be seen in tumours that have undergone pathological fracture.

Histopathology

Tumours consist of bland, spindle-shaped cells that are arranged in a storiform growth pattern. Mitotic activity is generally low. Osteoclast-type giant cells are scattered throughout the lesion. Reactive features include haemosiderin deposition and collections of foamy macrophages. Reactive woven bone formation and cystic change may occur focally. In cases with pathological fracture, areas of necrosis can be present. Tumours with morphology similar to that seen in NOF but occurring at sites such as pelvic bones and epiphysis of long bones, and in age groups unusual for NOF, have formerly been designated as benign fibrous histiocytoma of bone. Current concepts indicate that benign fibrous histiocytoma probably constitutes a heterogeneous group of lesions, with the majority of cases representing giant cell tumours of bone with regressive changes (see *Giant cell tumour of bone*, p. 440).

Cytology

Not clinically relevant

Diagnostic molecular pathology

KRAS and *FGFR1* mutation testing can be considered in ambiguous cases.

Essential and desirable diagnostic criteria

Essential: bone tumour with compatible imaging findings.
Desirable: storiform proliferation of plump spindle cells; metaphyseal location in long bones in skeletally immature patients; intermingled giant cells, haemosiderophages, and clusters of foamy histiocytes.

Staging

Not clinically relevant

Prognosis and prediction

The prognosis of NOF is excellent. Asymptomatic lesions detected incidentally do not require biopsy confirmation in cases with typical imaging. Treatment is not necessary as long as there is biomechanical stability of the involved bone. When ≥ 50% of the bone width is replaced or in case of pathological fracture, the lesion can be curetted. Local recurrences are rare; malignant transformation has not been reported.

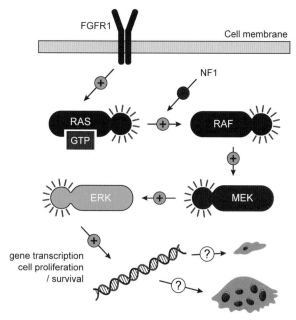

Fig. 3.147 Non-ossifying fibroma. Schema of signalling pathways involved in the pathogenesis of non-ossifying fibromas.

Benign notochordal cell tumour

Yamaguchi T
Inwards CY
Tirabosco R

Definition
Benign notochordal cell tumour (BNCT) is a benign tumour showing notochordal differentiation.

ICD-O coding
9370/0 Benign notochordal tumour

ICD-11 coding
2E89.Z & XH7MT7 Benign mesenchymal tumours of uncertain differentiation, unspecified & Benign notochordal tumour

Related terminology
Not recommended: notochordal hamartoma; giant notochordal rest.

Subtype(s)
None

Localization
BNCTs occur in the skull base, vertebral bodies, and sacrococcygeal spine. Occasionally they can be multiple and may be associated with chordoma {799}. Small numbers of extraskeletal BNCTs have been reported in a number of sites, including the lung {1621}. Ecchordosis physaliphora spheno-occipitalis (EPS) represents extraosseous intradural residual embryonic notochordal tissue sited in the region of the clivus.

Clinical features
Signs and symptoms
BNCTs are usually found in adults but have been reported in children. Most BNCTs are found incidentally on imaging, although they may be associated with pain. EPS may produce neurological deficits such as diplopia and visual field defects.

Imaging
Radiographs may reveal mild sclerosis within a vertebral body or the clivus, although they usually fail to demonstrate any abnormality. CT may show an intraosseous sclerotic lesion without bone destruction or extraosseous tumour extension, or it may fail to demonstrate a lesion. MRI reveals homogeneously low signal intensity on T1-weighted imaging, homogeneously high signal intensity on T2-weighted imaging, and no contrast enhancement on gadolinium-enhanced T1-weighted imaging. In some cases, foci of T1-hyperintensity are seen within the lesion, which correspond to fatty bone marrow. Technetium bone scans usually do not demonstrate any abnormal uptake. On PET-CT studies, the tumour usually shows low avidity for FDG. Occasionally, tumours may be extremely sclerotic, showing the radiographic appearance of an ivory vertebra {3333}.

Epidemiology
The incidence of BNCTs found incidentally is uncertain, although an autopsy study indicates a high incidence (~20%)

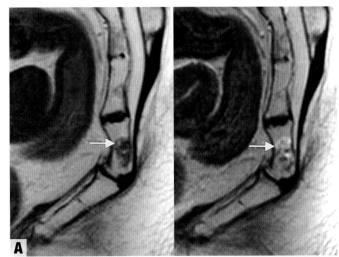
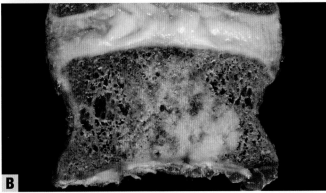

Fig. 3.148 Benign notochordal cell tumour. **A** Sagittal T1-weigthed MRI (**left**) and T2-weighted MRI (**right**) show a well-defined, intraosseous lesion in the first coccygeal vertebra, containing several small foci of hyperintense T1 signal, suggesting fat (arrow). Histological diagnosis was confirmed after coccygectomy for pain. **B** Vertebral body with dense white lesion.

of microscopic BNCT among Japanese individuals aged 7–82 years {3334}. EPS is found in 0.6–2.0% of autopsy cases and in 1.7% of patients on MRI {2052}.

Etiology
Unknown

Pathogenesis
The embryonic protein brachyury (encoded by *TBXT*) is expressed in BNCTs and EPS.

Macroscopic appearance
BNCTs are located within bone. The cut surfaces reveal a firm, well-demarcated but unencapsulated bright-tan tumour lacking any lobular configuration. EPS is a gelatinous polypoid lesion attached to the dorsal surface of the clivus.

Chapter 3

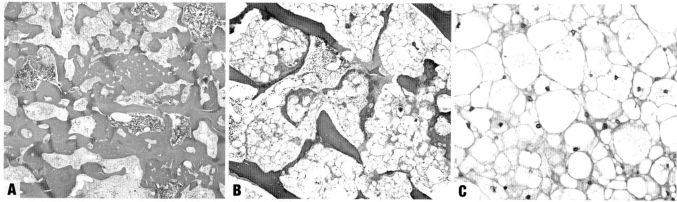

Fig. 3.149 Benign notochordal cell tumour. **A** Benign notochordal cell tumour reveals scattered residual bone marrow islands within the lesion. **B** The affected bone trabeculae show appositional bone formation and no osteolytic process. **C** Benign notochordal cell tumour consists of solid sheets of vacuolated tumour cells with bland nuclei. The tumour cells mimic mature fat or brown fat cells.

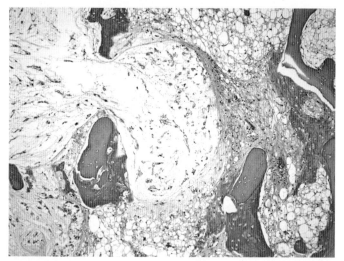

Fig. 3.150 Benign notochordal cell tumour coexisting with conventional chordoma. This tumour shows a focus of benign notochordal cell tumour (right) coexisting with conventional chordoma (left).

Histopathology

BNCT consists of solid sheets of adipocyte-like vacuolated tumours cells and eosinophilic, less-vacuolated tumour cells. The nuclei are usually bland and mitotic figures are absent. Some cystic spaces filled with colloid-like eosinophilic material may be present. The tumour often contains isolated islands of bone marrow. The involved bone trabeculae are usually viable and may be woven but show little evidence of excessive bone resorption or formation. Unlike chordoma, BNCT lacks a lobular architecture, fibrous septa and capsule, extracellular myxoid matrix, and tumour vasculature.

Immunohistochemistry
Both BNCT and EPS are immunoreactive for brachyury (encoded by *TBXT*), cytokeratin, EMA, and (variably) S100.

Differential diagnosis
BNCT and chordoma can be difficult to distinguish, particularly on a biopsy: the juxtaposition of a chordoma with BNCT confounds the challenge {3332}. Atypical notochordal cell tumour is a recently described entity, but the criteria distinguishing it from BNCT and chordoma are ill defined. Atypical notochordal cell tumour is considered a controversial and challenging diagnosis and may reflect a transition from BNCT to chordoma {498,1698}.

Cytology
Not clinically relevant

Diagnostic molecular pathology
Not clinically relevant

Essential and desirable diagnostic criteria
Essential: bone tumour with compatible radiology; notochordal differentiation without atypia; brachyury (encoded by *TBXT*) and cytokeratin immunohistochemistry.

Staging
Not clinically relevant

Prognosis and prediction
Prognosis is excellent and BNCTs do not require any surgical procedure. Malignant transformation to chordoma is rare, but the incidence is unknown. There is no consensus in terms of clinical surveillance {1698}.

Conventional chordoma

Tirabosco R
O'Donnell PG
Yamaguchi T

Definition
Conventional chordoma is a malignant tumour with a phenotype that recapitulates notochord and that usually arises in bones of the axial skeleton.

ICD-O coding
9370/3 Chordoma NOS

ICD-11 coding
2B5K & XH9GH0 Unspecified malignant soft tissue tumours or sarcomas of bone or articular cartilage of other or unspecified sites & Chordoma NOS
2B5K & XH17D8 Unspecified malignant soft tissue tumours or sarcomas of bone or articular cartilage of other or unspecified sites & Chondroid chordoma

Related terminology
None

Subtype(s)
Chondroid chordoma

Localization
Chordomas are chiefly located in the axial skeleton, involving bones from the base of the skull to the coccyx, the frequency being 32% skull-based, 32.8% in the mobile spine, and 29.2% in the sacrum and coccyx, according to the SEER Program {2042,2213}. Only a small number of extra-axial and extraskeletal chordomas are reported {3076,1774,2632}. Tumours in children and young adults have a greater propensity to occur in the base of the skull and upper cervical sites.

Clinical features
Signs and symptoms
Chordomas most commonly present with pain and site-related neurological symptoms.

Imaging
Chordoma is typically a lytic, destructive lesion arising in the midline. It grows slowly, expanding the bone, and is frequently associated with a large mass. It is not mineralized, but bone fragments are often seen within and at the periphery of the mass {2305}. On MRI, the mass is lobular, septated, and heterogeneous, showing low signal on T1-weighted images (but frequently containing high-signal foci) and hyperintensity on T2-weighted images {2995}. Enhancement after gadolinium administration is also heterogeneous and often septal {2995}, with myxoid areas enhancing poorly. The tumour shows low activity on technetium isotope bone scans {2672}, but there may be uptake at the margin and there is moderate avidity for FDG on PET studies {2445}.

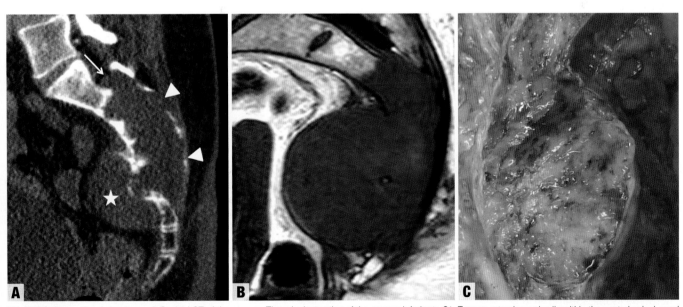

Fig. 3.151 Conventional chordoma. **A** Sagittal CT of the sacrum. There is destruction of the sacrum inferior to S1. Tumour extends proximally within the central spinal canal posterior to S1, the proximal level indicated (arrow). Bone fragments (arrowheads) remain visible anterior and posterior to tumour in the central spinal canal, which is expanded. Distally, there is an anterior extraosseous presacral mass (asterisk). **B** Sagittal T1 MRI shows a heterogeneous mass arising from the distal sacrum, extending within bone from S2 to the coccyx. There is a large anterior and small posterior extraosseous mass. **C** Sacrectomy specimen showing a large lobulated mass with a gelatinous appearance, invading and destroying the distal sacrum.

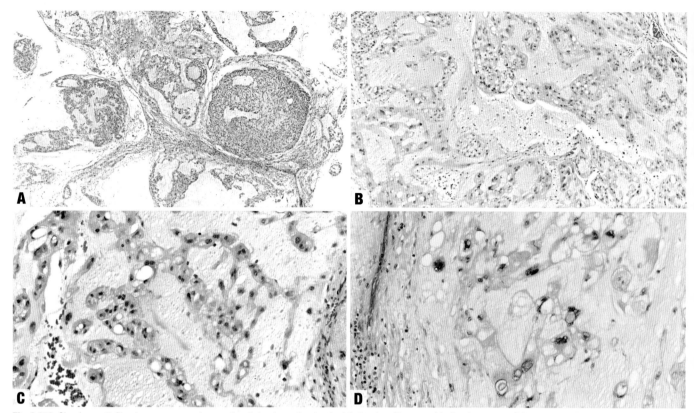

Fig. 3.152 Chordoma. **A** Classic appearance of conventional chordoma showing the lobulated architecture with abundant extracellular matrix. **B** Tumour cells are arranged in cords and nests. Note the typical light basophilic appearance of the myxoid matrix. **C** Cords of tumour cells with mixed physaliphorous and epithelioid features. **D** Cytological atypia including multinucleated cells with bizarre nuclei and pseudonuclear inclusion.

Epidemiology

The incidence of chordoma is 0.08 cases per 100 000 person-years, with an M:F ratio of approximately 1.8:1. Chordoma rarely occurs in the black African population but appears to be represented equally in people of other ethnic groups. However, in one review African-Americans were more represented in the paediatric cohort than in the adult cohort {2802}. All ages are affected, but chordoma most commonly occurs in the fifth to seventh decades of life.

Etiology

In rare cases, chordoma is associated with a germline tandem duplication of *TBXT* {1609}, and rare cases of childhood chordoma occur in the setting of tuberous sclerosis, caused by germline loss-of-function mutations in the tumour suppressor gene *TSC1* or *TSC2* {1820,2043}.

Pathogenesis

The hallmark of chordoma is the expression of brachyury (encoded by *TBXT*) {3210,3076}: in 27% of cases, this is associated with copy-number gain of *TBXT*, a transcription factor required for notochordal development {2539,3052}. This recapitulates the tandem duplication of *TBXT* that underlies familial chordoma {3052,3354}. The strong association of rs2305089 in *TBXT* in patients with chordoma makes a strong case that this SNP contributes substantially to the development of chordoma {2512}. Brachyury has also been shown to act as a master regulator of an elaborate oncogenic transcriptional network encompassing diverse signalling pathways, including components of

the cell cycle and extracellular matrix {2263}. Finally, growth arrest and senescence upon silencing of *TBXT* in chordoma cell lines adds to the critical role of *TBXT* in chordoma {2539}. In addition, PI3K signalling mutations have been reported in 16% of cases, and mutations (always inactivating) of *LYST* have been described in 10% of cases {3052}. Phosphorylated and total EGFR (HER1) appears to play an important role in the disease, because it

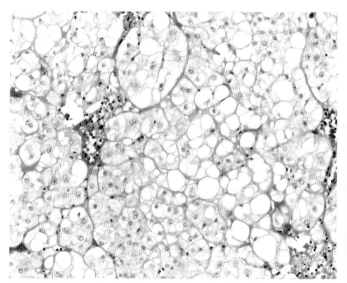

Fig. 3.153 Chordoma. Tumour cells arranged in a pseudoalveolar pattern, mimicking renal cell carcinoma.

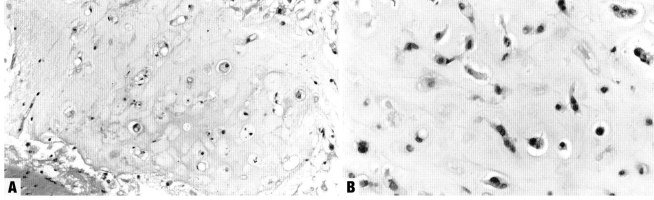

Fig. 3.154 Chondroid chordoma. **A** Lobules of tumour cells within a hyaline matrix. **B** Small clusters and cords of cells. This feature may be helpful in cases with widespread chondroid matrix.

is expressed in 47% and 67% of chordomas, respectively, and EGFR (HER1) inhibitors reduce cell survival {2823,2761}.

Macroscopic appearance

Chordoma presents as a lobular solid mass with a gelatinous appearance, destroying bone and extending into surrounding soft tissue. Sacrococcygeal tumours tend to be larger than those at other sites, most likely related to a longer symptom-free period.

Histopathology

Conventional chordoma is composed of large epithelioid cells with clear to light eosinophilic cytoplasm, separated into lobules by fibrous septa. The tumour cells may have bubbly cytoplasm (physaliphorous cells). They are arranged as cords and nests embedded within an abundant extracellular myxoid matrix, or as more-densely arranged epithelioid packets. Chordomas often show a substantial degree of intratumoural cytological heterogeneity, with features including nuclear atypia and pleomorphism ranging from minimal, usually associated with a low mitotic activity, to (less commonly) severe, in which bizarre nuclei or cell spindling can be seen. In the latter, mitotic figures can be easily detected and large areas of tumour necrosis may be present. The term "chondroid chordoma" refers to chordoma in which a large area of the matrix mimics hyaline cartilaginous tumours {2659,1384}.

Immunohistochemistry

The tumour is diffusely immunoreactive for cytokeratin and EMA and shows variable S100 positivity.

Differential diagnosis

The diagnostic hallmark is the expression of brachyury, which helps to distinguish chordoma from chondrosarcoma, carcinoma, and chordoid meningioma. The differential diagnosis includes metastatic carcinoma, chondrosarcoma, chordoid meningioma, and myoepithelial tumour of bone.

Cytology

Not clinically relevant

Diagnostic molecular pathology

No diagnostic molecular markers have been reported.

Essential and desirable diagnostic criteria

Essential: bone tumour compatible with imaging; voluminous epithelioid cells exhibiting notochordal differentiation embedded in copious myxoid matrix; brachyury and cytokeratin expression.

Staging

Staging is according to bone sarcoma protocols (see *TNM staging of tumours of bone*, p. 339). See also the information on staging in *Bone tumours: Introduction* (p. 340).

Prognosis and prediction

The overall median survival time is 7 years. As many as 40% of chordomas arising at sites other than the base of the skull metastasize. Metastatic sites include lung, bone, lymph nodes, and subcutaneous tissue. It is unclear whether chondroid chordomas behave differently than conventional chordomas; previous literature on the subject is no longer reliable, because data were derived from the pre-brachyury era, and therefore some cases coded as chondroid chordoma may have in fact been low-grade chondrosarcoma.

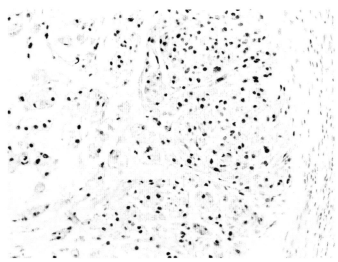

Fig. 3.155 Chordoma. Nuclear immunoreactivity for brachyury.

Dedifferentiated chordoma

Tirabosco R
Hameed M

Definition
Dedifferentiated chordoma is a chordoma with a biphasic appearance, characterized by conventional chordoma and high-grade sarcoma.

ICD-O coding
9372/3 Dedifferentiated chordoma

ICD-11 coding
2B5Z & XH7303 Malignant mesenchymal neoplasm of unspecified type & Dedifferentiated chordoma

Related terminology
None

Subtype(s)
None

Localization
The locations are similar to those of conventional chordoma, predominantly in sacrococcygeal sites {2213}.

Clinical features
Signs and symptoms
The symptoms are similar to those of conventional chordoma, although progression may be more rapid. Pain and site-related neurological symptoms are common. Dedifferentiated chordoma may present de novo or at a location of a previously resected conventional chordoma.

Imaging
Dedifferentiated chordomas show morphology similar to that of conventional tumours and cannot be distinguished on radiographs or CT. A bimorphic appearance may be appreciated on MRI, with the dedifferentiated component suggested by areas of tumour that are relatively hypointense on T2-weighted imaging / fluid-sensitive studies, distinct from the typically T2-hyperintense conventional chordoma {1294}.

Epidemiology
Dedifferentiated chordoma is the rarest notochordal tumour subtype, with only case reports and small series published {1294,2061,330,2127}.

Etiology
Unknown

Pathogenesis
See *Conventional chordoma* (p. 451).

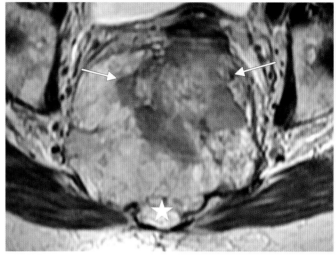

Fig. 3.156 Dedifferentiated chordoma. Axial T2-weighted MRI of the pelvis shows a biphasic tumour. A large, heterogeneous, hyperintense mass has destroyed the sacrum (asterisk) and extended into the presacral space. Within the anterior aspect of the mass, there is a well-defined, relatively hypointense component (arrows) consistent with dedifferentiated tumour (high-grade pleomorphic spindle cell sarcoma showing smooth muscle differentiation).

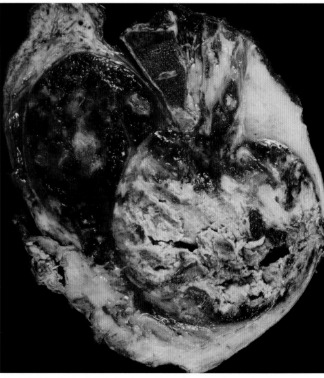

Fig. 3.157 Dedifferentiated chordoma. Sacrectomy specimen showing a large destructive tumour: the haemorrhagic area represents the conventional component, and the more solid fleshy larger area is a dedifferentiated tumour.

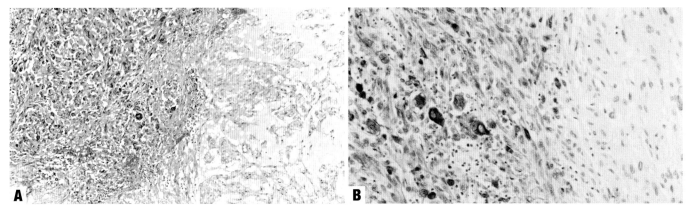

Fig. 3.158 Dedifferentiated chordoma. **A** Typical features of a chordoma (right), with an abrupt change to a high-grade pleomorphic sarcoma showing rhabdomyoblastic differentiation (left). **B** Rhabdomyosarcomatous differentiation highlighted by desmin immunostain. The tumour was also positive for myogenin (not shown).

Macroscopic appearance

The tumour presents as a large mass with a biphasic appearance. The dedifferentiated component has the gross features of a high-grade sarcoma with a solid surface, juxtaposed to a gelatinous and myxoid conventional chordoma.

Histopathology

The distinguishing characteristic is the simultaneous presence of a conventional chordoma and a high-grade spindle and/or pleomorphic sarcoma. Osteosarcomatous and rhabdomyosarcomatous differentiation can be seen. The two components are usually abruptly separated, but they can be intermingled.

Immunohistochemistry

The dedifferentiated component can show focal cytokeratin expression but does not express brachyury {3210}. Specific lineages, such as rhabdomyoblastic, should be supported by immunohistochemical expression of desmin and myogenin.

Differential diagnosis

The differential diagnosis includes dedifferentiated chondrosarcoma.

Cytology

Not clinically relevant

Diagnostic molecular pathology

No diagnostic molecular markers have been reported.

Essential and desirable diagnostic criteria

Essential: bone tumour with compatible imaging; conventional chordoma (histologically or by history) plus high-grade sarcoma.

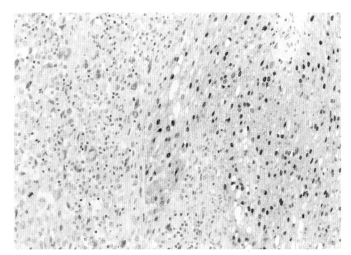

Fig. 3.159 Dedifferentiated chordoma. Immunoreactivity to brachyury is lost in the dedifferentiated component (left).

Staging

Staging is according to bone sarcoma protocols (see *TNM staging of tumours of bone*, p. 339). See also the information on staging in *Bone tumours: Introduction* (p. 340).

Prognosis and prediction

The prognosis is poor; the metastatic rate and mortality are high. The benefits of chemotherapy or radiotherapy seem negligible. Surgery is the only option.

Poorly differentiated chordoma

Nielsen GP
Dickson BC
Tirabosco R

Definition
Poorly differentiated chordoma is a poorly differentiated neoplasm with notochordal differentiation, usually arising in the axial skeleton, and characterized by loss of SMARCB1 expression.

ICD-O coding
9370/3 Chordoma NOS

ICD-11 coding
2B5Z & XH9GH0 Malignant mesenchymal neoplasm of unspecified type & Chordoma NOS

Related terminology
None

Subtype(s)
None

Localization
The most common location is the skull base (clivus), followed by the cervical spine and rarely the sacrococcygeal region {2607, 2843,2166,123,441,527,2402,2612,3326,546,1384}.

Clinical features
Signs and symptoms
Patients generally present with nonspecific symptoms such as headache, pain, cranial nerve symptoms, and weight loss.

Imaging
On imaging, the tumours are destructive, arise in bone, and extend into adjacent soft tissues. By CT, the tumours are lytic, and they are heterogeneous on T1- and T2-weighted MRI.

Epidemiology
This is a rare type of chordoma, with approximately 60 cases reported in the English-language literature. Tumours typically arise in children and occasionally in young adults; they occur in females roughly twice as frequently as in males. In the largest series to date, the age range was 1–29 years (median: 11 years) {2843}.

Etiology
Unknown

Pathogenesis
In most cases, cytogenetic studies have identified deletions involving *SMARCB1* {2402,1434}; these may be heterozygous or homozygous and of variable size, and they can be detected by DNA sequencing {2612,1201}. There is no evidence to date of single-nucleotide variants accounting for loss of SMARCB1 protein {2166,1318,2842}. A subset of cases also show heterozygous co-deletion *of the EWSR1* locus, which lies in close proximity to *SMARCB1* {527,2402,1434}. A minority of cases

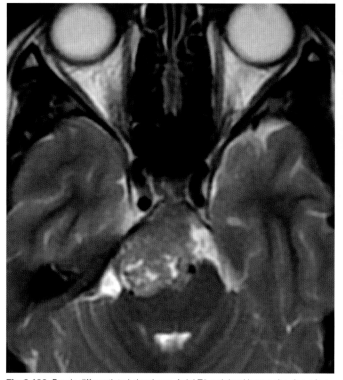

Fig. 3.160 Poorly differentiated chordoma. Axial T2-weighted image showing a large enhancing tumour arising in the skull base.

appear to have intact *SMARCB1* and loss of SMARCB1 expression {2166}, but the mechanism by which this is brought about is presently unclear {2402}. Unsupervised clustering analysis of DNA promoter methylation profiles indicates that the presence of *SMARCB1* deletions in these tumours readily distinguishes them from conventional chordoma, as well as the atypical teratoid/rhabdoid tumour {1318}.

Macroscopic appearance
The size of tumours generally ranges from 2.0 cm to > 10 cm, although most are about 5.0 cm at presentation {123,2402, 2843}. Descriptions of the cut surface are, to date, lacking; poorly differentiated chordomas are destructive and may be well demarcated and multilobulated {2607}.

Histopathology
Poorly differentiated chordoma is composed of cohesive sheets or nests of epithelioid cells, often with a focal rhabdoid morphology. There is relatively abundant eosinophilic cytoplasm and scattered cytoplasmic vacuoles reminiscent of signet-ring cells. The nuclei are round to ovoid, with vesicular chromatin, and they reveal mild to moderate pleomorphism; mitotic activity is increased. The physaliphorous cells typical of chordoma with classic features are absent. Similarly,

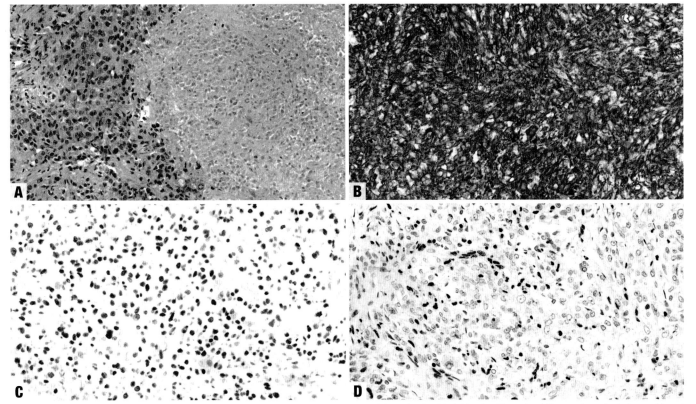

Fig. 3.161 Poorly differentiated chordoma. **A** The tumour is composed of sheets of poorly differentiated epithelioid cells with eosinophilic cytoplasm, irregular nuclei, and prominent nucleoli. There is a central area of necrosis, but no myxoid stroma is present. **B** Poorly differentiated chordoma demonstrating diffuse immunohistochemical staining for keratin. **C** Poorly differentiated chordoma demonstrating diffuse immunohistochemical nuclear staining for brachyury. **D** Poorly differentiated chordoma demonstrating lack of staining for (i.e. loss of) SMARCB1 (INI1).

extracellular myxoid stroma, if present, is generally no more than focal. Geographical necrosis is often conspicuous {1384, 2402,2843}.

Immunohistochemistry
The tumours are immunoreactive for cytokeratin and brachyury (encoded by *TBXT*), with variable positivity for S100. A diagnostic feature is the loss of SMARCB1 (INI1) expression {2166, 1318,2843}.

Differential diagnosis
The differential diagnosis includes malignant rhabdoid tumour and rhabdoid meningioma.

Cytology
Not clinically relevant

Diagnostic molecular pathology
FISH can be used to identify deletions in *SMARCB1*, and these may be associated with a co-deletion of the *EWSR1* locus. FISH for *EWSR1* in such tumours may exhibit a complex pattern that

is generally unlike the typical *EWSR1* rearrangements and must be interpreted with caution {1434}.

Essential and desirable diagnostic criteria
Essential: bone tumour with compatible imaging; poorly differentiated malignant neoplasm arising in the axial skeleton; positive immunohistochemical staining for keratin and brachyury; loss of SMARCB1 (INI1) expression.

Staging
Staging is according to bone sarcoma protocols (see *TNM staging of tumours of bone*, p. 339). See also the information on staging in *Bone tumours: Introduction* (p. 340).

Prognosis and prediction
Treatment consists of a combination of surgery, radiation therapy, and chemotherapy. Fewer than 60 cases have been reported in the literature, but this subtype of chordoma is associated with a poor prognosis – worse than that of conventional chordoma {2843,2402,3326,1384,1318}.

Chondromesenchymal hamartoma of chest wall

Fritchie KJ
Gambarotti M

Definition

Chondromesenchymal hamartoma of chest wall is a benign bone tumour arising from the ribs, composed of hyaline cartilage, woven bone, bland spindle cells, and blood-filled cystic spaces.

ICD-O coding

None

ICD-11 coding

None

Related terminology

Not recommended: chest wall hamartoma; vascular and cartilaginous hamartoma of the chest wall; giant chondromatous hamartoma; cartilaginous hamartoma; benign mesenchymoma.

Note: Nasal chondromesenchymal hamartoma most likely represents a distinct entity from chondromesenchymal hamartoma of the chest wall and is discussed in the head and neck volume.

Subtype(s)

None

Localization

Lesions arise from either the medullary cavity or the surface of the rib and may extend to involve multiple ribs simultaneously {845,104,634,187,2027}. The lateral or posterior aspects of the ribs are involved most frequently {845}. The majority of patients present with a solitary mass, but bilateral or multicentric tumours have been reported {1235,1400,2338,2350,3106,1346}.

Clinical features

Signs and symptoms

Patients often present with a slow-growing palpable mass, with or without clinical symptoms {104,1235,187}. Larger lesions result in respiratory distress, scoliosis, and chest wall deformity {187}.

Imaging

X-ray and CT usually show an expansile rib lesion with well-defined sclerotic margins and extrapleural extension containing mineralization and cystic regions with fluid-fluid levels {1235, 1632}. The mineralization is predominantly chondroid but may show osteoid or mixed features {1235}. MRI shows solid and cystic components, with heterogeneous signal intensities on T1- and T2-weighted images {1235,1632}.

Epidemiology

The reported incidence is 1 case in 3000 among primary bone tumours and < 1 case per 1 million person-years in the

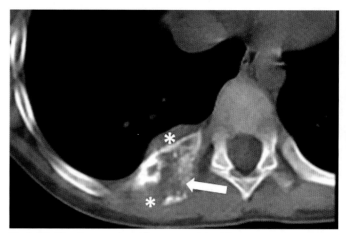

Fig. 3.162 Chondromesenchymal hamartoma. Axial CT of a chondromesenchymal hamartoma shows an expansile lytic lesion involving a right posterior rib with internal chondroid matrix (arrow) and an associated extrapleural and posterior soft tissue mass (asterisks).

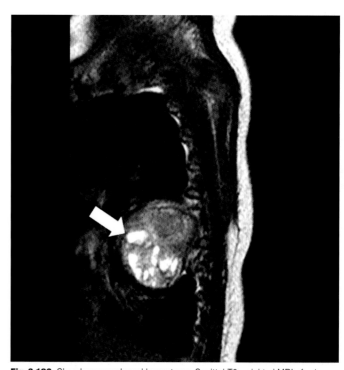

Fig. 3.163 Chondromesenchymal hamartoma. Sagittal T2-weighted MRI of a 1-year-old girl shows a large mass arising from a posterior rib with a large heterogeneous extrapleural soft tissue mass. The mass is associated with deformity of the adjacent rib (not shown) and contains multiple internal fluid-filled spaces (arrow), some of which contain fluid-fluid levels indicative of intralesional haemorrhage.

general population, with approximately 100 cases reported in the literature {2579,395,3170}. The majority of tumours appear to arise congenitally and are noted at birth, and almost all are

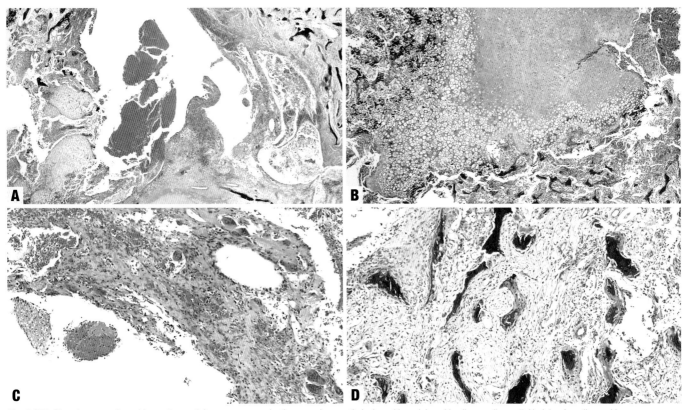

Fig. 3.164 Chondromesenchymal hamartoma. **A** Low-power examination reveals a cystic lesion with nodules of hyaline cartilage. **B** Nodule of cartilage with an appearance similar to the epiphyseal growth plate. **C** The cyst walls are composed of a loose arrangement of bland spindled cells and multinucleated giant cells. **D** Foci of immature bony trabeculae are also present.

diagnosed by the end of the first year of life {634,845}. Rare cases present in older children {845,3039}. There is a male predominance (M:F ratio: 2:1) {467,845}.

Etiology
Unknown

Pathogenesis
Unknown

Macroscopic appearance
Gross examination reveals a well-circumscribed multinodular or lobulated mass with a variably solid and cystic cut surface, typically ranging from 5 to 10 cm, although tumours > 15 cm have been reported {845,634}. The cystic component often contains blood-filled spaces, and the solid areas exhibit a reddish-brown or tan appearance with foci of cartilage.

Histopathology
Histological examination reveals a variably cystic lesion containing nodules of hyaline cartilage, often with enchondral ossification similar to the epiphyseal growth plate, surrounding blood-filled spaces. The walls and septa of the cystic component are composed of reactive-appearing bone, bland spindled cells, and multinucleated giant cells, often resembling aneurysmal bone cyst. The spindle cell component does not show substantial cytological atypia or nuclear hyperchromasia.

Cytology
Not clinically relevant

Diagnostic molecular pathology
Not clinically relevant

Essential and desirable diagnostic criteria
Essential: well-circumscribed mass arising from the rib; variable solid and cystic components; nodules of hyaline cartilage admixed with blood-filled cystic spaces, reactive bone, bland spindle cells, and osteoclast-like giant cells.
Desirable: paediatric presentation.

Staging
Not clinically relevant

Prognosis and prediction
Although chondromesenchymal hamartoma of chest wall is a benign entity, rare cases of death have resulted from respiratory insufficiency {2040,1346,634}. Surgical excision is typically curative, but postoperative complications may include severe scoliosis and chest wall deformity. There is some evidence that these lesions decrease in size after the second year of life, and conservative treatment may be an option if the patient is not in danger of respiratory compromise and can be routinely monitored {1873,187,1614,2277}.

Osteofibrous dysplasia

Nielsen GP
Hogendoorn PCW

Definition

Osteofibrous dysplasia (OFD) is a benign fibro-osseous tumour of long bone that typically arises in the anterior cortex of the tibia and/or fibula during childhood.

ICD-O coding

None

ICD-11 coding

2E83.5 & XH6M86 Benign osteogenic tumours of bone or articular cartilage of limbs & Ossifying fibroma

Related terminology

Not recommended: ossifying fibroma of long bones; Kempson–Campanacci lesion.

Subtype(s)

None

Localization

OFD typically arises in the proximal or middle third of the tibial cortex. Lesions can be bilateral with ipsilateral or contralateral involvement of the fibula. Ipsilateral involvement of the fibula is seen in approximately 20% of patients. Very rarely has it been reported to involve other long bones such as the radius, ulna, and humerus, although the documentation of these reports is not convincingly diagnostic for OFD.

Clinical features

Signs and symptoms

Patients report pain, localized swelling, and bowing deformity; rarely does it cause a pathological fracture. The tumour may also be discovered incidentally on X-rays taken for other reasons.

Imaging

OFD is typically epicentred in the cortical bone, but it may focally involve the underlying medullary cavity. Although slow growth is characteristic of OFD, some lesions may be periodically aggressive and may involve the entire bone with a substantial anterior bowing deformity. Often well demarcated, it is associated with a thinning, expanding, or even missing cortex. The expanding cortex is frequently sclerotically rimmed near the medullary bone. Separate or confluent oval, scalloped, saw-toothed or bubbly multiloculated, lytic lesions are often noted, oriented parallel to the shaft of the bone. Perilesional sclerosis may be considerable. The interior of the lytic foci is typically more radiodense than soft tissue. Bone scans are typically hot. CT delineates the cortical epicentre of the lesion not breaking through into the soft tissue and demarcated from medullary bone by sclerosis. MRI findings show intermediate to high signal intensity on T2-weighted images, with diffuse enhancement on postcontrast images and mixed signals on T1-weighted and fat-suppressed images. Radiological differentiation from adamantinoma may be difficult, but young age, presence of anterior bowing with ground-glass appearance and absence of multilayered periosteal reaction, and absence of moth-eaten destruction favour OFD {344}.

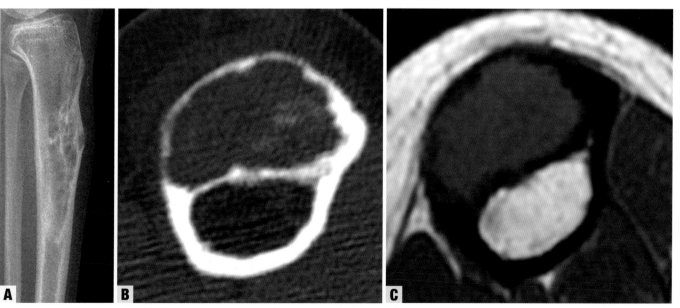

Fig. 3.165 Osteofibrous dysplasia. **A** Plain radiograph shows a mixed lytic and sclerotic lesion that is causing endosteal scalloping and cortical expansion of the proximal tibial diaphysis. **B** Axial CT shows that the tumour is confined to the cortex of the tibia and surrounded by a rim of bone, without involvement of the medullary cavity or soft tissues. **C** Axial T1 MRI demonstrates an expansile intracortical tumour causing cortical thinning, without periosteal reaction. There is no infiltration of the adjacent medullary cavity.

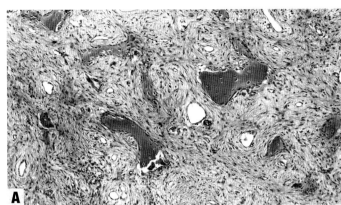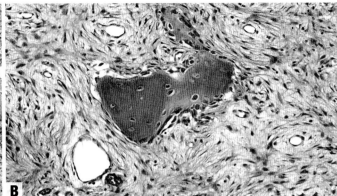

Fig. 3.166 Osteofibrous dysplasia. **A** Osteofibrous dysplasia composed of trabeculae of woven bone with osteoblastic rimming and fibrous tissue. **B** Higher-power view of osteofibrous dysplasia demonstrating the woven bone with osteoblastic rimming, surrounded by spindle-shaped cells.

Epidemiology

OFD is a very rare tumour, accounting for approximately 0.2% of all primary bone tumours. It typically develops during the first and second decades of life, which is younger than patients with adamantinoma. OFD is rare after the age of 15 years.

Etiology

The etiology is unknown. Rare familial cases have been reported {1211}.

Pathogenesis

Recurrent cytogenetic and FISH findings in OFD include trisomies of chromosomes 7, 8, and 12 that have been identified in both adamantinoma and OFD {1334}. The genetic abnormalities are found in a minority (5–10%) of spindle-shaped cells and not in the osteoblasts or osteoclasts, indicating that a large portion of the tumour is non-neoplastic in nature; it has been hypothesized that the stromal cells showing epithelial differentiation might be the neoplastic component {1168}. Causative molecular genetic aberrations have not been identified, but the proto-oncogenes *FOS* and *JUN* are expressed. Additionally, *GNAS* mutations (seen in fibrous dysplasia) are absent in OFD {3018}. Germline mutations involving *MET* (encoding a receptor tyrosine kinase) are seen in hereditary forms of OFD {1211}.

Macroscopic appearance

OFD is a solid, white or yellow, gritty tumour. It is confined to the cortex, rarely with minimal involvement of the adjacent medullary cavity. Although the cortex may be thinned, the overlying periosteum is intact.

Histopathology

Histologically the tumour is composed of an admixture of bone and fibrous tissue. The bone is composed of trabeculae of woven bone with prominent osteoblastic rimming. The intervening fibrous stroma is composed of bland-looking spindle-shaped cells embedded within an extracellular collagenous or sometimes myxoid matrix. Osteoclasts may be present. Mitoses are extremely rare. Zonal architecture is delineated with thin spicules and woven bone or even fibrous tissue predominating in the centre of the lesion with more-abundant anastomosing and lamellar bone peripherally, the latter often blending into the surrounding host bone. Hyalinization, haemorrhage,

xanthomatous change, cyst formation, and foci of giant cells are rare. Cartilage is absent.

Immunohistochemistry

Immunohistochemical staining for keratin shows no or only single keratin-positive stromal cells. Clusters of keratin-positive cells as seen in OFD-like adamantinoma are not present. Typically these individual cells express CK14, CK19, and to a lesser extent CK5 and CK17 {1331}. Additionally, OFD shows positive staining for p63 and occasionally S100 {2713}.

Differential diagnosis

OFD should be distinguished from fibrous dysplasia. The stroma in fibrous dysplasia is more cellular and collagenous than in OFD, and the woven bone in fibrous dysplasia does not show prominent osteoblastic rimming; additionally, mutations in the *GNAS* gene are found in most cases of fibrous dysplasia but are absent in OFD. Immunohistochemically, there are no keratin-positive epithelial cells in fibrous dysplasia, and this tumour is epicentred in the medullary cavity of the bone. The distinction from OFD-like adamantinoma, which also preferentially occurs

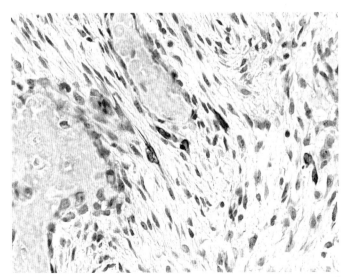

Fig. 3.167 Osteofibrous dysplasia. Osteofibrous dysplasia shows single scattered keratin-positive stromal cells. Clusters of keratin-positive cells (as seen in osteofibrous dysplasia–like adamantinoma) are not seen.

in the tibia, can be difficult and depends on the extent of the epithelial component. Classic adamantinoma can be distinguished by the presence of easily identifiable clusters of epithelial cells.

Cytology
OFD cannot and should not be diagnosed on the basis of FNA.

Diagnostic molecular pathology
Not clinically relevant

Essential and desirable diagnostic criteria
Essential: bone tumour with compatible imaging; almost exclusively in the tibia and/or fibula, always involving cortex; a fibro-osseous tumour of bone in which the woven bone shows prominent osteoblastic rimming; absence of keratin-positive clusters of cells.

Staging
Not clinically relevant

Prognosis and prediction
The tumour may gradually grow during the first decade of life. Most undergo spontaneous regression after puberty. It is controversial whether OFD may progress into OFD-like adamantinoma {2778}, and it is possible that some reported cases of this progression represent sampling issues or that series reporting the absence of progression lack prolonged follow-up. Most patients can be treated conservatively with close observation, patient/parent education, and no surgery. In the presence of substantial deformity or pseudoarthrosis, impending or existing pathological fracture, the desire for definitive diagnosis, or severe symptoms, surgical intervention may be warranted {3278}.

Adamantinoma of long bones

Nielsen GP
Hogendoorn PCW

Definition
Adamantinoma is a biphasic locally aggressive or malignant tumour characterized by a variety of morphological patterns, with a variable epithelial component within a bland osteofibrous component.

ICD-O coding
9261/1 Osteofibrous dysplasia–like adamantinoma
9261/3 Adamantinoma of long bones

ICD-11 coding
2B5J & XH1SV4 Malignant miscellaneous tumours of bone or articular cartilage of other or unspecified sites & Ameloblastoma NOS

Related terminology
Not recommended: well-differentiated adamantinoma.

Subtype(s)
Classic adamantinoma (malignant); osteofibrous dysplasia–like adamantinoma; dedifferentiated adamantinoma

Localization
The tibia, in particular the anterior metaphysis or diaphysis, is involved in 85–90% of cases. Multifocal involvement of the tibia is frequently present {3155}. In as many as 10% of patients, this is combined with one or more lesions in the ipsilateral fibula. Adamantinoma involving other bones has very rarely been reported, including the radius, ulna, calcaneus, femur, humerus, olecranon, ischium, rib, spine, metatarsals, and capitate {2778, 1606}; however, one should be very careful about making the diagnosis of adamantinoma outside the tibia and fibula.

Clinical features
Signs and symptoms
The main symptom is painful or painless swelling. Adamantinoma often displays a protracted clinical behaviour. Clinical symptoms such as swelling or radiographic abnormality may last for > 30 years before diagnosis, whereas local recurrences or metastases may develop years after primary, intralesional, or marginal surgical treatment {1606}.

Imaging
On X-ray, the tumour is typically well circumscribed, cortical, multilobulated, and osteolytic (soap bubble appearance). Intralesional opacities, septation, and peripheral sclerosis may also be seen. Multifocality within the same bone is regularly observed. The lesion commonly remains intracortical and extends longitudinally along the bone, but it may also destroy the cortex and invade the medullary cavity or adjacent soft tissue. This is usually accompanied by lamellar or solid periosteal reaction. Aggressive tumours occasionally present as a single, large, lytic

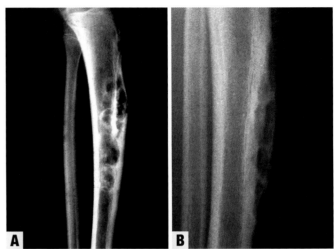

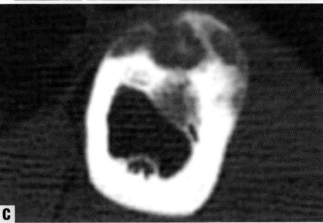

Fig. 3.168 Osteofibrous dysplasia–like adamantinoma. **A** Osteofibrous dysplasia–like adamantinoma presenting as numerous lytic areas involving the cortex and medullary cavity. The tumour has distorted the tibia, which demonstrates some anterior bowing. **B** In the anterior cortex of the mid-tibial shaft there is an intracortical, multiloculated lytic lesion with surrounding sclerosis. **C** Axial CT demonstrating lytic lesions with surrounding sclerosis involving the anterior cortex.

lesion. MRI is useful to document multicentricity, the extension of the lesion, and possible soft tissue involvement {3155}.

Epidemiology
Adamantinoma accounts for about 0.4% of all primary bone tumours. Patients present with this tumour at an age of 3–86 years, with a median age of 25–35 years. The youngest age group predominantly includes patients with osteofibrous dysplasia (OFD)-like adamantinoma, but young children with classic adamantinoma and adults with the OFD-like subtype have been reported {1333,2182,3010}. It is more common in males. Rarely, at middle and advanced age, further progression into dedifferentiated adamantinoma may occur {1332, 1499}.

Etiology

Unknown

Pathogenesis

Rare cases of OFD-like adamantinoma seem to arise from pre-existing OFD. OFD-like adamantinoma may also rarely progress into classic adamantinoma. Dedifferentiated adamantinoma arises in the setting of pre-existing classic adamantinoma {1332}.

A recurrent pattern of numerical abnormalities featuring extra copies of chromosomes 7, 8, 12, 19, and/or 21 has been detected in classic as well as OFD-like adamantinoma {1168,1565}. Extra copies of one or more of these chromosomes (except for chromosome 19) have also been identified in OFD, supporting a related pathogenesis {1168,411}. In addition to trisomy 19, structural abnormalities including translocations and marker chromosomes have been reported in adamantinoma, but not in OFD {1334,1565}. The progressive complexity of the karyotypic aberrations observed in OFD, OFD-like adamantinoma, and classic adamantinoma may be indicative of a multistep transformation process {1168}.

Trisomies 7, 8, and 12 have not been observed in osteoblasts or osteoclasts, suggesting that the osseous component is reactive and non-neoplastic, in contrast with the presence of these trisomies in the spindle cell stroma component of the same lesions {1168}. DNA index studies have shown

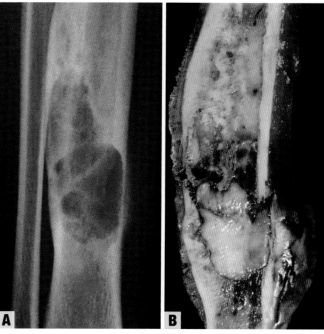

Fig. 3.169 Classic adamantinoma. **A** Classic adamantinoma demonstrating a large expansile osteolytic lesion with soap bubble appearance involving the distal tibia and causing cortical thinning. **B** A resection specimen from the tibia shows a tan mass involving the medullary cavity associated with a pathological fracture. Proximal to the main tumour there are smaller nodules of tumour associated with sclerosis.

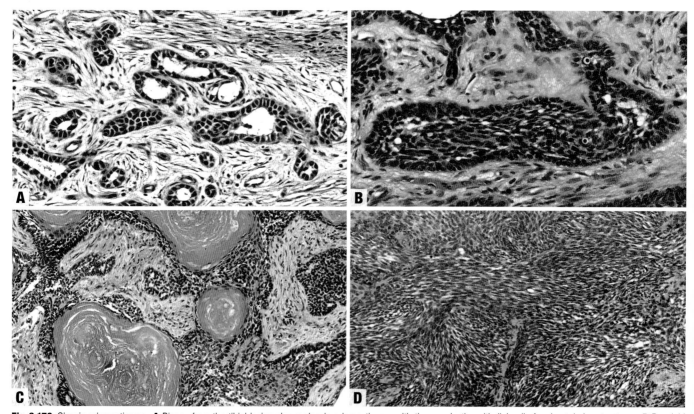

Fig. 3.170 Classic adamantinoma. **A** Biopsy from the tibial lesion shows classic adamantinoma with the neoplastic epithelial cells forming tubular structures. **B** Basaloid pattern with the peripheral palisading of the tumour cells surrounding inner spindle-shaped cells. **C** Squamous differentiation, where the centre of the epithelial islands shows obvious keratinization, is the rarest subtype of adamantinoma. **D** Spindle cell subtype of adamantinoma with tumour cells arranged in intersecting fascicles. This subtype must be distinguished from intraosseous synovial sarcoma.

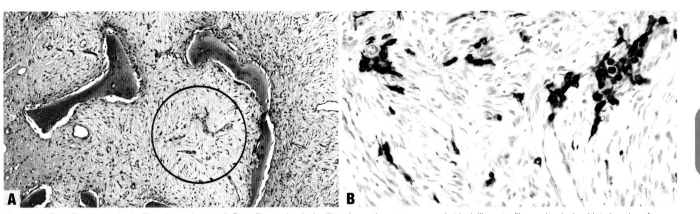

Fig. 3.171 Osteofibrous dysplasia–like adamantinoma. **A** Osteofibrous dysplasia–like adamantinomatous areas that look like osteofibrous dysplasia with trabeculae of woven bone rimmed by plump osteoblasts. Within the fibrous stroma there are small nests of epithelial cells (inside circle) that are hard to see on H&E-stained slides and may mimic endothelial cells. **B** A keratin stain highlights the small clusters of epithelial cells.

that in aneuploid adamantinomas, the aneuploid population is always restricted to the epithelial component {1330}. *TP53* aberrations are also restricted to the epithelial component.

Macroscopic appearance

Classic adamantinoma usually presents as a cortical, well-demarcated, lobulated, whitish-grey gritty tumour with peripheral sclerosis. It may be a single lesion or occasionally multifocal. Small lesions remain intracortical. Larger tumours may show intramedullary extension and cortical breakthrough, with soft tissue invasion in a minority of cases. Macroscopically detectable cystic spaces are common, filled with straw-coloured or blood-like fluid. The tumour varies in size from < 1 cm to > 10 cm.

Histopathology

The distinction between OFD-like and classic adamantinomas depends on the extent of the epithelial component. OFD-like adamantinoma contains a predominance of OFD-like areas with only small nests of epithelial cells; the epithelial nests may be difficult to see or to distinguish from endothelial cells by light microscopy. In classic adamantinoma, the epithelial component is prominent, with inconspicuous OFD-like areas. The epithelial component may be tubular, squamous, basaloid, or

spindle-shaped. The basaloid cells usually have peripheral palisading and central stellate or spindle-shaped cells {1606}. By far the rarest subtype is dedifferentiated adamantinoma. In these tumours, areas of classic adamantinoma gradually merge with a diffuse growing proliferation in which the characteristic epithelial differentiation is lost and instead pleomorphic cells are present, with a high mitotic count. Chondroid differentiation, osteoid deposition, and clear cell changes can be seen {1332,1499}.

Immunohistochemistry
Immunohistochemically, the fibrous tissue is positive for vimentin. The epithelial cells show coexpression of keratin, EMA, vimentin, p63, and podoplanin {822,1589}. Chain-specific keratin expression reveals a predominantly basal epithelial cell differentiation, regardless of subtype, with widespread presence of basal epithelial cell keratins CK5, CK14, and CK19 {1331}. CK1, CK13, and CK17 are also variably present. CK8 and CK18 are virtually absent.

Electron microscopy
Electron microscopy studies have confirmed the epithelial nature of adamantinoma, showing intracytoplasmic hemidesmosomes, tonofilaments, and microfilaments. Irrespective of histological subtype, the epithelial cells are bound by desmosomes, and

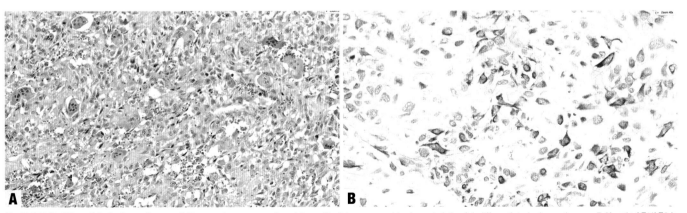

Fig. 3.172 Dedifferentiated adamantinoma. **A** Sarcomatous progression of the epithelial component is characteristic of dedifferentiated adamantinoma. **B** Keratin AE1/AE3 is positive in dedifferentiated adamantinoma.

Table 3.04 Adamantinomas and osteofibrous dysplasia (OFD)

	OFD	OFD-like adamantinoma	Classic adamantinoma	Dedifferentiated adamantinoma
Light microscopy	Osteofibrous lesion	Osteofibrous lesion, small clusters of epithelial cells	Biphasic lesion, epithelial component easily identified	Loss of epithelial differentiation, sarcomatoid change
Keratin staining	Single positive cells, no clusters	Small clusters of keratin-positive cells	Highlights the epithelial component	Sarcomatoid elements may or may not show some keratin positivity
Behaviour	Benign	Locally aggressive	Malignant	Malignant, high-grade

basement membranes have been found to surround the epithelial nests.

Differential diagnosis

The main differential diagnosis includes OFD, which may be difficult to distinguish from OFD-like adamantinoma. In OFD-like adamantinoma, there are small nests of epithelial cells, whereas in OFD, only single keratin-positive cells are seen. See also Table 3.04. Additionally, classic adamantinoma composed predominantly of a spindle cell epithelial component must be distinguished from synovial sarcoma, because the treatment is very different {1416}. Occasionally there is morphological and immunohistochemical overlap between Ewing sarcoma and adamantinoma, in the so-called Ewing-like adamantinoma. However, the specific gene fusions that characterize Ewing sarcoma are absent {1320}.

Cytology

Not clinically relevant

Diagnostic molecular pathology

Not clinically relevant

Essential and desirable diagnostic criteria

Essential: bone tumour with compatible imaging; primary biphasic fibro-osseous tumour of bone, almost exclusively of the tibia and/or fibula; always involves cortex; OFD-like adamantinoma: inconspicuous clusters of epithelial cells, embedded in the fibro-osseous stroma; classic adamantinoma: obvious epithelial elements embedded in fibro-osseous stroma; dedifferentiated adamantinoma: classic adamantinoma in which the epithelial component has progressed to high-grade sarcoma.

Staging

Staging is according to bone sarcoma protocols (see *TNM staging of tumours of bone*, p. 339). See also the information on staging in *Bone tumours: Introduction* (p. 340).

Prognosis and prediction

Risk factors for recurrence are intralesional or marginal surgery and extracompartmental growth. In OFD-like adamantinoma, recurrence rates are about 20% {2778}. OFD-like adamantinomas may rarely metastasize after recurrence and subsequent progression to classic adamantinoma. In classic adamantinoma, the recurrence rate after non-radical surgery may be as high as 90%. Recurrence is associated with an increase in the ratio of epithelium to stroma and with more-aggressive behaviour. Additionally, male sex, female sex combined with young age, pain at presentation, short duration of symptoms, young age (< 20 years), and lack of squamous differentiation of the tumour have been associated with increased rates of recurrence or metastasis {1606,1333,1555,2563,1420}. Classic adamantinomas metastasize in 12–29% of patients, with comparable mortality rates {1333,1606}. The tumour spreads to regional lymph nodes and the lungs, and infrequently to the skeleton, liver, and brain. Dedifferentiated adamantinoma has an aggressive clinical course {1332,1499}.

Simple bone cyst

Reith JD
Bloem JL
Forsyth RG

Definition
Simple bone cyst is an intramedullary, usually unilocular, cystic bone lesion lined by a fibrous membrane and filled with serous or serosanguineous fluid.

ICD-O coding
None

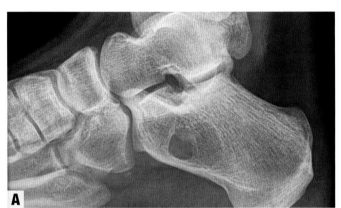

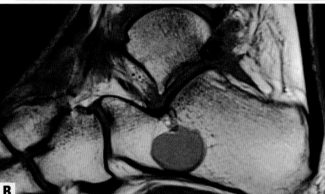

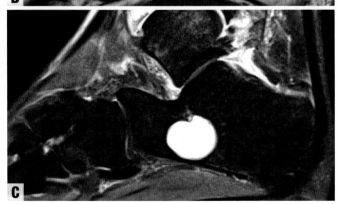

Fig. 3.173 Simple bone cyst. **A** Simple bone cysts may occur in the calcaneus in older patients. **B** T1 MRI highlights the circumscribed borders of the cyst and the low signal intensity of its contents. **C** MRI highlighting the increased signal intensity of the cyst contents on T2-weighted images.

ICD-11 coding
FB80.5 Solitary bone cyst

Related terminology
Acceptable: solitary bone cyst.
Not recommended: unicameral bone cyst.

Subtype(s)
None

Localization
Most simple bone cysts arise in the proximal humerus (50%) and proximal femur (25%), followed by the proximal tibia and other long tubular bones. The pelvic bones and calcaneus are less frequently involved, and patients with lesions in these bones are often slightly older. Rare cases have been described in other locations, including the spine and small bones of the hands and feet. Similar lesions in the jaws have been termed traumatic bone cysts.

Clinical features
Signs and symptoms
Patients may be asymptomatic or present with mild pain, swelling, or limitation of motion. Many simple bone cysts are discovered after pathological fracture {2541}.

Imaging
Roentgenograms show a central, radiolucent lesion that initially abuts the growth plate. As the skeleton grows, the cyst appears to migrate away from the growth plate. The cyst is well circumscribed from the adjacent bone, and it may cause mild expansile remodelling, thinning of the cortex, and endosteal scalloping. However, a periosteal reaction is seldom present unless a pathological fracture is present. In the presence of a fracture, fragments of cortical bone may float freely in the cyst fluid, a pathognomonic finding referred to as the fallen fragment sign {2966}. The finding of a gas bubble in the most non-dependent portion of a solitary bone cyst, referred to as the rising bubble sign {1549,1271}, has also been described as pathognomonic. MRI confirms the high water content of the cyst fluid, which shows low signal intensity on T1-weighted images and bright, homogeneous signal intensity on T2-weighted or other fluid-sensitive sequences {2982}. Repeated fractures may cause trabeculations to form or result in a multiloculated appearance, mimicking aneurysmal bone cyst.

Epidemiology
The majority of simple bone cysts are identified during the first two decades of life. Males are more commonly affected than females (M:F ratio: 2:1).

Etiology
Unknown

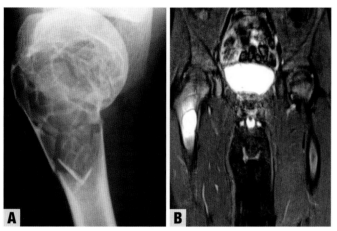

Fig. 3.174 Simple bone cyst. **A** X-ray demonstrating the fallen leaf sign of a fractured lesion, which when present is highly suggestive of a hollow lesion. **B** The contents of the cyst are bright on T2-weighted MRI.

Pathogenesis

Unknown

Macroscopic appearance

It is extremely rare to examine intact simple bone cysts. The unilocular cysts are lined by a thin, smooth layer of tan fibrous tissue and contain serous or serosanguineous fluid. Small bony ridges may be present in the cyst. After pathological fracture, the cyst may contain thickened reparative foci or brownish haemorrhagic foci similar to aneurysmal bone cyst.

Histopathology

The wall of a simple bone cyst is composed of a thin layer of fibrous tissue and lacks a true lining. Foci of chronic inflammation, multinucleated giant cells, haemosiderin, cholesterol clefts, and reactive bone may be present in the wall. Commonly, fibrin-like collagen deposits are seen on the cyst surface and within the wall {240}. These deposits may become mineralized, resulting in a cementum-like or ossified appearance.

Differential diagnosis

In the presence of a pathological fracture, multiloculated foci containing reactive bone, multinucleated giant cells, and haemosiderin may develop, which are difficult to distinguish from aneurysmal bone cyst. Simple bone cyst may also be difficult to distinguish from cystic fibrous dysplasia histologically. Calcaneal lipoma with cystic degeneration is also in the differential diagnosis.

Cytology

Aspiration generally yields a colourless to amber fluid with scant cellularity that may include histiocytes, chronic inflammatory cells, and giant cells {1291}. In the absence of a confirmatory curettage, if the fluid has the above characteristics and the clinical and radiological features are consistent with solitary bone cyst, FNA may be considered diagnostic. However, the presence of bloody fluid mandates further investigation.

Diagnostic molecular pathology

Not clinically relevant

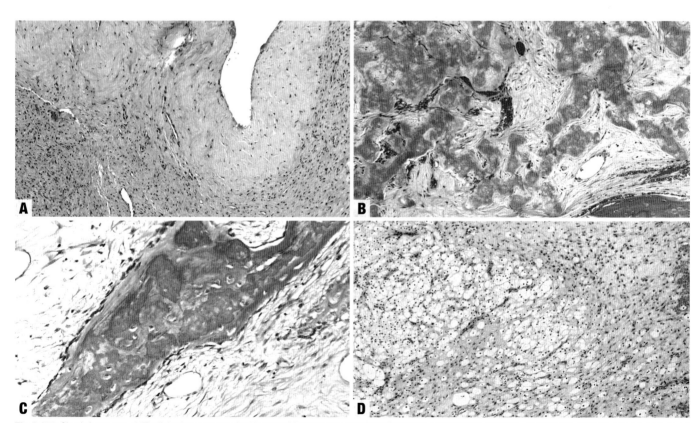

Fig. 3.175 Simple bone cyst. **A** The lining is composed of a thin layer of fibrous tissue containing fibroblasts and small blood vessels. **B** Fibrin-like deposits are commonly found in the cyst wall. **C** The fibrin-like deposits in the wall can calcify and ossify. **D** Foci of foamy histiocytes are commonly found in the cyst wall.

Essential and desirable diagnostic criteria

Essential: bone tumour with compatible imaging; a simple cyst lacking a true lining.

Desirable: often containing fibrin-like deposits, which may organize and mineralize, resulting in cementum-like structures.

Staging

Not clinically relevant

Prognosis and prediction

Local recurrence rates are typically reported in the 10–20% range {3389}. Factors that increase the likelihood of local recurrence include patient age ≤ 5 years, large cyst size, and fracture {3061}. Spontaneous healing after pathological fracture occurs in approximately 10% of patients {1213}. Simple bone cysts have been treated with a variety of injectables, including steroids and demineralized bone marrow, decompression techniques, and curettage {2541}. Complications of large cysts and pathological fracture include growth arrest of the affected bone and avascular necrosis.

Fibrocartilaginous mesenchymoma

Gambarotti M
Inwards CY

Definition
Fibrocartilaginous mesenchymoma is a locally aggressive neoplasm composed of spindle cells with mild cytological atypia, nodules of hyaline cartilage–containing areas resembling growth plate-like cartilage, and bone trabeculae.

ICD-O coding
8990/1 Mesenchymoma NOS

ICD-11 coding
2F7C & XH2AD1 Neoplasms of uncertain behaviour of connective or other soft tissue & Mesenchymoma NOS
2E8A & XH7AA3 Other mixed or unspecified benign mesenchymal tumours & Mesenchymoma, benign

Related terminology
Not recommended: fibrocartilaginous mesenchymoma with low-grade malignancy.

Subtype(s)
None

Localization
Fibrocartilaginous mesenchymoma most frequently occurs in the metaphysis of long tubular bones (61%), followed by the iliac-pubic bones (18%), vertebrae (15%), and metatarsus and rib (3% each) {1113,3027,445}.

Clinical features
Signs and symptoms
Fibrocartilaginous mesenchymoma can be asymptomatic or can present as a painful lesion with localized swelling.

Imaging
Radiologically, fibrocartilaginous mesenchymoma has the appearance of an aggressive benign or low-grade malignant tumour. Radiographs and CT show a lytic, expansile lesion with calcifications. Thinning of the cortex with areas of cortical destruction and soft tissue extension is common. On MRI, fibrocartilaginous mesenchymoma shows low signal on T1-weighted images and high signal on T2-weighted images, with very strong contrast medium uptake {1113}.

Epidemiology
Fibrocartilaginous mesenchymoma is very rare, with < 40 reported cases. It tends to affect young patients (age range: 3 months to 27 years; median: 13 years), with a slight male predominance {1113}.

Etiology
Unknown

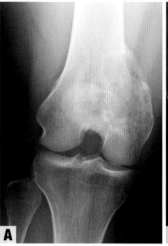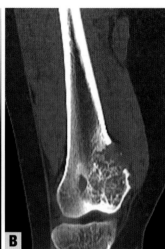

Fig. 3.176 Fibrocartilaginous mesenchymoma. **A** Anteroposterior radiograph shows an eccentric, lytic lesion in the metadiaphysis and epiphysis of the distal right femur, containing a punctate and hazy internal matrix. **B** Coronal CT shows an eccentric, lytic, expansile lesion in the distal right femoral metadiaphysis with extension into the epiphysis. The lesion contains a punctate and hazy internal matrix and is associated with cortical destruction and a soft tissue mass along the proximal aspect of the lesion medially.

Pathogenesis
Unknown

Macroscopic appearance
Fibrocartilaginous mesenchymoma is composed of tan-white fibrous tissue with scattered pale, bluish-grey, glistening areas corresponding to cartilaginous tissue. Resected specimens may show areas of cortical destruction.

Histopathology
Fibrocartilaginous mesenchymoma is characterized by a population of spindle cells, hyaline cartilage nodules, and trabeculae of bone. The hypocellular to moderately cellular spindle cell component contains elongated cells with slightly hyperchromatic, mildly atypical nuclei arranged in bundles or intersecting fascicles. Cellular areas may resemble a low-grade spindle cell sarcoma, but mitotic figures are rare or absent. Benign-appearing cartilaginous nodules of varying size and shape are scattered throughout the tumour. They often contain zones mimicking epiphyseal growth plate characterized by chondrocytes arranged in parallel columns and areas of enchondral ossification. Bone is present as long or short trabeculae. Woven bone rimmed by osteoblasts can be seen emerging from enchondral ossification of the cartilaginous nodules. Both the spindle cell and the cartilaginous components often infiltrate host bone, at times extending into surrounding soft tissues. Clusters of osteoclast-type giant cells may be found.

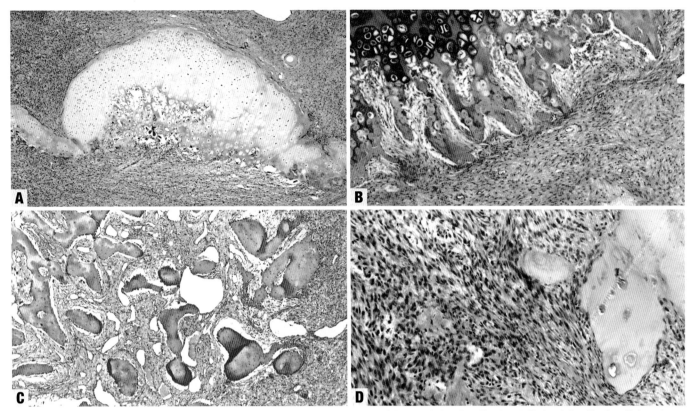

Fig. 3.177 Fibrocartilaginous mesenchymoma. **A** Epiphyseal growth plate–like cartilaginous nodule in a spindle cell proliferation. **B** Enchondral ossification with bone formation at one edge of a cartilaginous nodule. **C** Long and short bony trabeculae are present. **D** High-power view showing a highly cellular spindle cell component that can resemble fibrosarcoma.

Immunohistochemistry
Immunohistochemistry is not helpful.

Differential diagnosis
The main differential diagnosis is with fibrous dysplasia containing cartilage (fibrocartilaginous dysplasia). The cartilage in fibrous dysplasia can have a growth plate–like appearance, but in fibrocartilaginous mesenchymoma it is a more prominent feature. Moreover, the spindle cells in fibrous dysplasia contain small bland nuclei, unlike those in fibrocartilaginous mesenchymoma with mild hyperchromasia. Desmoplastic fibroma of bone and low-grade fibrosarcoma lack cartilaginous nodules. Unlike fibrocartilaginous mesenchymoma, dedifferentiated chondrosarcoma is characterized by a high-grade sarcomatous component. Chondromesenchymal hamartoma shows similar cartilaginous nodules, but these occur in the chest wall of infants and usually contain an aneurysmal bone cyst–like component.

Cytology
Not clinically relevant

Diagnostic molecular pathology
Mutations in *GNAS*, *IDH1*, and *IDH2* and amplification of *MDM2* were absent in the few tumours tested {1113}.

Essential and desirable diagnostic criteria
Essential: bone tumour with compatible imaging; spindle cells with mild cytological atypia, nodules of hyaline cartilage–containing areas resembling growth plate–like cartilage, and bone trabeculae.
Desirable: young patient (aged < 30 years).

Staging
Not clinically relevant

Prognosis and prediction
No metastatic spread or tumour-related deaths have been reported {1113}. Local recurrences tend to occur after intralesional excision, although the literature describes some patients who were disease-free many years after incomplete surgery {445,3027}. Surgical removal with a wide margin is generally the best treatment {1113}.

Fibrous dysplasia

Siegal GP
Bloem JL
Cates JMM
Hameed M

Definition

Fibrous dysplasia is a benign, medullary, fibro-osseous neoplasm that can be multifocal and is characterized by distorted, poorly organized and inadequately mineralized bone and intervening fibrous tissue.

ICD-O coding

8818/0 Fibrous dysplasia

ICD-11 coding

FB80.0 Fibrous dysplasia of bone

Related terminology

Not recommended: liposclerosing myxofibrous tumour; fibro-cartilaginous dysplasia.

Subtype(s)

None

Localization

Craniofacial bones and the femur are the two most common sites, both in monostotic and polyostotic forms, but every bone can be affected {311}. In the monostotic form, a substantial number of cases involve the femur, skull, tibia, and ribs. In the polyostotic form, the femur, pelvis, and tibia are involved in most cases {1306}.

Clinical features

Signs and symptoms

Fibrous dysplasia can be monostotic or polyostotic; in the latter case it can be confined to one extremity or one side of the body, or it can be diffuse. The monostotic form is 6–10 times as common as the polyostotic form. Fibrous dysplasia presents in childhood or adolescence, but the monostotic form may remain asymptomatic until adulthood. The polyostotic form often manifests earlier in life than the monostotic form {1306}. The lesion is often asymptomatic, but pain and fractures are common presenting features {542}. Fibrous dysplasia infrequently produces excess FGF23, causing osteomalacia similar to tumour-induced osteomalacia {2449,2634}. Fibrous dysplasia occurs in association with endocrinopathies and abnormalities of cutaneous pigmentation in McCune–Albright syndrome, as well as with intramuscular myxomas in Mazabraud syndrome {954,1527}.

Imaging

Radiographs often show a non-aggressive geographical lesion with a ground-glass matrix. However, radiographic findings can be substantially altered by changes in longstanding lesions (e.g. cyst formation and fracture). A cartilaginous component can sometimes be identified. Shepherd's crook deformity of the proximal femur is highly diagnostic when present. Generally, there is neither soft tissue extension nor periosteal reaction

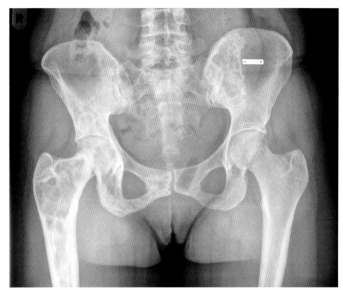

Fig. 3.178 Polyostotic fibrous dysplasia. Polyostotic fibrous dysplasia with localizations in proximal femur, pubic bone extending through inferior ramus to acetabulum, and left iliac bone. The lesions have sclerotic, well-defined, lobulated margins and a geographical pattern of destruction, and they exhibit a combination of osteolysis, ground-glass opacities, and sclerotic septations. Also note the varus deformation (shepherd's crook) of the right femur, which eventually resulted in a fracture.

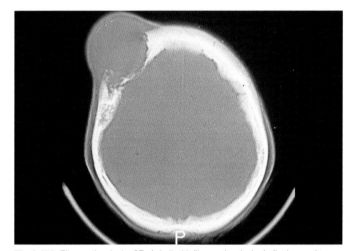

Fig. 3.179 Fibrous dysplasia. CT of skull with fibrous dysplasia. In flat bones the process is often expansile.

unless there is a complicating fracture. Bone scintigraphy, CT, and MRI best delineate the extent of polyostotic disease {706, 1518,3081}.

Epidemiology

Fibrous dysplasia occurs in children and adults worldwide and affects all racial groups with an equal sex distribution.

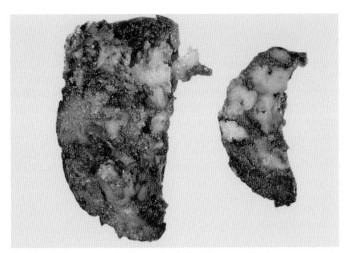

Fig. 3.180 Fibrous dysplasia. Fibrous dysplasia with gross cartilaginous components.

Etiology

Fibrous dysplasia is caused by postzygotic activating missense mutations in the *GNAS* gene (20q13.32), which encodes the alpha subunit of the stimulatory G protein ($G_s\alpha$) {1813,1553}.

Pathogenesis

GNAS activating mutations are detected in 50–70% of fibrous dysplasia samples, with p.Arg201His (66%) and p.Arg201Cys (31%) as the most commonly identified mutations {1813,1553}. $G_s\alpha$ proteins increase WNT/β-catenin signalling, which inhibits terminal maturation/differentiation of osteoprogenitor cells {1619}. Studies of transgenic mice constitutively expressing $G_s\alpha$ p.Arg201Cys replicate the human disease and show that fibrous dysplasia develops through three distinct histopathological stages {2705}. However, we do not typically recognize these stages in routine histology. *GNAS* mutations have also been associated with McCune–Albright syndrome and nonskeletal isolated endocrine lesions, suggesting a spectrum of phenotypic expression {310}.

Macroscopic appearance

The bone is often expanded and the lesional tissue has a tan-grey colour with a firm to gritty consistency. There may be cysts, which may contain some yellow-tinged fluid {2857}. When cartilage is present (a rare event), it often stands out as sharply circumscribed, blue-tinged, translucent material {3132}.

Histopathology

Fibrous and osseous tissues are present in varying proportions. The fibrous tissue is composed principally of bland fibroblastic cells. Mitoses are uncommon but are more often seen in the setting of a fracture. The osseous component consists of irregular, curvilinear trabeculae of woven (or rarely lamellar) bone in the majority of cases, but other appearances including cementum-like bone deposition, and rounded psammomatous calcification can be seen, particularly in the jaw {2877}. In some cases, the bony spicules assume a pagetoid appearance, with interconnecting thickened trabeculae and intervening fibrous tissue. Nodules of benign hyaline cartilage, which undergo endochondral ossification, can be seen in rare cases. Osteoblasts are present but inconspicuous and sometimes spindle-shaped. Other changes include aneurysmal bone cyst–like changes, foam cells, multinucleated osteoclastic giant cells, and extensive myxoid change (particularly in longstanding cases) {839}.

Cytology

Not clinically relevant

Diagnostic molecular pathology

The mutation discovery rate in *GNAS* is dependent on the technology used and is adversely affected by sample decalcification. Somatic mosaicism may also account for the reported variability in mutation detection rates in the literature {1553}. These molecular assays are diagnostically useful, because occasionally fibrous dysplasia can be confused histologically with low-grade central osteosarcoma {2724}. The only recurrent clonal chromosome aberrations described to date include trisomy 2 and structural aberrations of 12p13 {719}.

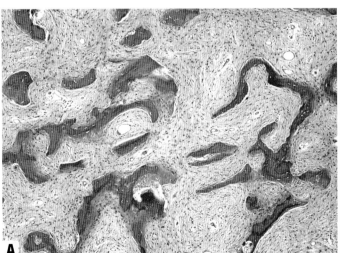
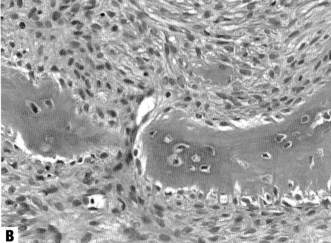

Fig. 3.181 Fibrous dysplasia. **A** Typical deposition of woven bone in a background of bland spindle cell proliferation. **B** Higher power showing Sharpey-like fibres, a typical finding in fibrous dysplasia.

Essential and desirable diagnostic criteria

Essential: bone tumour with compatible imaging; osseous component composed of irregular, curvilinear trabeculae of woven bone without conspicuous osteoblastic rimming; fibrous component composed of bland fibroblastic cells.

Desirable (in selected cases): activating missense mutations in *GNAS* (p.Arg201His, p.Arg201Cys) present.

Staging

Not clinically relevant

Prognosis and prediction

The prognosis for many patients with fibrous dysplasia is excellent. However, monostotic fibrous dysplasia can cause skeletal deformities or leg-length discrepancies, or it can impinge on cranial nerves, and extensive polyostotic disease may be crippling. Malignant transformation very rarely occurs {1894}.

Lipoma and hibernoma of bone

Rosenberg AE
Bloem JL
Sumathi VP

Definition
Lipoma and hibernoma of bone are benign neoplasms composed of white adipocytes (lipoma) or brown adipocytes (hibernoma) that arise within or on the surface of bone.

ICD-O coding
8850/0 Lipoma NOS
8880/0 Hibernoma

ICD-11 coding
2E80 & XH1PL8 Benign lipomatous neoplasm & Lipoma NOS
2E80 & XA5GG8 Benign lipomatous neoplasm & Bones
2E80 & XH1054 Benign lipomatous neoplasm & Hibernoma

Related terminology
None

Subtype(s)
None

Localization
Lipomas commonly arise in the calcaneus and metaphysis of long tubular bones, especially the femur, tibia, and humerus, and infrequently in the skull, pelvis, vertebrae, sacrum, mandible, maxilla, and ribs; approximately 70% involve the lower limb {1289,471}. Parosteal lipoma develops on the diaphysis of long tubular bones, especially the femur, radius, humerus, and tibia {234}. Hibernoma often affects the axial skeleton {1710}.

Clinical features
Signs and symptoms
Lipoma may be asymptomatic (30%) or produce aching pain (70%) {1710}. Parosteal lipoma may be painful and can produce a palpable mass {234}. Hibernoma is usually asymptomatic and detected during evaluation for an unrelated disorder {1710}.

Imaging
Intraosseous lipomas occur mainly (71%) in the lower extremity (calcaneus) and exhibit low density on plain radiographs, high signal on T1-weighted images, and low signal on fluid-sensitive fat-suppressed images {471}. Calcifications in the well-defined margin and within the lesion are seen as high density on radiographs and CT, and they show signal void on MRI. Fat necrosis and cystic degeneration occur more frequently in the calcaneus and have high signal on fluid-sensitive sequences. Parosteal lipomas display the same fatty characteristics on imaging, but the lesion is superficial to and in continuity with the periosteum. Bone formation can be seen in the centre of the lesion at the surface of cortical bone {2222}. Underlying cortical bone and bone marrow are not involved. Hibernoma is characterized by a combination of imaging features: high uptake of FDG on PET-CT, uptake on bone scintigraphy, sclerotic ill-defined appearance

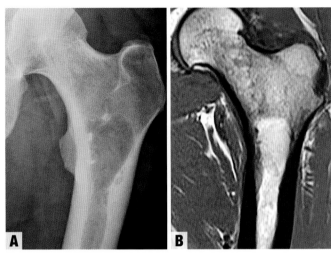

Fig. 3.182 Lipoma of bone. **A** Radiograph shows well-circumscribed oval radiolucency, with calcifications. **B** Coronal T1-weighted MRI demonstrates the lipoma that has high signal intensity and is longer than appreciated on the plain film.

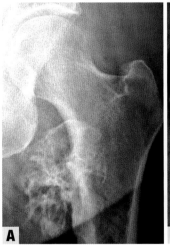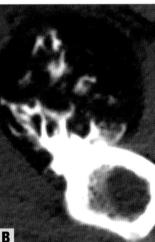

Fig. 3.183 Parosteal lipoma. **A** Juxtacortical mass is well circumscribed and bubbly in appearance. It contains linear mineralization that is most prominent at its site of attachment to the bone. **B** Axial CT shows bone at base of parosteal lipoma surrounded by oval well-circumscribed mass of fat that is dark with low density. Cortex is intact and there is no continuity between the lesion and the bone marrow of the diaphysis.

on CT, low signal on T1, slightly increased heterogeneous signal on fluid-sensitive MRI sequences, and mild enhancement on gadolinium chelate–enhanced MRI {362}.

Epidemiology
Lipoma is rare and accounts for < 0.1% of primary bone tumours. The patient age range is from the second to eighth decades of life (mean age: 50 years). Males are affected more frequently than females (M:F ratio: ~1.3:1) {1568}. Parosteal

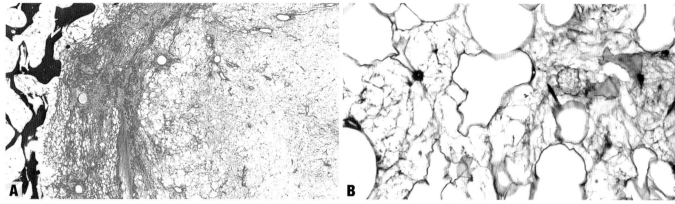

Fig. 3.184 Lipoma of bone. **A** Lipoma within the medullary cavity is well circumscribed. **B** Large white adipocyte with crescent-shaped nucleus containing intranuclear inclusion.

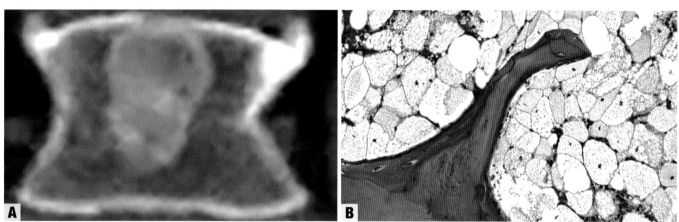

Fig. 3.185 Hibernoma of bone. **A** Coronal CT shows well-circumscribed hibernoma that is mineralized. **B** Brown fat cells of hibernoma have multiple small clear vacuoles enmeshed in eosinophilic cytoplasm.

lipoma accounts for 15% of bone lipomas and develops during the fifth to sixth decades of life. There is a slight male predominance (M:F ratio: ~1.3:1). Hibernoma is very rare, develops in patients aged 40–80 years, and shows a female predominance {1710}.

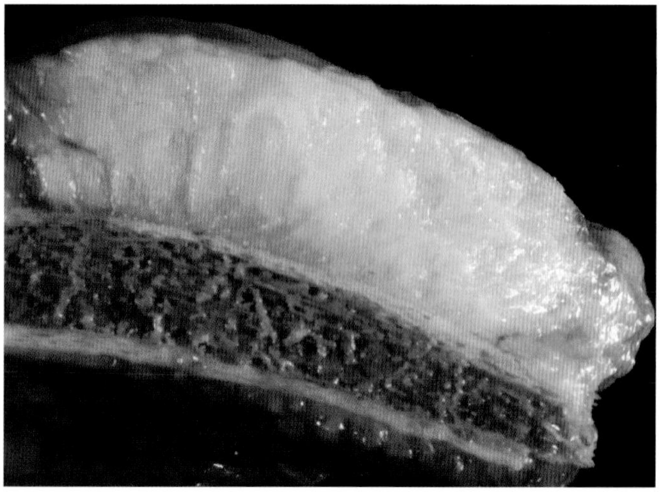

Etiology
Unknown

Pathogenesis
The pathogenesis is unknown, but it is presumably related to genetic abnormalities and activation of specific cell signalling pathways.

Macroscopic appearance
Intramedullary lipoma is well defined, soft but sometimes gritty, and yellow; tumours containing brown adipocytes are yellowish-brown in colour. Tumours are usually 3–5 cm in size; exceptional cases are > 10 cm {1568}. The bone surrounding the tumour is often sclerotic. Parosteal lipoma is 4–10 cm in greatest dimension, well defined, soft, and yellow. Some cases contain gritty spicules of bone or firm nodules of cartilage in the base or scattered throughout the mass.

Histopathology
Lipoma is composed of lobules of mature-appearing adipocytes. Delicate trabeculae of woven and lamellar bone may be present throughout the tumour. The adipocytes have a single, large, clear cytoplasmic vacuole that displaces the crescent-shaped nucleus to the periphery. Some tumours may demonstrate necrosis with foamy macrophages and fibrosis. Parosteal lipoma is a well-defined mass of white fat. Its base, adjacent to

Fig. 3.186 Parosteal lipoma. Parosteal lipoma of rib composed of a juxtacortical, well-defined mass of yellowish fat.

the cortex, may have bone trabeculae or hypocellular hyaline cartilage, which undergoes endochondral ossification. Brown fat cells in hibernoma are large, have numerous clear vacuoles that scallop central nuclei, and are surrounded by eosinophilic cytoplasm; the cells may be admixed with haematopoietic elements.

Immunohistochemistry
Adipocytes are positive for S100 and negative for CD68. Hibernomas strongly express the brown fat marker UCP1 {2319}.

Differential diagnosis
Bone marrow infarction with dystrophic calcification is distinguished from lipoma by the presence of pre-existing necrotic bone throughout the lesion and the lack of a discrete mass on imaging studies.

Cytology
Cytology shows adipocytes with vacuolated cytoplasm; there is no cytological atypia.

Diagnostic molecular pathology
Not clinically relevant

Essential and desirable diagnostic criteria
Essential: lipoma of bone: aggregates of mature-appearing adipocytes, presenting as a bone tumour with compatible imaging; parosteal lipoma: aggregates of mature-appearing adipocytes, presenting as a bone tumour on the surface of the bone; hibernoma of bone: aggregates of brown fat cells, presenting as a bone tumour with compatible imaging.

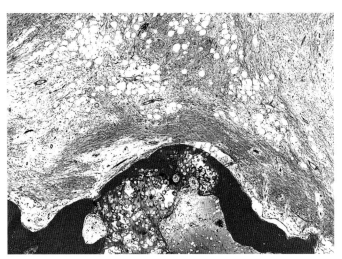

Fig. 3.187 Parosteal lipoma. Woven bone with a small amount of cartilage at the base beneath lobules of white adipose tissue.

Staging
Not clinically relevant

Prognosis and prediction
The prognosis is excellent. Symptomatic intraosseous tumours are curetted, and parosteal lipoma is marginally excised. Recurrence rates are extremely low.

Leiomyosarcoma of bone

McCarthy EF
Antonescu CR

Definition
Leiomyosarcoma (LMS) of bone is a primary malignant neoplasm of bone showing smooth muscle differentiation.

ICD-O coding
8890/3 Leiomyosarcoma NOS

ICD-11 coding
2B58 & XH7ED4 Leiomyosarcoma & Leiomyosarcoma NOS
2B58 & XA5GG8 Leiomyosarcoma & Bones

Related terminology
None

Subtype(s)
None

Localization
Most lesions occur in the lower extremity around the knee (distal femoral or proximal tibial metaphysis), followed by the craniofacial skeleton {131,1194,2606}.

Clinical features
Signs and symptoms
Patients typically report pain and occasionally present with pathological fracture. Metastatic disease from extraosseous primary lesions (uterus, bowel, soft tissue) should be excluded, because this is much more common than primary LMS of bone.

Imaging
There are no specific imaging features. Radiographically, they are lytic, aggressive lesions, with a permeative growth pattern

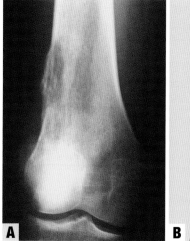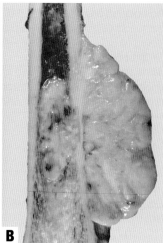

Fig. 3.188 Leiomyosarcoma. **A** X-ray of a tumour in the distal femur showing an aggressive, permeative lytic lesion with cortical destruction. **B** Femoral macroscopy. Note both an intraosseous and an extraosseous component of the white fleshy tumour.

and cortical destruction. MRI shows soft tissue extension, and signal intensities are nonspecific {2832,181}.

Epidemiology
There is a wide age distribution (9–87 years), with a peak incidence in the fifth decade of life and a slight male predominance.

Etiology
A small subset of LMSs of bone are associated with prior exposure to radiation therapy or with bone infarcts {147,2504}. LMS of bone related to EBV infection in immunocompromised patients has been reported {811}.

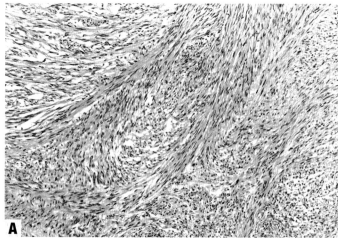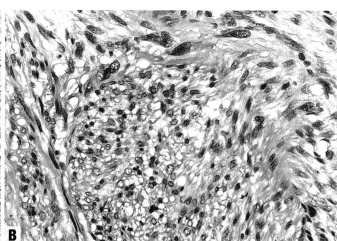

Fig. 3.189 Leiomyosarcoma. **A** Low-power image showing bundles of spindle cells. **B** On high power, cellular pleomorphism of the tumour cells is seen.

Pathogenesis

Similar to deep soft tissue LMSs, intraosseous lesions show genomic losses and absence of phosphorylated RB1 {3194}.

Macroscopic appearance

The lesions vary widely in size. On cut surface, they show a tan, fleshy, creamy appearance, with obvious areas of necrosis.

Histopathology

The lesions resemble LMSs from other locations, with cells arranged in long, intersecting fascicles, growing in an infiltrative pattern. The tumour cells have fibrillary, eosinophilic cytoplasm and elongated, cigar-shaped nuclei with blunted ends. The tumours are associated with variable degrees of necrosis, nuclear pleomorphism, and mitotic activity.

Immunohistochemistry

Smooth muscle differentiation is demonstrated by diffuse staining with desmin and/or h-caldesmon, as well as SMA {2606}. LMP1 immunohistochemistry can be used to document the EBV protein {811}. Positivity for ER or PR in female patients strongly suggests a primary uterine origin.

Cytology

Not clinically relevant

Diagnostic molecular pathology

Not clinically relevant

Essential and desirable diagnostic criteria

Essential: bone tumour with compatible imaging; exclusion of other primary sites; intersecting fascicles of fusiform cells with eosinophilic fibrillary cytoplasm and elongated cigar-shaped nuclei, with variable nuclear pleomorphism; SMA and desmin and/or h-caldesmon immunoreactivity.

Staging

Staging is according to bone sarcoma protocols (see *TNM staging of tumours of bone*, p. 339). See also the information on staging in *Bone tumours: Introduction* (p. 340).

Prognosis and prediction

Histological grade correlates with clinical outcome {131}. High-grade lesions are highly aggressive, with a high index of distant spread (often to the lung) and a 5-year disease-free survival rate of < 50% {18,2195}.

Undifferentiated pleomorphic sarcoma

Inwards CY
Czerniak B
Dei Tos AP

Definition

Undifferentiated pleomorphic sarcoma (UPS) is a pleomorphic malignant neoplasm of bone with no identifiable line of differentiation; this is a diagnosis of exclusion.

ICD-O coding

8802/3 Pleomorphic sarcoma, undifferentiated

ICD-11 coding

2B54 & XH0947 Unclassified pleomorphic sarcoma, primary site & Malignant fibrous histiocytoma

Related terminology

Not recommended: malignant fibrous histiocytoma of bone; pleomorphic fibrosarcoma of bone.

Subtype(s)

None

Localization

UPS has a predilection for long tubular bones, particularly around the knee {315,2302}. The most frequently involved bone is the femur, followed by the tibia and humerus. Among the bones of the trunk, the pelvis is most commonly affected. UPS rarely occurs in the spine.

Clinical features

Signs and symptoms

Symptomatic patients typically report pain and occasionally swelling. Pathological fractures are common, particularly in weight-bearing long tubular bones.

Imaging

The radiological features of UPSs are nonspecific, but the majority of cases demonstrate an aggressive osteolytic neoplasm with ill-defined margins, cortical destruction, and an associated soft tissue mass {1684}. Periosteal reaction is an infrequent finding, and mineralized matrix is absent. The tumours are usually centred in the metadiaphyseal region of long bones and occasionally extend into the epiphysis.

Epidemiology

UPS of bone is rare, representing < 2% of all primary malignant bone tumours. Males are more frequently affected than females. There is a broad age distribution, from the second to

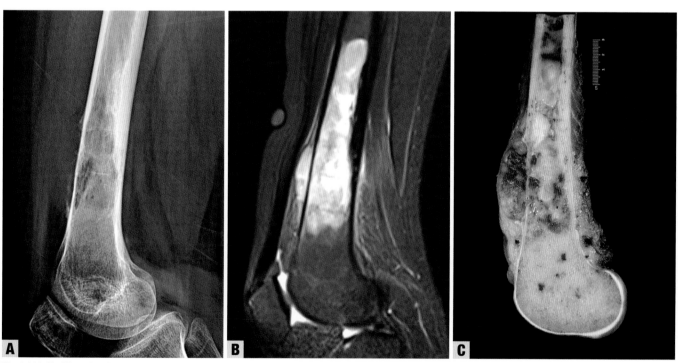

Fig. 3.190 Undifferentiated pleomorphic sarcoma of bone. **A** Lateral radiograph shows a predominantly osteolytic lesion in the distal femoral diaphysis, with malignant periosteal new bone formation. **B** Sagittal T2-weighted fat-suppressed MRI shows a predominantly osteolytic lesion in the distal femoral diaphysis, with malignant periosteal new bone formation and soft tissue mass anteriorly. **C** Cut surface of the resected tumour shows a yellowish-grey tumour with areas of reddish-brown haemorrhage and soft tissue extension.

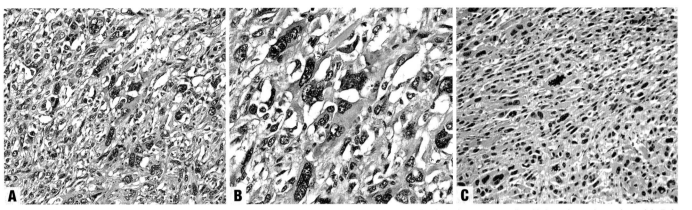

Fig. 3.191 Undifferentiated pleomorphic sarcoma of bone. **A** Marked cytological pleomorphism characterized by giant tumour cells with large hyperchromatic nuclei. **B** At higher power. **C** Marked cytological pleomorphism characterized by giant tumour cells with large hyperchromatic nuclei and atypical mitoses.

eighth decades of life, but most patients are aged > 40 years. Only 10–15% of cases occur in patients aged < 20 years.

Etiology

The etiology of primary UPS of bone is unknown. Secondary UPS, representing approximately 28% of cases, arises in association with a pre-existing bone condition or disease {2302,2432,1448}. The majority of secondary UPSs are associated with a bone infarct, Paget disease, or prior irradiation in the field of the affected bone {1452,836,2933}. Rare examples of UPS of bone occur at the site of a metallic orthopaedic prosthesis or hardware {1604,1903}. Diaphyseal medullary stenosis, a rare autosomal dominant bone dysplasia, is another less common setting associated with UPS of bone {172,1300}. This disorder is characterized by cortical growth abnormalities, including diffuse diaphyseal medullary stenosis with overlying endosteal cortical thickening, metaphyseal striations, and scattered infarctions {846}. Approximately 35% of patients with this syndrome develop UPS of bone {1987, 2218,466}. The disorder is caused by mutations in the gene encoding methylthioadenosine phosphorylase, *MTAP* {466}.

Pathogenesis

UPS of bone is highly aneuploid and shows complex chromosomal complements with numerous structural aberrations and marker chromosomes {2865}. These cytogenetic observations are confirmed by array hybridization studies, which reveal frequent losses of 8p, 9p, 10, 13q, and 18q and gains of 4q, 5p, 6p, 7p, 8q, 12p, 14q, 17q, 19p, 20q, 22q, and X {2295}. Homozygous deletions of *CDKN2A*, *RB1*, *TP53*, and *ING1* are present in a subset of UPSs {2295}. Mutations in *TP53* (~30%) and/or chromatin-remodelling genes (~40%) are most frequent {68}. In general, the copy-number alterations in UPS of bone overlap with those identified in the same tumours originating in soft tissue {68,472}. UPS of bone exhibits multiple somatic gene fusions, two of which, *CLTC-VMP1* and *FARP1-STK24*, appear to be recurrent and were reported previously in multiple cancers {68,1145}. RNA sequencing expression data indicate that UPS has an expression profile distinct from that of its soft tissue counterpart and is characterized by activation of the FGF23 pathway {68}.

Macroscopic appearance

The gross appearance of UPS is quite variable. The cut surface texture ranges from fibrous to soft. Areas of necrosis and haemorrhage are frequently present. The tumours exhibit a range of colours, including greyish-white, yellow, and brownish-tan. Cortical destruction and a soft tissue mass are commonly present.

Histopathology

The tumour is diffusely composed of spindle-shaped and epithelioid or polygonal cells with marked pleomorphism arranged in a haphazard, storiform, and fascicular growth pattern. Variable numbers of large, bizarre multinucleated giant cells and numerous typical and atypical mitotic figures are readily identified. The tumour cells are often embedded within a collagen-rich stroma, which may be hyalinized. A background population of scattered foamy histiocytes and inflammatory cells can be seen among the neoplastic cells. Importantly, the tumour lacks any evidence of malignant osteoid or cartilage, thus necessitating thorough sampling in order to rule out osteosarcoma and dedifferentiated chondrosarcoma. Trabeculae of reactive woven bone are occasionally present, particularly at the periphery or in the setting of a pathological fracture {2239}.

Immunohistochemistry

Immunohistochemistry is an essential part of the diagnosis because, by definition, UPS lacks an identifiable line of differentiation and is a diagnosis of exclusion. Caution is required when interpreting myogenic markers, because approximately 50% of UPSs of bone show focal positivity with a single myogenic marker {3123,2651}. SMA positivity with an additional myogenic marker (desmin or h-caldesmon) supports leiomyosarcoma in an appropriate histological context. Desmin, myogenin, and MYOD1 aid in ruling out rhabdomyosarcoma. SATB2 immunoreactivity can be seen in UPS, a limiting factor when exploring the possibility of osteosarcoma {742}. H3.3 p.Gly34Trp (G34W) expression is occasionally seen in bone sarcomas without associated giant cell tumour histology; these are usually sited in the epiphysis in young people, suggesting a relationship with a giant cell tumour. Therefore, there is a move to expand the definition of primary malignant giant cell tumour on the basis of an *H3-3A (H3F3A)* or *H3-3B (H3F3B)* p.Gly34 mutation {2358, 2630,91,3337}. Focal cytokeratin positivity can be seen in UPS, but abundant expression should raise concern for metastatic sarcomatoid carcinoma. Several melanocytic markers are indicated in the setting of focal S100 expression in order to exclude melanoma.

Differential diagnosis
The differential diagnosis is broad, including a variety of high-grade sarcomas, metastatic carcinoma, and metastatic melanoma. When features are similar to those of high-grade myxofibrosarcoma of soft tissue, some pathologists favour a diagnosis of high-grade myxofibrosarcoma of bone {2651}.

Cytology
Not clinically relevant

Diagnostic molecular pathology
The absence of *IDH1* or *IDH2* mutations in UPS of bone can be used in the differential diagnosis with dedifferentiated chondrosarcoma {558}. Similarly, the presence of an *H3-3A* (*H3F3A*) or *H3-3B* (*H3F3B*) p.Gly34 mutation may suggest a relationship with giant cell tumour of bone, and there is a move to expand the definition of primary malignant giant cell tumour of bone on the basis of an *H3-3A* (*H3F3A*) or *H3-3B* (*H3F3B*) p.Gly34 mutation {2358,2630,91}.

Essential and desirable diagnostic criteria
Essential: bone tumour with compatible imaging; pleomorphic spindle-shaped and epithelioid cells in a storiform or fascicular growth pattern; no malignant cartilage or bone production by the tumour cells; no specific line of differentiation.
Desirable: atypical mitotic figures; necrosis.

Staging
Staging is according to bone sarcoma protocols (see *TNM staging of tumours of bone*, p. 339). See also the information on staging in *Bone tumours: Introduction* (p. 340).

Prognosis and prediction
Patients with UPS of bone are generally treated with chemotherapy and complete en bloc resection {3365,198,1525}. Patients with localized disease and adequate therapy have a 5-year survival rate of 50–67% {399,2432,315}. Pulmonary metastases are common, occurring in approximately 35–50% of cases. Secondary UPS and metastatic disease are associated with a poorer prognosis. Incomplete expression of myogenic markers is not thought to affect the prognosis {2651}.

Bone metastases

Kalil RK
Bloem JL
Hornick JL
Righi A

Definition
Bone metastases are tumours involving bone as a result of haematogenous spread from malignancies at distant sites.

ICD-O coding
None

ICD-11 coding
None

Related terminology
None

Subtype(s)
None

Localization
Any site can be involved. Common sites are long bones such as femur and humerus and the axial skeleton. There is a predilection for more-vascularized areas of bone like the metaphysis of long bones and vertebrae. Lung cancer is the most common primary malignancy that metastasizes to acral sites {2611,3264}.

Clinical features
Signs and symptoms
Pain is usually the first symptom and is almost always present. Pathological fracture is common and may cause abrupt pain. Sometimes metastasis is the first manifestation of cancer. A primary tumour cannot always be identified (a so-called unknown primary).

Imaging
Radiographically, metastases can be lytic, sclerotic, or mixed. Typical lytic metastases include primary renal cell, lung, and thyroid carcinomas. Sclerotic metastases suggest primary prostate, breast, and neuroendocrine carcinomas. Bone scintigraphy has been the method of choice to detect bone metastases because of its high sensitivity to osteoblastic activity, which is almost always present to some degree. FDG PET has largely replaced bone scintigraphy because it directly shows tumour in any location rather than host bone reaction only. However, this functional technique is dependent on glucose metabolism and is only reliable if the primary tumour takes up FDG. Whole-body MRI is an alternative, depending on the morphological features of the tumour deposits.

Epidemiology
Metastatic carcinoma lesions constitute the more common type of osseous tumour in elderly patients. The more frequent primary sites are lung, breast, prostate, kidney, thyroid, pancreas, and liver. Other common primary tumours are lymphoma and melanoma. Metastases in young patients are much less frequent and are usually due to neural, renal, or soft tissue and bone tumours, such as neuroblastoma, rhabdomyosarcoma, Ewing sarcoma, and osteosarcoma.

Etiology
Bone metastases result from metastatic spread of a primary malignancy elsewhere in the body.

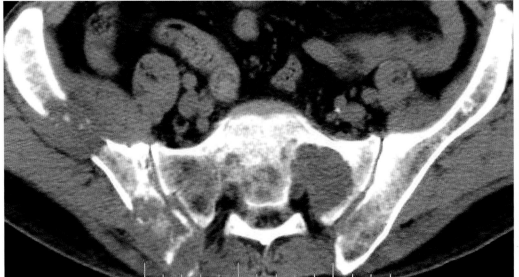

Fig. 3.192 Metastatic carcinoma in pelvic bone. Multiple skeletal lesions in elderly patients are suggestive of metastatic spread.

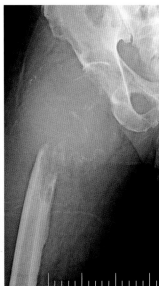

Fig. 3.193 Metastasis from renal carcinoma. Radiography of hip with large solitary skeletal lesion.

Pathogenesis

Involvement of bone by these tumours is the result of haematogenous spread (metastasis) from the site of the primary malignancy.

Macroscopic appearance

Usually, metastases have haemorrhagic and friable tissue, especially if they are from thyroid or kidney. Metastases from prostate and breast can be hard due to reactive bone sclerosis. Melanoma can produce dark, pigmented metastases.

Histopathology

Metastases present with histological features similar to those of the primary lesions, the most common being adenocarcinomas and squamous cell carcinomas. Osteoblastic metastases contain abundant reactive woven bone and must be distinguished from osteosarcoma. Haemorrhage, fibrosis, and osteoclast-like giant cell reactions are frequent and can sometimes obscure the metastatic cells.

Immunohistochemistry

Immunohistochemistry should be used to suggest or confirm a possible primary origin {3180,2940}. See Table 3.05.

Differential diagnosis

Primary vascular tumours of bone can very closely simulate metastatic carcinoma on radiology and histology, and they may also be positive for epithelial markers {3189,3197}.

Cytology

Not clinically relevant

Diagnostic molecular pathology

Molecular diagnostics related to the primary tumour may be of diagnostic or prognostic relevance {3295,360}.

Essential and desirable diagnostic criteria

Essential: malignant growth at distance from a primary site elsewhere; correlation with imaging and clinical history.
Desirable (in selected cases): immunohistochemistry, as indicated, is frequently necessary.

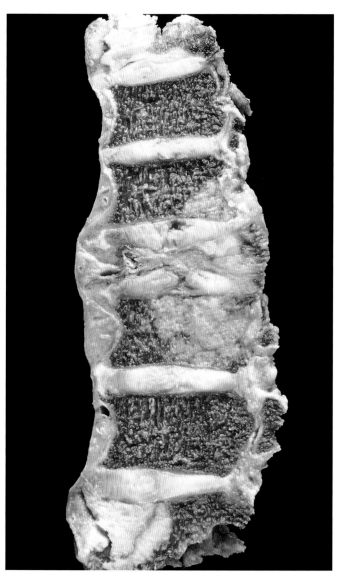

Fig. 3.194 Metastatic carcinoma in the spine. Gross photography showing a solid vertebral lesion involving multiple levels.

Table 3.05 Immunohistochemical markers for the most common metastatic carcinomas to bone: primary site determination

Primary site	CK7 and CK20 (most-common patterns)	Other markers	
		Cytoplasmic or membranous	Nuclear[a]
Breast	CK7+, CK20–	GCDFP-15, mammaglobin	ER, GATA3, SOX10 (triple-negative)
Kidney (renal cell carcinoma)	CK7–, CK20–	RCCm	PAX8
Liver (hepatocellular carcinoma)	CK7–, CK20–	Arginase-1 (ARG1), CPS1 (Hep Par-1)	Arginase-1 (ARG1)
Lung (adenocarcinoma)	CK7+, CK20–	Napsin A	TTF1
Pancreas	CK7+, CK20–		SMAD4 (loss)
Prostate	CK7–, CK20–	PSA, PSAP	NKX3-1
Small cell carcinoma[b]		Chromogranin, synaptophysin	TTF1, RB1 (loss)
Squamous cell carcinoma[c]		High-molecular-weight cytokeratins (e.g. CK5)	p63, p40
Thyroid	CK7+, CK20–	Thyroglobulin	PAX8, TTF1

[a]Nuclear markers are particularly susceptible to decalcification; the possibility of false-negative results (when relevant) should be included in a disclaimer in pathology reports. [b]Immunohistochemistry cannot distinguish among metastatic small cell carcinomas (i.e. pulmonary vs extrapulmonary origin). [c]Immunohistochemistry cannot distinguish among metastatic squamous cell carcinomas (other than p16 – diffuse staining suggests a high-risk HPV–associated squamous cell carcinoma, such as from the oropharynx, anal canal, or uterine cervix).

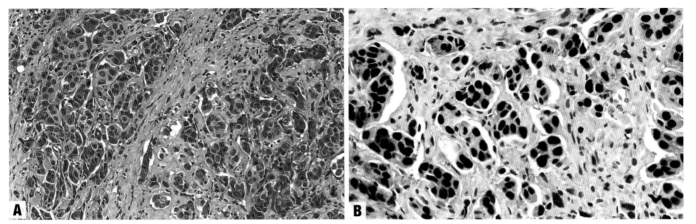

Fig. 3.195 Metastasis from breast carcinoma. **A** Medium-power microscopic view showing small infiltrating glands. Comparison with the specimen from the original cancer site is often necessary. **B** Staining for ER is positive.

Staging
Not clinically relevant

Prognosis and prediction
The prognosis is predominantly defined by the primary tumour {358}. The overall median survival time for patients with spinal metastases in one series was 5.1 months {359}.

Solitary plasmacytoma of bone

Ferry JA
Deshpande V
Lorsbach RB

Definition

Solitary plasmacytoma of bone (SPB) is a localized, intraosseous neoplasm composed of clonal plasma cells, with no evidence of other bony lesions and no evidence of plasma cell myeloma (PCM).

ICD-O coding

9731/3 Plasmacytoma of bone

ICD-11 coding

2A83.2 & XH4BL1 Solitary plasmacytoma & Plasmacytoma NOS

Related terminology

Not recommended: osseous plasmacytoma.

Subtype(s)

None

Localization

The axial skeleton is affected more often than the appendicular skeleton; other bones commonly affected include the pelvis, ribs, skull, and long bones {3250,1656,2071,2978}.

Clinical features

Signs and symptoms

Patients typically present with localized pain, sometimes accompanied by fracture. Vertebral SPB with fracture can be associated with spinal cord compression {2978}. SPB may present occasionally as a soft tissue lesion in cases with localized extraosseous extension. Patients commonly have a serum or urine M component {2978,233}.

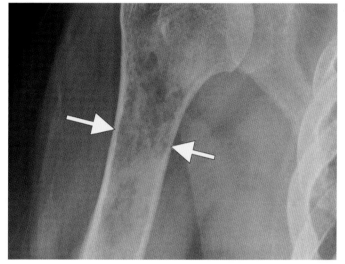

Fig. 3.197 Solitary plasmacytoma of bone. Anteroposterior radiograph of the right humerus shows geographical destruction consisting of patchy bone lysis. There is no surrounding sclerosis and the cortex is mildly thinned (arrows) but intact.

Imaging

Radiographically, SPB manifests as a well-circumscribed geographical lytic bone lesion without identifiable matrix {1622, 3255}.

Epidemiology

SPB affects men more often than women (M:F ratio: 2–3:1) {3250,1656,1622,1139}, and its incidence is higher in black people than in white people {1622}. Most patients are middle-aged and older adults (median age: 55–60 years) {1622,1139, 3255,233}. Young adults are occasionally affected {3250,1656}.

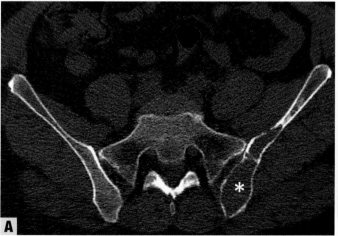 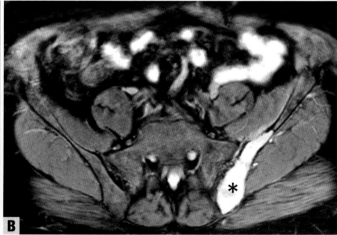

Fig. 3.196 Solitary plasmacytoma of bone. **A** Axial CT image of the pelvis shows a well-defined lytic lesion (asterisk) in the posterior aspect of the left ilium. The cortex is thinned and there is mild expansile remodelling. **B** Proton density MRI with fat saturation image of the pelvis shows a well-defined lytic lesion (asterisk) in the posterior aspect of the left ilium, with homogeneous, hyperintense marrow infiltration.

Table 3.06 Solitary plasmacytoma of bone: differential diagnosis

Diagnosis	Clinical features	Morphology	Immunoglobulin (Ig) expressed	Immunophenotype, additional features	Cytogenetic/genetic features
Solitary plasmacytoma of bone	Isolated lytic lesion of bone, often painful, +/− fracture; no association with immunodeficiency	Diffuse, destructive infiltrate of mature, immature, lymphocyte-like, plasmablast-like, or rarely anaplastic plasma cells	Monotypic cytoplasmic Ig light chain; IgG > IgA > light chain only; others rare	As for plasma cell myeloma	Similar to plasma cell myeloma, but not as extensively studied
Chronic osteomyelitis	Fever, local pain	Mature plasma cells, +/− lymphocytes, granulocytes, fibrosis, and necrotic bone	Polytypic cytoplasmic Ig light chain	CD138+, CD38+, CD19+, CD56− plasma cells	No abnormalities
Plasmablastic lymphoma	Immunosuppressed patient with extranodal lesion (oral cavity, gastrointestinal, others; bone involvement is uncommon), usually without lymphadenopathy	Diffuse infiltrate of plasmablasts +/− differentiation to more-mature plasma cells; high mitotic count; may have starry-sky appearance	Monotypic cytoplasmic Ig light chain +/−	CD138+, CD38+, IRF4 (MUM1)+, MYC+, CD45+/−, CD79a+/−, CD56+/−, CD20−, PAX5−, BCL6−, ALK−, HHV8−, Ki-67 high; EBER usually positive	Complex karyotype; MYC often rearranged, less often amplified
Lymphoplasmacytic lymphoma	Symptoms usually related to anaemia and paraprotein, +/− autoimmune phenomena or cryoglobulinaemia; lymphadenopathy and/or splenomegaly may be present; discrete bone lesions are rare	Diffuse, interstitial, or patchy involvement by small lymphocytes, plasma cells, and plasmacytoid lymphocytes	Monotypic surface and cytoplasmic Ig light chain; IgM+, almost all cases	CD19+, CD20+, CD5−, CD10−, BCL6−, CD23− clonal B cells and clonal plasma cells	MYD88 p.Leu265Pro point mutation
Plasma cell myeloma	Most patients have symptoms related to CRAB, infections, and bleeding; some are asymptomatic and may have smouldering myeloma	Diffuse, interstitial, or patchy marrow involvement by mature, immature, lymphocyte-like, plasmablast-like, or rarely anaplastic plasma cells	Monotypic cytoplasmic Ig light chain; IgG > IgA > light chain only; others rare	CD138+, CD38+, IRF4 (MUM1)+, CD45− or dim, CD19−, CD56+; cyclin D1+ (in cases with CCND1 rearrangement); minority: CD20+, KIT (CD117)+, CD10+; Ki-67 usually low; EBER almost always negative	**Hyperdiploid cases (~45%):** 48–75 chromosomes; gains of ≥ 3 of odd-numbered chromosomes: 3, 5, 7, 9, 11, 15, 19, 21 **Non-hyperdiploid cases (~50%):** Translocation of IGH with CCND1 (most common), MAF, or FGFR3/NSD2 (FGFR3/MMSET); rare IGH partners (≤ 2% of cases): CCND3, CCND2, MAFA, or MAFB **Other changes:** Activating mutations of KRAS, NRAS, or BRAF; mutations activating NF-κB; MYC translocation; TP53 abnormalities

CRAB, hypercalcaemia, renal insufficiency, anaemia, and bone lesions. EBER, EBV-encoded small RNA.

SPB accounts for < 5% of all plasma cell neoplasms {2071, 3255}. Most cases of SPB progress to PCM, a condition that is much more common than SPB. In the USA, there are an estimated 22 350 new cases of PCM diagnosed per annum and 10 710 deaths each year due to PCM {2859}.

Etiology
Unknown

Pathogenesis
Changes in SPB are similar to those in PCM (see the volume *WHO classification of tumours of haematopoietic and lymphoid tissues* {3011}. Genetic and cytogenetic abnormalities are heterogeneous. Immunoglobulin (Ig) heavy and light chain genes are clonally rearranged, with a heavy load of mutations in the variable region of the Ig heavy chain gene, without ongoing mutations. Complex karyotypes are common. FISH is much

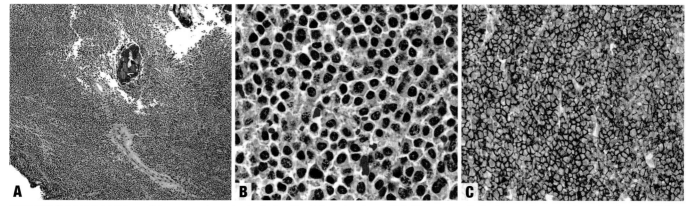

Fig. 3.198 Plasmacytoma of bone. **A** Low power shows sheets of cells without intervening stroma. **B** In this case, neoplastic plasma cells are mostly small and mature. **C** Neoplastic plasma cells are CD138-positive on immunohistochemistry. They were also positive for CD56 and monotypic kappa (not shown).

more sensitive for detecting cytogenetic abnormalities than routine karyotyping. Two main groups of PCM are defined by cytogenetic abnormalities: hyperdiploid and non-hyperdiploid (see Table 3.06, p. 487) {570}.

Macroscopic appearance
SPB is a gelatinous, haemorrhagic lesion.

Histopathology
SPB is composed of sheets of neoplastic plasma cells, which can be small and mature or enlarged, immature, and atypical. Infrequently, the tumour cells are large and poorly differentiated, rarely with anaplastic morphology. SPB may be associated with amyloid deposition {1139} and rarely with crystal-storing histiocytosis {1918}. Immunophenotyping can be performed by flow cytometry or immunohistochemistry. The immunohistochemical profile of the neoplastic cells in SPB is as follows: CD138+, CD38+, IRF4 (MUM1)+, CD45– or dim, CD19–, monotypic Ig+, and usually CD56+ and CD20–. Cyclin D1 is expressed in a subset of cases. SPB may resemble large cell lymphoma, plasmablastic lymphoma, round cell sarcoma, germ cell tumour, or metastatic carcinoma or melanoma {1139,2245}. Occasional tumours are composed of small lymphocyte-like plasma cells and may mimic a low-grade lymphoma.

Cytology
Not clinically relevant

Diagnostic molecular pathology
There is rearrangement of Ig heavy and light chain genes.

Essential and desirable diagnostic criteria
Essential: single osseous lesion on skeletal survey; diffuse, destructive infiltrate of clonal plasma cells; no evidence of PCM on staging iliac crest bone marrow biopsy; no related end-organ damage (e.g. hypercalcaemia, renal insufficiency, anaemia, and bone lesions [CRAB]).

Staging
Bone marrow biopsy and radiographic studies are required. Additional plasmacytoma(s) and/or > 10% clonal plasma cells in a random bone marrow biopsy is diagnostic of PCM and excludes SPB {3250}.

Prognosis and prediction
Radiation provides excellent local control. Local recurrence is frequent without radiation {1656,2978,1622,233}. Radiation does not prevent progression to PCM {1656,2978,3255,233}. Approximately two thirds of cases of SPB progress to PCM within 5 years {3250,1622}. SPB > 5–6 cm has been associated with recurrence or local progression of disease {3255}, higher risk of PCM, and worse overall survival {1656,1622,233}. Progression to PCM is more likely among SPB patients with minimal bone marrow involvement by clonal plasma cells (< 10%, so-called plasmacytoma plus) than among patients with negative marrows (60% vs 10% within 3 years) {2568}. Older age and persistence of serum M component after treatment (probably representing persistent disease) are associated with higher risk of PCM {3255}. Elevated B2M is associated with worse overall survival {2978}. As many as one third of SPB patients have long survival (> 10 years) without progression to PCM {1622, 233}. SPB is associated with substantial morbidity {3250}. Mortality usually results from progression to PCM. The 5-year and 10-year overall survival rates of patients presenting with SPB (most of whom develop PCM) are in the range of 70–80% and 40–60%, respectively {1656,2978,1622,233}.

Primary non-Hodgkin lymphoma of bone

Cleven AHG
Ferry JA

Definition
Primary non-Hodgkin lymphoma of bone is a neoplasm composed of malignant lymphoid cells, producing one or more lesions within bone, with no (supraregional) lymph node involvement or other extranodal lesions.

ICD-O coding
9591/3 Malignant lymphoma, non-Hodgkin, NOS
9650/3 Hodgkin disease NOS
9680/3 Diffuse large B-cell lymphoma NOS
9690/3 Follicular lymphoma NOS
9699/3 Marginal zone B-cell lymphoma NOS
9702/3 T-cell lymphoma NOS
9714/3 Anaplastic large cell lymphoma NOS
9727/3 Malignant lymphoma, lymphoblastic, NOS
9687/3 Burkitt lymphoma NOS

ICD-11 coding
2B33.5 & XH0L78 Malignant lymphoma, not elsewhere classified & Malignant lymphomas NOS or diffuse

Related terminology
Acceptable: primary bone lymphoma.

Subtype(s)
None

Localization
Primary bone lymphomas most frequently occur in the femur, followed by the pelvis, vertebrae, and humerus, usually arising in the metadiaphyseal region of the bone {302}. Approximately 10–40% of cases are multifocal, producing several lesions in one bone or involving multiple bones concurrently (polyostotic).

Clinical features
Signs and symptoms
The majority of patients with primary bone lymphoma present with pain in the affected bone but rarely with systemic symptoms such as fever, weight loss, or night sweats.

Imaging
Although there is no specific radiological appearance for primary bone lymphomas, imaging frequently shows a large, lytic, and destructive tumour that may erode the involved bone cortex and extend into the adjacent soft tissue {3256}. Borders of the lesion are often moth eaten or permeative, and an onion-skin periosteal reaction may be present. In some cases, the tumour may elicit extensive medullary sclerosis {259,893}.

Epidemiology
Primary lymphoma of bone is not a common disease, constituting approximately 7% of all malignant bone tumours, 5% of all

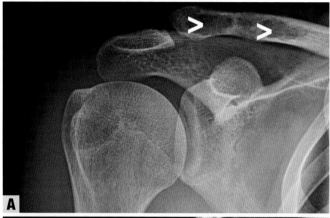
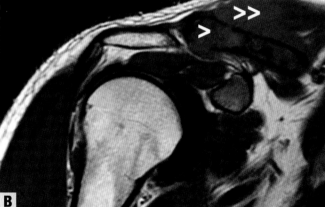

Fig. 3.199 Diffuse large B-cell lymphoma of bone. **A** A lesion in the right clavicle (arrowheads) on conventional X-ray. **B** MRI of the right clavicle (single arrowhead) shows soft tissue extension (double arrowhead).

extranodal lymphomas, and < 1% of all non-Hodgkin lymphomas {301}. Almost 50% of patients with primary lymphoma of bone are aged > 40 years; only a minority of cases arise in children {301,1361}. Importantly, primary nodal lymphomas frequently involve the skeletal system; bone involvement is seen in as many as 20% of patients and may be indistinguishable from primary lymphoma of bone on biopsy {301}.

Etiology
Primary lymphomas of bone typically arise sporadically, with a few exceptions: rare HIV-positive patients with primary lymphoma of bone are reported {757,798}. In rare patients, lymphoma has arisen on a background of longstanding osteomyelitis {2394,658} or Paget disease of bone {2394}.

Pathogenesis
Although the pathogenesis and role of the microenvironment in primary bone diffuse large B-cell lymphoma (DLBCL) are not fully elucidated, clinical and molecular genetic data suggest

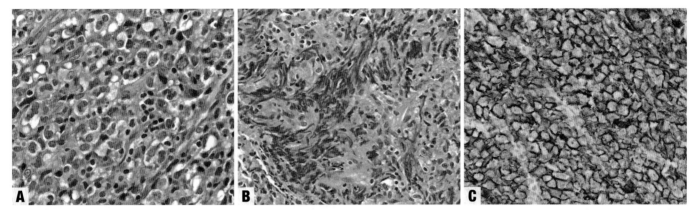

Fig. 3.200 Primary bone diffuse large B-cell lymphoma. **A** Pleomorphic B cells with large irregular multilobulated nuclei and prominent nucleoli. **B** Crush and smear artefacts are frequently observed in primary bone diffuse large B-cell lymphoma. **C** Extensive immunoreactivity for CD20, a pan–B-cell marker, in tumour cells of this primary bone diffuse large B-cell lymphoma.

that primary bone DLBCL probably arises from centrocytes. Naïve B cells in the bone may enter lymphoid follicles as part of an inflammatory/immunological response and undergo IGH somatic hypermutation to become centrocytes in the germinal centre light zone {1847}. Primary bone DLBCL may originate from these centrocytes. Alternatively, the centrocytes from which the lymphoma originates may also derive from extraosseous lymphoid tissue, migrate to the bone, and give rise to lymphoma {1847}.

Macroscopic appearance

It is uncommon to see gross specimens of primary bone lymphomas, because diagnosis is made on biopsy material and treatment consists of chemotherapy and radiotherapy without surgery. If available, macroscopy shows a greyish-white and fleshy tumour in the bone, frequently with areas of necrosis.

Histopathology

The majority (> 80%) of primary bone lymphomas are diffuse large B-cell lymphomas. Follicular lymphoma, marginal zone lymphoma, lymphoblastic lymphoma, Hodgkin lymphoma, ALK-positive and ALK-negative anaplastic large lymphomas, and other B-cell and T-cell lymphomas only rarely originate primarily within the bone {1646,2103}.

DLBCL is characterized by a diffuse growth pattern of large atypical lymphoid cells filling the marrow space, sometimes with prominent fibrosis. Bony trabeculae show reactive changes. Neoplastic cells have large, round or irregular nuclei, often with a cleaved or multilobated (or occasionally pleomorphic) appearance and variably prominent nucleoli. Cytoplasm may be amphophilic but is not abundant. Crush artefact is common; this histological finding should raise the possibility of a lymphoma. Typically the tumour cells are accompanied in areas by many reactive, non-neoplastic lymphocytes and histiocytes. The crush artefact, admixture of reactive cells, and reactive bone may obscure the neoplastic population, sometimes necessitating rebiopsy to obtain diagnostic tissue.

The rare cases of lymphoblastic lymphoma, ALK-positive and ALK-negative anaplastic large cell lymphomas (ALCLs), Burkitt lymphoma, low-grade B-cell lymphomas, and other peripheral T-cell lymphomas have pathological features similar to those seen in extraosseous sites. ALCL in bone is very rare, but it is the most common primary T-cell lymphoma of bone. Tumour cells are large, with characteristic irregular, eccentric kidney-shaped nuclei. Uncommonly, classic Hodgkin lymphoma presents with bony involvement, probably reflecting extranodal localization of a primary nodal Hodgkin lymphoma in most cases, although

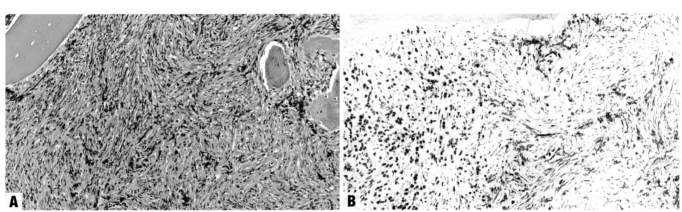

Fig. 3.201 Primary bone diffuse large B-cell lymphoma. **A** Extensive sclerosis with crush artefact in a case of primary bone diffuse large B-cell lymphoma mimicking sarcoma. **B** PAX5 immunoreactivity highlights the spindle cell appearance of the neoplastic B cells.

rare cases of classic Hodgkin lymphoma primary in bone are described {2393}.

Immunohistochemistry

The diagnostic work-up for primary lymphomas of bone includes a combination of light microscopy and a panel of immunohistochemical markers as used to evaluate other lymphoproliferative disorders. Most primary bone lymphomas are DLBCLs that express CD20, PAX5, and CD79a {617}. Optimally, an immunohistochemical panel to evaluate cases thought to be DLBCL includes CD20, PAX5, CD3, CD5, CD10, BCL6, BCL2, IRF4 (MUM1), MYC, and Ki-67, as well as in situ hybridization for EBV using EBV-encoded small RNA (EBER). Selected markers may be added in cases with unusual features. With this panel, primary bone DLBCL can be further subdivided into germinal-centre B-cell (GCB) type and non-GCB type using BCL6, CD10, and IRF4 (MUM1) immunohistochemistry (the Hans algorithm) {73}: CD10+ or CD10–, BCL6+, IRF4 (MUM1)– supports GCB type, whereas CD10–, BCL6– or CD10–, BCL6+, IRF4 (MUM1)+ supports non-GCB type. Non-GCB type suggests an inferior prognosis {2663}. ALCLs are diffusely positive for CD30 and are usually positive for at least one pan–T-cell marker such as CD3, CD2, CD4, or CD5. In cases with an *ALK* translocation, expression of ALK protein is observed (ALK-positive ALCL).

Cytology

Not clinically relevant

Diagnostic molecular pathology

Clonal rearrangements of immunoglobulin heavy and light chain genes are detectable in primary bone DLBCL, whereas clonal rearrangement of the T-cell receptor genes are detectable in T-cell lymphomas. In primary bone DLBCL, *BCL2* translocation was found in approximately 20% of cases, *BCL6* translocation in 14%, and *MYC* translocation in 10%. High-grade B-cell lymphomas with *MYC* and *BCL2* and/or *BCL6* rearrangements (double-hit lymphomas) {3011} primary in bone are rare {1861}. Recently, the genomic landscape of DLBCL has been evaluated by extensive next-generation sequencing studies in large cohorts of B-cell lymphomas, identifying frequent driver mutations in genes such as *MYD88*, *CD79A/CD79B*, *CARD11*, and *TP53* that are associated with an adverse prognosis and resistance to therapy {2588}, although such studies focusing on primary lymphoma of bone are limited. In parallel with the recommendation for performing triple (*BCL2/BCL6/MYC*) FISH in DLBCL, it is likely that a targeted next-generation sequencing approach will become part of the routine DLBCL diagnostics in the near future, in order to better characterize the lymphomas and tailor therapeutic choices {3196}.

Essential and desirable diagnostic criteria

Essential: lymphoma identified by histology and immunohistochemistry; only bone affected, with no previous or concurrent extraosseous disease except in regional lymph nodes.

Staging

Not clinically relevant

Prognosis and prediction

Primary bone DLBCLs have a favourable prognosis. With current treatment protocols (chemotherapy followed by radiotherapy), overall survival is excellent {1360}. Age is a significant factor associated with survival, with age > 60 years indicative of inferior survival {1361}. In general, GCB-type primary bone DLBCLs are associated with a better survival than the non-GCB type {1847}.

Langerhans cell histiocytosis

Pileri SA
Cheuk W
Picarsic J

Definition
Langerhans cell histiocytosis (LCH) is a clonal neoplastic proliferation of myeloid dendritic cells expressing a Langerhans cell (LC) phenotype. LCH can be unifocal or multifocal within a single system (usually bone) or it can be multisystem {3078}.

ICD-O coding
9751/1 Langerhans cell histiocytosis NOS
9751/3 Langerhans cell histiocytosis, disseminated

ICD-11 coding
2B31.2 & XH1J18 Langerhans cell histiocytosis & Langerhans cell histiocytosis NOS

Related terminology
Not recommended: Langerhans cell granulomatosis.

Solitary lesion
Not recommended: histiocytosis X; eosinophilic granuloma.

Multiple lesions
Not recommended: Hand–Schüller–Christian disease.

Cases with disseminated or visceral involvement
Not recommended: Letterer–Siwe disease.

Subtype(s)
None

Localization
Single-system LCH predominantly involves the bone (skull, femur, vertebrae, pelvis, ribs, and mandible) and less commonly lymph node, skin, and lung. In multisystem LCH, the skin, bone, liver, spleen, and bone marrow are preferentially involved.

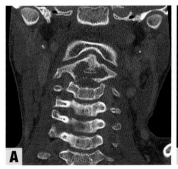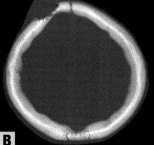

Fig. 3.202 Langerhans cell histiocytosis. **A** CT with a C2 vertebral lytic lesion of Langerhans cell histiocytosis. **B** CT of the skull without contrast. Lytic lesion in the right frontal bone with associated soft tissue component. Margins should be left intact for proper healing in cases of bone Langerhans cell histiocytosis.

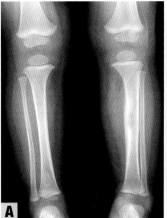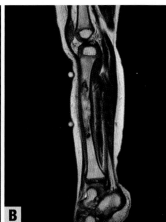

Fig. 3.203 Langerhans cell histiocytosis involving diaphysis of the left tibia. **A** Plain X-ray shows a radiolucent lesion in the left tibia, with periosteal new bone formation. **B** In the same case, MRI shows an intramedullary lesion in the tibial diaphysis with erosion of the adjacent cortex.

Clinical features
Signs and symptoms
Patients with single-system LCH are usually older children or adults with a painful lytic lesion eroding the bone cortex. Solitary lesions at other sites present as masses. Patients with multifocal single-system LCH are usually young children with multiple or sequential destructive bone lesions, often associated with adjacent soft tissue masses. Diabetes insipidus follows cranial bone and parenchymal involvement. Patients with multisystem LCH are infants presenting with fever, cytopenias, skin and bone lesions, and hepatosplenomegaly {167,75}.

Epidemiology
The annual incidence in children is about 5 cases per 1 million population {1264}. The M:F ratio is 1.2:1 {75}. The annual incidence in adults is 1–2 cases per 1 million population. The disease is more common among individuals of European descent and Hispanics. LCH can also be associated with Erdheim–Chester Disease, either concomitantly or preceding, with shared molecular alterations {901}.

Etiology
Unknown

Pathogenesis
The cell of origin is closer to a myeloid dendritic cell than to an epidermal LC {74}. MAPK pathway activation plays a central role in LCH pathogenesis {75}. A misguided myeloid differentiation model has been proposed, in which activating MAPK mutations at a pluripotent haematopoietic, tissue-restricted, or local precursor level give rise to high-risk multisystem, multifocal low-risk, or unifocal LCH, respectively {75}. These mutations,

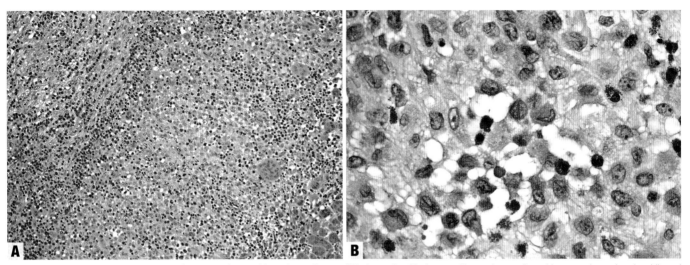

Fig. 3.204 Langerhans cell histiocytosis. **A** Low-power image of bone Langerhans cell histiocytosis with clusters of Langerhans cells and large numbers of eosinophils and osteoclast-like giant cells. **B** High-power image of Langerhans cell histiocytosis showing distinctive morphology of intermediate-sized cells with nuclear grooves, irregular nuclear contours, and pale eosinophilic cytoplasm.

especially *BRAF* p.Val600Glu, may confer an advantage for tissue site accumulation via disrupted cell migration and apoptosis inhibition {1393}. Rare familial cases are reported {168}. About 30% of cases show clonal IGH, IGK, and/or TR gene rearrangements {561}.

Macroscopic appearance
Not clinically relevant

Histopathology
Diagnostic LCH cells are oval and measure about 10–15 μm. They are recognized by grooved, folded, indented, or lobed nuclei, as well as fine chromatin, inconspicuous nucleoli, and thin nuclear membranes. Nuclear atypia is minimal, but mitotic activity is variable and can be high without atypical forms. The cytoplasm is moderately abundant, slightly eosinophilic, and devoid of dendritic processes. The characteristic milieu includes variable numbers of eosinophils, histiocytes (both multinucleated LCH-type and osteoclast-type cells, especially in bone), neutrophils, and small lymphocytes. Plasma cells are usually sparse.

Occasionally, eosinophilic microabscesses with central necrosis are found. LCH cells predominate in early lesions. In late lesions, they are decreased in number, with increased foamy macrophages and fibrosis. The ultrastructural hallmark is the cytoplasmic Birbeck granule, which is 200–400 nm long and 33 nm wide, with a tennis-racket shape and a zipper-like appearance.

Immunohistochemistry
LCH cells express CD1a, CD207 (langerin), S100, CD68, and HLA-DR {75}. CD45 expression is low. The *BRAF* p.Val600Glu mutation can be identified by a specific antibody {2246,214}. The Ki-67 proliferation index is highly variable (typically < 10% by double staining) {2511,1393}. Rare cases associated with follicular lymphoma or B- or T-lymphoblastic leukaemia are considered a transdifferentiation phenomenon and behave more aggressively {3274,981,512}.

Differential diagnosis
The differential diagnosis includes osteomyelitis and chondroblastoma.

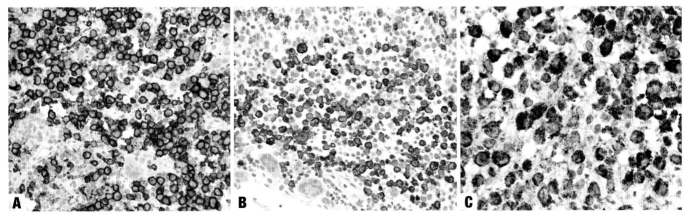

Fig. 3.205 Langerhans cell histiocytosis. **A** Langerhans cell histiocytosis with surface CD1a immunoreactivity on the majority of cells. **B** Langerhans cell histiocytosis with cytoplasmic granular positivity for CD207 (langerin) in the majority of Langerhans cells. **C** Langerhans cell histiocytosis with molecularly confirmed *BRAF* p.Val600Glu mutation showing strong diffuse cytoplasmic granular VE1 positivity in Langerhans cells.

Cytology

Clusters of LCH cells are diagnostic, but caution is needed in lymph nodes because paracortical dendritic/Langerhans cells cannot be distinguished from sinus-based LCH cells.

Diagnostic molecular pathology

MAPK pathway gene mutations are recorded in > 85% of cases. They affect *BRAF* or alternatively *MAP2K1* or much more rarely *ARAF*. *ERBB3*, *NRAS*, and *KRAS* mutations can also occur in adults {75}.

Essential and desirable diagnostic criteria

Essential: typical LC morphology.
Desirable: CD1a, CD207, and S100 positivity; detection of MAPK pathway mutations.

Staging

According to the Histiocyte Society's 2009 evaluation and treatment guidelines, single-system LCH is defined by the involvement of one organ/system (unifocal or multifocal), and multisystem LCH is defined by the involvement of two or more organs/systems (± risk-organ involvement).

Prognosis and prediction

The clinical course is related to staging at presentation, with a ≥ 99% survival rate for unifocal disease and < 20% mortality in risk-organ multisystem LCH with prolonged therapy {1101,2151, 3078,75}. Progression from initially focal to multisystem LCH can occur, most commonly in infants with hypothalamic pituitary involvement. Patient age is a less important indicator than disease extent {2151,3078}. Multisystem LCH can be complicated by macrophage activation syndrome {974}. *BRAF* p.Val600Glu mutation correlates with increased relapse risk {282,1351} and potentially worse clinical parameters, including resistance to first-line therapy and neurodegenerative CNS LCH {1351}. In previously diagnosed LCH patients with *BRAF* p.Val600Glu mutation, additional lesions demonstrating BRAF p.Val600Glu–positive, CD1a/CD207-negative histiocytes may still represent active disease {1810}.

Erdheim–Chester disease

Emile JF
Haroche J
Picarsic J
Tirabosco R

Definition

Erdheim–Chester disease (ECD) is a clonal systemic histiocytosis with inflammation and fibrosis.

ICD-O coding

9749/3 Erdheim–Chester disease

ICD-11 coding

2B31.Y & XH1VJ3 Other specified histiocytic or dendritic cell neoplasms & Erdheim–Chester disease

Related terminology

None

Subtype(s)

None

Localization

ECD is a multisystem disease. Long bones are involved in > 90% of cases. Infiltration of the retroperitoneum (58%) or around aorta (46%) is also frequent {635}. Neurological or pituitary involvement occurs in 20–50% of cases. Infiltration of lungs, heart, skin (xanthelasma), or any other organ or soft tissue may also occur, but the spleen, lymph nodes, and liver are generally spared.

Clinical features

Signs and symptoms

ECD may be asymptomatic; however, most patients have general, inflammatory, or site-related symptoms, most of which are considered to be related to the inflammation and fibrosis associated with the histiocytic infiltration of the tissues and organs. Bone pain (37–50%), exophthalmos (25%), xanthelasma (19–26%), and diabetes insipidus (28%) are frequently reported. CNS disease presents with either tumour-like or neurodegenerative-type symptoms. Involvement of the basilar arteries can lead to stroke. Pulmonary, renal, endocrine, or cardiac dysfunction may also be responsible for clinical manifestation, and 25–50% of patients die from disease progression before treatment.

Imaging

As many as 95% of patients with ECD have a symmetrical osteosclerosis of the leg bones, best visualized by PET with bilateral uptake of FDG. Bone lesions may be visualized on CT or MRI, but they are often missed on plain X-rays. Bilateral perinephritic infiltration, responsible for a hairy kidney aspect on CT, is noted in 66% of cases. Imaging may also disclose a coated aorta, corresponding to an infiltration of soft tissues surrounding abdominal or thoracic aorta. Detection of mass-like infiltration of the right atrium by MRI (33%) is highly suggestive of ECD. CT of the chest may show pleural and septal thickening, as well as serosal effusions. Infiltration of other organs is less

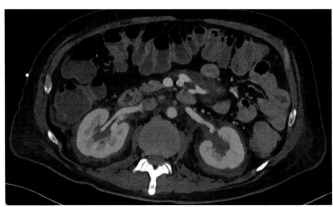

Fig. 3.206 Erdheim–Chester disease. The hairy kidney sign. CT showing perirenal infiltration by Erdheim–Chester disease.

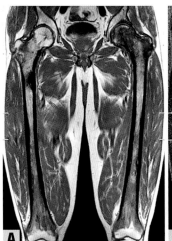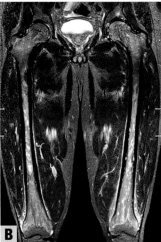

Fig. 3.207 Erdheim–Chester disease. Coronal T1-weighted spin echo MRI (**A**) and short-tau inversion recovery (STIR) MRI (**B**) showing heterogeneous marrow abnormality throughout both femoral shafts in a 46-year-old man..

specific. It is also noteworthy that 10–20% of cases of ECD are associated with other forms of histiocytosis, such as Langerhans cell histiocytosis {1354,901}.

Epidemiology

ECD is a rare but probably underdiagnosed disease. The median age at diagnosis is 55 years, with an M:F ratio of 3:1. Cases in children aged < 15 years are very rare and overlap with systemic juvenile xanthogranuloma.**Etiology**
Unknown

Pathogenesis

Most cases have an activating mutation of the MAPK pathway. This mutation may also be present within bone marrow progenitors, and some patients may have an associated

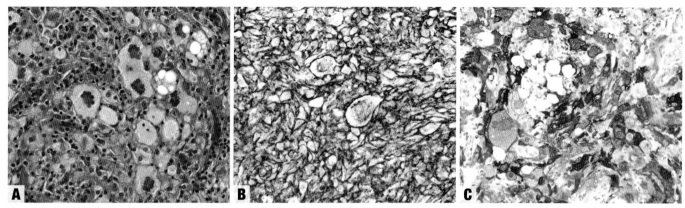

Fig. 3.208 Erdheim–Chester disease. Brain xanthogranuloma in a patient with typical bone lesions. **A** H&E staining. **B** Diffuse immunoreactivity for CD14. **C** Immunoreactivity for factor XIIIa.

myeloproliferative or myelodysplastic neoplasm {2433,50}. Recent data suggest that some cases of ECD result from tissue accumulation of histiocytes derived from mutated bone marrow progenitors {875}.

Macroscopic appearance

Most of the samples obtained for diagnosis correspond to biopsies of perirenal fat, bone, or skin. They are usually firm and sclerotic.

Histopathology

Lesional tissue demonstrates infiltration of foamy, lipid-laden, and/or small mononuclear histiocytes associated with variable proportions of Touton giant cells, small lymphocytes, plasma cells, and neutrophils, which is indistinguishable from xanthogranuloma. Fibrosis is usually present and sometimes predominant, leading to misinterpretation of the lesion as a reactive fibroinflammatory process. Admixed Langerhans cell histiocytosis may be present in the same biopsy.

Immunohistochemistry

The immunohistochemical profile is similar to that of xanthogranuloma, with ECD histiocytes positive for CD163, CD68, and CD14 and negative for CD1a and CD207. They may also be positive for factor XIIIa and fascin, and less commonly for S100.

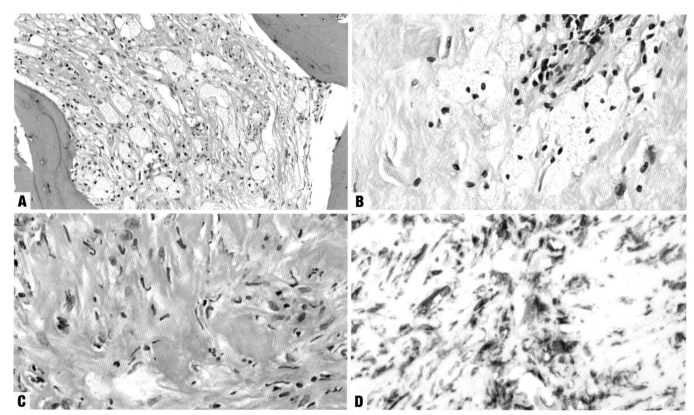

Fig. 3.209 Erdheim–Chester disease. **A** Characteristic bone infiltration by the histiocytic proliferation. **B,C,D** Retroperitoneal (perirenal) biopsy showing infiltration by foamy histiocytes (**B**) or predominant fibrosis (**C**); immunohistochemistry shows expression of CD163 (**D**).

Expression of phosphorylated ERK is frequent in ECD histiocytes, and strong diffuse cytoplasmic VE1 monoclonal antibody overexpression may signal a *BRAF* p.Val600Glu mutation.

Differential diagnosis
Disseminated xanthogranulomas with the relevant mutation of the MAPK pathway are now considered part of the same syndrome {901}. The differential diagnosis mainly includes xanthogranuloma, as well as other inflammatory processes.

Cytology
Not clinically relevant

Diagnostic molecular pathology
A *BRAF* p.Val600Glu mutation is present in 50–60% of cases of ECD {1304}. This frequency may be underestimated, because the mutant allele frequency is < 5% in a quarter of cases {2069}.

Patients without *BRAF* p.Val600Glu frequently have other mutations (also activating the MAPK cell signalling pathway) on *ARAF*, *NRAS*, *KRAS*, or *MAP2K1* {817}. *PIK3CA* may also be mutated {903}.

Essential and desirable diagnostic criteria
Essential: collections of bland foamy histiocytes in the appropriate clinical and radiological context.
Desirable: mutation analysis of the MAPK pathway.

Staging
Not clinically relevant

Prognosis and prediction
CNS and cardiovascular involvement is associated with a worse prognosis {635}. *BRAF* mutations do not have a prognostic value, but targeted therapies might improve the prognosis.

Rosai–Dorfman disease

Rosenberg AE
Demicco EG

Definition
Rosai–Dorfman disease (RDD) is a histiocytic proliferation characterized by large S100-positive histiocytes with emperipolesis.

ICD-O coding
None

ICD-11 coding
EK92 Histiocytoses of uncertain malignant potential

Related terminology
Not recommended: sinus histiocytosis with massive lymphadenopathy.

Subtype(s)
None

Localization
Primary intraosseous RDD most commonly affects the metaphysis of long bones and craniofacial skeleton {2204}. In 71% of cases, one bone is affected; the remainder involve multiple bones {2204}.

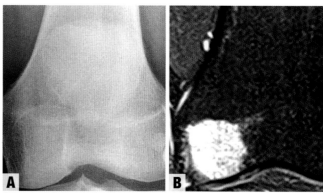

Fig. 3.210 Rosai–Dorfman disease. **A** Radiograph showing distal femur that appears unremarkable. **B** Tumour in medial femoral condyle that is bright on coronal fat-saturated T2-weighted image.

Clinical features
Signs and symptoms
Patients usually present with pain localized to the involved anatomical site; pathological fracture is rare.

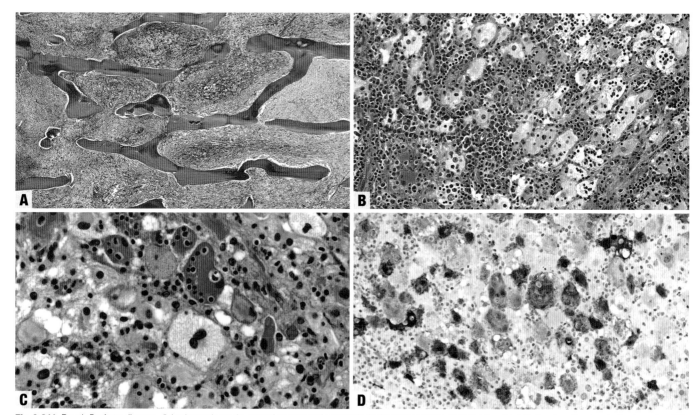

Fig. 3.211 Rosai–Dorfman disease. **A** Lesion replaces the normal marrow and surrounds the bony trabeculae. **B** Numerous large histiocytes with abundant pale eosinophilic cytoplasm are surrounded by chronic inflammatory cells. **C** Rosai–Dorfman histiocytes with emperipolesis. **D** Rosai–Dorfman histiocytes are strongly immunoreactive for S100.

Imaging

Imaging studies reveal a well-defined lytic, sometimes expansile, septated mass. Cortical thickening and periosteal reaction are present in a minority of cases {789}.

Epidemiology

RDD is a rare disease that usually presents in the lymph nodes, but it may affect extranodal sites in > 40% of cases; bone involvement occurs in 2–10% of patients {901}. Primary bone involvement is very rare, is associated with equal sex distribution, and may affect patients of any age (mean: 31 years) {2204}.

Etiology

Unknown

Pathogenesis

Constitutive activation of the RAS/MAPK pathway probably plays a role in a subset of cases, because this pathway is important in monocyte maturation {457}. Mutually exclusive missense mutations in *NRAS*, *KRAS*, *MAP2K1*, *ARAF*, and *BRAF* have been reported in 33–40% of tumours and are considered driver genetic aberrations {6,2622,973}. Germline mutations in *SLC29A3* and *FAS* (*TNFRSF6*) are associated with patients who have the rare familial form of the disease {6}.

Macroscopic appearance

Tumours range in size from 1 to 7 cm; most are < 5 cm and are well defined and tan-grey, with a soft or gritty texture.

Histopathology

The tumour is poorly defined, replaces the marrow, infiltrates haversian systems, and is associated with local bone resorption {789}. The mass is characterized by sheets and clusters of large histiocytes with nuclei that range from round or oval to reniform, with fine or vesicular chromatin and prominent eosinophilic nucleoli. The cytoplasm is abundant and pale eosinophilic, and it demonstrates conspicuous emperipolesis (lymphocytophagocytosis) of lymphocytes, plasma cells, or neutrophils. The tumour cells are enmeshed in a fibrotic stroma that contains a prominent mixed inflammatory infiltrate composed of lymphocytes, plasma cells (often containing Russell bodies), neutrophils, foamy macrophages, and rare eosinophils. Microabscesses may be present. The neoplastic histiocytes are variable in number and distribution, and they may be undersampled on biopsy.

Immunohistochemistry

The histiocytes express S100 and are negative for CD1a and CD207 {901}.

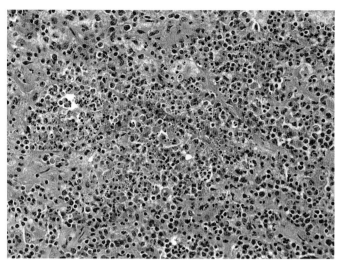

Fig. 3.212 Rosai–Dorfman disease. Numerous neutrophils are present, which can lead to a misdiagnosis of osteomyelitis.

Differential diagnosis

The differential diagnosis includes osteomyelitis, Langerhans cell histiocytosis, Erdheim–Chester disease, and IgG4-associated sclerosing lesion because RDD may also contain numerous IgG4-positive plasma cells {901}.

Cytology

FNA reveals large histiocytes in a mixed inflammatory background. Emperipolesis of inflammatory cells can usually be seen in the cytoplasm of the tumour cells {1959}.

Diagnostic molecular pathology

Not clinically relevant

Essential and desirable diagnostic criteria

Essential: large S100-positive, CD1a-negative histiocytes with cytoplasmic emperipolesis; plasma cell–rich inflammatory infiltrate.

Staging

There is no applicable staging system. Imaging studies (e.g. FDG PET-CT) to identify additional sites of disease should be considered {6}.

Prognosis and prediction

Prognosis is good; one or more other organs become involved in 58% of patients {2204}. Bone lesions are effectively treated for local control by curettage {789}.